Praise for Jax Peters Lowell

"Lowell covers every aspect of living wheat- and gluten-free."
—*The New York Times*

"Be forewarned: This book is addictive. Jax inspires, educates, entertains. You'll laugh, you'll learn, you'll discover the abundant life that can be yours—gluten-free."
—*Living Without* magazine

"A lot of attitude and a terrific sense of humor."
—*New York Daily News*

"Just what the doctor ordered."
—ALESSIO FASANO, MD, director, Center for Celiac Research and Treatment, Massachusetts General Hospital for Children

"Aren't we lucky this talented writer is one of us!"
—ALICE BAST, founder, National Foundation for Celiac Awareness

"The definitive guide to coping with wheat allergy and celiac disease . . . the author has left no resource untapped."
—*Science News*

"This book will bring tears of joy . . . a treasure . . . a must. No library is complete without *The Gluten-Free Bible*, the ultimate resource for all things gluten-free."
—ELAINE MONARCH, founder, Celiac Disease Foundation

"Her writing is conspiratorial, her research vast . . . I have never read an allergy book that I could say had a heart, but this one does."
—JIM BURNS, food editor, *Los Angeles Times* syndicate

"With her trademark cheekiness and deep-hearted wisdom, Jax Lowell serves up another celiac classic."
—DIANE EVE PALEY, past president, Celiac Support Association

"A primer for the wheat intolerant."

"Informative . . . extensive . . . written by someone who knows what it's like to live with a difficult condition. Highly recommended."

"Lowell has succeeded in creating a work that will inspire the patient, dietician, and doctor—RUN, don't walk, to pick up your copy!"

"A book that nurtures as it advises."

"Jax Lowell proves it's possible to live *and* eat happily ever after!"

The Gluten-Free Revolution

The Gluten-Free Revolution

Absolutely Everything
You Need to Know
About Losing the Wheat,
Reclaiming Your Health,
and Eating Happily Ever After

Jax Peters Lowell

Foreword by Anthony J. DiMarino Jr., MD

A HOLT PAPERBACK   HENRY HOLT AND COMPANY   NEW YORK

Holt Paperbacks
Henry Holt and Company, LLC
Publishers since 1866
175 Fifth Avenue
New York, New York 10010
www.henryholt.com

A Holt Paperback ® and ⓗ ® are registered trademarks of Henry Holt and Company, LLC.

Library of Congress Cataloging-in-Publication Data

Lowell, Jax Peters.
  [Against the grain]
  The gluten-free revolution : absolutely everything you need to know about losing
the wheat, reclaiming your health, and eating happily ever after / Jax Peters Lowell ;
foreword by Anthony J. DiMarino, Jr., MD. — First Holt Paperbacks edition.
      pages cm
  "A Holt Paperback."
  Previous title: Against the grain.
  Includes bibliographical references and index.
  ISBN 978-0-8050-9953-9 (paperback) — ISBN 978-0-8050-9954-6 (electronic copy)
  1. Wheat-free diet.   2. Gluten-free diet.   I. Title.
  RM237.87.L68 2015
  641.5'638—dc23
                                                                    2014006764

Henry Holt books are available for special promotions and premiums. For details contact:
Director, Special Markets.

Originally published in hardcover in 1995 as *Against the Grain* by Henry Holt and
Company and in paperback in 2005 as *The Gluten-Free Bible* by St. Martin's Griffin.

First Holt Paperbacks Edition 2015

Designed by Meryl Sussman Levavi

Printed in the United States of America

10 9 8 7 6 5 4 3 2 1

In memory of the angels at my table:

Kay and Jack Peters, Catherine Petitpain

For John, always

Gluten-Free Poem

There is no wheat in this poem,

no barley, rye or derivatives thereof.
I can't say why, but it doesn't involve
any sort of nut. Cross contamination
is not an issue here. These words are

100% safe to eat.

There is longing, though. And heat.
A phantom crumb lingers on the tongue,
buttered with hungry eyes. Jam sticky lust
licks its finger and thumb, some sugar

to swallow down with the losses.

One in 132 poets experience the urge
to fondle dinner rolls, swoon
at the sight of a batter-coated spoon,
slow walk past the patisserie,
breathe from the knees

sweet burnt air to last a lifetime.

While these lines contain absolutely no lactose,
high fructose corn syrup, casein, palm kernel oil
or genetically modified ingredients,
they do possess a prayer,
a memory, a wish, the taste

of every forbidden dish.

—Jax Peters Lowell

Contents

A Birthday Party: *Banana Split Cake* • A Hanukkah Celebration: *Sweet Potato, Pumpkin, and Sage Latkes* and *Harvest Tzimmes* • A Dickens Christmas • *Nigella Lawson's Proper English Trifle* • A Gathering of Gifts: Incredibly *Rich Date Nut Loaf, Walnut Cherry Chocolate Bark, Tarragon Mustard,* and *Cranberry Chutney* • Entertaining Cookbooks and Web sites

Foreword

The Importance of a Well-Informed Patient

When I first met Jax Peters Lowell in September 1996, it was clear I was in the presence of one of the most highly motivated patients I'd met in my many years of practice. Here was someone possessed of enormous energy with great respect for knowledge. She was willing and able to do her homework, assessing treatment options so that her decisions were always well informed. It was apparent to me from the start that we would be more like colleagues in our joint effort to understand and overcome the medical obstacles and complications presented by long-standing celiac disease.

But that's only half the story. The other side of this highly motivated, smart, and courageous woman is that of a skilled communicator, first-rate writer, and gifted speaker. I have asked Jax to apply her quietly persuasive humor to more than one recalcitrant gluten-intolerant patient and she has done so with tact, charm, and her trademark resourcefulness. Add to this her great generosity and a powerful desire to use her talent to help others, and it's no surprise that her first book, *Against the Grain*, and its second edition, *The Gluten-Free Bible*, became bestsellers.

When she asked me to write the foreword for *The Gluten-Free Revolution*, her definitive work on the gluten-free lifestyle, I felt like the village painter summoned by Michelangelo to paint his house. She's that good. Not only has she produced another important resource for those with celiac disease and varying degrees of gluten intolerance and sensitivity;

she has chronicled the choices and challenges we all face in the post-gluten age.

The detail, specificity, and scope of *The Gluten-Free Revolution* is on a par with what a medical specialist would provide, but in her hands, complicated issues are accessible and easy to understand. As complete and instructive as the chapters dealing with the various and sometimes-serious aspects of celiac disease and gluten intolerance are, it is her keen intelligence and ability to see how the gluten-free diet affects every aspect of life—and how we see ourselves within its parameters—that separates this work from other self-help books. Never content to give us a simple how-to with lists of dos and don'ts, this award-winning poet and novelist captures our hearts once again with stories that inspire, make us laugh, make us rethink, and resonate with the narratives of our own lives. With great skill, compassion, and wit, those stories lead us back to our tables and traditions, families, and friends.

Much has been learned about celiac disease in the years since Jax Lowell first gave the gluten-free community a much-needed voice. Once thought to be present in approximately 1 in 10,000 North Americans, we have seen that this immune response to the gluten in common grains was merely the tip of the iceberg. Landmark work done by Dr. Alessio Fasano and others at the Center for Celiac Disease at the University of Maryland and ongoing at the center's new home at Boston's MassGeneral Hospital for Children suggests that the condition may occur in a quiescent but insidious form as frequently as 1 in 133 individuals in the United States.

Whatever the prevalence, what we do know is that the symptoms of frequent diarrhea, malodorous/fatty stools, extreme weight loss, and subsequent malnutrition occur only in the minority of patients. The more subtle presentations of this genetic disease include unexplained bone loss, anemia—especially iron-deficiency anemia—or any number of autoimmune or allergy-like disorders, including a blistering itchy rash called dermatitis herpetiformis, headaches, dental enamel defects, fatigue, and aphthous ulcers, among other wide-ranging symptoms. For a few young women, miscarriage or the inability to become pregnant exposes the underlying problem. These atypical presentations make up the majority of celiacs, many of whom report having vague symptoms for many years prior to diagnosis. Others pick up an incorrect diagnosis of wheat allergy or irritable bowel disease along the way.

In recent years, there has been a virtual explosion of scientific literature describing the increased incidence of allergic conditions, especially celiac disease. We have determined that there has been a fourfold to five-fold increase in celiac disease over the last fifty years by comparing the serum from allegedly healthy blood donors collected from 1948 to 1954 to a comparable group of blood donors today. This interesting study from the Mayo Clinic offered by Joseph Murray and colleagues helped us understand that celiac disease is truly increasing rather than simply being better diagnosed. Furthermore, in the follow-up of many of the original 9,133 subjects from the 1954 group, there was an increase in all-cause mortality in individuals who had undiagnosed celiac disease, further emphasizing the importance of early diagnosis and adoption of a gluten-free diet.

Why celiac disease has increased so dramatically over the past fifty years is not known. Perhaps it is due to a change in the type or concentration of gluten in the wheat we are ingesting, the introduction of synthetic yeast products into baked goods, or the widespread introduction of gluten into our food products resulting in a marked increase in the consumption of gluten. It may be the altered genetic structure of the wheat itself. Whatever the reason, clearly celiac disease is increasing throughout the world. Recently, in Finland, it was estimated that approximately 2.5 percent of the population has celiac disease.

Physicians can establish a diagnosis simply and easily by testing for antibodies to celiac disease. Subsequent biopsy of the small intestine or duodenum showing atrophy, or damage to the intestinal villi, confirms it. Serological screening of the immediate family is important as well, with as many as 10 percent of first-degree relatives testing positively.

In addition to the known increase in incidence of true celiac disease throughout the world, there has also been a concomitant upsurge of information concerning the presence of so-called non-celiac gluten sensitivity (NCGS). Non-celiac gluten sensitivity is characterized by symptoms that mimic the gastrointestinal complaints of those with celiac disease, including abdominal bloating, gas, and altered bowel habits, but without the abnormalities in the intestinal biopsies or blood tests. NCGS patients do not appear to have the same increased risk of complications that celiac patients have, including cancer and autoimmune conditions, anemia, bone disease, and so on. To further complicate matters, many individuals are following a gluten-free diet even if they do not have gluten sensitivity. This growing group has voluntarily given up gluten without consulting their physicians and claim they feel better without it. Fact or fad? The jury is still out.

Helpful as this new definition may be, trying to identify and diagnose non-celiac gluten-sensitive patients remains a challenge. There are no reliable blood tests at the current time. Much work is being done in this area, but in the absence of newer ways to screen, gluten sensitivity is still basically a diagnosis of exclusion. While it is much easier today to observe a gluten-free diet than it was when Jax Lowell was diagnosed over twenty years ago, many gluten-free products continue to be higher in fat and calories than their glutenous counterparts. Therefore a gluten-free diet is not a weight-reduction diet, as some in the media say. In addition, many gluten-free cereals and breads are less vitamin-fortified than gluten-containing products and are frequently more expensive than non-gluten-free products.

While the celiac population in the United States continues to be approximately 1 percent, it is estimated that as many as sixfold to eightfold more individuals may be gluten-sensitive. As a result of the dramatic increase in numbers of gluten-free consumers, the gluten-free food business has grown dramatically, up to $2.5 billion by some accounts, and many of them, well ahead of government-mandated gluten-free standards, have voluntarily labeled their products, making it easier and easier for patients to find foods that are safe to eat.

Indeed, in August 2013, after nine years of lobbying by the gluten-free community, the Food and Drug Administration has stepped in with strict guidelines to help clarify the standard of what *gluten-free* means and limiting this label to those foods containing less than 20 parts per million of gluten or less. American food companies have one year to fully comply with this requirement. This is a real boon, not only for gluten-free consumers, but for their physicians as well, now able to offer their patients real choices and sending them out into a much friendlier gluten-free marketplace.

There's more good news on the horizon. I venture that in the not-too-distant future there will be medications or vaccines that may prevent or lessen the negative impact of ingestion of gluten-containing foods. We are getting there, but much work has yet to be done. It may be possible for a medication to be taken either with a meal or before eating to "tighten the gut" and prevent the absorption of gluten. Other areas of investigation include ways to either break down gluten into a more digestible protein or prevent its absorption through the intestinal cells. Jax Lowell participated in one such trial herself here at Thomas Jefferson University Hospital. When I asked her if she was sure she wanted to take a chance of being placed in the control group and getting a placebo, which would do nothing to counter the effects of the gluten she needed to consume for several weeks, she did not hesitate. "If not me," she said, "who?"

These attempts at a medication for celiac disease are not designed to replace a gluten-free diet but rather to allow celiac patients or those with non-celiac gluten sensitivity the freedom and flexibility to try a new restaurant, or to have a meal with well-intentioned friends or coworkers, or to attend a family holiday gathering with confidence. I am optimistic that by the time Jax is ready to write another book, advances will have continued and we will have a gluten-blocking option as well as the best and most nutritious gluten-free food possible.

The future is bright.

Still, despite all these advances, the fact remains that many patients with celiac disease and gluten intolerance, especially those with classic presentations, are fearful of ingesting hidden gluten, and with good reason. Others are in denial, especially those with few symptoms or who have been diagnosed through family screening; they tolerate abdominal bloating and gaseousness out of a mistaken belief that it is impossible to enjoy life without gluten. Many ignore the increased risk of other serious complications that can be associated with failing to strictly observe the gluten-free diet, such as autoimmune problems like diabetes mellitus, rheumatoid arthritis, and Sjögren's syndrome, and even some cancers.

As physicians, we must reassure and rigorously pursue follow-up care for our celiac patients—identifying and treating nutritional deficiencies; monitoring bone density and calcium absorption; assessing vitamin and mineral levels; offering dietetic education; and using periodic serological screenings and/or repeat biopsies to check for compliance and healing. For now there are no magic pills, and we must remind ourselves and our patients that food is our medicine and lifelong adherence to the gluten-free diet is the only path to good health. Education and confidence are paramount, too, as is the physician's attitude toward the diet. If he or she delivers the news with gloom and doom, the patient will respond accordingly. It is incumbent on all of us to communicate the accessibility and rewards of truly satisfying gluten-free living.

Inspiring this kind of educated optimism is where Jax Lowell is at her best and where *The Gluten-Free Revolution* offers the greatest reward to the reader. This comprehensive edition is as much a literary gift as it is an invaluable resource. That she is an incredibly talented writer is apparent in every paragraph. The chapter headings alone make you laugh out loud, but there is real insight behind the author's humor. You know you are in the hands of someone who's been there and doesn't take no for an answer.

Lowell's witty and wise advice on the doctor-patient relationship can make visits with willing and cooperative physicians much more pleasant and informative. Other chapters offering commonsense tips on general health, sexual matters, and tough situations like college, dating, and family holidays exude optimism, creativity, gratitude, and grace. From nitty-gritty label reading and shopping to traveling and negotiating safe restaurant meals, this is an invaluable resource for newcomers and veterans alike.

Nowadays, many of us are trying to eat well and consciously. The gluten-free diet is not the only one we have tried. By choice or necessity we follow low-fat, low-sugar, meat-free, dairy-free, egg-free, and cruelty-free diets. Some diets are associated with gluten intolerance, some not. Lowell addresses the multiplicity of our preferences with a thorough grounding in popular diets and other food intolerances and how the gluten-free diet fits into this complex picture. And her approach is by no means one of deprivation. In fact, everywhere in this book is fantastic food. Jax gives us a veritable *Who's Who* of five-star chefs, fabled restaurants, master bakers, food writers, and gluten-free-cookbook authors.

This is an indispensable reference, not only for those who have celiac disease and gluten intolerance, but also for the physicians who care for them. I have recommended *Against the Grain* and *The Gluten-Free Bible* to my patients for many years, along with my encouragement to find community in local and national support groups in order to learn more and become active in the gluten-free life. Now we have the new *Gluten-Free Revolution*, twenty years in the making and in my opinion one of the most valuable, comprehensive, and well-written of the numerous "self-help" books I have ever read. A must for every serious gluten-free library.

Jax Lowell has written a road map, really, of an ever-changing, ever-growing world in which living gluten-free is not only understood, it is celebrated as a healthy way of life. It is no accident that her incredible energy, enthusiasm, and wonderful outlook have enabled her to overcome every challenge life has thrown her way. That she continues to guide others to do the same is an extraordinary gift to an entire new generation of Americans and their families.

Once again, thank you, Jax Peters Lowell.

ANTHONY J. DIMARINO JR., MD
Director, Jefferson Celiac Center
William Rorer Professor of Medicine
Chief, Division of Gastroenterology and Hepatology
Thomas Jefferson University Hospital, Philadelphia

Introduction

The Gluten-Free Revolution

Twenty years ago, *Against the Grain: The Slightly Eccentric Guide to Living Well Without Wheat or Gluten*, with its cheeky tone and iconic toaster cover, made its debut into an America still in the dark about the gluten-free diet. I could not have imagined then a world where millions would gladly embrace life without gluten; where the Food and Drug Administration (FDA) would dispense with grocery shopping Russian roulette and actually standardize labels on gluten-free products.

I would have laughed if you'd told me a waiter would one day be informed enough to tell me that though the buckwheat polenta I was considering was gluten-free, the buckwheat itself was milled in a facility that also processed wheat. Or that beyond full-blown celiac disease, there would be many shades of gray on the spectrum of gluten sensitivity.

It seems quaint now in the explosion of all things gluten-free that my first editor, the formidable Beth Crossman, taking a chance on a new author convinced celiac disease wasn't as rare as experts believed, felt most readers would not know what gluten is, much less why we shouldn't eat it, and hedged her bets with a subtitle that put the word *wheat* before *gluten*.

Not in my wildest dreams could I have envisioned the reception that first book would receive. Long marginalized by this strange ailment, the gluten-free community responded with laughter and tears to my quirky way of managing what was then a daunting diet and felt a new assertiveness in negotiating not just a safe meal, but also a darn good one.

To my everlasting surprise, this newcomer was quoted in *Newsweek*, reviewed in the *New York Times*, and invited to speak on what was then a little-known condition on National Public Radio and at support groups and conferences all over the country. I am grateful for the outpouring of friendship and gratitude from fans in every city and town in the United States and Canada who shared their amazing stories of courage and resourcefulness with me. In times of great personal challenge, I have been buoyed and blessed by the kindnesses of my extended gluten-free family. Job satisfaction doesn't get better than this.

In the hungry years of blank stares from waiters and bread that tasted more like spackling compound than food, I had no idea *Against the Grain* and its second edition, *The Gluten-Free Bible*, would become bestsellers, or that I would play a part in inspiring a new generation of gluten-free Americans, as well as chefs and entrepreneurs who have swept us all from the culinary fringes to the beating heart of today's food culture, ushering in the gluten-free revolution.

My mother taught me never to make reciprocation a term for giving. She always said, "A gift will come back to you on its own." My small contribution to the gluten-free community has come back to me a hundredfold and, with it, joy beyond measure.

There has never been a better time to forgo gluten or a culture more conversant in what that means. From haute to down home cuisine, the best of the best are turning their attention to high-quality offerings that do not apologize for their lack of the offending grain. Quite the opposite.

Thomas Keller, celebrated chef and owner of the legendary French Laundry, Per Se, and Bouchon, has set a new standard with his gluten-free flour blend, Cup4Cup, and his line of Ad Hoc Gluten-Free mixes. The Bouchon Bakery Gluten-Free Brioche Rolls he shares with us (page 163) are nothing short of spectacular. Nowadays, all it takes is a gentle request and many fine restaurants will begin the meal with a warm gluten-free dinner roll, Parmesan crisp, or other form of amuse-bouche. And this is occurring up and down the food chain.

More and more fast-food and chain restaurants offer gluten-free options. In stores, refrigerated cases boast fresh pasta—spaghetti, linguine, lasagna noodles, and tagliatelle—that tastes like homemade and cooks up, light and airy, in minutes. Just the other day, I discovered fresh, gluten-free three-cheese ravioli in the supermarket, of all places. Dried pastas in infinite varieties are a far cry from their soggy forebears and are as good as, if not better than, those made with semolina. Healthier, too, with rice bran and whole grains like quinoa, millet, sorghum, and amaranth. English muffins, breads, bagels, brownies, crackers, cake mixes, and piecrusts, even panko bread crumbs abound.

Is the whole world gluten-free?

Some days, it seems that way.

Tate's Bake Shop in Southampton, New York, once a place any sane gluten-free citizen would avoid, has made a gluten-free variation of its legendary chocolate chip cookie that melts on the tongue and flies off the shelf faster than the original. A Philadelphia baker takes on the classic French baguette with extraordinary results. Gone are frozen cardboard pizzas; we find real takeout, cheesy and sublime, popping up in cities all over the country, along with gluten-free cupcakes, biscotti, and cookies for whiling away an afternoon with a latte and laptop.

Babycakes, a tiny bakery on New York's Lower East Side, has quickly become the epicenter of gluten-free vegan delights and home to a cookbook empire. Erin McKenna's Meyer Lemon and Bing Cherry Cupcakes with Vanilla Frosting (page 196) are a taste of how sinful healthy gluten-free can be. Some savvy businesses are making their goodies lactose-free, casein-free, and sugar-free as well, because today we know food sensitivities often come in multiples.

To the French, pastry isn't just food, it's a form of worship. And yet, Helmut Newcake, the first gluten-free patisserie in Paris, bucks centuries of tradition with glorious versions of every classic. I am honored to say they have made their American debut on these pages with a sublime fondant for you to make at home. Waiters in four- and five-star restaurants no longer sniff at special requests; they offer customers gluten-free alternatives that not only live up to every star but inspire envy in other guests.

Once upon a time, there was a kind of feeding frenzy around gluten-free treats. We ate more than we wanted or was good for us because a slice of peach pie or a fudge brownie was rare; better to eat it now than never see it again. I love the idea that in the abundance of today's gluten-free choices, there can be moderation. When I'm offered a slice of pizza, I can say, "No thanks, I'm on a diet," knowing there's more where that came from.

This is no small thing.

While there is only one gluten-free diet, one that needs to be followed scrupulously and for life, there are delicious variations on the path to healthy eating. With a little homework, and a solid grounding in the essentials, vegan, vegetarian, paleo, Mediterranean, lactose-free, casein-free and/or dairy-free, old-fashioned omnivore, *and* gluten-free all have a place at the table.

In fact, a growing number of us are eating locally and going organic, passing up processed, GMO (genetically modified organism), and factory-farmed foods along with gluten. The gluten-free path is now synonymous with vibrant good health. Gwyneth Paltrow is a glowing example of this and proves it with her recipe for vegan Sweet Potato and Five-Spice Muffins (page 194); as does Jennifer Katzinger, founder of Flying Apron Bakery (Sweet Potato Rosemary Bread, page 156; Fresh Strawberry and Blueberry Fruit Tart, page 185; and Banana Split Cake, page 236), among others earning their places among the best of the best baking today.

This kind of conscious eating is giving the processed, high-fructose-corn-syrup world of the supermarket a run for its money. We are learning one can eat sustainably and well and still be gluten-free. There are many reasons for choosing to give up meat or dairy; we no longer have to worry about how this will work with a gluten-free diet. We've got options galore. In Chapter 2, "The New Food Hyphenate," I've covered the basics and suggested some further reading material, so you can explore a way of eating that's right for you.

Every day someone tells me they've sworn off gluten.

"I feel less tired," declares a new mother of twins.

"It helps my candida," says the punked-out drummer down the block.

And there is the world-class tennis player who swore off gluten and rocked his game straight to Wimbledon.

"Humans were not designed to digest gluten," the hostess of a dinner party tells me, showing off her fresh gluten-free ravioli con funghi as if I lived on the moon.

Even the UPS guy gets in on the act. "That stuff'll kill you," he says.

My own publisher is gluten-free.

We are in good company.

Fifteen million Americans follow a gluten-free diet, of which three million, myself included, are gluten-intolerant with documented celiac disease. And there is a broad spectrum of sensitivity. It is estimated that as many as 30 to 40 percent of the US population have non-celiac intolerance and sensitivity in the absence of this serious autoimmune condition, and up to 8 percent of American children under eighteen have food allergies. Even more amazing, over forty million of us buy gluten-free products, not only for ourselves but also for our friends and families, creating a $4.2 billion market, which is expected to swell to $6 billion by the year 2017. And that's a modest assessment. One market research firm says those numbers are even higher at $10.5 billion last year and $15 billion in sales of all things gluten-free predicted by 2016. Given the added cost of gluten-free products, we are generous, too.

Thanks to a landmark study funded by the National Institutes of Health and spearheaded by the best minds in the international celiac research community, what many of us only knew in our gut has been confirmed. A staggering 1 in 133 otherwise healthy people have celiac disease, even more among those with affected first- and second-degree relatives. According to the University of Chicago Celiac Disease Center, these numbers are rising sharply, fourfold in the last fifty years.

I wonder if this is not just because of greater awareness or better diagnoses but also due to the widespread theory that changes to the wheat crop, especially a new super-drought-resistant and bug-resistant, genetically engineered variety containing higher amounts of gluten, are wreaking havoc with human digestion.

Even bees can't handle the stuff. A recent *New York Times* article on a new mystery malady killing bees points to pesticide-containing GMO crops (see Chapter 22, "Food Fights") as a possible cause for the worst thing to hit the apiary since colony collapse. Some say it's because food companies are adding vital wheat gluten to already glutinous grains. Others point to artificial yeast. Still more cite the dramatic increase in all food allergies and blame a food supply being systematically tainted by frankenfoods. Maybe, too, as boomers age, those who have eaten gluten safely all their lives may be losing their immunological tolerance for the stuff. What we do know is that we are eating wheat our grandparents wouldn't recognize.

But whatever the reason, we know that gluten intolerance and its many variations are far more common than we ever thought. Who could have predicted a time when Lady Gaga would tweet that she'd gone gluten-free and expected to lose ten pounds by month's end? Or that Miley Cyrus would exhort us to lose the gluten and watch our skins glow.

Most would agree that the gluten-free diet per se is not a great way to lose weight, unless you swear off *all* refined carbohydrates and eat only whole grains packed with nutrition. In fact, once we eliminate the absorption issues caused by gluten, we may even gain a pound or two as we relearn how much we can eat to maintain a healthy weight.

But if certain pop stars consider carbohydrate-free a synonym for gluten-free, we want to gently set them straight and welcome them to the club. The more, the merrier, I say.

* * *

The explosion in all things gluten-free irks some in the celiac community and may even strike fear into the hearts of those who have brought us to this tipping point, selfless souls who have worked long and unflaggingly for awareness of celiac disease as a bona fide disease. Many would dismiss the sudden popularity of the gluten-free diet as a fad and, admittedly, for some it certainly is. But that would underestimate the plain truth that every day more and more of us have good reasons to swear off gluten.

Instead of looking for purity, we should be asking ourselves why so many feel better without wheat, barley, rye, and their derivatives. Is celiac disease merely the tip of the gluten iceberg, as some in the scientific community say? Is the human immune system under assault? Is our food supply compromised? Is that compromise environmental or manufactured, as some suspect? Are we the canaries in the coal mine?

Food for thought.

The good news is that the gluten-free revolution is many millions strong and, as a massive consumer group, we are demanding new regulation and transparency about the safety of our food supply. We have insisted on a high and uniform standard for gluten-free labeling. It took nine years but, in the summer of 2013, we got a long-overdue final ruling from the FDA. Is the ruling perfect? No. Will we continue to press for mandatory labeling rather than the current voluntary rules? I hope so.

Our voices rise again for full disclosure about GMOs and additives in the food we eat. Powerful, vocal, and growing in number, we are able to bring pressure to bear on the food industry and government agencies to disclose their practices and fund more research. At this writing, deadly trans fats, deemed unsafe for human consumption, may soon be a danger we no longer have to worry about, with the FDA moving toward significantly limiting, or more or less banning, their use in processed foods.

As a group, we get things done.

Personally, I'm thrilled to be part of such a large and diverse family. I'm not worried about overexposure or that those of us with celiac disease will suffer somehow. The more of us there are, the better we all eat. As consumers, we have given the gluten-free market critical mass and have encouraged entrepreneurs to abandon the tried and true and dedicate themselves to building new business models that embrace the fact that gluten-free is here to stay. But abundance also brings challenge.

Not all of us have a zero-tolerance mind-set when it comes to gluten. Should we treat with suspicion the safety of food offered by those who may have a laissez-faire attitude about what constitutes a gluten-free meal, and especially those in a position to instruct our children? Absolutely. Do we have to double-check meals served by well-meaning but undereducated newcomers? We certainly do. Must we take with a grain of sea salt the health claims of this growing group? You betcha.

Vetting becomes even more important in a world where not everyone is sensitive to the same degree and there is not as much at stake when mistakes are made. A little knowledge can be a dangerous thing.

Recently I walked into one of those big chain pasta restaurants to ask if there were any gluten-free options on the menu; I was hoping for pizza or ready-made ravioli close to home.

The pretty blond greeter's smile was electric.

"Oh, yes," she gushed. "We have quite a few gluten-free customers who LOVE the whole-wheat pasta."

Seriously?

Notoriety never comes without its challenges and foods, like health conditions, all have their moments—remember Swedish meatballs, chicken fricassee, fondue, the South Beach Diet, Atkins, the year everyone in America was in the Zone?

Will the Rastafarian macrobiotic down the street fall off the gluten-free wagon and jump on some other food fad? It goes without saying. Will the frenzied writing of cookbooks, blogs, and building of gluten-free empires abate?

Of course.

But when the wave finally breaks, we will be left with a world that takes gluten-free in its stride, equal to low-fat and cholesterol-, salt-, and sugar-, preservative-, peanut-, pesticide-, GMO-, and lactose-free, as valid options for those with celiac disease, gluten sensitivity, food allergies, and other sensitivities. We will be healthier, wiser, and far more assertive about what we put in our mouths than ever before in history. And science will have found out why so many millions of us react badly to wheat and gluten.

For some, a gluten-blocking pill or patch is a long-held dream, and I wouldn't mind popping something myself, then having a nice gooey cheesy slice. But who knows, in the post-gluten age the hunt for the magic bullet for when we just want the real thing may be beside the point because the alternative is so good and so much healthier—it *is* the real thing.

How did I become so passionately involved in the issue of gluten-free, or, as my friends have adorably said, become a gluten-free goddess?

I come from a family of writers and painters who believe that the artist's job is to bear witness to their circumstances. As a poet and novelist, I believe in the power of story to show us another way to handle our circumstances. My circumstances included celiac disease and the very primal hunt for food on a daily basis. I am interested in the gray areas and in the soft, emotional ground we all stand on, where so much of how we feel about food rests. I could care less about lists of what we should and should not do. I became an activist and author because I wanted to give voice to a group who once upon a time had none and to do it in a way that took into account the real lives of my readers.

It doesn't get more personal than food. How we eat is inexorably intertwined with how we live. It is the sensory thread that runs through the narrative of our lives.

Genes and destiny had something to do with it, too.

My mother's maiden name was Petitpain, French for "little bread."

Her people were originally from Nantes and Paris, and settled in the Caribbean city of Saint-Domingue, where, according to family legend, my ancestor, a young widow named Marguerite, was trying to figure out how to get her late husband's bakery out of debt just as the uprising that would birth the nation of Haiti was beating a bloody path to her door. She fled back to France, but her sons made for America and New Orleans, where one of them opened a bakery whose beignet recipe survived straight down into my own childhood.

Given this heritage, it was a great surprise that after years of puzzling and increasingly troublesome symptoms, my own classic presentation of celiac disease was diagnosed, and among the first and second cousins in my generation, there are four more cases, as well as my mother, who demonstrated all the signs at the age of eighty-three. Another cousin, long plagued with plumbing problems, now sees her tricky digestion in terms of our family gene pool.

I'm a believer in the idea that where we are injured is where we shine the brightest. Heal yourself first, then help others do the same. A gift for story and a keen sense of connecting the dots allowed me to do just that.

Revolutions move fast and in unexpected ways. A book big enough to capture all the choices in our rapidly expanding gluten-free universe was a daunting proposition, one that is ultimately impossible. My goal is to instead arm you with the latest information and put you on the path to the good life without gluten, able to navigate any situation with knowledge, confidence, and joie de vivre. Because change is a fluid, vibrant thing, I want you to know how to look for the new products, services, and medical break-throughs that will inevitably come after this book goes to press.

On these pages you will learn how to find caterers, chefs, cooking teachers, dieticians, and culinary schools specializing in gluten-free cook-ing and baking, as well as ballparks with gluten-free hot dogs and buns. Gluten-free cookbooks abound, and I include a sampling of recipes from the best ones. There are gluten-free-friendly inns, hotels, and luxury resorts, as well as cruises, travel companies, and summer camps.

In our increasingly connected world, community is crucial. I've included a guide to blogs, travel sites, bulletin boards, forums, gluten-free workshops and conferences, magazines full of articles and mouthwatering recipes, res-taurant reviews, new product information, and articles for the allergic.

A stroll through any farmers' market will net bread, rolls, cookies, muffins, scones, and often something to nibble on while shopping. In Chapter 5, "Marketing 101," I've listed the best places to meet your fellow travelers. There are smartphone apps to check product ingredients while shopping, others to give an overview of fast-food and chain restaurants' menu choices, and still others, through GPS mapping technology, that make it possible to find the nearest gluten-free bakery or restaurant. Still more offer a list of GMO-free products and those free of common aller-gens. With so many resources, this vastly expanded edition captures the complexity and enormity of the choices before you.

Of course, food is always paramount. The food in this special anni-versary edition showcases the range and excellence of gluten-free cuisine: Chapter 6, "Essential Skills," with its uncomplicated kitchen techniques and recipes, makes the point that the more we know about the simple preparation of food, the more control we have over our health and the less dependent we are on foods that come out of a box, bag, pouch, or frozen slab full of additives and artificial ingredients.

Chapter 7, "Cooking With the Stars," proves that America's favorite chefs—celebrities and soon-to-be—are the most generous in the world. Among them are Alice Waters, Thomas Keller, Traci Des Jardins, Katy Sparks, Bobby Flay, Molly O'Neill, Marcie Turney, Kelli and Peter Bronski, Rick Bayless, Steve DiFillippo, and Kristine Kidd.

Chapter 8, "A Baker's Dozen," offers recipes from America's best gluten-free bakers and one from as far away as Paris, from buttery pas-tries to extraordinary dairy-free and vegan concoctions.

Chapter 9, "You Gotta Have It," speaks to the hunger for foods associated with childhood, love, and comfort, the times we remember most, the very ones usually loaded with gluten. Here you'll find recipes for guilty pleasures like Grown-Up Macaroni and Cheese (page 208), Pizza Just Like Mama Makes (or Wishes She Could) (page 209), French Onion Soup with Gruyère-Smothered Crostini (page 213), Spiced Carrot Cake with Sweet Mascarpone Frosting (page 215), Oh, Mama! Meat Loaf (page 211), and more, with the gluten-free versions of products like Oreo cookies, ice cream sandwiches, and licorice, comfort foods you thought you'd never eat again.

In Chapter 10, "Gather," we look at all the ways, large and small, we break bread together and bind ourselves to something much bigger than our dietary restrictions.

For ordering a great meal anywhere in the world, provided your server is literate, see Chapter 14, "Sprechen Sie Gluten?" You'll find simplified and all-new foreign dining cards, twenty-three in all, including English— Arabic, Thai, Hindi, and Swahili, along with French, Spanish, German, Croatian, Hebrew, Swedish, Russian, Polish, Portuguese, Czech, Italian, Japanese, Danish, Dutch, Greek, Korean, Vietnamese, and Chinese—to take abroad or to the nearest ethnic restaurant. You can pack as many as you need for any given adventure.

I've tackled the tough issues, too, ones that go well beyond the problem of what's for dinner. I have consulted with the experts to bring to you the newest tests, what to do, and who to see if you suspect you are gluten-intolerant. I offer a recipe for disaster and what to keep on hand for emergencies. How do we survive childhood? College? Dating?

In Chapter 17, "Sex and the Celiac," I'll take on both the lighter and more serious side of reproduction, followed by some thoughts on raising happy, healthy, gluten-free kids, which includes an important discussion of childhood gluten intolerance by Ritu Verma, pediatric gastroenterologist and director of the Center for Celiac Disease at the Children's Hospital of Philadelphia.

Later you'll find answers to many other questions of concern to newcomers and veterans alike, such as where to find support groups, expos, and conferences, and, if you lean toward activism, how to get involved in the politics of lobbying for healthier food and GMO labeling.

If you want to read this book from cover to cover, I won't complain, but I've structured it for you to dip into as situations arise. You may want to try a certain chef's recipe before you invest in his or her cookbook, find a gluten-free bed-and-breakfast, plan a Paris or Rome itinerary around the best gluten-free bakeries or gelaterias, or maybe you need to make or bake something special for a dinner party or picky eater. You may be thinking about becoming a vegan and wonder how that squares with the gluten-free diet. Or you're looking for a smartphone app, or just jonesing for something from your glutenous past. Maybe you want to read more about a particular subject or find a blogger who shares your worldview. I've ended every chapter with a way to learn more.

I have signed more soup-stained editions than I can count, which thrills me beyond words. You might want to put a plastic cover on this one. It's going to get a lot of wear.

The Gluten-Free Revolution, like my previous books, celebrates the whole person, not just the one sitting at the dinner table. A cheeky attitude and a healthy sense of humor help; I've learned this from long experience, and it's something I will never change. While I have focused on the new, I have not fiddled with what many of you now consider classic wisdom.

I offer comfort, strategies for every occasion, and proactive approaches for everyone who has ever faced a howling hunger, an empty plate, a non-compliant waiter, or, worse, a member of the family who just doesn't get it. And believe me, despite national awareness of gluten intolerance and all the attention given to the gluten-free diet, there are still pockets of indifference and scorn. Those unenlightened souls are in the minority now, but still. There are those who dismiss us as faddists, but more often than not we find ourselves the focus of well-meaning questions and a genuine need to please. We must guard against being the recipients of attention spurred on by good intentions and not enough know-how. Like it or not, we must educate as well as negotiate. All these years later, I do know that nothing is more difficult than giving up the deep pleasure and satisfaction of one's favorite foods, even if avoiding them is purely voluntary.

I still remember in piercing detail the aching sense of loss that accompanied my own diagnosis. How sick I was. How thin I got. How everywhere I looked I saw evidence of other people's pleasure. I grieved for the foods I thought I could never enjoy again and did what most people in denial do: I cheated every chance I could get.

What saved me then and what will save you now is the thrill of discovery—a richly satisfying pumpkin and sage risotto, gnocchi light as clouds, Thai rice noodles, a pear and fig crisp still warm from the oven, a vegetarian or dairy-free dish that can't be, but is, the best meal you've ever had.

Your own discoveries will lead you out of the kitchen and into the world of dinners, brunches, lunches, parties, weddings, holidays, vacations, and business trips. Creativity, emotional directness—a sense of fun; not gloom and doom—and a good bit of chutzpah will soon have your friends fussing, hostesses adjusting, and chefs gladly rising to the culinary challenge you offer. As you develop skills in your own kitchen, and cook for friends and family, you may even find you've got more gluten-free company than you bargained for. So easy will you make it look.

My purpose is no different today than it was when I first started. I am convinced that nothing is beyond the person who can conquer the loss of something as important, as primal, and as basic to one's comfort as food. I present my case for choosing joy over sorrow, self-assertion and resourcefulness over scarcity and negative thinking, pleasure over regret, generosity over self-absorption, and health over what I call *Industrial Eating*.

Whether you are a veteran or a newcomer, have endured a lifetime of being sick or just feel better without gluten, my modest hope is that you will find on these pages one of life's most transforming lessons: imperfection is what makes us interesting, injury the motive that makes us shine. And if by chance you miss a meal, there's always another one coming. Not to mention two snacks. Tomorrow you get to start all over.

What follows is the only way I know to live: with a glad heart, a wise head, and a full stomach. Chapter and verse, this special anniversary edition chronicles this remarkable gluten-free revolution of ours. It is my proof that living without gluten has never been easier or more satisfying, a piece of cake, actually. With all that is available to us today, no one should go hungry, miss a celebration, be ignored, or have to eat something underwhelming just because it's gluten-free.

Know that you join a large, boisterous, and sometimes fractious family; we have walked in your gluten-free shoes. No road is long in good company and no day that includes laughter is ever wasted. Armed with information, a good sense of humor, and food you never thought you'd eat again, there's no reason this can't be one of life's excellent adventures.

Welcome to the gluten-free revolution.

JAX PETERS LOWELL
Philadelphia, 2014

Part I

Me,
Gluten-Free?

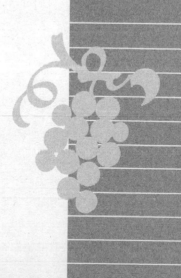

Gluten-Free Nation

Home of the brave, land of the gluten-free.

—WITH APOLOGIES TO FRANCIS SCOTT KEY

◆ What Exactly Is Gluten?

◆ What Is Celiac Disease vs. Non-Celiac Gluten Sensitivity?

◆ The Good News, the Bad News, the Basics

Symptoms: Puzzling and Protean

Yes, No, Maybe Foods

Alcohol

Oats

◆ Do I Still Have to Read Labels?

◆ Ten Basic Rules to Help You Cook and Eat Safely

Congratulations.

You have just joined the biggest food movement since soup in a can.

After months or even years of not feeling quite right or in downright misery, you may have recently discovered you're the 1 in 133 of the general population of otherwise healthy Americans who have celiac disease or CD, sometimes referred to as gluten-sensitive enteropathy, the quaintly archaic celiac sprue, or, even more remote, nontropical sprue, an inherited condition that triggers an autoimmune response that causes damage to your small intestine when you consume any grain containing gluten, which includes wheat, rye, barley, and oats from fields and mills contaminated with wheat.

If you've had the classic symptoms related to celiac disease (diarrhea; weight loss; abdominal distention; flatulence; frequent bulky, foul-smelling stools; vomiting; nausea; anemia) and if one of your parents, children, or siblings are celiacs, your chances of gluten intolerance could be as low as 1 in 56.

If any of your first-degree relatives are celiacs, the University of Chicago Celiac Center says chances are 1 in 22 that you've got it. Among second-degree relatives, it's 1 in 39. If you are African, Hispanic, or Asian American, you could be the 1 in 236 people genetically unable to digest gluten. A landmark study published by Dr. Alessio Fasano and colleagues in the *Archives of Internal Medicine* in February 2003 proved once and for all that celiac disease is not and never has been rare, just underdiagnosed. Even more remarkable, 60 percent of children and 41 percent of adults diagnosed during that study had absolutely no symptoms.

Subclinical or atypical symptoms include bone and joint pain, thyroid problems, osteoporosis, osteopenia, ataxia, dental enamel defects, brain fog, fatigue, irritability, weakness, weight gain, constipation, spontaneous miscarriage, infertility, intensely itchy and burning rash, depression, muscle cramps, peripheral neuropathy, even memory loss and seizures. And if you think you're the only one in the family with problems, guess again. Remember skinny Uncle Max with the delicate stomach; Grandma Reilly, stooped over with osteoporosis, who always fell asleep after a spaghetti dinner; the extremely small, fussy baby your nephew was; or your cousin Minnie, who couldn't get pregnant even if she stood on her head, which she tried, too? And come to think of it, there's poor Cousin Fred who just can't seem to ever get out of the bathroom and Uncle Harry whose foot slaps when he walks. Shake the CD family tree, and chances are others will fall. It's just a matter of time and testing.

But that's only the tip of the iceberg.

Millions of you, more and more every day, are sick and tired of feeling lousy every time you eat a piece of wheat bread or a bowl of pasta. You've decided to give up gluten on your own, even though you have tested negative for celiac disease, even if you haven't yet been tested. You fall somewhere on the spectrum, from mild to full-blown non-celiac gluten sensitivity, which causes bloating, gastrointestinal distress, fatigue, headaches, and mental fogginess among other nasty symptoms when you eat something glutenous or, as we insiders like to say, when you get "glutened."

You may be dealing with multiple food allergies and intolerances, of which gluten is only one. In the last decade there has been a precipitous rise in your ranks. An increasing number of you have simply come to realize that you feel better without it and have gotten rid of gluten on your own. You think more clearly, have more energy, don't feel as weighed down by processed wheat, and, frankly, are suspicious of the genetic structure of grains grown today.

So, you've got a lot to digest. Your odd little immune system, leaky gut, and the pool in which your particular genes are swimming have tricked your body into thinking bread and other foods containing gluten are poison. Foods as seemingly basic to human life as breathing are off-limits. Suddenly the stuff of life is life's big stiff.

It doesn't matter how you got here; you're here now.

What Exactly Is Gluten?

Forgive the bare-bones simplicity of this, but lately too many people say they're gluten-free, then order the barley soup and the seitan steak. Gluten, a mixture of two proteins—gliadin and glutenin—is found in wheat, rye, and barley, and a long list of derivatives thereof, which are described in this chapter. This is the stuff that gives dough its elasticity and causes digestive problems and disorders from mild to serious in those sensitive to it. That's you.

What Is Celiac Disease?

Celiac disease is a serious inherited autoimmune condition in which there is an immune reaction to eating gluten, which causes the immune system to attack the walls of the intestine as gluten proteins travel through the intestinal tract. This inflames the lining of the small intestine (villi), causing the small bowel to atrophy, rendering the intestine permeable. In turn, this prevents the absorption of important nutrients, depriving the bones, brain, liver, and other organs of vital nourishment. This causes multiple deficiencies such as osteoporosis and anemia and can lead to infertility, miscarriage, neurologic problems, and cancer if not diagnosed. Celiac disease is also associated with many other autoimmune conditions, such as asthma, autoimmune thyroid problems, diabetes, lupus, and Sjögren's syndrome. The need for testing cannot be emphasized enough.

What Is Non-Celiac Gluten Sensitivity?

This is a condition, newly recognized by the medical community, in which the individual cannot tolerate gluten and experiences symptoms similar to those with celiac disease, but lacks the antibodies, intestinal damage, and risk for complications seen in CD. Gluten sensitivity is not associated with the destruction of the lining of the small intestine, but it does cause inflammation and mimics many of the symptoms of celiac disease. As of now, there is no accurate test for the condition, nor does anybody have a clue as to exactly how many people are affected by this, except that they are probably in the millions. By conservative estimates over 20 percent of the population has non-celiac gluten sensitivity, a group far larger than those who have celiac disease, and growing every day. Diagnosis at this point is really just a description of someone who does not have celiac disease, but whose health improves on a gluten-free diet and worsens if gluten is reintroduced. That would be you, too.

To Confuse Things Further

In addition to the above-described conditions, researchers, physicians, nutritionists, and allergists are noting that incidences of wheat allergy, which is typically a pediatric disorder that tends to peak and subside by age one, are increasing daily. There is an uptick in cases of exercise-induced wheat allergy, as well as an itchy rash among food handlers, bakery workers, and restaurant personnel, who are all in frequent contact with uncooked wheat. In a double-blind Australian study published in the *American Journal of Gastroenterology*, Dr. Peter Gibson tested patients with irritable bowel syndrome (IBS) who do not have celiac disease but were on a gluten-free diet. One group was given gluten-containing bread and muffins to eat for six weeks, and the other, gluten-free bread and muffins. Those who ate gluten suffered considerably worse pain, bloating, nausea, and fatigue. There is more research to be done, but experts concluded that IBS is also a very big part of the gluten iceberg.

Even more puzzling, researchers say it is entirely possible that many of you who are sensitive to gluten and embark on the gluten-free diet are really responding to FODMAPs—foods that include gluten, lactose, and fructose, or a protein in wheat that naturally protects the plant against pests. And some speculate that the increase in gluten-related heath issues is because of the way wheat is grown today.

It's a big iceberg under the surface. In my view, it's one that comes down to troubling changes in our food supply. We are learning more about it every day, but we certainly don't yet know everything. So for now, let us fully understand the gluten-free diet.

The Good News, the Bad News, the Basics

The good news is that you can eat rice and corn, millet and quinoa (if you're not allergic to them for different reasons), and exotic grains like amaranth and teff, as long as they are pure and untainted by wheat. The good news is that gluten-free food is really good nowadays. So good, everybody wants some. There is more of it than you'll have time to eat.

More good news: you're not dead.

Not only are you not dead, even if you have celiac disease, you don't have anything that could be even remotely construed as fatal, life-threatening, degenerative, or even chronic. (Unless you cheat constantly, and you're not going to do that, are you?) Unlike other conditions that involve serious drugs, frequent doctor visits, and expensive hospital stays, gluten intolerance requires no surgery, no nasty procedures, no prescription drugs with side effects printed in minuscule type, only that you remain scrupulously gluten-free. The right food is your medicine. How many conditions can claim that?

All those years of terrible, puzzling, and conflicting symptoms are over. Gone. History. Outta here. This is very good news.

Better still—if you stay on your diet, you will feel good again. Not only good, better than you've ever felt. Even if you have no symptoms and took the blood test only to humor your grain-challenged sister, your sharper, more energetic new normal will have you wondering why it took you so long.

Great news.

Be Advised!

Get tested for celiac disease before you start a gluten-free diet. You need to be eating gluten in order to get an accurate diagnosis. If you don't have celiac disease, fine. But if you do and don't get tested, CD will be much harder to detect, as will connecting the dots for the many and sometimes serious conditions associated with it. Fair warning: I will say this many times before I'm through and you will be sick of hearing it.

Now that the whole world knows what gluten-free is, you are in good company. If you have CD, know that it affects 1 percent of healthy average Americans. That's three million of us with documented celiac disease. That leaves 97 percent of us undiagnosed. Which may account for the untold millions like you who are mildly to not so mildly sensitive to gluten but have no diagnosis.

Despite the fact that more and more cases are being caught through family screening, and more of us are seeking the services of a gastroenterologist sooner rather than later, according to the University of Chicago Celiac Disease Center most people knock around from doctor to doctor for an average of four years before somebody figures out what's wrong. That's down from an average of eleven years. This is really good news. The faster you pinpoint the problem and lose the gluten, the better your chances are of not acquiring any condition related to undiagnosed celiac disease.

SYMPTOMS CAN BE PUZZLING AND PROTEAN

My own battle with gluten took a huge toll on my health. Most of my life I suffered stomach pains but never got sick enough to seek help. Then, in my late twenties, during a particularly stressful period, I expressed full-blown celiac syndrome, losing as much as five pounds a week and developing everything from gigantic hives to bone pain and a constant low-level nausea that seemed to point to serious illness.

My hair lost its shine and fell out in clumps. My muscles had begun to atrophy from a lack of protein. I suffered from anemia. Two bones fractured from lack of calcium absorption. For a New Yorker, there was suddenly such a thing as too thin. I weighed an astonishing ninety pounds, which at five foot eight gave me the look of a mobile cadaver.

My heart developed a murmur. (What was it saying?) I stopped counting how many trips to the bathroom I made and had to nap to recover from taking a nap. The smart money was on lymphoma, a cancer of the lymphatic system that reveals itself in many of the same ways as celiac disease. I was given a bed in a section of the hospital grimly dubbed "the bone yard."

Happily, the smart money lost.

Suddenly, everything made sense.

As I have said, gluten damages the ability of the villi to absorb vital nutrients; mine were so thickened and scarred that I'd literally stopped absorbing. My long history of painful and overly long periods was due to my inability to absorb vitamin K, which is necessary in the coagulation of blood. This, too, was the reason for my puzzling resistance to healing.

A lack of vitamin B$_{12}$ was the culprit in the anemia department, and zero calcium absorption, not a forgotten fall as one X-ray technician had insisted, was the reason for the fracture, the constant pain in my joints, and the onset, much later, of osteoporosis.

All the years spent doubled over with what I repeatedly described as the feeling of "ground glass in my gut" were not due to a teenager's panic over the SATs or, later, the adrenaline rush of an advertising career or a nervous temperament. It wasn't PMS, or the push and shove of a marriage settling in, or because it was Thursday, or because I was "neurotic," as one baffled diagnostician suggested, playing a pernicious form of "blame the victim" when her search for the cause stalled.

It wasn't a case of simple blood work then. A battery of medieval tests no longer performed showed a seriously diminished ability to absorb foods, particularly those with a high fat content. A surgical biopsy or upper endoscopy (still the gold standard for a definitive diagnosis) was done and my besieged intestinal villi showed the doctor everything he needed to know.

I was told I could thank my father's Irish roots. It would be years before I stopped blaming the folks from Donegal and looked to my mother's French forebears for the real culprit.

"Go home, take your supplements, and live a normal life," the doctor told me, bursting with pride at having detected what most believed then was a disease rare in adults.

"Just don't eat any bread, pasta, cookies, sandwiches, tarts, croissants, bagels, granola, cereal, cakes, pies, muffins, pastries, sauces, soufflés, stuffing, prepared gravies, crab cakes, pancakes, carrot cakes, birthday cakes, frozen dinners, canned soup.

"And oh, by the way, Happy Thanksgiving."

There were no gluten-free cartoons in the *New Yorker* then. No gluten-free bakeries on every corner. No jokes on late-night TV. Gluten-free labels on food were unheard of. People stared. Waiters glared. Hostesses greeted my presence at their tables with weak smiles. I was the object of rude questions, questionable dinner conversation, and bad jokes. Gluten-free products did not exist. There were no gluten-free options in restaurants, no gluten-free muffins to nibble in the coffee shop. Al Gore had not yet invented the Internet.

What could I do?

I stayed home, ate tuna fish, and avoided the whole thing.

While my family shed tears of relief and told embarrassing stories about how as an infant I refused to be weaned and clung to my mother's

My People/Your People

Legend has it that early invaders poisoned the wheat harvest. Who were they—Goths, Huns, the Uncle Ben's people? As the myth goes, succeeding generations adapted by reacting to gluten as the poison it was meant to be. While there is no basis for this in scientific fact, I like this theory because it allows me to imagine that I am from a fierce tribe that would not be conquered, adapting instead and becoming the first people to exhibit passive-aggressive behavior.

breast as if my little intestines *knew*, and how, the summer that I was four, I threw every bit of food I was given against our cottage's knotty pine wall, I felt selfish and petty.

How could I complain about a meal when so many face real illness in their lives?

It became clear that I had to make a choice. I could feel sorry for myself or I could turn that attention into a positive and teach myself how to enjoy life again. I didn't know then that one day I would share these hard-won lessons with others. I resolved to see the good news, but it wouldn't be good news until I said it was.

We all get here via different routes.

For many of us, the path is painful and confusing. For others, it is a journey marked by challenge, determination, and courage. Maybe you had to confront the insurance company and demand to be referred to the right people. Or had to face up to derision and teasing, were accused of being neurotic, a sucker for the latest fad. Whether it took years or a few miserable months, you hung in there. You asked questions, kept pushing despite the fact that you may have been told your only problem was an overactive imagination. Maybe you just woke up one morning and said, "Today is the day I get healthy," and made a serious commitment to a gluten-free diet.

The point is, something happened.

Whether it was a long battle or a brief skirmish, your journey needs to be acknowledged before you move on. This may come as a surprise to some of you, especially those who were taught to keep a stiff upper lip, but you really don't have to feel better because other people say you do. Not that you need it, but you have my permission to whine a little.

An entire food group is missing from your life. It deserves its own mourning period.

Tell your story, as I have told you mine, until you no longer need to tell it. This may take longer than the time allotted to you by others, even friends and family. Never mind. Find somebody who hasn't heard it yet.

Lord knows, I love a good joke, but Jimmy Fallon aside, the gluten-free diet is not a laughing matter. Nor is it a passing fad for the nuts-and-sprouts-diet-du-jour crowd. It is a serious commitment to health.

Whether you have celiac disease, are intolerant, or are mildly sensitive, getting rid of gluten can be the difference between feeling so-so and positively glowing. It is possible to save your own life and eat happily ever after.

I am living proof of this.

Best news of all—with sophisticated gluten-free baking formulas and mixes, sauces, breads, and sweet treats made with a myriad of high-fiber, protein-packed, and good-for-you grains, gluten-free foods are so delicious, not only is it hard to tell the difference, more often than not they are better. In side-by-side comparisons, a surprising number of gluten-eating citizens prefer the gluten-free version.

BAD NEWS

You knew there'd be some.

The change is swift and terrible. A bagel eaten one day is verboten the next. Unless it's gluten-free, of course. You've ordered your last slice with everything on it, as well as your last cheeseburger on a brioche roll, you've buttered your last croissant and bought your last frozen dinner, ice cream cone, slice of apple pie.

Some of you will eat the things that make you feel sick until you realize this is true. This is not a good idea, especially if you have undiagnosed celiac disease, but you know that.

Spontaneity is out. Planning is in.

From now on you have to think about every bit of food you put in your mouth. No more aimless grazing, nibbling, or grabbing something, anything, when you're famished.

Even in a gluten-free-friendly world, you've got to plan meals and snacks and restaurant dinners, especially on road trips. You are on a diet that allows no slack. It will test your resolve and turn even the meekest among us into a serial killer (which, in your case, is spelled "cereal").

More bad news.

There is no such thing as a casual gluten-free diet. You can't be good at lunch and succumb to the garlic bread at dinner. You're either off gluten or you're not. And not everybody agrees about what is and what is not gluten-free.

Did I say this would be a walk in the park?

THE BASICS

Here's the basic gluten-free diet as described by the Mayo Clinic, *The Merck Manual*, *Living Without* magazine, expanded upon by the Gluten Intolerance Group and the American Dietetic Association. Look carefully. Some foods require explanation.

How Did Gluten Intolerance Come to Be?

The scientific explanation is that when the discovery of nuts and seeds turning into edible plants ushered in the Paleolithic Age, the first food intolerance was born. Given the popularity of the modern paleo diet, maybe the cave people knew something we don't.

NATURALLY GLUTEN-FREE FOODS

Beans

Butter

Cheese, natural, aged

Chocolate

Cocoa and cocoa powder

Coffee

Corn

Dairy products

Eggs

Fruits

Meats, fish, and poultry that have not been breaded, battered, or marinated in gluten-containing sauces or ingredients

Milk and milk products

Nuts in their natural, unprocessed form

Oils, shortening, olive oil

Rice

Tea

Vegetables

Seeds

NOTE: The above foods are gluten-free only if they are in their fresh, natural forms and have not been processed or mixed or in any way contaminated with gluten-containing grains, additives, or preservatives.

ALWAYS AVOID

Barley

Barley enzyme

Barley extract

Barley grass

Barley malt sweeteners

Barley pearls

Bran (unless rice bran)

Bulghur wheat

Durum

Einkorn

Emmer

Farina

Farro

Graham

Graham Flour

Hydrolyzed wheat

Kamut

Malt flavoring

Malt vinegar

Rye bread or rye crisp

Seitan (wheat gluten)

Semolina

Spelt

Tabbouleh

Triticale

Udon noodles (unless certified gluten-free)

Wheat

Wheat berry

Wheat bran

Wheat germ and wheat germ oil

Wheat starch

AVOID UNLESS CERTIFIED GLUTEN-FREE

Baked goods

Beer

Bread

Breading and coating mixes

Cakes and pies

Candy

Cereal

Communion wafers

Corn muffins

Crab cakes

Cream soups

Gravies

Imitation meat, bacon, or seafood

Marinades

Oats

Pastas

Pizza

Processed cheese spreads

Processed luncheon meats

Salad dressings

Sauces

Seasoned rice mixes

Self-basting turkeys

Stuffing

Vegetables in sauce

NOTE: *Wheat-free* does *not* mean *gluten-free!*

Living Without magazine tells us that wheat is wheat, no matter what aliases it assumes, namely einkorn, emmer, durum, farina, farro, graham, semolina, spelt, rye, and triticale, a cross between wheat and rye.

Allowed grains and flours are rice, corn or maize, cassava, soy, potato, tapioca, beans, garfava, sorghum, quinoa, millet, buckwheat, arrowroot, amaranth, teff, montina, flax, and nut flours.

Should you photocopy this list and stick it on your refrigerator door? Not so fast.

In a perfect world, everyone would agree on what is and what is not gluten-free.

In the gluten-free world, the issue is how a particular grain is grown, milled, or otherwise mixed (the term we use is contaminated) with forbidden grains. Further, not all organizations, Internet sources of nutritional information, and medical practitioners offer the same guidelines for safe eating. Even in the new world of FDA-mandated and -standardized gluten-free labeling, you must be prepared to do your homework on any given food item and make an informed decision.

This is especially important for the newly gluten-free whose bodies are still on the mend. To complicate matters, what we know about the presence or absence of gluten in food is evolving as research catches up with our diet.

ALCOHOL

The American Dietetic Association (*Manual of Clinical Dietetics*, 6th ed.) considers distilled alcoholic beverages not fortified or otherwise flavored or enhanced—gin, whiskey, and vodka (but not beer, which contains malt)—and other products that contain distilled alcohol, such as vinegar and vanilla and other flavored extracts—safe to consume on a gluten-free diet.

The science is clear; the distilling process itself renders the end result safe and microscopically free of gluten.

You may have other reasons to avoid alcohol, but gluten is not one of them.

Still, some prefer to avoid these products. While you're making up your mind what's best for you (discuss it with your doctor, assuming he or she is up on all the new research), there is always wine, potato vodka, and gluten-free cider vinegar, balsamic vinegar, or rice vinegar.

OATS

Oats are gluten-free.

The Seattle-based Gluten Intolerance Group (GIG) reports the discovery of the specific reactive peptide involved in gluten intolerance. Research conducted by Dr. Don Kasarda, on the amino acid sequencing of oats versus the reactive peptide sequence known to be a problem for gluten intolerance, put oats in the clear. Based on numerous recent studies like this one, the group clearly states that oats are safe to eat on the gluten-free diet.

The consensus is that oats are fine for all but the most sensitive to enjoy in moderation. Many of us eat oatmeal for breakfast on a regular basis. This is a conversation you need to have with your doctor (my own doctor warns his CD patients not to try oats for at least a year or until the villi are completely healed).

If you are mildly sensitive to gluten, have a small amount and see how you feel.

BUT.

Before you grab the nearest oatmeal cookie—

It is virtually impossible to find commercial oats that have not been contaminated by wheat or other toxic grains in the milling process or in the manufacturing of the food itself.

When and if you decide to add oatmeal to your diet, opt for gluten-free oatmeal from companies like Glutenfreeda, Bob's Red Mill, or one of the other excellent gluten-free companies that certify that their oats are gluten-free, grown in dedicated fields, and not cross-contaminated with wheat at any time in the milling process.

Never buy a quick-cooking or processed domestic brand like Quaker. These are always mixed with wheat or other unsafe grains.

Never consume a product that lists oats among the ingredients. You have no idea what form it's in or where it's from.

For you, the expression "feeling one's oats" takes on a whole new meaning.

PROCEED WITH CAUTION

Buckwheat. Pure buckwheat is gluten-free but, like oats, is almost always contaminated (there's that scary-sounding word again) by unsafe grains at the growing, milling, or processing stage. If you love the stuff, find a company like Bob's Red Mill or Pocono that gets it from dedicated fields and mills it in a safe facility.

Flaxseed or -meal, or nut flours are a great way to get gluten-free protein and fiber, provided they are not mixed with unsafe ingredients.

Legumes such as lentils, beans, soy, and peas are a safe choice, as long as you know what else has been cooked with them and you are not allergic to soy products.

Millet. This is another grain that is gluten-free, but often mixed or milled with wheat. Always consider the source and make sure a millet product is not being baked or processed in a facility that handles unsafe flours or grains.

Montina is the brand name of a type of gluten-free flour created from milled Indian ricegrass grown by Native Americans for thousands of years. Today ricegrass, which is not rice, is grown by local farmers, the majority of whom use no GMOs in the growing or in the processing in a certified gluten-free facility. As a precaution, though, check other ingredients in foods made with this flour.

Quinoa, amaranth, and teff. These grains are naturally gluten-free, but always make sure they have not been mixed with couscous, wheat flour, barley syrup, or other unsafe ingredients, as they often are, either in the recipe or in the milling process.

Roots and tubers such as tapioca, potatoes, sweet potatoes, yams, arrowroot, and manioc or cassava are quite safe.

White and brown rice, corn, wild rice, and sorghum. These grains are gluten-free as well, as long as they haven't been "enhanced" in any way.

MAYBE/MAYBE NOT

Every day we discover gluten-free beer, hard cider, bagel chips, croutons, and other products formerly off-limits on the gluten-free diet. Before you rule out the following, read the ingredients carefully, or call the company. You may be pleasantly surprised. Or not.

Products that are labeled vegan are often gluten-free.

In the case of Communion, always check with the priest or minister and, depending on your personal relationship, make special arrangements for yourself and others to partake during services.

Here is a short list of products that may seem on the surface off-limits but may not be, as more and more companies are making gluten-free alternatives:

Bagels and bagel chips	Bread	Candy
Beers, ales, lager	Breading, coating mixes,	Cereals
Biscotti	and panko	Croutons
Biscuits	Cakes and pies	Custards

Dressings

Energy bars

French fries

Granola

Ice Cream

Jelly beans

Licorice

Marinades

Matzo

Pastas

Pizza

Potato, corn, and tortilla
  chips

Pretzels

Puddings

Soups

Soy Sauce

Stuffing and dressings

Tortilla and wraps

Veggie burgers

At the Drugstore

All over-the-counter medication, vitamins and minerals, prescription drugs, nutritional and herbal supplements, shakes, cold and flu products, toothpaste, mouthwash, and so on, must be verified gluten-free.

Bottom Line?

+ Ask questions first. Eat later.

+ Always check ingredients, and look for products labeled gluten-free in accordance with the new FDA guidelines. (More about that in Chapter 22.)

+ Better yet, look for products certified by national organizations, like the Gluten Intolerance Group, that hold food companies to a stricter standard.

+ Press food companies to use gluten-free ingredients. Be patient, persistent, and polite. Food giants like Betty Crocker and General Mills have responded to the demand for gluten-free products. Letters, calls, e-mails, tweets, and blog posts work. If you have the time or inclination, lobby for food safety.

+ Buy organic and local.

+ Say no to hormones and antibiotics in your food.

+ Push for full disclosure about how your food is grown, processed, or otherwise genetically engineered.

+ In the meantime, if the kid in the health food store tells you it's okay to have spelt because it is a more digestible form of wheat, walk away. It's only more digestible if you're not sensitive to gluten. I was once told by a zealous macrobiotic counselor that if I ate seaweed and brown rice and ground my own gomasio (roasted sesame seeds and salt) while facing east and standing on my left foot, my celiac disease would go away. Don't fall for that, either.

✦ Eating whole, unrefined, unprocessed, un-engineered foods is a great way to get real quality and vitality from what you eat, and it may even hasten the healing process, but it won't *cure* gluten intolerance.

Facts, Tips, and Other Important Things to Remember

✦ Forget kamut bread or cereal on the gluten-free diet.

✦ Go with peanuts, almonds, cashews, pecans, or other tree nuts unless you are allergic, in which case, don't you dare.

✦ To further confuse the issue, those on a gluten-free diet often have allergies, lactose intolerance, peanut allergy, carbohydrate intolerance, casein allergy, and chemical sensitivities. It's important to sort out where the reaction is coming from before you blame it on gluten.

✦ It's a good idea to avoid processed cheeses and spreads and dips and other flavored, herbed, and otherwise enhanced products, which can contain gluten. Best to buy natural cheeses such as cheddar, Swiss, mozzarella, and ricotta and imported cheeses like Brie, Camembert, chèvre, and Gouda.

✦ It is said that richly veined cheeses like Maytag blue and Stilton are off-limits because the culture that makes them so rich and gorgeous is made with bread mold. Nobody really knows how much, if any, gluten is broken down in the aging process, but most experts advise caution. Better to be safe than sorry.

✦ Many candy bars are not gluten-free, even though there is no gluten in the ingredients. Wheat flour is often used on the gooey confections to help mold them into shape or to keep them from sticking to each other and gumming up the works on the conveyor belts.

✦ Did you know that licorice contains wheat flour? Ditto for many brands of jelly beans and other jelly candy. But take heart: there are several brands of gluten-free licorice, jelly beans, and enough gummy candy to keep a dentist busy for years.

✦ Strange as this may sound, not all turkeys are gluten-free. It's not because the turkey may have eaten wheat in his or her lifetime; it's because pre-basted turkeys and other poultry products may contain gluten in the "butter" mixture injected into the bird.

What's a consumer to do?

Oh, Henry, What's a Girl to Do?

Contact the company that makes a candy bar you really love and ask how it's made, then give yourself a Hershey's Kiss and a big box of Goobers—they're both gluten-free.

Why Do I Still Have to Read Labels?

As of August 2, 2013, the FDA joined Europe, Brazil, Argentina, Canada, Australia, and the UK in mandated, standardized gluten-free labeling. But government regulations are as good as their policing (look how well they've kept Wall Street in line). Come to think of it, the FDA hasn't exactly stamped out salmonella or E. coli. Not reading a label is like using spell check but never really learning to spell. Label reading is a skill every gluten-free citizen needs to know.

Ten Basic Rules to Help You Cook and Eat Safely

Basic Rule No. 1

> Never forget that you are the customer and, as
> such, you are entitled to a complete explanation
> of a food manufacturer's process.

Without you, companies are out of business. They are not doing you a favor by answering your questions or complaints. They want you to tell them what you think. That's why they post their Web sites, e-mail, and snail-mail addresses prominently on their packages. It's why they put "cookies" on your tail when you go browsing. It's why they send you free stuff when you find a piece of gravel in your soup or a pit in a box of pitted prunes. It's why McDonald's finally downsized its portions, why you can now bake a gluten-free version of the same Betty Crocker toothachingly sweet cake mix you enjoyed as a child.

If you really love a product and are not sure how it's made, call, write, or e-mail the manufacturer's customer service department and find out.

Don't stop at gluten. Demand to know if you are eating GMOs, and while you're at it, lobby for zero trans fats and zero high-fructose corn syrup. If they give you a hard time, tell them you and your friends and family, and everyone you've ever met in this life and the next will boycott their products.

If what you are told meets with your satisfaction and you get a clear answer regarding the status of the product, call back every few months. Manufacturing standards and formulas change. Standardized definitions of gluten-free notwithstanding, labels, which are extremely expensive to reprint and apply, often lag behind in this process.

If you run into trouble, make sure to mention that you got very sick eating something the company made.

Basic Rule No. 2

*Take food company disclaimers with
a grain of salt.*

We live in litigious times. People sue companies because they got fat eating too many French fries or because they ate thirty-seven jelly doughnuts and went into a diabetic coma.

Soon Oreo cookies will be on a government watch list. It's sad but true. Americans have learned to blame somebody else for every dumb thing they do. The downside for the gluten-avoidant is that even though the product is gluten-free, there will be some legal gibberish attached to the answer. Stuff like "There could be gluten or other allergens in this product . . . made in a facility that also processes wheat." It is impossible to say positively that gluten or any other offending substances may not have entered the manufacturing process . . . someone who touched your food may have once eaten a slice of bread.

One company, in an inspired burst of obfuscation, actually sent as its response a list of products that were definitely not gluten-free. They fudge, they are ambiguous, they cover their you-know-whats. Don't take these responses literally. These are not dire warnings. This is simply a sign of our lawsuit-happy society.

Bottom line: use common sense. If you are seriously sensitive, buy only certified gluten-free products made in a dedicated facility or grown in a dedicated field.

If you have a reaction, stop using the product.

Basic Rule No. 3

*Never eat a meal or a packaged food
if you don't know what's in it.*

If there's no label, ask for it. It it's not available, don't risk it.

This can be a problem on airlines, at salad bars (there are lots of reasons to avoid them), and catered affairs, school cafeterias, and some weight-loss programs such as Jenny Craig, LA Weight Loss, Nutrisystem, and other companies that sell frozen meals and products directly to clients.

Such programs are not required by law to disclose any nutritional information, including calories and fat content and ingredients, which is probably why so many people fail on these plans and regain the weight. They have no idea what they've eaten and the minute they resume eating normal food, they overeat.

The point is, whenever you are a captive audience—where you have not specifically requested a gluten-free meal, or the chef is unavailable for consultation, or the ingredient label is missing—you are in real danger of getting glutened.

Try not to go anywhere without a banana, a Kind protein bar, or a bag of nuts. It'll be better than what they give you anyway.

Basic Rule No. 4

Look for gluten in unexpected places.

Gluten intolerance doesn't just pose a problem at mealtimes, but on Sunday mornings as well. My doctor told me about a patient of his who continued to feel lousy even though she followed the gluten-free diet scrupulously. Just as more tests were ordered to rule out something more serious, the devout Catholic volunteered that she attended Mass and took Communion every day. Bingo.

Some other little-known facts:

The glue used on some envelopes and mailing labels (most of them imported) may contain wheat. Since glue is not a food to those of us over the age of four, this source is easily overlooked. It's smart to use a damp sponge, self-sticking envelopes, and to buy self-stick US postage stamps, or forget the whole thing and let somebody else in the family pay the bills.

Many of us are sensitive to chemicals as well as to gluten. Those with dermatitis herpetiformis (a skin reaction to gluten described in Chapter 19) should be careful using furniture refinishers, craft kits, paste and spray waxes, and cleaners. Try to avoid using these substances and, if you must, only do so wearing a mask and work in a well-ventilated area.

It's important for those who are highly sensitive, especially those with sensitive skin, to avoid wheat germ oil in cosmetics and in many personal products such as skin creams, lotions, and potions that could end up being swallowed. Even toothpaste and false teeth fixatives must be scrutinized.

Watch out for imitation seafood commonly found in many take-out food stores, salad bars, and restaurants. These products often start out gluten-free, but binders are added to help mold the product into shrimp, crab, lobster, or scallop shapes. Look for gluten-free imitation seafood and always ask in a restaurant or deli if the shrimp or lobster salad is mixed with imitation seafood. Better yet, eat real fish.

Don't forget to ask the dental hygienist what's in the prophy paste used to clean your teeth.

On the plus side, a trip to a winery will be a special joy for the gluten-impaired because pure wine in all its glorious variety is gluten-free. This includes pure sherries, ports, cognacs, brandies, and sake, Japanese rice wine.

Watch out for fortified and flavored wines. Just as food companies use wheat in the manufacturing process, wineries use additives, too.

Beer is a no-no. Gluten-free beer and hard ciders abound.

Before you start licking your lips, make sure your lipstick is gluten-free, too.

Basic Rule No. 5

If you don't understand it, don't eat it until you do.

This is especially true in restaurants. You don't understand a menu term, but you remember the time you asked for steak tartare medium well and you never want to be that embarrassed again. This is one time that ignorance is not bliss, not to mention fiscally irresponsible. Why spend your hard-earned money on foods that could make you sick? (For a full list of menu terms that may pose problems, refer to page 275.)

In the age of globalization, and the increased availability of foreign products, knowledge is power. Let's review some basic food additives:

Caramel coloring. In the United States and Canada, caramel coloring is the dark brown liquid that results from heating dextrose, invert sugar (a mixture of dextrose and levulose found in fruits or that is produced artificially by the process of inversion), lactose, molasses, or sucrose from beet or sugarcane. This ingredient should always be questioned, as it may be made from malt syrup or wheat. When in doubt, consider the country of origin and contact the company for specifics.

Dextrin. Not as common as maltodextrin made from corn, dextrin is an incompletely hydrolyzed starch that can be made from corn, potato, arrowroot, rice, tapioca, and/or wheat. It's used as a thickener, prevents caking of sugar in candy, and encapsulates flavoring in mixes. It is wise to question an imported product containing dextrin or that which is not labeled corn dextrin, tapioca dextrin, and so on.

Glutinous rice. The word *glutinous* just means "sticky" or "gummy" and should not be taken to mean containing gluten, as in *glutenous*.

Guar gum. According to *Webster's New Collegiate Dictionary*, guar gum is "a gum that consists of the ground endosperm of guar seeds and is used especially as a thickening agent and sizing material." Basically, this is the edible stuff used on your sheets and shirts to make them feel crisp and in foods to make them feel fuller. Icky, but totally gluten-free.

Hydrolyzed vegetable protein (HVP), hydrolyzed plant protein (HPP), or textured vegetable protein. Attention vegans and vegetarians! These additives can be made from soy, corn, rice, peanuts, casein, or wheat. Always check with the manufacturer of a product containing HVP or HPP for the source of the protein. These are commonly found in canned foods like soups, sausages, hot dogs, and "mock" meats.

Malt or malt flavoring. These are made from barley malt or syrup and are often found in cereals, cookies, and candies. They are not gluten-free. If made from corn, of course, these flavorings are gluten-free.

Maltodextrin. Not to be confused with malt or malt flavoring (yes, it is easy to be led to conclusions by the word *malt*), the FDA describes this stuff as "non-sweet white powder or concentrated solution made from corn, potato, or rice." American products containing maltodextrin are gluten-free by regulation. However, it is always good to check the source when considering imported products.

Maltol. While its name may be misleading, it is a synthetic flavoring that contains no malt or gluten.

Mannitol. Used as an anti-caking, flavoring stabilizer and thickener in foods, Rx medications, and sugar-free candies, this sweet substance is made most commonly from seaweed.

Modified food starch. This can be made from corn, tapioca, potatoes, wheat, or other starches, but in North America, corn is almost always used.

MSG or monosodium glutamate. Unless you are allergic to MSG (Chinese Restaurant syndrome), you need not worry about this additive made from sugar beet or molasses.

Sorbitol. This sweet-tasting, poorly absorbed sugar alcohol is used in many sugar-free or "dietetic" food products. It is gluten-free, but even the tiniest amount can cause bloating, diarrhea, and abdominal pain in sensitive individuals, especially in those who are still feeling the effects of gluten.

Starch. When you see "starch" listed on an American food manufacturer's label, it means it is made from cornstarch only, in keeping with FDA requirements. If another starch is used—for example, wheat starch or tapioca starch—it must be disclosed. No such rule exists for imported products.

Triticale. This grain is a cross between wheat and rye and, as such, it's doubly toxic for people like us.

Wheat starch. This substance is a part of wheat considered by some to be less toxic than flour for gluten-intolerant people. It is considered unsafe in the United States and Canada, but in Great Britain and Europe, in accordance with the Codex Alimentarius, it is considered acceptable for those on the gluten-free diet. Check the country of origin.

Vegetable gums. Avoid any product that contains oat gum. But if a vegetable gum is made from carob bean, guar gum, gum arabic, gum acacia, locust bean, cellulose gum, gum tragacanth, or just plain gum, while it may sound unappetizing, it's fine.

Basic Rule No. 6

It's better to look silly than to get sick.

There are worse things to be called than "fussy."

Only a crumb would ask you to share a toaster. Newton's law of physics applies here. A toaster oven is a better choice than a conventional toaster because it allows your bread to toast flat, clear of the crumbs that normally drop off breads, muffins, and bagels and collect on the bottom, mixing with your gluten-free toaster delights.

Likewise, do not assume a French fry is just potato.

Yes, I know it's embarrassing to ask the restaurant to clean the grill and wash the utensils used to toss your salad. It may sound pushy to ask for special treatment, but do it anyway. For those not blessed in the self-assertion department, it may be tempting to succumb to the pressure of eating an unsafe meal a friend has cooked you. Refusing is awkward, yes; impossible,

Travel Advisory

In 2008, the Codex Alimentarius, which sets international standards for food and food safety, revised its guidelines for gluten-free as that which contains no more than 20 ppm (parts per million) of wheat, rye, barley, or oats in keeping with the FDA standard of what constitutes gluten-free in America. This is good news for Americans on a zero-gluten diet. According to an article in the *Journal of the American Dietetic Association*, "Wheat starch used in European gluten-free foods is specially formulated to comply with the Codex Alimentarius Standard for gluten-free foods." Especially gluten-free-friendly: the United States, Brazil, Argentina, Canada, Australia, and the UK with standardized labeling laws in place. "¿Se habla gluten?"

no. Say, "I love you for making this and I'm sorry for not explaining my diet properly."

And by the way, if your sweetie has just had two pieces of apple pie, no kissing until he or she has brushed and flossed.

Basic Rule No. 7

Make sure you know who or what is touching your food at all times.

People can spread gluten just like viruses, and, in fact, you can make yourself sick by not washing your hands after handling wheat flour.

Watch inanimate sources of contamination, too, such as deep-fat fryers and grills and ice cream scoops. Always ask the clerk at Baskin-Robbins to rinse the scoop before serving your cup (or the cone you've supplied) to avoid getting some cookie dough or other unsafe flavor mixed with yours. Find out if your French fries have been "beer-battered," coated in some other way, or cooked in the same oil as the breaded onion rings. Is the hamburger patty all beef or has it been mixed with bread crumbs? (Many establishments do this to stretch profits.) Find out before ordering. By all means, bring your favorite pasta to your neighborhood Italian restaurant (only after you've asked if you can), but don't forget to ask that it be cooked in a pot of fresh water. When you barbecue at home or with friends, always make sure your food is first up on the grill; this way, you won't end up with bits of grilled buns and other glutenous food on yours.

You wouldn't slice a peach on a cutting board used to cut up raw chicken. Same goes for gluten.

Basic Rule No. 8

Live by the Boy Scout motto—Be Prepared!

Right about now you're wondering if you'll ever eat again.

The answer is a resounding yes. Life will be full and rich and fragrant with glorious foods you can't imagine are gluten-free. There's a whole world of bakeries, pizza parlors, restaurants, sports stadiums, fast-food chains, and even food trucks and farmer's markets ready to ply you with everything you loved before, only without the gluten.

But for now, as you get used to your gluten-free training wheels, you may prefer to eat at home. You'll want to stock the pantry with the staples listed below. If space allows, set aside a place apart from the family's provisions. This way you'll always know what you've got in stock, and you will limit the possibility of mixing things up.

A revolutionary thought: Given that today's gluten-free foods are world-class and, in many ways, better for us than the wheat based versions and so readily available, why not simplify and run a gluten-free household? Think about it.

For now, these products should help with the transition:

Alternative grains. Amaranth, buckwheat, mesquite, millet, Montina, quinoa, sorghum, and teff are full of nutrients, either ground as flour or whole grain. These give a nutrient-dense bang for your buck.

Arrowroot. This thickening agent blends well with most gluten-free flours and makes for silky gravies.

Baking mixes. There are many wonderful commercial gluten-free baking mixes to substitute cup for cup for wheat flour in your favorite recipes—Bob's Red Mill, King Arthur All-Purpose Blend, Cup4Cup (more in Chapter 5, "Marketing 101")—or you can make your own. Start with ½ cup rice flour, ¼ cup corn starch or potato starch, ¼ cup tapioca flour, and double or triple as needed. Blend well and keep on hand for baking.

Bean flours. Garfava and Romano are packed with protein.

Brown and white rice flours. Keep these on hand and use them for dusting, dredging, flouring hands, and mixing with other gluten-free flours for cooking and baking.

Cereals. Breakfast is no longer grab-a-Danish-and-go, so always keep a box of gluten-free granola bars, cold cereal, hominy grits, instant gluten-free oatmeal, millet, and hot rice cereal on the shelf. There are pancake mixes, gluten-free waffles, and don't forget gluten-free bagels and English muffins. These freeze especially well. It's a good idea to keep individual bags of G/F snacks at the office and in your workbag as well. Add your own nuts and raisins, mix with G/F pieces, and you've got a quick-energy snack far better than any found in the vending machine.

Corn flour. This smoother version of cornmeal is the right texture for corn muffins and other baked goods or recipes requiring a lighter result than cornmeal alone can achieve.

Cornmeal. You'll need to keep this staple on hand for cereals, crusts, accompaniments to roasts, soft or grilled polenta, and gluten-free batters. Corn bread makes an excellent addition to stuffing, meat loaf, and other ground meat dishes and can often replace bread crumbs in standard recipes. There is nothing like cornmeal-crusted fish or soft-shell crabs sautéed in a little butter and olive oil.

Cornstarch. Like arrowroot, this is a great thickening agent for sauces and gravies and is less prone to lumps than wheat flour.

Crackers and biscuits. Always keep a quantity of whole-grain gluten-free crackers on hand for cheese, dips, crusts, munching, and taking to friends' houses, parties, and so on.

Gluten-free breads, muffins, bagels, and toaster cakes. Fresh, in mixes or premade, these are available in specialty stores, gluten-free bakeries, large chains like Whole Foods, farmers' markets, and, of course, via mail order online. Experiment with small orders until you find your favorites. Many of these breads freeze well, so stock up.

Gluten-free pastas. Gone are the gooey, limp pastas of yesterday. Gluten-free dried pastas such as spaghetti, lasagna, penne, fettuccini, ziti, and manicotti are here. These are a must for any gluten-free pantry. Try fresh pastas in small quantities, since these can be pricey and do not freeze well, but they are well worth the occasional expense in terms of taste and texture.

Legume flours. Garbanzo, chickpea, lentil, and pea flour are great for baking and provide protein and fiber.

Oriental rice sticks, rice wrappers, and noodles. These are available in Asian markets and in the international sections of many supermarkets and specialty stores and require very little preparation, usually no more than soaking, for use in gluten-free cooking.

Potato flour. Don't confuse this with potato starch flour. Potato flour is made from the whole potato. A small amount goes a long way to refine the texture of coarser rice flours. For example, 1 teaspoon potato flour is enough to redefine the texture of ½ cup rice flour, or as little as 1 tablespoon can retexturize 1 to 2 cups rice flour.

Potato starch flour. This thickener is interchangeable with cornstarch and can be found in most supermarkets, health food stores, or whole-food markets.

Rice. Stock up on white rice, brown rice, wild rice, sweet basmati rice, arborio rice, the highly absorbent risotto rice, and all the gorgeous varieties of this delicious grain as you can afford. Play. Experiment. But avoid commercial rice mixes, which may be mixed with other grains.

Rice bran. This is the bran that comes from polishing brown rice. It's loaded with minerals, vitamins B and E, and fiber. Add it to cereals, muffins, cookies, smoothies, and other baked goods. The oil content makes it fragile, so store it in the freezer.

Rice polish. This is soft flour made from the hulls of brown rice. Like rice bran, it's fragile, so buy a little at a time.

Soy or soya flour. This can have a heavy flavor when used alone, so it should be used in conjunction with other, milder flours. Since it is high in fat and protein, it can add nutrients and needed moisture to an otherwise dry recipe. For example, if a recipe calls for 2 cups wheat flour, use 1 cup rice flour, ¾ cup potato starch flour, and ¼ cup soy flour.

Specialty flours. You may want to keep on hand small amounts of flours made from artichokes, acorns, beans, coconut, mung beans, almonds, hazelnuts, pistachios, sweet potatoes, and even cabernet grapes, but unless you are going to use them consistently, they are best bought fresh. It is best to buy fresh nuts to make your own nut flours—used in many "flourless" cake and torte recipes, especially for the paleo dieters among you. Grind them yourself because the high oil content means that commercial flours can turn rancid when stored for long periods.

Sweet rice flour. This is usually found in Asian food markets and international sections of stores like Whole Foods. Because it has more starch than regular rice flour, it makes an excellent thickening agent.

Tapioca flour (or starch) a.k.a. cassava or manioc. Use this flour in recipes where a light texture is required, as in pancakes and waffles. It is on a par with and, in some cases, superior to wheat flour.

Xanthan gum. This is used as a binder, thickener, or stabilizer. It is used commercially as a suspension agent in salad dressings and in pie fillings, canned gravies, and sauces to give these products a smoother texture. It is made by using the bacteria *Xanthomonas compestris* to ferment corn sugar. If you are planning to make your own gluten-free breads and baked goods, you'll need to lay in a supply.

Yeast. Never buy synthetic yeast. Fresh, slow-rising yeast is the key.

Don't Be a Mealy Mouth!

All flours and meals should be tightly sealed and kept in the refrigerator to avoid rancidity and mealybugs. Purchase them where the turnover is high to avoid rancidity. Most flours and meals freeze well and can be kept for months this way. Date everything you freeze.

A WORD OF ADVICE

Whether you have celiac disease or gluten sensitivity, get thee to a registered dietitian who can assess your nutritional status and deficiencies, if any, design a well-rounded and nutritious eating plan, and get you off to a healthy start. Many hospital gastroenterology departments offer nutritional counseling to their patients after diagnosis. Or contact the Academy of Nutrition and Dietetics (page 583) for a referral.

Basic Rule No. 9

> I'll say it again. Never, never assume the words
> *wheat-free* on a label mean *gluten-free*.

Wheat-free products may contain rye, oats, barley, or other unsafe ingredients. And some product labels are just Greek to you. The more you know about unusual or exotic foods, the better you'll eat. Here's a little homework before you head out to the store.

Amaranth. *Webster's* defines this ancient Aztec grain now enjoying a comeback as "from the Greek *amaranton* meaning unfading; any of a large genus of coarse herbs including pigweed which is also known as tumbleweed in certain parts of the country, and various forms cultivated for their showy flowers." In its commercial form as a breakfast cereal, amaranth is tasty, full of fiber, and gluten-free, as long as it isn't mixed with any other unsafe grains.

Buckwheat. Some things bear repeating. Despite its unfortunate name, this gluten-free plant bears no relationship to wheat. It's a fruit, really, and it comes closer to the density of animal protein than any other plant. Consume it *only* if you are sure it has been milled in a dedicated facility and is not contaminated with other glutenous grains.

Kamut. Pronounced *KA-moot*, this ancient Peruvian member of the wheat family is low in gluten and is often touted as something tolerated by those who are allergic to wheat, but don't try this on a gluten-free diet.

Mochi. This sticky Japanese sweet rice cake is gluten-free as long as it does not contain any other unsafe grains or flavorings. Scored, cut into squares, and baked, mochi puffs up as individual rolls or can be cut into strips and made into waffles.

Quinoa. Pronounced *keen-WAH*, this is Incan for "the mother grain." According to legend, it was so crucial to the Incan diet that the king planted the first row of quinoa each season with a solid gold spade. Royal traditions aside, this tiny, slightly nutty-tasting grain that is no bigger than a mustard seed dates back over five thousand years. Is it gluten-free? Absolutely.

Spelt. This is another way of saying a split piece of wood and the British past tense of the word *spell*. *Webster's* tells us it is also a form of wheat called *Triticum spelta*. Wheat by any other name is just as glutenous.

Teff. Not the stuff in your nonstick pan, this is the smallest grain in the world and has, for thousands of years, been the grain of choice for the baking of the traditional Ethiopian flat bread called injera (see the recipe on page 293). As long as it isn't mixed or milled with forbidden grains, it's gluten-free.

Tempeh. Not the city in Arizona, this is a low-fat, vegetarian source of protein made from soybeans that can be sautéed, steamed, baked, barbecued, used as a bread substitute in meatballs, or diced and simmered in soups and stews. It is gluten-free as long as it is sold in its natural state and is not mixed with other grains or wheat-containing soy sauce.

Basic Rule No. 10

Whether it's gluten-free or not, if a food won't rot
or sprout, throw it out.

A Final Note: Get on the Gluten-Free Grapevine

Look for online newsletters, recipe sharing, support and announcements of celiac-friendly restaurants, medical information, and the latest on everything. You can Walk for the Cure, learn how to become a lobbyist, sample new products, or attend gluten-free gatherings; it depends on how involved you want to be. Community is especially important just after going gluten-free: to have a place to network, share information, and learn the ropes from the veterans. See Chapter 23 for community, networking, and resources.

2 | The New Food Hyphenate

Hyphenate/noun: a person who has more than one job
or function, as in the film industry's producer-writer-director.

—*AMERICAN ENGLISH DICTIONARY*

Gone are the days of simple, one-size-fits-all eating. There are more ways to be gluten-free than varieties of heirloom tomatoes. Many of us have multiple food sensitivities and allergies beyond gluten. Our diets may be medically mandated, or undertaken for optimum health, weight loss, or the wish to eat more consciously; how we shop and eat may also be motivated by environmental issues or by our passion for the cause of anti-animal cruelty.

You may be gluten-lactose-nut-free or, in the case of one friend, able to eat only nuts that start with the letter *p*. You may be gluten-free-paleo, gluten-free-vegan, or gluten-dairy-free-vegetarian. Some of you are gluten-free-no-carbs-no-hormones carnivores. Or gluten-sugar-dairy-free. Or gluten-casein-free. If you're like me, you're gluten-preservative-processed-high-fructose-corn-syrup-free-preferably-organic.

You try to avoid GMOs, but with no real disclosure, that's a crap-shoot. Ditto for chemical ingredients and additives—one particular cable comedian calls the processed foods found on supermarket shelves "food-like substances." If you are a carnivore, you may eat only grass-fed, hormone- and antibiotic-free beef. You maybe be a locavore, doing your best to eat local and organic from farm to table, which means eating only seasonal produce. Not so easy in the long, cold gulag of root vegetables when you'd kill for a kiwi.

Some of you have dispensed with fire altogether and embraced the ethos of raw. Others stop short at hitting dinner over the head. Even if you are a red-blooded American omnivore and eat everything but gluten, chances are someone in your household or at your dinner table is intolerant, either by choice or by diagnosis, to one or more foods.

You may still be trying to find out what, other than gluten, causes you problems, in which case your diet is gluten-free-elimination-to-be-determined. For all I know, up to now you've happily lived on chia seeds and toast and the gluten thing has thrown a real monkey wrench into the works. In short, you are the new food hyphenate and you've got a lot on your plate.

I'm often asked how the gluten-free diet fits in with lactose-free, casein-free, vegetarian, vegan, Mediterranean, paleo, and the like. I've set forth the basics of each path, pluses, and pitfalls with as little personal opinion as I can muster, so you can see for yourself how you need to tailor your current or aspirational diet to the requirements of eating gluten-free.

Let's review.

Gluten-Free Mediterranean

Grilled fish. Beans. Yogurt. Lentils. Fresh greens. Sardines. Feta. A nice hunk of gluten-free artisanal bread to mop up the olive oil. As my hero, Mark Bittman, says in the *New York Times* article "When Diet Meets Delicious," "The Mediterranean diet prohibits nothing that was recognized as food by your great-grandmother."

A February 25, 2013, NYTimes.com article reports on a new study that finds that 30 percent of heart attacks, strokes, and deaths from heart disease can be prevented in high-risk people if they switch to a Mediterranean diet. This comes as great news to those of us who already eat meals rich in olives, nuts, beans, fresh fruits and vegetables, and fish and enjoy a glass or two of good wine in the bargain.

The Spanish study, published on the *New England Journal of Medicine*'s Web site, measured the Mediterranean diet's effect on heart risks, and the magnitude of the positive, heart-protective benefits shocked the researchers. The study was shut down after five years because it was considered unethical to continue. Not only that; the Mediterranean diet is associated with a lower incidence of Parkinson's disease, Alzheimer's, and other dementias.

So, too, its emphasis on nuts, seeds, fish, and olive oil is just what the doctor ordered for pain and inflammation.

So what exactly is the Mediterranean diet?

Think Spain, France, Italy, Greece, Turkey, the Middle East, and the North Africa of fifty years ago before highly processed foods, high-fructose corn syrup, and fast foods sullied the land of lavender, olive groves, oranges, and saffron. Think fresh, whole, rarely processed food; wild-not-farmed fish; meats grilled, baked, braised, or roasted in a bath of olive oil, garlic, and lemon. Not a lot of overeating. Small portions intensely flavored and infused with fresh herbs.

If you were to draw a Mediterranean pyramid, you'd put fruits, vegetables, whole gluten-free grains, olive oil, beans, nuts, legumes, seeds, herbs, and spices at the bottom, forming the base on which to design every meal. Next, grilled, baked, or roasted fish and seafood to enjoy often, at least twice a week. On the third and even smaller step up are eggs, cheese, and low-fat yogurt to be eaten with moderation. At the very top, meat and sweets to be eaten in slivers and bits.

Mediterranean desserts are often fresh fruit or a wedge of good cheese drizzled with honey, nuts, or chocolate. Olive oil is the primary source of fat, and pastas, gluten-free, of course, are more often dressed in garlic, olive oil, and anchovies or capers instead of the heavier sauces used elsewhere in the region.

Ripe tomatoes are served à la caprese with fresh mozzarella, basil, and a dollop of the savory olive, caper, and anchovy paste called tapenade. Bouillabaisse, pistou, tagine, paella, aioli, escarole, cannellini and red lentil soup, and the ever-present chickpea are mainstays.

Small plates called *mezze* pack a flavor wallop with slivers of meat, olives, maybe a lentil salad, cheeses, and tomatoes. This is a diet high in healthy omega-3 fats and antioxidants.

What with all the good gluten-free pasta and breads, focaccia and pizzas, eating like a Greek fisherman or an Italian farmer is pretty much a slam dunk, as long as you stay away from glutenous soups and sauces like the béchamel used in moussaka and dishes and desserts wrapped in phyllo or filo dough. (It doesn't matter which spelling you use; you can't have it.)

Talk About Being Ahead of the Curve

Archeologists just discovered the skeleton of a woman who lived in Tuscany 2,000 years ago that showed signs that she tried to adapt her diet to cope with gluten sensitivity. Gold and bronze jewelry buried alongside her pointed to a relatively cushy existence, and yet her remains bore evidence of malnutrition and osteoporosis, which can be signs of celiac disease. DNA analysis showed the woman carried two copies of an immune system gene variant associated with CD, and an analysis of carbon and nitrogen isotopes in her bones, which can relate to food intake, make the case that she attempted to avoid wheat. Imagine telling a Tuscan waiter to *"Render unto me a Caesar salad with no croutons."*

MEDITERRANEAN BEAN SOUP

½ package of dried gluten-free penne, about 8 ounces
3 tablespoons extra virgin olive oil, plus more to moisten the pasta
2 teaspoons garlic, finely chopped
1 cup celery, diced
1½ cups yellow onions, diced
1 tablespoon fresh rosemary, chopped
1 tablespoon fresh thyme, stripped from stem and chopped
2 tablespoons fresh basil, chopped
2 cups carrots, diced
1 14-ounce can diced, fire-roasted organic tomatoes, such as Muir Glen or Whole Foods 365 Everyday Value brand
1 15.5-ounce can organic kidney beans, well rinsed and drained
1 15.5-ounce can organic cannellini beans, well rinsed and drained
1 15.5-ounce can garbanzo beans (chickpeas), well rinsed and drained
6 cups gluten-free chicken stock, or vegetable stock, if you prefer
8 ounces fresh baby spinach, triple washed
Salt and freshly ground black pepper to taste
1 cup homemade or store-bought pesto
6 fresh basil leaves
Wedge of good medium-aged pecorino for garnish

This recipe originally came from one of my cousins who married a Sicilian who introduced the family to pasta e fagioli, spaghetti alla puttanesca, and the other glories of Italy. In my kitchen this zuppa has morphed into something thoroughly modern and in constant demand. If summer had a taste, this would be it.

Because there is a lot of chopping and the soup freezes well, I double it and keep an extra batch on hand. Buy fresh herbs or grow your own. No need to soak beans overnight as long as you buy the organic canned variety and rinse them thoroughly. Serve it for a simple supper with a gluten-free baguette or a warm dinner roll in a puddle of rosemary olive oil, and a simple salad. In smaller portions, it makes a spectacular first course.

SERVES 6

1. Prepare the penne al dente according to the package directions, moisten the pasta with a little olive oil, and set it aside.
2. In a large soup pot (especially if you are doubling the recipe), heat the olive oil over medium-high heat.
3. Add the garlic, celery, and onions to the pot and sauté until transparent, about 4 minutes.
4. Add the rosemary, thyme, and basil to the pot. Stir the vegetables until they are fragrant, 1 to 2 minutes.
5. Add the carrots, tomatoes, kidney beans, cannellini beans, chickpeas, and stock. Bring the mixture to a boil, cover, reduce the heat to low, and simmer for 10 to 15 minutes, or until the vegetables are tender.
6. Add the spinach and cover the pot to wilt the spinach, 1 to 3 minutes.
7. Season with salt and pepper to taste.
8. Place a small amount of pasta in each bowl and ladle the soup over it. Add a dollop of pesto and a basil leaf on each serving. Using a vegetable peeler, finish with a few curls of cheese.

NOTE: Do not freeze the soup with the penne. The pasta will suck up all the liquid and get mushy. Better to boil up a fresh batch when you defrost the soup. If you don't eat dairy or nuts, skip the pesto and cheese curls or substitute vegan pesto and nondairy cheese.

MEDITERRANEAN COOKBOOKS

Mediterranean Light by Martha Rose Shulman (Bantam Books)
The New Mediterranean Diet Cookbook: A Delicious Alternative for Lifelong Health by Nancy Harmon Jenkins (Bantam Books)
Williams-Sonoma Essentials of Mediterranean Cooking by Charity Ferreira (Oxmore House)

Gluten-Free Paleo

Followers of the paleo diet, so named for the Paleolithic Age, believe our bodies were not designed to handle excessive sugar, refined carbohydrates, processed foods, and grains of any kind. They posit that by eating what our ancestors did, which is only what they could gather, grow, forage, fish out of a stream, and hit over the head, we can wipe out obesity, heart disease, type 2 diabetes, and other chronic and degenerative conditions associated with the modern world.

Given that wheat entered the human diet a mere 10,000 years ago and for the previous 250,000, humans evolved very nicely without it, this makes a great deal of sense. The human intestines never quite got used to digesting the stuff. Today, with pesticides and drought resistance engineered right into the DNA of the seed, wheat is giving us an even bigger bellyache.

The modern paleo diet is based on a simple idea: if Fred Flintstone and his family didn't eat it, we shouldn't either.

Since grains didn't exist until the rise of modern-day agriculture, all grains are verboten. Eating paleo also involves grass-fed (not grain-fed) meat; wild (not farmed), fish; fowl; omega-3-enriched eggs; leafy greens, nuts, seeds, and local seasonal vegetables (early humans were a long way from the luxury of flying in out-of-season food). No bread, pizza, pasta, muffins, turkey stuffing, piecrust, or croissants, gluten-free or not, unless made with nut, legume, or coconut flours.

There seems to be some disagreement regarding dairy. Paleo purists say humans were designed to drink mother's milk only as infants. After that, no butter, whole milk, ice cream, Greek yogurt, or cappuccino. However, heavy cream is called for in some paleo cookbooks I've reviewed, so I suspect there is room for interpretation.

No matter, there is a lot of beef, venison, bison, elk, and other esoteric proteins, both fresh and cured. Lard and duck fat play a prominent role (ghee and tallow, too), which means there's quite a bit of fat in this diet—39 percent, which is beyond the 35 percent maximum recommended by the FDA, according to U.S. News & World Report. The jury seems to be out as to whether eating paleo is good or bad over time for cardiovascular health and health in general.

PREHISTORIC DIET PLAN: PROS AND CONS

In an article in *Real Simple* magazine, Mike Roussell, PhD, says that when we stop consuming starchy carbohydrates, saturated fats have less of a negative impact on the heart. Other experts disagree and see a real risk for getting too much fat from protein. They warn of developing deficiencies of vitamin B and thiamine from an absence of fortified grain, and calcium and vitamin D deficiencies from a lack of dairy products, something those with both gluten and lactose intolerance already have to deal with.

Critics say that studies have been too small to conclude that the paleo path leads to lower cardiovascular risk, and they have called for following a larger number of dieters for longer periods. No matter the outcome, some find this diet overly restrictive and not easy to sustain. Not everybody can get used to breadless sandwiches and crustless pies.

But just as gluten-free chefs and bakers have gotten around the rules with wonderful non-glutenous grains and nut flours, so have paleo chefs worked wonders that include pigs in a blanket and Yorkshire pudding with absolutely no forbidden grain, gluten-free or otherwise.

Even better, those who eat paleo are more likely to meet the recommended nine to twelve servings of fruits and vegetables a day.

Eating no processed foods is also a very good thing.

It's possible to drop weight fast on this diet and that's a big plus given that many modern American Homo sapiens are overweight, overtired, and as out of shape as the wooly mammoth.

It is said that paleo enthusiasts started the growing trend of do-it-yourself butchering. One can only wonder how much more weight would come off if we actually had to burn the enormous number of calories involved in tracking, stalking, killing, and dragging home our dinner, too.

Nobody really knows what the long-term effects of the paleo diet will be, and this could just be another, more interesting spin on the Atkins diet and other low-carb or no-carb programs like it, but if you have a lot of weight to lose and are at risk for all the problems associated with that, *and* you remember to take your vitamins, it just may blast away the belly fat and get you back on the right track.

On a compatibility scale of 1 to 10, 10 being the most compatible, and with all the appropriate caveats, the gluten-free diet combined with the paleo diet is about a 12.

No grain, no gluten.

A Typical Day Eating Like a Cave Person

Breakfast: Mushroom, spinach, and lox omelet (egg whites for the diehards), fresh figs on the side, coffee, with or without cream depending on your interpretation.

Lunch: Big steak salad, lots of greens, avocado chunks and veggies, iced tea.

Snack: Two hard-boiled eggs or a handful of nuts or lean turkey rolls with mustard.

Dinner: Rosemary roasted chicken, carrot salad, and cauliflower puréed with a little white truffle oil and a glass of wine. You've earned it.

NOTE: Kitchen skills are crucial on this program. The best paleo cookbooks do wonders with gluten-free nut crusts and crustless crusts and breads, even wonton-less wontons and Yorkshire pudding. Yes, you can entertain. You just have to learn how.

Learn More

PALEO COOKBOOKS AND COMMUNITY

Gather: The Art of Paleo Entertaining by Hayley Mason and Bill Staley (Victory Belt Publishing)

Paleo Cooking from Elana's Pantry: Gluten-Free, Grain-Free, Dairy-Free Recipes by Elana Amsterdam (Ten Speed Press)

The Paleo Diet, rev. ed., by Loren Cordain (Wiley)

The Paleo Solution: The Original Human Diet by Robb Wolf (Victory Belt Publishing)

Well Fed: Paleo Recipes for People Who Love to Eat by Melissa Joulwan (Smudge Publishing)

DIET BASICS, RECIPES, RESOURCES, COMMUNITY

www.paleoleap.com

www.rawpaleodiet.com

Gluten-Free Vegetarian

According to the Vegetarian Society, a vegetarian is someone who lives on grains, nuts, seeds, and vegetables and fruits with or without the use of dairy products and eggs. A vegetarian does not eat meat, poultry, game, fish, shellfish, or crustaceans of any kind or the by-products of slaughter.

So no flesh eating whatsoever.

Many of us have found within this strict definition our own interpretations, including my own lazy approach, which calls for a few meatless days a week.

Here's the skinny:

Lacto-ovo vegetarians eat eggs and dairy.

Lacto-vegetarians eat dairy but draw the line at eggs.

Pescatarians won't eat meat but enjoy fish and other types of seafood.

Vegans are the sticklers. This principled group, which is gaining in popularity, refrains from dairy products and eggs, and are also committed to a philosophy that respects animal life and the ecology of the planet. Cane sugar is out because it is prepared in a process that uses animal bone. Ditto for honey because bees are killed by way of forced procreation to maintain the hive and honey production. Vegans also avoid gelatin, which is made from the bones, skin, and connective tissue of animals. Now that I know this, I may avoid it, too. Vegan purists do not wear or use leather, wool, silk, fur, goose down, or any goods that have been processed using animal products.

Fruitarians, as their name implies, eat mainly fruit and some vine plants considered fruit, such as cucumbers, tomatoes, avocados, bell peppers, nuts, and seeds, as well as green, leafy vegetables. They do not eat grain and therefore have no problem with being gluten-free.

Raw foods advocates do not cook their food above 118°F and eat them as close to their natural state as possible. Along with fruits, vegetables, nuts, and seeds, there are many soaked and sprouted grains, which makes it challenging to give up gluten and still get enough nutrition from the remaining allowable grains.

This is the kale crisp crowd—totally gluten-free and delish, I might add.

Excepting those who do not get enough protein and calories to meet the daily requirements to maintain health, the vegetarian diet, while difficult in some cases to accommodate gluten intolerance, is hands down a healthy way of life. For weight loss, cardiovascular health, for preventing and controlling diabetes, this is the gold standard.

Some famous examples come to mind: Bill Clinton, poster boy for resurrection, greyhound lean and with the gleam of enlightenment in his eye; Gwyneth Paltrow, svelte, positively glowing with optimum health and energy thanks to her low-fat, zero-processed, no-refined-sugar, often gluten-free, vegan diet. Paltrow's mostly gluten-free, mostly vegan cookbook with Julia Turshen, *It's All Good*, is an appetizing argument for clean eating.

There are some caveats.

As a vegetarian, you must always be mindful that many meatless dishes rely on seitan (pure wheat gluten) and various other textured proteins as a way of adding the flavor of meat or poultry, often to tofu, without the meat itself. While seitan is obviously not gluten-free, many other proteins must also be thoroughly vetted. Some are gluten-free; some are not. Homework is in order. Good sources of vegan protein are oatmeal (gluten-free, of course), soy milk, peanut butter, vegetarian beans, tofu, almonds, and brown rice.

Getting enough iron is another issue, especially for young women. Find it in soybeans (with no wheat added), lentils, blackstrap molasses, kidney beans, beet greens, raisins, gluten-free millet, prunes, and green leafy vegetables like bok choy, Swiss chard, and kale.

Vegetarians must also be vigilant about getting enough omega-3s and vitamin B_{12}, which poses a challenge for the newly gluten-intolerant, especially those with celiac disease. Anemia is often a problem, so you may be coming from behind as you embark on the veggie gluten-free path. Expand your repertoire of gluten-free grains and those foods that function like them.

It's always a good idea to check in with your doctor to measure B_{12} levels and other important vitamins and minerals to make sure you are absorbing properly. This is doubly important if you are a vegetarian.

Adding gluten-free eating into the mix isn't easy, especially for strict vegans. Learning to cook instead of relying on hydrolyzed wheat protein helps enormously. So, too, does learning what to substitute for what.

For now the basics:

✦ **Butter** 1 stick = 8 tablespoons Earth Balance Non-Dairy Buttery Spread
  – 8 tablespoons Spectrum Organic Shortening

Gluten-Free-Vegan Wrapsody

Blanch (see page 145 for instructions) several large, organic collard green leaves. Carefully cut out the thick spine and overlap the two halves horizontally. Place the gluten-free vegan filling of your choice down the center. Roll tightly, tucking in the ends. Gorgeous.

= 8 tablespoons coconut, vegetable, or olive oil

= 1/3 cup organic canola oil

= 1/3 cup coconut oil

= 1/3 cup olive oil (not for baked goods)

= 6 tablespoons unsweetened apple sauce plus 2 tablespoons fat of choice above

✦ **Buttermilk** 1 cup = 1 cup soy milk plus 1 tablespoon lemon juice or cider vinegar*

= 1 cup coconut milk plus 1 tablespoon lemon juice or cider vinegar*

= 7/8 cup rice milk plus 1 tablespoon lemon juice or cider vinegar*

= 1 cup plain dairy-free yogurt plus 1 tablespoon lemon juice or cider vinegar*

* Allow to sit and "sour" for 5 minutes before using

✦ **Milk** 1 cup = 1 cup soy milk

= 1 cup rice milk

= 1 cup fruit juice

= 1 cup coconut milk

= 1 cup hemp milk

= 1 cup almond milk

✦ **Cream** 1 cup = 1 cup So Delicious creamer

= 1 cup full-fat coconut milk

= 2/3 cup dairy-free milk

= 1/3 cup melted vegan butter, canola oil, or coconut oil

= 1 cup Silk soy creamer

✦ **Sour Cream** 1 cup = 1 cup Tofutti Better Than Sour Cream

= 1 cup Follow Your Heart Vegan Gourmet Sour Cream Alternative

✦ **Egg** 1 whole egg = 4 tablespoons puréed silken tofu plus 1 teaspoon baking powder

= 4 tablespoons unsweetened applesauce or other fruit purée plus 1 tablespoon baking powder

= Egg Replacer per package directions

✦ **Egg** 1 white = 1 tablespoon agar powder (vegetable-based gelatin) dissolved in 1 tablespoon water, beaten, chilled for 15 minutes, and beaten again

✦ **Yogurt** 1 cup = 1 cup soy yogurt

= 1 cup coconut milk yogurt

= 1 cup rice milk yogurt

= 1 cup unsweetened applesauce, banana, or other fruit purée

✦ **Cheese** 1 cup = 1 cup vegan cheese alternative
  = 1 cup Redwood Foods Cheezly
  = 1 cup Daiya vegan cheese
  = 1 cup Follow Your Heart vegan cheese
  = 1 cup Parma! vegan Parmesan

✦ **Sugar** l cup = ¼ cup agave nectar. When using agave nectar in baking, decrease the liquid ingredients by ¼ cup for every cup of liquid ingredients, mix the agave nectar with the liquid ingredients instead of the dry ingredients, and reduce the oven temperature by 25 degrees because baked goods brown faster with agave.

✦ **Good sugar substitutes** Depending on your sweet tooth and what you are baking, good choices include maple syrup, sorghum molasses, brown rice syrup, coconut sugar, palm sugar, maple sugar, date sugar, yacon syrup, stevia, puréed raisins, applesauce, or bananas.

✦ **Not-so-good sugar substitutes** High-fructose corn syrup, anything with aspartame and artificial sweeteners like Splenda, and sorbitol, maltilol, or mannitol, which can cause uncomfortable cramping.

Note: Aspartame by any other name is still aspartame. Producer Ajinomoto has rebranded and remarketed NutraSweet under the healthy-sounding name AminoSweet.

✦ **Nuts** Replace tree nuts and peanuts with equal amounts of crushed crispy quinoa, flax or amaranth cereal, pumpkin or sunflower seeds, toasted sesame seeds, or toasted coconut.

VEGETARIAN AND VEGAN COOKBOOKS

The Gluten-Free Vegan: 150 Delicious Gluten-Free, Animal-Free Recipes by Susan O'Brien (Da Capo Press)

Great Gluten-Free Vegan Eats by Allyson Kramer (Fair Winds Press)

The Heart of the Plate: Vegetarian Recipes for a New Generation by Mollie Katzen (Rux Martin/Houghton Mifflin Harcourt)

It's All Good by Gwyneth Paltrow and Julia Turshen (Grand Central Life and Style)

125 Gluten-Free Vegetarian Recipes by Carol Fenster (Avery Trade)

Vedge: 100 Plates Large and Small That Redefine Vegetable Cooking by Rich Landau and Kate Jacoby (The Experiment)

Vegetable Literacy by Deborah Madison (Ten Speed Press)

The American Vegan Society, www.americanvegansociety.org
The American Vegetarian Association, www.amerveg.com

Lactose-Dairy-Gluten-Free

For some of you, giving up dairy is not voluntary. If you have a problem with gluten, you may find that you don't do well with lactose, the sugar component of milk and other dairy products. Sometimes lactose intolerance precedes gluten sensitivity by months or years.

Symptoms of lactose intolerance or disaccharidase deficiency include bloating, gas, and urgent trips to the bathroom—not pleasant. Sometimes a problem with lactose is permanent. Sometimes it's not.

Lactose intolerance can be a condition on its own. Or it can be the temporary consequence of villous atrophy from the long-standing insult of gluten. Once gluten is removed and the intestine heals, lactose problems often disappear for many—myself included, a little over a year after my diagnosis.

For others, lactose intolerance is permanent, a separate issue standing alongside the new challenge of a gluten-free diet. There are many lactose-free ice creams and cheeses, and there is Lactaid milk, as well as a pill that can be taken before eating dairy.

While lactose problems stem from the part of the milk that is sugar, allergies to milk and other dairy products require that you avoid *all* dairy, which includes casein and whey, and products labeled lactose-free. There is no magic pill for this. In addition to gluten-free, you must ensure that the products you buy are dairy-free or vegan, as long as those products contain no gluten.

To further complicate things, there is a difference between dairy-free and nondairy. While there is no FDA definition of the term *dairy-free*, you can pretty much expect a product labeled dairy-free or vegan will be just that. Nondairy is trickier. FDA regulation allows for the presence of milk protein, such as casein, whey, and other derivatives in products labeled "nondairy." Despite misleading labels, commercial nondairy creams and cheeses actually do contain casein, and whey and other derivatives are not milk-free.

Why?

As the story goes, the term came into being because the dairy industry did not want products that were dairy substitutes to be mistaken for pure dairy products. This makes no sense, but who am I to argue with the dairy lobby? Perhaps this kind of lobbyist-skewed decision making is why so many of you are swearing off eating dairy products and becoming vegan in the first place.

Confusing? Yes. Impossible? No.

Just as you scrutinize labels for gluten ingredients, you need to memorize dairy-derived ingredients. Many labels will list the allergens the product contains. Even better, more and more products list the common allergens the products do *not* contain.

It should go without saying. Identify products you can trust. Buy whole, unprocessed food and cook it yourself. Identify vegan products that are also gluten-free. See the frozen gluten-free, dairy-free, casein-free veggie burger (page 217) and enjoy more foods like it.

Nut Alert!
Those allergic to nuts must read labels carefully. Many dairy-free products contain nuts.

VEGETARIAN, DAIRY-FREE, SOY-FREE, AND EGG-FREE COOKBOOKS

The following books will get you doing gluten-free, dairy-free, and lactose-free like a pro:

Cooking for Isaiah: Gluten-Free and Dairy-Free Recipes for Easy, Delicious Meals by Silvana Nardone, foreword by Rachael Ray (Reader's Digest)

The Diary-Free and Gluten-Free Kitchen by Denise Jardine (Ten Speed Press)

The Healthy Gluten-Free Life: 200 Delicious Gluten-Free, Dairy-Free, Soy-Free and Egg-Free Recipes by Tammy Credicott (Victory Belt Publishing)

Casein-Free Gluten-Free

While many adults follow the dairy-free and casein-free diet because of a real food allergy or intolerance, there is another group whose parents have long believed that this particular diet could possibly provide relief from some of the debilitating and often isolating symptoms of a serious neurologic condition: those with autism spectrum disorder (ASD) or Asperger's syndrome. These are the littlest hyphenates of all.

Science may be catching up. According to a 2012 study conducted at Penn State and published in the journal *Nutritional Neuroscience*, "a gluten-free casein-free diet may lead to improvements in behavior and psychological symptoms in some children diagnosed with an autism spectrum disorder (ASD)."

This is the first research study to actually draw on parents' observations. In an online survey, the researchers asked parents and primary caregivers of 387 children to complete a ninety-question survey and to report their children's gastrointestinal (GI) and allergy symptoms, along with the degree to which they adhered to a gluten-free, casein-free diet.

The Penn State team observed that a greater proportion of the children in their study reported GI and allergy symptoms that are normally seen in the general population. The study group then found that among children with symptoms of GI and food allergies, as compared to those with no symptoms, there was an improvement in social behaviors, language, eye contact, attention span, and other problems when there was strict adherence to the diet.

A more recent study conducted at Columbia University Medical Center found that a subset of autistic children showed higher immune activity to gluten, but with no link to celiac disease. Of 37 children with autism and 103 without, 20 percent of the autistic children had significantly elevated levels of gluten antibodies compared to those without autism, pointing to immunologic and/or intestinal permeability abnormalities in these children. It's possible that a better understanding of the immune response to gluten may offer clues about autism and help identify those children who would respond positively to dietary treatment. Clearly, these are promising developments.

Up to now, there has been much disagreement in the scientific community and only anecdotal evidence from parents about whether or not the gluten-free casein-free diet really helps children with this condition. Obviously, more research is necessary. In the meantime, there is hope for parents who must make informed choices about whether or not the gluten-free casein-free diet is right in their particular situation.

For many fine articles on the possibility of a link between autism and gastrointestinal problems, tips on coping strategies, and a more comprehensive look at this challenging diet, as well as interviews with parents who have found a way forward, see:

Autism Parenting Magazine
AutismWeb.com
Gluten-Free Living magazine
Living Without magazine

A CASEIN-FREE PRIMER

Foods that contain casein are milk, cream, half-and-half, yogurt, sour cream, cheese, butter, creamed vegetables and soups, white or milk chocolate, ice cream, ice milk, sorbet, puddings, and custards.

In other words, anything from a cow.

Foods that may or may not contain casein and must be investigated further are margarine, tuna, dairy-free cheeses, artificial flavorings, semi-sweet chocolate, hot dogs, lunch meats, sauces, and ghee (the clarified butter used in Indian cooking), including many foods that carry a nondairy label.

Only those kosher foods labeled "kosher parve" contain no casein.

Cooking for the Littlest Hyphenates

The Autism and ADHD Diet: A Step-by-Step Guide to Hope and Healing by Barrie Silberberg (Sourcebooks)

Getting Your Kid on a Gluten-Free Casein-Free Diet by Susan Lord (Jessica Kingsley Publishing)

The Kid-Friendly ADHD and Autism Cookbook, updated and revised, by Pamela Compart and Dana Laake (Fair Winds Press)

The Simple Way to Start the GF/CF Diet: An Easy Guide to Implementing the Gluten Free/Casein Free Diet for Your Child with Autism by Natalie A. Kulig (Trafford Publishing)

Learn More

ANDI (Autism Network for Dietary Intervention. www.autismndi.com

Autism Spectrum Disorder Foundation. www.myasdf.org

The GFCF Diet Support Group. www.gfcfdiet.com

National Institute of Mental Health Publications. http://www.nimh.nih .gov/health/publications/a-parents-guide-to-autism-spectrum -disorder/index.shtml

The Gluten-Free-And-I'm-Not-Sure-What-Else Diet

Something besides gluten is bothering you. How do you find out what? Process of elimination.

According to the Mayo Clinic, there is no standard test to rule out food allergy and this is where the elimination diet comes in. A true elimination or exclusion diet should be undertaken temporarily and in concert with your doctor. Ideally, it should be used to confirm allergy testing.

An elimination or exclusion diet completely eliminates a food or a small group of suspected foods, then reintroduces them if symptoms improve.

Think of it as a kind of take-home test, which looks for the most common food allergens—milk, eggs, nuts, wheat, and soy, and after that, corn and sesame and potatoes, tomatoes, peppers, eggplant, or whatever it is you think you may be allergic to.

The elimination diet can be time-consuming but is well worth it. Buy yourself a journal or use the Note function on your smartphone and write down everything you put in your mouth. No shorthand.

WRITE EVERY BITE
If you've had pasta for dinner, write:

Pasta (even if gluten-free)
Tomatoes
Basil
Olive oil
Cheese

Make note of what time you had it and how you felt afterward.
If lunch was a meatball sandwich, write:

Ground beef
Ground veal
Ground pork
Egg
Bread crumbs (even if gluten-free)
Tomato ketchup
White bread (even if gluten-free)
Sandwich bread (even if gluten-free)

Don't forget to observe your reactions to foods throughout the day.
Record the obvious and not-so-obvious symptoms.
Diarrhea, obvious.
Coughing, not so much.
Nothing is off the table—observe feelings as well as foods. Fatigue, jumpiness, and depression are all suspects, too. If you're going to be a food detective, you've got to have all the clues.

Once a few suspects arise, eliminate that food or foods for at least two weeks, while continuing to make note of what you are eating. And what you are *not* eating.

During this phase, you may want to consult with a dietician to make sure you are replacing those foods with a substitute that offers the same nutrients.

Feel better?

No?

Observe again. Rethink the list of foods that may be causing the problems and eliminate those.

If you do feel better, your doctor will most likely ask you to challenge the list of suspects by putting problem foods, one at a time, back into your diet. Carefully record any allergy symptoms you experience as you add each food. This is where you narrow down the culprits to a shorter list.

As a final step, you will be asked to stop eating those foods that are causing symptoms one at a time. The goal is to find out if your symptoms clear up for good.

Food Allergy Alert

Never undertake an elimination diet challenge if a certain food causes hives, swelling of lips and throat, or, God forbid, anaphylaxis.

AN IMPORTANT NOTE

You may have found that you have a problem with wheat or gluten by process of elimination. For some of you, this may not be an allergy at all but rather non-celiac gluten sensitivity or full-blown celiac disease. This requires a consultation, not with an allergist, but with a knowledgeable gastroenterologist. Do yourself and your whole family a favor and get tested for celiac disease.

To learn more about a medically supervised elimination diet and to find a specialist in food allergy or a registered dietician or a knowledgeable gastroenterologist, see Chapter 20, "The Doctor Will See You Now."

CLASSICS FOR EVERY FOOD HYPHENATE'S LIBRARY

The Art of Simple Food: Notes, Lessons, and Recipes from a Delicious Revolution and *The Art of Simple Food II: Recipes, Flavor, and Inspiration from the New Kitchen Garden* by Alice Waters (Clarkson Potter)

The Conscious Cook by Tal Ronnen (William Morrow)

Cooked: A Natural History of Transformation by Michael Pollan (Penguin)

Food Matters by Mark Bittman (Simon and Schuster)

The Omnivore's Dilemma: A Natural History of Four Meals by Michael
    Pollan (Penguin)
One Big Table: A Portrait of American Cooking by Molly O'Neill (Simon
    and Schuster)

Learn More

Academy of Nutrition and Dietetics. www.eatright.org/programs
    /rdfinder
American Academy of Allergy, Asthma, and Immunology. www.aaaai.org

3

Necessary Losses

For every action
there is an equal
and opposite reaction.
—NEWTON'S THIRD LAW OF MOTION

- First You Mourn
- Acceptance
- The Resourceful Bird Gets the Bagel
- Communicate—Negotiate
- Pity Is Not Positive
- The Harder You Work, the Better You Eat
- Assume Nothing and Never Take Yes for an Answer
- No One Knows More About Your Diet Than You Do
- Ideas to Ease the Transition

You tell yourself that with so many amazing gluten-free foods arriving literally every day, restaurants becoming fluent, instant access to recipes, smartphone apps, cookbooks, blogs, and bakeries on every corner, not to mention friends and family asking how they can help, this will all be a slam dunk, right?

Wrong.

Before we move on from the basics to the next level of learning how to live a totally successful, healthy, food-centered, and satisfying gluten-free life, let's pause for a reality check: giving up gluten is a big deal, and for most of you it's forever. This may be a good time to acknowledge you may be having a slightly emotional reaction.

If you've just been diagnosed with celiac disease, you may be having a *big* emotional reaction. You're not alone.

A friend of mine, a well-known gluten-free cookbook writer, acquired her skills, not because she had to be gluten-free, but so she could cook for her dad who did. There is nothing she doesn't know about this diet. For most of her life she was able to commute between the two worlds. When she received her own diagnosis right before Christmas, she went into shock. Depression set in. Something major would always be missing from her diet, even though she is one of the country's finest gluten-free cooks.

If you are feeling less than thrilled right now, you are in good company. Loss gives rise to longing; we want what we cannot have.

Don't think that just because you are mildly sensitive, you're off the hook. Even if going gluten-free was solely your decision, undertaken for many good and sound reasons, you may be wondering why you're so out of sorts. A little snarky, even. Yes, it was your choice. But choices have consequences and one of them is wondering what you've gotten yourself into and how you'll manage to go without something you've eaten all your life.

We mistakenly believe that if we rush into action, we can circumvent the discomfort. We become dervishes of doing. We power through the learning curve, trying to master everything we need to know in our new gluten-free, possibly multi-hyphenated lives. We don't take the time to attend to the inevitable feelings of loss that come with such a change. We do not allow the grieving process to take place. And believe me, there is one.

No matter that glutenous foods make us sick. No matter the degree of sick we experience. No matter that yearning for something that hurts us doesn't make sense. We miss them. It's important to allow ourselves to feel their absence until we don't miss them anymore.

When we pay attention to ourselves and not just to all of the information we need to acquire, we may find we are overwhelmed. Questions arise.

How do I *really* feel about having to be gluten-free every day for the rest of my life?

Am I comfortable with being self-assertive? Or am I a shrinking violet who would rather avoid asking for what I need?

How will I manage to get what I need?

Do I see two perfectly poached eggs slathered in silky hollandaise beckoning from matching slabs of honey-baked ham?

Or do I see only the English muffin I can't have?

Do I feel I deserve serious attention?

How you answer these and other important questions will determine how hard or easy it's going to be to make your way through the gluten-free maze.

You wonder how you will cope with those who have only a fuzzy idea about what a zero-tolerance gluten-free diet is and would rather dismiss you as neurotic or trendy. Will you be able to navigate situations where you are not taken seriously? How will you cope with people who find it easier saying no than yes, possibly members of your own family? Will you be a casualty of all of the recent press attention, celebrity hype, and general fuss? Or will you thrive in the gluten-aware culture?

You worry that people will make assumptions about your diet, get it wrong, and possibly make you sick. They may.

The other day, as I was asking the deli person at Whole Foods if a certain item was gluten-free or not, a woman stood alongside me waiting at the counter for her vegan General Tso's chicken (100 percent texturized wheat protein) and said, "I'm gluten-free, too." You may remember the perky greeter in an Italian restaurant who responded to my question about gluten-free menu options by saying that their gluten-free customers loved the whole-wheat pasta.

Where once we had to explain what a gluten-free diet is and is not, then convince people to help us get a good and safe meal, now we wonder if we can depend on the information we're getting. How will we wade through all the degrees and definitions? We're faced with a different set of challenges. We've gone from *Ripley's Believe It or Not* to *Fad du Jour*. Let's call it the too-much-of-a-good-thing syndrome.

So, yes, getting the diet down cold is a given. But just as important is learning to be our own best advocate, to develop resourcefulness, creativity, and a can-do attitude, even if these qualities don't come naturally. If we see the diet as an obstacle to pleasure, it will be.

Looking back at the New Year's Eve when I slipped a demitasse spoon out of my evening bag, headed for the caviar, and ate my fill seems silly now with all the choices available today. But seeing yourself as special and, by virtue of that, allowed to reinvent the rules is as relevant now as it was then. If my attitude had been less positive and did not allow for this exercise in creative problem solving, I might have rung in that year with a big helping of self-pity.

By seeing my situation in a new way, I was able to draw on my sense of self-reliance, adventure, and fun. By giving myself permission to be creative about my problem, I was able to apply the principle of old-fashioned positive thinking and come up with an elegant solution that fit the festive tone of the occasion. I venture that if you tried this today, you'd find your fellow guests wishing they'd followed your lead—how smart to skip the carbohydrates and go straight for the protein! You would also learn an invaluable lesson: people see you through the prism of their own self-interest.

The point is, how tough an adjustment this is depends on how willing you are to move out of your comfort zone, negotiate past "no," and find the kind of resourceful and self-reliant spirit others cannot resist. How seriously do you take yourself and your dietary circumstances, and how willing are you to appear assertive, self-indulgent, even foolish, to strangers? How good are you at asking for what you need?

For now, it comes down to how willing you are to honor the empty place that has just opened up in you, to acknowledge and examine it without judgment and give it its due.

First You Mourn

Mourning may sound a bit dramatic when there are more important things in life to lose than a food group. After all, the whole world seems to be gluten-free, and with more goodies arriving every day, it just gets easier and easier, doesn't it? There is starvation in the world and all you have is a little problem with grain. It's only a meal.

Not quite. You are saying good-bye to a way of life, and even if that way of life included less than optimum health, it's tough to say good-bye to something forever.

I know you're going to be fine, more than fine, actually. I am certain you will discover so many gluten-free pleasures, you'll wonder why you ever made such a big deal of the diet in the first place. You'll feel better than you ever have. You'll be healthier. Maybe even slimmer.

But what I think doesn't matter. I am years into this, an expert, thrilled at how easy it is to be gluten-free at this moment in our culture. I've already done my share of whimpering and whining, of refusing to be in the same room with spaghetti—even if today's gluten-free version is so good, no one can tell which is which anyway.

Now it's your turn.

To use food terms, if you don't attend to your feelings and allow yourself to grieve for the freedom of being able to eat anything, anytime, anywhere, the spontaneity of that—even if going gluten-free was your choice—resentment will simmer and eventually boil over, scalding everyone in its path. We all know people who'd have a great smile if it were not for the blood on their teeth.

When you're ready to move forward knowing you have put the past to rest and have done the emotional homework that will pave the way for a healthy and self-affirming new chapter, you will take on the challenge with optimism and delight.

Accept That You Are Powerless over Your Diet

To borrow a bromide from Alcoholics Anonymous, beyond pain is acceptance and beyond that is recovery. I'm not talking about recovery in the look-Ma-I-can-eat-grain-again sense. I'm talking about recovering your balance, your good humor, your ability to see yourself as a creative person who uses his or her natural optimism to enjoy life and maintain health, someone who can say, "It's no big deal" and mean it.

As long as I'm in the AA mode, you can't develop a healthy attitude toward your food intolerance until you admit that you are powerless over it.

The sooner you accept the unalterable fact that some days you will not get what you need and some days you will sail through fully sated and you can't control which is which, the sooner you can move beyond it to coping with the ups and downs resourcefully, responsibly, and positively.

Put another way, it takes energy to deny, ignore, trivialize, pretend, and otherwise delude yourself into thinking you are in charge, even though you know what and what not to eat. This is energy best put to a more satisfying purpose.

The Resourceful Bird Gets the Bagel

To live well on the gluten-free diet requires thinking outside the box. Even more important, it requires a certain comfort level with creativity, bending the rules, and shifting the focus from the problem to a satisfying solution.

The operative words here are *What if?*—as in what if I bring my favorite gluten-free bread or roll to a restaurant and ask the server to ask the chef to grill it (and could the chef please scrape the grill before he plunks my bread on it), then order a hamburger the way I like it (as long as I can be sure the other ingredients are gluten-free)?

What if I ask the chef to boil, in a fresh pot of water, thank you, the spaghetti I called ahead to say I'd supply? Or maybe the *fresh* ravioli, so I don't hold them up in the kitchen?

What if I ask them—*after* I've called ahead and explained how to keep my food safe from cross-contamination with other foods—to make veal Parmesan with my gluten-free bread crumbs or buttery garlic bread with my gluten-free baguette, enough for the whole table to enjoy?

What if I ship my suitcase, packed with all I need including enough gluten-free food for the business meeting, long weekend, or conference, addressed to me care of the hotel, and marked HOLD FOR ARRIVAL?

And what if by doing that I avoid the baggage fee and, for the same amount of money, I could guarantee my bag would get there on time and with all of my stuff still in it?

And what if the next time we have company for the weekend, I make absolutely everything gluten-free, showing off the wonders of what's available, knowing they will ask for the recipes and names of the products, virtually ensuring that my next stay at *their* house is a win-win for everyone?

Answers are limited only by the questions asked.

Don't Complain—Explain

When the gluten-free gods are not smiling, it's tempting to complain to the management, walk out in a huff, and leave it at that, then post something snarky about the restaurant on Yelp. But if you adjust your thinking slightly, you'll find every missed or less-than-perfect meal is an opportunity to explain what you need next time, a chance for people to get it right with a little help from you.

It's unproductive to complain that the gluten-free cookies brought along for you are not up to snuff. Why not tell friends where to find the really good ones and oh, by the way, they are so good, you'll never know they're gluten-free? Why complain to your sister that she didn't get it right when she had you over for dinner? Show her how to do it next time. At your house.

We don't ask a person who is trying to quit smoking to empty the ashtrays, do we? We don't send a person on a diet out for a gallon of ice cream. We don't send the problem drinker to the liquor store for wine. So why do you have to make the lasagna for your big Italian family? You don't as long as you explain why.

Waiting for people to magically understand your needs is always unrealistic. Expecting your spouse, your children, your friends, and your coworkers to know at any given moment which food cues upset you is asking for trouble. And it's not fair to them. Explanations are in order.

I am reminded of the old story about the man who is working up the courage to ask his neighbor if he can borrow a ladder. He thinks about the chances of his neighbor lending it to him with generosity and thinks, "Well, after all, I loaned him my electric drill."

A little while later he remembers the time the neighbor took a month to return a barbecue fork. Even later, still worrying about whether his request will be met with a negative response, it occurs to him that his auto-buffing attachment has never been returned. After several hours stewing, the man marches across his neighbor's lawn and rings the bell.

When the unsuspecting fellow comes to the door, he shouts, "I don't want your damn ladder anyway!" and stomps off.

It's tempting to find fault with the people who disappoint us. After all, that's selfish, isn't it?

Not really.

The blame lies not with those who fall short, but with us for failing to explain why things need to change. Adjusting to the gluten-free diet is tough enough; suffering in silence is self-defeating.

Communicate—Negotiate

If you are the cook in the household, it's your responsibility to let your family know, and not theirs to guess, how crucial it is to your well-being and long-term health to eliminate wheat and gluten from your diet. People, even those who love us, just want things to stay the same. It's up to you to let them know what foods are safe for you to eat and how best to ensure that you enjoy your time together as much as everyone else. Give them practical information, but also be honest about your feelings.

Let them know how hard it is for you to make sandwiches for everyone or to watch them eat pizza during Monday night football. Tell them how you feel when you watch them nibble a brioche. For a long time I unconsciously chewed along with people, like a passenger who brakes from the backseat.

Communication works both ways. Listen carefully to how they feel about this change in their lives and try to be just as understanding and accommodating when they express sadness or anger at losses resulting from your diet. Pay close attention to the smallest members of the family. What about Sunday morning bagels or baking holiday cookies together? If Mom or Dad or Billy or Jane can't eat lobster rolls, does this mean we can't go to Maine next summer?

This is where negotiating comes in.

Ask the kids to take charge of making their own breakfasts for a while. Maybe family pizza night moves to a pizza parlor that offers gluten-free options. Maybe you take responsibility for finding new gluten-free recipes for the family's traditional holiday treats.

Never Trivialize Your Diet or Allow Others to Do So

This should go without saying.

But you may have a hard time asking for special treatment. You don't want to make waves. You say it's no big deal. It's just a little gluten problem. It's just my wheat allergy. Belittling the importance of your diet is a cue for others to do the same. Besides, gluten intolerance is not a little problem or an allergy.

This sort of self-effacement reminds me of an old joke:

How many martyrs does it take to change a lightbulb?
None.
They'd rather sit in the dark.

Or, as Dolly Parton is fond of saying, "Get down off the cross, honey. We need the wood."

Of course you want special treatment. You *need* special treatment. And in this growing gluten-free culture of ours, a gentle and assertive request usually nets something memorable to eat. If not now, next time.

Words such as *just*, *only*, and *merely* signal the listener to turn off and not take your request seriously. This is very much like going to the doctor, being asked if your joints hurt, and saying, "Yeah, well, I'm not getting any younger." You've just guaranteed that the doctor will move on, perhaps missing a serious issue.

Let's face it. Some of us are pretty darned uncomfortable calling attention to ourselves. It could be that someone in your past wanted you to believe that you don't deserve the full attention of others, or that your problems are not as important. Or you fear that if you ask others to meet your needs, they won't love or like you.

I am sorry to open up Pandora's box, but when we fully examine our response to a change as important as this one, we see that our reactions have very little to do with food at all.

The next time you feel you are about to trivialize your needs or your commitment to your health, or you reject special attention, write out the following affirmation on an index card or, better yet, type it into your smartphone and say it aloud until you believe it.

Yes, it sounds silly. But it works.

I, _____, am a unique and special person worthy of all the special attention, love, and understanding I ask for from those around me.

Strike When the Iron Is Cold

Not properly mourning the feelings that come up, not accepting them as your own with equanimity and kindness, and not kissing them good-bye easily turns to anger. The experts call this projection, which goes like this:

I feel bad, so now I'm going to get rid of the bad feeling, by making you feel bad.

It's not so much fun to be on the receiving end of this.

Let's say someone who should know better has failed to remember your diet. You're so mad, you're sure your head will blow off. Jet fuel is less volatile than you are at this moment. You haven't done the emotional work, and your lizard brain wants to crush the person responsible for the uncomfortable feelings that have come up in you.

If you don't want to spend the rest of your life mending fences or running the risk of losing a friend you otherwise love, breathe, count to ten,

Vérité
If food is love, love is never having to say you're sorry for, or otherwise defend, your gluten-free diet.

leave the room, splash water on your face, until the choke hold your anger has over you has let go.

When the anger has cooled, and you can see the offender as the fallible human being he or she is, not the perpetrator of your unhappiness, express your disappointment with kindness and respect, preferably much later or the next day. Calmly and with compassion, be clear about the behavioral change you are asking for. Say, "I was disappointed last night, and I need to know there's something safe for me to eat when I come to your house. Maybe you could call me before we get together next time, so I'll know what to bring for myself."

Notice that this request is in first person. You are not verbally pointing the finger. You haven't said, "*You* forgot my food. I can't rely on *you*."

It's amazing how easy it is to resolve conflict, and how apologetic and accommodating others can be when they're not looking down the barrel of unexpressed anger.

Pity Is Not Positive

The other side of this coin is *too* much attention.

After giving yourself enough time to feel sorry for yourself, make it clear that you will reject the poor-you stuff politely and firmly. Excess concern isn't healthy. Nor does it inspire confidence. If anything, it can erode self-esteem and may even contribute to a victim mentality. You may find yourself presenting that needy side of yourself to the person who encourages it, and it also may result in being treated less than equally in other areas of the relationship.

Beware the saboteur who does not encourage you or offer ways to help you get back to your old/new self. This is the one who whispers to others about how hard it is for you to live on this diet, who is always there to pat your hand and remind you how badly you feel about pasta, and who, whether consciously or not, keeps you in that swamp so long, you start to see yourself only as the one who can't eat gluten. Pretty soon, you are forgetting all the wonderful things you are besides being someone who gets sick after eating gluten.

Naturally, you need to distinguish negativity from genuine concern. The fastest way to do this is to see what action follows the talk. People who use pity to keep the people in their lives feeling bad never follow through with positive action. And they don't seem as happy as they should be for you when you have a triumph to report. True compassion and healthy caring usually results in wonderful surprises, special foods, generous ideas, pantries permanently stocked with goodies for you, and very little talk about your diet beyond learning more about how to make it easier and more pleasant for you.

Whether we like it or not, gluten intolerance and the profound change it brings to our everyday lives can lay bare a relationship. We pay dearly for being coddled. You don't need it. But you know that.

The Harder You Work, the Better You Eat

From here on in, you have to participate in the process. Every meal at home, every breakfast, lunch, and dinner out, every bite on the road, every snack at the movies, at work, at the mall, on a plane, at the park, on a date in a dark, glutenous bar. Every time.

You can't just hand your friends and family a list of gluten-free foods. You have to teach them how to properly prepare the foods you can eat, where to buy them, and how to keep them from touching that which you can't eat.

You have to verify they're using the right thickeners, ice creams, spreads, and dips, that their corn bread is all corn, that their barbecue sauce is safe, that their soy sauce is gluten-free. If necessary, you must supply these things.

Suddenly, you can't just dash to the market for a few things. You have to take the time and extra expense to bake or buy or otherwise prepare gluten-free foods. Not only do you have to master the Thanksgiving stuffing; some of us have to render it vegan or dairy or nut-free as well.

You can no longer just show up, sit back, and be served. The desire to give up and eat something out of a can or a box will be very strong. Maybe you weren't such a good cook to begin with, someone whose idea of dinner is takeout or something frozen to pop into the microwave. Gluten-free cooking isn't always convenient, but it can be a whole lot healthier and more satisfying. You're going to have to acquire some skills, be willing to prepare the meal, host the party, do the dessert, and even cook the entire holiday dinner if that's what it takes to show everyone how it's done. On the following pages you will find real inspiration.

Yes, it takes some work, but the rewards are huge.

For every dish you master, every gluten-free ravioli, fruit tart, cookie, and bread crumb you share with others, the better you eat.

Simple as that.

Assume Nothing and Never Take Yes for an Answer

Whether you like it or not, you must learn to press the waiter for assurance that your meal is safe.

By this I don't mean grilling in an adversarial way, but politely asking for the list of ingredients and how the dish is prepared. Likewise, it is no longer possible to nibble the offered energy bar until you read the ingredients. Or assume, because people know about your intolerance to gluten, that the food they are serving or how they are serving it will not make you sick.

Periodically phone, write, or e-mail any company that makes a gluten-free product you really like. Just because it was gluten-free when you read the label doesn't mean it will always remain so. Many companies buy their ingredients from different suppliers, and changes may not be reflected on labels that are printed well in advance of any such reformulation. You don't have to be paranoid, but you do need to be careful, especially if said product is a big part of your diet.

The operative attitude, cloaked in gracious words and polite requests, is: *I'm the customer and you are in business to please me and I need to make sure I don't get sick from something you have not told me about.*

While this may sound confrontational, it really isn't. The people who make your food have an obligation to tell you what it contains. Competition for your gluten-free dollar is fierce. As more and more food marketers are making gluten-free products and labeling them accordingly, companies not willing to answer your questions deserve to lose your business.

Honey Beats Vinegar Hands Down

If you don't believe me, ask a stranger, in a self-entitled way, that you need to use their copier. You may get lucky, but most likely you will be politely told to go to Kinko's.

Now go somewhere else and ask the same question, this time starting with, "I hope you can help me. I really am in a tight spot and I wonder if you would be kind enough to allow me to make a copy of this." Chances are the person will offer to do it for you.

The lesson is simple. The better your ability to ask a question in a way that encourages the other person to do the right thing, the better your chances of hearing the answer you want. The trick is asking it in a way that brings out the other person's natural instincts to help you.

"You have no idea what a treat it would be for me to have your wonderful Bolognese sauce on my gluten-free pasta."

"I love your burgers, but I'm afraid to order one unless you scrape the grill where you cook it. Is that too much trouble?"

Practice on your family:

Darling, it would mean so much to me if you took out the trash/changed the cat's litter/passed that math test/didn't text at dinner.

No One Knows More About Your Diet Than You Do

You are the expert.

When it comes to your diet, no one will ever be as clever, as resourceful, as smart about it, or articulate its requirements as clearly as you will soon be able to.

No one has a better reason to be.

All too often, we sell ourselves short because we take the word of someone we presume to have authority. When the waiter tells us that the chef uses flour to coat a cutlet or a plate of scallops, we can suggest with authority that the dish be prepared with cornstarch or cornmeal or simply grilled, baked, sautéed, or roasted unadorned.

If we understand that chefs have reputations to uphold, we can ask with all deference if that change is okay and doesn't hurt the integrity of the dish. It is important to remember that the chef is an expert on the preparation of food, not necessarily on the preparation of *your* food. When you know what to ask for, more than likely you will be treated to a lightbulb moment when he or she realizes how a great meal can be adapted for you.

It should go without saying never to let someone speak, shop, or order for you unless, of course, that person is gluten-free as well and as exacting about it as you. And don't always assume that your doctor knows more about living with your condition than you do, either. With notable exceptions, most physicians don't spend five minutes understanding the conditions they diagnose so expertly, especially if those conditions require no medical intervention.

If you need proof of this, ask for his or her position on kamut or spelt. Better still, ask why, when you have had a short gastroenterological procedure like a colonoscopy or a follow-up small-bowel biopsy, you are handed a package of peanut crackers along with everyone else.

From now on, it's up to you to connect the dots.

Speaking up for yourself not only teaches you how much you know, but it also exudes confidence, takes responsibility, and affirms your intention to take charge of your health.

If the picture seems a bit bleak or confusing right now, that's normal. You still have much to learn.

For now, trust what you know. It's more than you think.

Some Ideas to Ease the Transition

If you are the primary chef in the family, opt out of preparing glutenous meals for a while. You may find that one meal is more difficult to prepare for others than another. Breakfast and brunch are the most brutal for me because, even after all this time and despite gluten-free versions, so much bread is involved. I will go out to brunch, but I still won't do it at my house.

Hold a family meeting to discuss food preparation options and develop a rotating schedule so that no one is ever stuck with fixing the same meal for longer than a week. Include everyone in the family, even the youngest members, so everyone plays a part. Review the schedule weekly or monthly as your own skills improve.

Review the family's social calendar. Talk about upcoming parties and holidays, barbecues and picnics, and ask everybody to think of ways they can be easier on you. If the whole tribe is on the same page, you're less likely to be blindsided by the birthday cake you can't eat or suffer a thankless Thanksgiving at your sister-in-law's.

If there is one food in particular, such as mac and cheese, cream of wheat, rye bread, or marble pound cake, that you can't stand to see being enjoyed, say so. Ask friends, family, and receptive coworkers not to eat these things in front of you for a while.

Don't prepare multiple versions of meals. Be very clear that your pasta or gravy or stuffing is really good and will have to be good enough for your family. Ask for their understanding about this. Experiment to find out what their favorite gluten-free brands are.

Master a few basic mixes. Offer manioc bread sticks still warm from the oven. Serve gluten-free ravioli with the tomato sauce you're famous for.

Make gluten-free brownies or pad thai. Who says selfishness is a bad thing?

⊷

When your family tells you they're going out for pizza and have not invited you so they can enjoy it without having to bear the guilt of gobbling it up in your presence, thank them for their consideration and mean it. Your new diet doesn't mean life is a one-way street in your direction. Try to be sensitive to the needs of others.

⊷

Talk to your children. Children have very strong feelings about being cared for and nurtured, and they really can't understand a parent's problem unless they are directly told. Consider this conversation a lesson in becoming an adult who isn't afraid to ask for special attention. If you honor your children with their own importance in your happiness, they will honor you. They will also grow up honoring themselves. Never underestimate them. They will surprise you.

⊷

When you're comfortable at home, broaden your audience to people with whom you are not necessarily intimate, but who may be in a position to cook or order food for you, such as the office lunch pool, cafeteria manager, secretary, or meeting planner.

It's important to state the problem and what you require of people without baring as much of yourself as you have to your immediate circle. Hint: your office rival is not the one with whom to discuss your deep sense of loss over cheese Danish.

⊷

Controlling someone's food is as close to controlling the person as it gets. Be prepared for some disappointments, even some nasty surprises. There will be people who will always find a reason to forget your special diet and never seem to have extra goodies on hand for you. Asking people to extend themselves may unearth some negative feelings toward you, ones that may have lain dormant until now.

Be direct. Ask why this person never remembers your problem. You may be surprised at the answer. Be willing to hear it.

⊷

Accept that some people fear and resist change. We've all seen this happen when there is a sudden shift in economic status or an illness or a life-altering disability. You will expect the best and discover inflexibility, perhaps even the inability to renegotiate the relationship in new terms. In

Vérité

Find the generosity in yourself before looking for it in others.

some cases the awakening will be rude. For every disappointment, someone you never expected to will come through and you will be blessed by a friend you never knew you had.

Try to accept with grace that some people will never be able to give you what you need and lower your expectations. If possible, continue to love them despite their limitations.

⌗

As sure as the sun comes up, you will find yourself in food situations where someone in your family or circle of friends has forgotten you completely. Most people will apologize profusely. You should accept it as graciously as you can.

Consider this: most people usually forget once. After all, this is new to them, too.

Some will forget twice before they get it.

If it happens a third time, it's probably not about food but about the relationship. This is a good time to reexamine and shore up the shaky ground upon which it stands.

⌗

Let the punishment fit the crime. Obviously you're not going to tell the recently bereaved at the funeral luncheon that she forgot to order you a gluten-free meal, nor are you going to tell the host of a surprise birthday party for someone else that it was tacky to serve cake.

Often well-meaning friends, after realizing they've served a slice of flourless chocolate cheesecake (safe) with a cookie crust (not safe), will make this common mistake. Instead of apologizing profusely and getting you a dish of ice cream or some fruit, they may suggest that you just eat the middle.

Never put your health at risk to avoid making waves. No matter how carefully you remove the crust, the middle will most likely be contaminated.

⌗

Conversely, you may find yourself with friends and family eager to go gluten-free with you. The idea is not to judge their intentions or knowledge of the diet. The idea is to instruct. Share what you know. Cook together. Be an example of zero-tolerance for gluten. If you have celiac disease, take seriously the friend who doesn't. He or she may and it's up to you to explain why testing is important for everyone.

Be glad for the company.

Gluten-Free Thinking

4

Living gluten-free isn't as hard as it may seem, but it does teach us to use our noodles, rice noodles, that is. It forces us to be organized, creative, inventive, ingenious, canny, curious, and clever. Once you get the hang of it, it becomes second nature.

You ask yourself: What can I do to make this diet easier, to save time and money, eat well, and, in the process, avoid getting glutened? The idea is to know how to do it so well that you hardly have to think about it.

Here are some shortcuts, ideas, strategies, and just plain smart thinking to help you feel better, organize, and plan for any eventuality including emergencies.

Organizational Thinking: The Gluten-Free Kitchen

Like that pesky sock drawer that we never seem to get around to, we're always promising ourselves we'll clean out the refrigerator, defrost the freezer, and throw away that petrified lump under the frozen peas. Someday, we say, we'll organize the cupboards, rearrange the drawers—Do I really need such a vast twist-tie collection?—replace the crummy old shelf liners, and throw out the canned beans that expired before the turn of millennium.

Well, someday is here. No better time than now to organize a smooth-functioning, safe cooking, separate but equal, gluten-free kitchen.

Let's start with a radical idea.

You may not be ready for this, but at some point you might consider a totally dedicated, gluten-free kitchen, especially if more than one of you is gluten-free. Of course, the non-gluten-free family members have to agree. If you are going to cook gluten-free for everyone, as I do, there's no need for separate equipment and pantry shelves.

My family and friends have grown quite fond of my food. These days, with high quality and taste defying us to tell the difference, it's not a big sacrifice.

As many people do, my husband reports feeling lighter after a gluten-free meal, especially those involving pasta. It's just not as heavy and sleep-inducing as the full-on gluten version.

When we have overnight guests or give a dinner party—as you will, too, eventually—it's always gluten-free. All recipes in my repertoire have been perfected over time: no learning curve required. Simplicity and practice are the keys to success.

✦ Ease into it with a store-bought chocolate flourless torte gussied up with a little whipped cream and a few raspberries. No special skills required.

✦ For something a little more impressive, but not difficult, see Chapter 6, "Essential Skills," for poaching pears or dried fruits.

✦ You're always covered with fresh fruit, a pint or two of ice cream or sorbet, and an assortment of gluten-free cookies in the freezer.

✦ Bagels and breads freeze well. Buy in bulk and defrost a quantity in the microwave before toasting. Ditto for fresh pasta and ravioli and a few containers of tomato sauce and some Mediterranean Bean Soup (page 46) ready to go on a moment's notice.

✦ Chēbē bread mix makes wonderful rosemary breadsticks or rolls. For a party, put them in small vases or little pots and hope they're not gone before you sit down.

✦ Serve cheese and other spreads on gluten-free crackers. No need to worry about putting away expensive cheese full of crumbs.

✦ For breakfast eat oatmeal, certified gluten-free only, or cold amaranth, quinoa, and flax cereal.

✦ Buy or make whole-grain gluten-free sandwich bread, waffles, granola, pizza, soups, bread crumbs, salad dressings, soy sauce, and veggie burgers. No need to worry about crumby toasters, toxic jam jars, suspicious skillets, and other forms of cross-contamination.

I acknowledge that this may be easier for someone like me with an empty nest and a willing adult who doesn't care what he eats as long as it's good. It's not so simple when you are a growing and diverse family. Something to think about.

Here are some rules to organize by.

Rule No. 1

Everybody learns the rules.

Right down to the littlest member, this is a family affair and nobody, not even Mom, should have to shoulder the entire burden alone. If everyone knows what foods and utensils should touch what, and takes responsibility for it, there's a better chance of avoiding a gluten accident, especially in the morning when breakfast and lunches are being fixed on the fly, and everybody has to be somewhere fast. Once you get the drill down, it's second nature and everyone learns the lesson about looking out for each other.

Think of your kitchen as a neighborhood where all the residents are watching out for shady characters and unusual activity instead of relying on the lone and usually overworked cop on the beat.

Rule No. 2

Establish "gluten-free only" equipment.

You may want to have two of the following in a mixed-use kitchen:

Cutting board
Toaster—to avoid extra expense and save space, many gluten-free cooks use toaster ovens because household crumbs drop to the bottom, away from gluten-free bread.
Flour sifter
Oven-safe casseroles and Pyrex dishes
Omelet pan
Colander
Cake knife
Baking sheet
Bread knife
Any pot or pan that isn't easy to clean
Cast-iron frying pan
Sugar bowl
Serving spoons
Wooden spoons and spatulas—it's time to dispose of old spoons that may have a lifetime of gluten in the cracks!
Honey pot
Storage jars
Lunch boxes or insulated travel containers

If Budget Allows:

Grill/panini maker
Bread machine
Electric rice cooker
Crock-Pot

While you're at it, this is a good time to invest in a label maker or big fat marker so you can remember which utensil is for gluten and which one is not. If labels do not fit in with your kitchen aesthetic, why not buy a pretty crock or pitcher and keep your gluten-free spoons, forks, spatulas, egg turners, tongs, and so on, away from the drawer that contains gluten-mixing utensils.

To save having to buy separate cookie sheets or baking pans, tin foil is your best friend. Keep an extra roll on hand for heating and baking gluten-free foods where pizza or cookies may have been baked.

If any utensil is regularly used for gluten-containing foods, buy a new one and use it only for gluten-free cooking. If it's glass or metal and washed properly in lots of hot water after each use, it's fine to use for both. Ditto for expensive pots and pans that are easy to clean.

Lose all the tubs of margarine, cream cheese, and hummus contaminated by knives and spoons carrying bread crumbs and start all over, buying two of each and clearly label: DADDY'S BUTTER, MOM'S CREAM CHEESE, FRED'S BREAD, MY MAYONNAISE!

If your fridge is big enough, dedicate a shelf as a gluten-free zone, preferably the top one so gluten can't drift downward.

Don't forget to label leftovers as gluten-free or not. You're going to forget which is which faster than ice crystals can form.

In a shared kitchen, where two versions of the same meal are being made, gluten-free always comes first. After you prepare a gluten-free meal, you can do the other without having to wash all the pots and utensils, griddle, cutting board, and so on, in between. Less work, less risk.

Another Reason to Wash Your Hands

It should go without saying that anyone touching food, especially raw poultry, should err on the side of too much hand washing. This is even more important now, because gluten travels from one set of sticky fingers to another. From now on, cleanliness is next to gluten-freeness.

Rule No. 3

When in doubt, wipe it down.

Even I will make the occasional sandwich, serve the odd croissant, and leave a basket of brioches and muffins on the kitchen counter for certain die-hard friends to nibble on when they get up. I put the jam in a little glass dish, to prevent a sticky spoon from leaving crumbs in the jar. Ditto for the butter. Butter is a crumb magnet and crumbs are the bane of any gluten-free kitchen. A small serving dish keeps the rest of the stick pristine.

This means cleaning counters, cutting boards, sinks, backsplashes, the rim of the olive oil bottle: anything that might have come in contact with gluten. Afterward, I wipe everything down, including the shelves in the refrigerator (it's amazing what ends up on them) and the revolving microwave plate. When I'm sure I have de-glutened the premises, I then put the contaminated sponge in the dishwasher.

The rule is simple and unbreakable.

Never spread butter, cut a sandwich, slice cheese, fry an egg, flip a burger, cut up a chicken, or scoop ice cream with the same utensil or in the same pan that has touched gluten. In my kitchen, any knife or spoon or plate that has come into contact with bread or flour, and so on, goes directly into the dishwasher or is promptly washed by hand. It is something we don't have to remember anymore. It's reflex.

Rule No. 4

Divide and conquer.

How separate should gluten-free food be from the rest of the family groceries?

Think Church and State.

A separate cupboard or shelf is a good idea. Keep a supply of gluten-free cereals, crackers, mixes, soups, special flours, cookies, pretzels, and other treats and snacks on hand. If space allows, dedicate a shelf of the freezer for individual gluten-free pizzas, frozen macaroni and cheese, and other entrées, bread, rolls, and muffins. This will help other family members understand that these foods are off-limits to them (unless invited to share), and you always know when it's time to restock.

In a big family, providing there's space and if budget allows, it's wise to buy duplicates of things like jam, peanut butter, mayo, and dips too easily contaminated by the spoons and knives and chips of gluten-consuming members.

This also makes keeping an inventory of your favorite products much easier. Tack a sheet of paper to the inside of the cabinet door and keep track of which ones you like best.

Even more important, cross off those you never want to buy again. Since gluten-free is not cheap, you might want to keep your coupons in the same place.

Rule No. 5

I love you, but stay out of my kitchen.

We were all taught to be good guests, gracious sisters and brothers, aunts and uncles. We arrive with flowers or a nice bottle of wine, maybe something homemade for the hostess just to show her you've got this gluten-free thing down. We write thank-you notes.

We do our part, especially at the holidays and other family events. Pitching in with the prep work to help move things along is a given. After dinner, we want to jump up and help with the cleanup. As gracious and helpful as friends and family are, they don't know the rules, and this could lead to a gluten disaster. No matter how well meant the offer is, firmly decline.

Be diplomatic. Tell them how wonderfully they treat you at their houses, so now it's your turn to wait on them. Or do as I do: say your kitchen is small and too many cooks throw off your timing.

Give them a harmless job, like opening the wine, setting the table, or reading a story to a fussy toddler.

Bless their hearts, they honestly don't know they can't flip the burgers with the same spatula, make sandwiches or cut vegetables with a knife that's been used to cut something glutenous. They have no idea you have a special place for gluten-free and glutenous leftovers in the refrigerator or that the plastic wrap they're using has already touched your food. If necessary, give these kind and gracious guests seats that are extremely difficult to get out of. A bench on one side of our dining table seats four and makes sliding out tricky unless everybody moves. This is where my helpers are always asked to sit.

Rule No. 6

If you finish it, you replace it.

In general, it pays to be generous with your goodies—after all, don't you want more family members eating your way?—but only to a point. At these prices, special foods are just that—special—too rich for the munching and grazing habits of ravenous teenagers, hungry toddlers, or the midnight prowling of snacking adults. Not to mention the personal cost of needing a handful of gluten-free pretzels and finding that they're gone. Grrrr.

Taking Stock: The Basic Starter Pantry

If you are not a cook and do not feel comfortable substituting gluten-free ingredients for those you are accustomed to, the first order of business is to buy one or two basic gluten-free cookbooks and maybe treat yourself to a subscription to one of the excellent gluten-free cooking magazines such as *Living Without, Gluten-Free Living,* or *Simply Gluten-Free Magazine* (See Chapter 23, "Community," for more books and magazines).

Nutrition is key and most gluten-free packaged food isn't enriched, so the first order of business is to stock up on foods that will supply enough B vitamins, fiber, and protein.

The idea is to choose fresh, naturally gluten-free foods bursting with nutrients. See Chapter 6, "Essential Skills," for some simple cooking techniques that will make all the difference between a fresh, whole-food diet and one that comes out of a box or a bag.

+ Beans pack a nutritional wallop and are always a great choice for any number of dishes.
+ Whole grains like quinoa and sorghum, wild and brown rice, and millet are good choices, easy to cook up as porridge or to add to soups and stews.
+ Stock up on whole-grain gluten-free bread, and bagels, tacos, tortillas, wraps, waffles, crackers, fruit and nut mixes, granola, protein bars, and soups.
+ Have on hand a few wholesome gluten-free treats.
+ This is the time to toss and replace items like soy sauce, marinades, sauces, and even seasoning blends full of hidden gluten. Any ice cream you have with mix-ins, like candy or cookie dough, need to go as well.

Where does it say you have to be a masterful baker to be gluten-free?

A good all-purpose gluten-free flour mix is all you need to substitute cup for cup in your favorite recipes and for thickening gravies, dusting pans, and coating oven-baked and fried foods. And with all of the wonderful gluten-free baking mixes out there, it really isn't hard to produce a few cookies, muffins, or even a cake occasionally. If you were comfortable using a baking mix before, you can do it now.

Baking from scratch has a bit more of a learning curve. Where once there was pretty much only brown or white rice flour, there are now as many specialty flours and formulas as you have purposes for them. The selection can be overwhelming. It's best to keep things simple and experiment before you make an investment. Or mix up your own blend using one of the recipes here before settling on the one that works best for you.

By all means, invest in a good gluten-free baking cookbook. You can bet the author has mastered the art of gluten-free baking by making all of the mistakes you will undoubtedly make on your own.

Always buy packaged mixes and flours made in a dedicated gluten-free facility. Some flours are milled and processed with wheat flour. Equipment is washed down between uses, but that's no guarantee.

Avoid open bins when buying flours. First, there's no way of knowing where these flours come from or how fresh they are or what they have been mixed with. Don't get me started on the germy, gluten-coated spoon dangling from the bin.

Note: Many specialty flours are expensive and fragile. In order to prevent mealybugs and to lengthen shelf life, always store in the refrigerator in airtight containers and include the purchase date on the label. Let flours come to room temperature before you use them and whisk out the clumps before you start measuring.

The Cost of Living Gluten-Free

No way around it: gluten-free food is still more expensive than non-gluten-free.

We are not going to have a European system in which medically mandated food is paid for by health insurance anytime soon.

For some, paying extra for special food is merely annoying. For others, it means scrimping on something else, and for still more, it is a downright hardship.

✦ Watch the papers for supermarket coupons. Whenever you go to stores like Whole Foods, grab a flyer with your cart. As often as not, some of the gluten-free foods you like will be on sale.

✦ Frequent-buyer cards and quantity discounts are making more and more competitive sense to gluten-free companies.

✦ Many of you belong to food co-ops and you buy in bulk, which really brings down prices. If you do this, remember the open-bin rule and verify the origin of gluten-free grains and flours.

✦ Gluten-free shopping Web sites compete with brick-and-mortar stores by offering deals. Many will waive shipping charges for an order over a certain total.

+ Ask your favorite market if they have a loyalty program.

+ For expensive imports, it pays to buy as a group to avoid the heavy freight costs and tariffs. This is sometimes done through a central drop-off point and a system for distributing the individual orders.

+ Another way to cut back on sticker shock on a product you love and use a lot is to convince a local retailer to give you a price close to wholesale if you buy a case.

+ These are tough times. Deals can be made.

If, despite your best efforts, the gluten-free diet is still too much of a burden, or if you feel that shouldering the extra expense adds insult to injury, and you are good at keeping track of details, you can always deduct the extra costs of these items from your income tax return.

Finally, those who are disabled, elderly, and otherwise down on their luck, and for whom buying gluten-free products is a serious hardship, may qualify for assistance under the US Department of Agriculture's Supplemental Nutrition Assistance Program (SNAP). Income and asset requirements vary from state to state; see www.fns.usda.gov/snap.

US Tax Regulations

Is the gluten-free diet tax deductible? Is it a medical expense?

If you avoid gluten voluntarily, the answer is no. If you have a medical diagnosis documented by your doctor, yes.

Need a good argument for getting tested? Look no further than your wallet. According to Publication 502 of the Internal Revenue Service and as of 2003, medical expenses are "the costs of diagnosis, cure, mitigation, treatment, or prevention of disease, and the costs of affecting any part or function of the body. Medical care expenses must be primarily to alleviate or prevent a physical or mental defect or illness. Medical expenses include dental expenses. Medical expenses do not include expenses that are merely beneficial to general health, such as vitamins or a vacation." Sorry Pilates people.

Most tax professionals agree that celiac disease, requiring special food in order to avoid disastrous consequences, definitely does qualify as a medical expense if you don't take the standard medical deduction but rather itemize your medical deductions—and until December 31, 2012, that meant *only* if your medical and dental expenses exceed more than 7.5 percent of your adjusted gross income, which means some years you'll deduct gluten-free expenses and some years you won't.

According to an amended IRS Publication 502, for the years beginning after December 31, 2012, "you may deduct only the amount by which your total medical expense exceeds 10% of your adjusted gross income." However, individuals age 65 or older (and their spouses) are temporarily exempt from the increase. The exemption for seniors applies to any tax year beginning after December 31, 2012, and ending before January 1, 2017, if the taxpayer or taxpayer's spouse attained the age of 65 for the tax year.

If you qualify, you are allowed to deduct the difference between so-called normal food and the higher-priced items only if the food is used for your sole consumption. If you share meals with those who consume gluten, you must determine the fraction you consume, then figure the price difference—an accounting nightmare, if you ask me. You may want to track purchases using a spreadsheet.

It's critical to save all receipts (and some register tapes showing the cost of non-gluten-free items against which to compare) and have a certified letter and a prescription from your doctor stating the medical necessity of your gluten-free diet and the consumption of special (and more expensive) foods.

I would add that it's a good idea to have that letter and prescription updated from time to time and rewritten if you change doctors, which is likely to happen in the course of a lifetime. Keep this documentation handy in case of an IRS challenge.

Most tax preparers will tell you that deducting a medical expense as esoteric and unfamiliar to the IRS as gluten-free food may flag your return for a closer look, which is why you may come to the conclusion, as I have, that deducting gluten-free food is more trouble than it's worth.

To order a copy of IRS Publication 502, contact the Internal Revenue Service, (800) 829-3676, www.irs.gov.

Flexible Spending Arrangements and Health Savings Accounts

Here's where things may get a little bit complicated. Certified public accountant Howard Kass writes in an article for Celiac.com that whether or not you can deduct the additional costs of gluten-free food under your

Think Like an Accountant

Don't wait until April 14 to organize your receipts. Set up a spreadsheet or a schedule of frequently purchased items. In one column, fill in the regular price, in another the cost of its gluten-free counterpart. Don't forget special flours and mixes for baking breads, cookies, cakes, muffins, and so on. As you put away groceries, scan all register tapes and receipts and highlight the gluten-free items in yellow. Use your price sheet to note the difference in cost. Toss the receipts in a shoe box or basket kept in the kitchen. At the end of the year, all you need is a calculator.

flexible spending plan depends on your adjusted gross income and whether or not you have accumulated enough in deductible medical expenses to be able to take the deduction.

If you participate in a Section 125 Plan with a flexible spending arrangement, and only if that plan allows it, you may be able to take a reimbursement for the costs associated with a medically mandated gluten-free diet and effectively reimburse yourself for the cost.

This may be possible as well for those with health savings accounts. These are available only to those who use them as part of a high-deductible health insurance plan. Before you check with your plan administrator, study your plan carefully. You may be talking to someone who is paid to say no.

While there was previously no limit on contributions to flexible spending accounts, the Affordable Care Act restricts flexible spending plans to contributions of no more than $2,500, which could put a serious dent in the amount available to you for other health expenses.

Think it over carefully and consult an accountant before you choose a plan that's right for you.

Canadian Tax Regulations

According to the Canada Revenue Agency, "persons who suffer from celiac disease or gluten intolerance are entitled to claim the incremental costs associated with the purchase of gluten-free products as a medical expense."

These individuals, as the CRA points out, are "not entitled to claim the disability tax credit on line 316 for the amount of time it takes to shop for or prepare gluten-free products."

The incremental cost is the difference between purchasing gluten-free products and the cost of similar non-gluten-free products. This is calculated by subtracting the cost of a non-gluten-free item from the cost of a gluten-free one.

Generally, the food items are limited to those produced and marketed as specifically gluten-free, like bread, bagels, muffins, and cereals. Intermediate items, such as rice flour and other gluten-free ingredients, will also be allowed where food is used to make gluten-free items for their exclusive use. The operative word here is *exclusive*. If several people consume the products, only the cost related to the parts of the product consumed by the individual with celiac disease are to be used for a medical expense tax credit.

All of this assumes you have a certificate from a medical practitioner stating that you require a gluten-free diet because of celiac disease or gluten intolerance. Without it, deductions are ineligible.

A receipt for every item purchased during the year is required to make your claim. For example, fifty-two loaves of bread, which should cost, let's say, $1.49 each but cost $3.45 each, would result in an incremental cost of $1.96, resulting in a total of $101.92 for bread for the year.

For more information and questions, contact the Canada Revenue Agency, (800) 959-8281, www.ccra-adrc.gc.ca.

Thinking Ahead: Disaster Plans

These are the days of monster hurricanes, tornadoes, raging wildfires, earthquakes, floods, ice storms, blizzards, heat waves, power failures, and sadly, post-9/11, all manner of man-made catastrophes. We live in a world where the weather is getting more and more extreme and anything can come out of a clear blue sky.

It's gratifying to know that in the aftermath of Hurricane Sandy the gluten-free community came together in record numbers to provide safe meals for gluten-free families left homeless. Manufacturers like Udi's and PB&J and folks up and down the East Coast donated gluten-free products to several of the organizations and food banks distributing food to the victims.

This is the power and the compassion of the gluten-free community.

We can't do anything about what we don't know is coming, but we can be reasonably prepared for most emergencies. Getting to a shelter only to find that there's nothing to eat but doughnuts, peanut butter crackers, and bologna sandwiches is a recipe for disaster. Ditto for being trapped at home with no way to shop for food.

With a little advance planning, you can leave the future to a higher power, knowing you've done all you can do to weather the storm.

When you remember your umbrella, it never rains.

With gluten-free adaptations, the American Red Cross suggests the following:

+ Have on hand one gallon of water per person per day (two quarts for drinking, two quarts for food preparation), at least a three-day supply, and don't forget to include pets.
+ Keep a three-day supply of nonperishable gluten-free food. Select

foods that require no refrigeration, preparation, or cooking and little or no water, such as gluten-free canned beans, tins of tuna fish or salmon, canned fruits, vegetables, shelf-stable soy milk, canned juices, protein bars, and gluten-free soups. If you must heat food, pack a can of Sterno. Don't forget sugar, salt, and pepper, and high-energy staples such as peanut butter (unless yours is a nut-free household), jelly, gluten-free crackers, gluten-free energy bars, cereal, and granola. Don't forget dog or cat food for the family pet. Check expiration dates and replace as needed.

+ Set aside a supply of vitamins, formula for infants, and special foods and medicines for any seniors in your household. Ditto for EpiPens, rescue inhalers, nitroglycerin, CPAP (continuous positive airway pressure) machines, blood pressure cuff, and other crucial medical equipment.

+ Tuck in a quantity of comfort/stress foods, such as gluten-free cookies, pretzels, candy, lollipops, instant coffee, and tea bags.

+ Assemble a first-aid kit for your home and one for your car with the following items: sterile adhesive bandages in assorted sizes, adhesive tape, scissors, tweezers, needle, moistened cleansing wipes, antiseptic, antibacterial cream, thermometer, petroleum jelly, safety pins, soap, two pairs of latex gloves, sunscreen, aspirin or non-aspirin pain reliever, anti-diarrhea medication, antacid, syrup of ipecac (used to induce vomiting if advised by the poison control center), laxative, and activated charcoal (if advised by the poison control center). Don't forget prescription medications, especially heart and blood pressure medications and insulin, contact lenses and supplies, extra eyeglasses, and denture supplies.

+ Assemble a quantity of necessities such as toilet tissue, liquid detergent, personal hygiene items, garbage bags and ties, a plastic bucket with a tight lid, disinfectant, and chlorine bleach.

+ Also good to have on hand are paper cups, plates, and plastic utensils, a battery-operated radio and extra batteries, a flashlight and extra batteries, cash or traveler's checks and change, nonelectric can opener, utility knife, small canister-type fire extinguisher, pliers, tape, compass, matches in a waterproof container, aluminum foil, plastic storage containers, a signal flare, paper and pencil, a medicine dropper, a shut-off wrench to turn off household gas and water, a whistle, plastic sheeting, and a map of the area.

+ Include at least one change of clothing, a pair of socks, and a pair of shoes for each person.

✦ Throw in a few niceties, such as games, puzzles, and books, and a chew toy for the dog.

✦ Keep wills, insurance policies, deeds, stocks, bonds, passports, Social Security cards, birth certificates, bank credit card account numbers, immunization records, and other important family documents in a waterproof portable container.

The American Red Cross further recommends that you keep all of these things in an easy-to-carry container in a place known to all family members, with a smaller version of your supply kit in the trunk of your car. A good container is a large, covered trash can, a camping backpack, or a duffel bag. Always keep the items in airtight plastic bags. Change your stored water supply every six months, and always rotate stored food at the same time.

Establish a family plan: how people will stay in contact, meeting places, emergency phone numbers, teaching children how and when to call 911 or other local emergency services. Practice the plan from time to time, and if you don't know your neighbors already, get to know them.

While you're at it, don't forget about your gluten-free kids at school, who may not be able to get home during an emergency. Give them an emergency supply of crackers, peanut butter (if their school is not nut-free), trail mix, juice boxes, gluten-free protein bars, a couple of cans of beans, beef stew, and tuna fish, to stash in their school lockers (don't forget the can opener).

It's up to you what story you tell the little ones about all this preparation. A snowstorm is always good, unless you live in Florida, in which case a hurricane will do. You don't want to scare them unnecessarily. Should you be evacuated, politely thank the Red Cross people for their snacks and give them to your neighbors to enjoy.

To learn more about how you can help or donate, or to find resources in your area, see Chapter 23, "Community."

Gluten-Free Doesn't Mean Home-Free

You've sought out and destroyed every molecule of gluten, but that doesn't mean your diet is ideal. In fact, banishing toxic grains won't do you much good if you replace them with equally empty calories and fat. Refined flour, bad fats, and sugar, whether gluten-free or not, can be just as health zapping as the other stuff.

Think Again!

If you are starting out on the gluten-free diet heavier than you should be, don't buy into the myth that gluten-free pastas and breads are less fattening. Eat only nutrient-dense foods and watch your servings. If portion control is a problem, use smaller plates.

Baseline Thinking

As you begin the gluten-free life, see your doctor and have a baseline bone density scan (dual-energy X-ray absorptiometry, or DEXA) if you haven't already gotten one. This is especially important if you have been diagnosed with celiac disease. If you are developing osteopenia or osteoporosis because of problems with absorption, you want to know now.

When you consider you're coming from behind and maybe haven't been optimally absorbing your vitamins and minerals, eating well becomes even more important.

SUGAR

While you're examining labels for gluten, ferret out excessive sugar, which is often listed as anything but. Corn syrup, fructose, dextrose, glucose, high-fructose corn syrup, fruit juice concentrate, high-maltose syrup, molasses, invert sugar, sucrose, and plain syrup are all synonyms for the sweet stuff. And just because the product is labeled "all fruit" or "no added sugar" doesn't mean it's good for you, says *Consumer Reports*. Artificial sweeteners are a billion-dollar industry. Do you really think anybody's going to tell you they're bad for you?

Consider the following substitutes: agave syrup, honey, coconut palm sugar, mesquite (this can be used as a sweetener or as a gluten-free flour, depending on how it's processed), blackstrap molasses, brown rice syrup, and stevia (some find this bitter, others do not).

CALCIUM

Bone up on the subject. Gluten insult can deplete this important mineral. Eat yogurt, low-fat cheese, and spinach and other greens such as kale and collards. Try to do some weight-bearing exercises every day. Talk to your doctor about supplementing calcium, magnesium, and zinc.

OTHER NUTRIENTS

We live in a society that's always looking for the quick fix.

For years, we drank black coffee and ate cottage cheese. Then there was grapefruit, and then hard-boiled eggs, an alternating exercise in heartburn and constipation. We ate enough fruit to found a banana republic. Some of us keeled over (literally) from high-protein drinks. We tried being macrobiotic, but who had time? The one-bowl movement took over, and then fermented foods, and we all tried to stay in the Zone. For almost a decade, we rid our lives of every ounce of fat.

It's amazing our systems worked at all. In order to get our collective cholesterol down to healthy levels, we ate so much pasta, we ended up with insulin resistance and worse. We got even fatter. Then we took it all off again with Atkins. Now we're gorging on ghee and duck fat in the name of our prehistoric ancestors. Recently we discovered the amazing chia seed.

There is no bad food and there is no one food that will save us. It's all good. I hope one day that we'll wake up to the idea of moderation in all things.

In the meantime, dear friend, think on this. Good health is not about gimmicks, even if those gimmicks contain not a scintilla of gluten.

Here are a dozen super foods that possess important disease-fighting properties. These should be the mainstays of any healthy diet. Eat some of these foods every day and limit the gluten-free treats.

They are:

+ **Blueberries**—These are good for the eyes, heart, immune system, brain, sweet tooth, waistline, and soul. Mix them with pretty much anything. Or freeze and eat them like candy. Raspberries, too.
+ **Broccoli, Brussels sprouts, bok choy**—These are the big three cruciferous vegetables and they're loaded with cancer fighters like beta-carotene, fiber, and vitamin C.
+ **Chia seeds**—These are a bone builder's secret weapon, loaded with calcium, phosphorus, and manganese, even more than flaxseeds, if that's possible. Buy them ground and sprinkle in everything. Or look for salba seeds, their lighter-colored cousin.
+ **Garlic**—One of the great health wonders of the world. Not only will it keep vampires and colds away, it can make blood less sticky and less likely to form clots. Smash it, mince it, or mash it to release its power, but don't overcook it. My favorite way to eat it is roasted with a little olive oil, then spread on a slice of toast (gluten-free, of course). If you take aspirin or other blood-thinning drugs, be careful. You can have too much of a good thing.
+ **Green tea, and to a lesser degree, black tea**—May help to prevent cancer, and some say it even inhibits cavity-causing bacteria. This is good news for those of us prone to dry mouth and other conditions related to celiac disease.
+ **Nuts**—If you are not allergic to them, nuts are full of fat (the good kind) and protein and can lower your LDL, or bad cholesterol, while raising the good HDL. Nuts trigger a process called apoptosis, in which cancer cells kill themselves. But don't go nuts—a handful a day is enough.
+ **Oats**—Oats may lower your blood pressure and contain a soluble fiber that makes short work of cholesterol. If your doctor thinks these are safe for you, use only oats certified gluten-free and grown in dedicated fields. The last thing you want to do is feel your oats.

Long-Term Thinking

Balance gluten-free indulgences with nutrient-dense super foods. Eat blueberries and ground chia seeds with your GF cereal. Stir broccoli or spinach into a frittata made with hormone-free eggs or fresh whole-grain GF pasta with olive oil and garlic. Reach for the almonds and a handful of pumpkin seeds instead of a cookie. Bake some, but not too much, rice bran into your brownies. Pour yourself a nice glass of pinot noir. You've earned it.

- **Pumpkin seeds**—These tasty little seeds are packed with tryptophan, an amino acid that aids in the production of serotonin, a neurotransmitter that regulates mood and wards off depression.
- **Rice bran**—With protein and all the essential amino acids, B-complex vitamins, as well as potassium, magnesium, manganese, and other minerals, this is one of nature's hypoallergenic foods and can help release endorphins and aid in the removal of environmental toxins from the body.
- **Salmon**—Bursting with omega-3 fatty acids that help keep arteries from developing plaque, salmon may protect brain cells from the diseases of aging. Ditto for bluefish, herring, and mackerel. Wild is always preferable to farmed.
- **Spinach**—Full of iron and folate, spinach can prevent neural-tube defects in newborns and lower levels of homocysteine, an amino acid linked to heart disease. This is especially important for those who have been and may still be deficient in this important B vitamin due to gluten intolerance. Spinach also contains phytochemicals that may ward off macular degeneration.
- **Teff**—This little powerhouse is the smallest grain in the world. High in protein and fiber and amino acids, its lysine levels are higher than in wheat or barley. Teff is available in whole grain or flours for gluten-free baking.
- **Tomatoes**—Rich in lycopene, these are the most powerful of the antioxidant carotenoid-containing fruits and vegetables.
- **Wine**—A few glasses of red wine per week can help raise good cholesterol (HDL) and may also help reduce the degenerative condition we call hardening of the arteries.

THINK OUT OF THE BOX
The cereal box, that is.

- Get a full serving of B vitamins with gluten-free whole grains like brown rice, wild rice, quinoa, and buckwheat, which pack a nutritional wallop.
- Look for gluten-free products that are enriched with B vitamins.
- Choose calcium-fortified milks and dairy products and lactose-free varieties.
- Pump iron by trading up on carbs—switch rice pasta for teff, quinoa, and beans.
- Eat fresh berries as a way to better absorb vitamin D.

Social Thinking

Twitter. Facebook. Instagram. Tumblr. Google+. YouTube. Pinterest. And the Next Big Thing to come down the pike after we go to press.

Find a new community and reach out to your own. Post and tweet your finds and best blogs. Collect and organize your gluten-free life. Follow gluten-free experts like yours truly. Send dispatches to your social network, both real and virtual. Inform, educate, and entertain. Let everyone know how this gluten-free thing is going for you. Tell them about making a little funeral for the Oreos (and how they came back to life as Joe-Joe's). Rave about the gluten-free cruise your hubby booked for your anniversary, and the totally gluten-free bed-and-breakfast you found in the Berkshires. Share how the kids brought your test results to show-and-tell and made a big sign designating the kitchen a GLUTEN-FREE ZONE.

While you're at it, brag about the Thanksgiving dinner that was so good, nobody noticed everything was gluten-free. Accompany this news with a picture of you tucking into the pumpkin pie, eating your first gluten-free pizza, posing with a pastry in front of Helmut Newcake in Paris. Post your mistakes as well as your triumphs, so others can learn from them. Pin your favorite restaurants and recipes. Change your Facebook status to *Committed Gluten-Free*.

The idea is that you want everyone to know how to help you, how to host you, what's safe and what's not, and have fun in the process. Use all available means to get the word out. Community is only a mouse click away. Who knows? You may make it big in the blogosphere.

Myths, Misconceptions, and Grains of Truth

Pioneer exercise guru and health nut Jack LaLanne said, "If it tastes good, spit it out."

That's the way this gluten-free life of ours can feel at first, confusing and dangerous, with gluten lurking in the oddest and most unsuspected places.

What's true? What isn't?

The gluten-free diet is confusing at best, and there is quite a bit of folklore out there, including some misconceptions coming from professionals who should know better. While there is solid research telling us how common celiac disease and gluten intolerance really are (and getting more common, it seems, every day), what it actually means to be gluten-free is often misunderstood. Some of us fret about the safety of tea bags, dental floss, dog food, airborne contaminants, cheese, sticky rice, and whether or not it is safe to breathe while passing a bakery.

Is the gluten-free diet really a way to lose weight? Is it healthier? Is there any truth to the rumors of a pill, patch, or vaccine in the pipeline? Is celiac disease a bona fide disability or is it just plain annoying? If it's possible for medication to get into the body via a skin patch, can gluten?

For starters, let's agree that we are among friends and there's no such thing as a dumb question. Here are some of the most commonly asked questions from newcomers and veterans alike. Herewith a few myths are debunked and misconceptions corrected, along with the addition of some grains of truth.

> Q: *I've heard that the gluten-free diet is great for weight loss. Is this true?*
> A: *It depends.*

If you were eating a lot of processed foods loaded with sugar and artificial junk before you began the gluten-free diet, *and* you trade those foods for more fruits and vegetables and nutrient-dense gluten-free whole grains and starches like brown rice, quinoa, and sweet potatoes, *and* you keep portion sizes modest, you will undoubtedly see a drop on the scale. But realize that not all the gluten-free foods on the market are healthy for you, especially when you are trading the old fat, carbohydrates, and sugar for the just-as-bad-for-you gluten-free version. On the other hand, if you were diagnosed with long-standing celiac disease and absorption problems, you may find that you gain weight on the gluten-free diet. Why? Your body is fully absorbing food, but your brain hasn't yet caught up to how much you can eat without gaining weight.

> Q: *My doctor says I'm not skinny enough to have celiac disease. Is that true?*
> A: *Absolutely not.*

According to the Celiac Disease Foundation's medical advisory board, 40 percent of people with celiac disease are overweight at the time of their diagnosis. Only 4 to 5 percent are underweight.

Q: Are gluten-free foods healthier than other foods?
A: Possibly.

Healthy choices are healthy choices, period. If you are eating fresh, organic, non-GMO whole foods that are naturally gluten-free, and occasional gluten-free treats made without excessive sugar and fats, the answer is yes. If, on the other hand, your diet consists of gluten-free versions of the same high-fat, high-sugar, high-calorie carbohydrate-dense foods you ate before, probably not. With notable exceptions coming from big industrial food processors and the high-fructose corn syrup crowd, many makers of gluten-free products are smaller companies that offer foods free of common allergens and often use organic ingredients. It depends on what you ate before and how you eat now.

Q: My blood tests were positive for celiac disease. Does that make it official?
A: Not quite.

Although positive blood work taken while eating gluten is a pretty good indicator, the only real way to get a definitive diagnosis is to undergo a small-bowel biopsy in order to assess the damage to the gut. Follow-up is important, too, to assess healing.

Q: I drink at least three cups of coffee a day. Now I'm getting coffee nerves about whether or not my jolt of java is gluten-free.
A: Maybe. Maybe not.

Coffee and tea are naturally gluten-free as long as you are a purist and drink plain, unflavored brews. However, many instant coffees and decaffeinated coffees contain cereal fillers, which make them unsafe. Be wary, too, of fancy coffee drinks, coolers, and teas. Many contain wheat-based flavorings and syrups. Do your homework before you shell out big bucks for a single-serving home coffee system. Starbucks offers a list of gluten-free blended drinks, which, as we go to press, includes its Frappuccino skinny and regular. Bottom line: ask before you imbibe and always, when in doubt, go without.

FYI, I've checked: there is no gluten in coffee filters, nor is there glue in tea bags. If they're not folded and stapled, they're pressure sealed. Of course, you could forget the whole thing, buy a nice pot, and brew leaf tea the old-fashioned way.

> **Q:** *I've got a hankering for a nice, big hunk of Maytag blue cheese, but I've heard it's not safe on a gluten-free diet. Why?*
> **A:** *You heard wrong.*

Not so long ago the gluten-free community avoided rich, veined cheeses like Maytag and Gorgonzola because of the blue mold, which is started from bread and inoculated into the cheese before aging. No more. In 2009, the Canadian Celiac Association released a study proving that blue cheese is, in fact, gluten-free. The study tested three blues where mold is harvested from gluten-containing media and tested two other blue cheeses where the mold was grown on gluten-free media. In all cases, the cheeses contained less than 1 part per million of gluten. The FDA's definition of gluten-free is 20 parts per million. Despite evidence to the contrary, there is still some controversy—all the more reason to buy natural, unprocessed varieties. Smile. Say cheese.

> **Q:** *Can I eat just a little gluten without getting sick?*
> **A:** *Not really.*

The FDA allows 20 parts per million of gluten in order for a food to be labeled gluten-free. According to experts, ingesting 50 milligrams of gluten per day is enough to cause intestinal damage in those with celiac disease. If you eat five pounds of gluten-free-labeled food a day containing under 20 parts per million of gluten, damage will occur. What better argument for eating naturally gluten-free food?

> **Q:** *I like a drink occasionally. Do I have to give up alcohol?*
> **A:** *Absolutely not.*

Distilled alcohol (as well as non-malt vinegar) is gluten-free: the gluten molecule is too large to be part of the end product. Wine is gluten-free, as well, as long as it isn't fortified in any way with gluten-containing ingredients. Beers, ales, lagers, and malt vinegar are not distilled and are made with non-gluten-free grains. Sorry. But there are some wonderful gluten-free beers and ales on the market now. Look for the gluten-free label.

Q: *Can I lick the icing off the cupcake or pick the cheese off the pizza?*
A: *Don't you dare!*

You may not see it, but the icing may contain cake crumbs. The pizza cheese may have a bit of dough clinging to it or a bit of meatball or non-gluten-free sausage. *Cross-contamination* is a scary term, but that is exactly what it is. So no, that innocent cream cheese frosting is enough to make you sick. Ditto for eating the middle of a non-gluten-free sandwich.

Q: *Is it possible to inhale gluten and have a bad reaction?*
A: *Yes and no.*

If you walk into a cloud of anything, you're going to sneeze, wheeze, or cough. You may even experience breathing problems. Let's say you're walking down the baking aisle and a bag of flour explodes (not likely) or you rear-end a flour truck and are buried in an avalanche of the stuff (even less likely). You may have a reaction, not because you're breathing gluten particles but because you've swallowed some. A big enough face full of any substance, such as pollen or dust, is going to cling to the back of your throat, and you're going to swallow. If you are cleaning up the mess yourself, a small amount may get under your nails and find its way, via a circuitous and completely unconscious route, into your stomach. This is something you shouldn't worry about, unless, of course, you work in a bakery, in which case I respectfully suggest a change of career. If you have a dog and you pour out a bowl of dry dog food every morning and routinely swallow small particles, you may want to consider gluten-free pet chow.

Q: *I thought tuna fish salad was safe to order out but heard that*
**   *some diners use white bread in preparing it. Is this true?***
A: *I'm afraid so.*

You've heard of hamburger helper? Well, this is tuna surprise. Or chicken surprise. Or even shrimp and crab or seafood surprise. The truth is that ingredients go farther when stretched with bread filler. Always, always, always ask how a dish is prepared before ordering any food that can be doctored, enhanced, or plumped in any way, even those that sound innocent enough.

The biggest offenders are diners, delis, food courts, and truck stops. Profit margins are very slim in these places. Other areas of potential problems are omelets in chains like International House of Pancakes (IHOP), which may contain batter. Do they do it to make the eggs go farther or to enhance the taste? Your guess is as good as mine. Batter on French fries is another potential pothole.

Q: *If food doesn't cause a reaction, does that mean it's gluten-free?*
A: *Nope.*

This should be obvious but isn't. Gluten may be present in such small amounts that it doesn't cause a reaction. But that doesn't mean the food is safe. Eating gluten can cause problems, whether you notice them or not. Always check and eat only those products or foods you know for sure are gluten-free. This is one time when a little bit can hurt.

Q: *I'm not severely sensitive to gluten. Can I cheat every now and then?*
A: *You'd only be cheating yourself.*

In order to be effective, the gluten-free diet should be *zero gluten*. This is crucial for those with celiac disease and non-celiac gluten sensitivity. Even if you are mildly sensitive, by continuing to eat gluten you may be worsening the problem. With no real tests for gluten sensitivity or to assess the damage, it just isn't smart. There are no half measures. You're either in or you're out.

Q: *My doctor says I'm too old to have celiac disease. Is this true?*
A: *Not on your life.*

The average age of onset of gluten intolerance is getting older. Some say this is due to changes in the growing of wheat, an aging population, and compromised immunity in older adults, but nobody really knows why. To compound the problem, few patients fit the classic picture. Complaints can be vague and seemingly unrelated to the gastrointestinal tract and can range from bloating, abdominal discomfort, or poor digestion to osteoporosis, problems easily dismissed as normal signs of aging. Stand your ground and insist on the proper blood tests and try not to fault your doctor for being wrong. Help him or her to get it right.

Q: If a dermal patch can deliver medicine through the skin, can gluten be absorbed the same way?

A: Sounds logical, but it doesn't work that way.

It's easy to make that assumption, but gluten and skin patches are apples and oranges in the highly engineered world of dermal drugs. Kays Kaidbey, MD, retired University of Pennsylvania adjunct professor of dermatology, explains that drugs delivered to the systemic circulation through the skin are usually small molecules incorporated in specially formulated and highly complex vehicle systems designed to maximize drug release to the stratum corneum (the skin's outermost layer) via patches. The ability of chemicals or molecules to penetrate the skin is determined by several factors, including the size of the molecule, its solubility in lipids or fats, and its physico-chemical properties. Most proteins, as well as glutens, are simply too large to penetrate the skin. Translation: gluten has to get into your gut to cause trouble.

Q: I've heard there are patents pending for pills, patches, and a vaccine for celiac disease. Is this true?

A: Close, but still no cigar.

As we go to press, four drugs are in development, each team of researchers racing to be first to deliver the magic pill. Perhaps the most exciting is an enzyme designed to break down the gluten protein, much the way enzymes work with lactose. Scientists Justin Siegel and Ingrid Swanson Pultz and their team engineered an enzyme called KumaMax that has successfully broken down more than 95 percent of gluten peptides in conditions that mimic stomach acid. Lead study author Siegel told WebMD that the plan is to incorporate the enzyme into a food additive like Beano or Gas-X and make it available without a prescription.

There is a vaccine in the pipeline, too, designed to help desensitize a person to gluten just like an allergy shot or flu shot. Another, according to About.com, is a medication to help prevent leaky gut, and a fourth actually binds to the gluten molecule in an effort, to put it delicately, to *escort* gluten safely from your body.

Each advance comes on the shoulders of the one before it, which is why I was part of a study a few years ago. Being a lab rat is not for everyone, but I was thrilled at the idea of being able to go to a party and pop a pill first. Not a cure, mind you, no one is offering that, but just a little something to make eating out easier and more spontaneous. I didn't have to ask whether or not I got the real deal or the placebo because I spent most of the two-week trial in the bathroom. If eating spaghetti for science can make a difference, why not?

FYI: The Celiac Disease Foundation tells us to avoid glutenase and other gluten-cutter products containing DPP-IV. They do not help digest gluten.

Q: *This is a tacky question, but is it normal to have a bowel movement every day?*
A: *Not necessarily.*

There's a lot of *toilet talk* in the gluten-free community, mainly because that's where many of us notice our first symptoms. According to the National Digestive Diseases Clearinghouse Web site, "The frequency of bowel movements among normal healthy people varies from three days a week to one a day, and some people fall outside both ends of this range." And guess who might typically fall outside both ends of the range? You, that's who. If diarrhea was your main problem when eating gluten, you may be prone to more frequent bowel movements than those who may have experienced constipation and bloating.

On the other hand, don't give yourself a hemorrhoid trying to force the issue. Self-medicating with laxatives or habitual use of enemas can, over time, impair the natural muscle action of the intestines, leaving them unable to function properly. Better to skip a day or to go after each meal than to obsess. If there's really a problem—and you will know it if there is—seek medical attention. Otherwise, accept that you are someone who cannot be quantified, categorized, and normalized.

Q: *Is my child entitled to a gluten-free lunch at school?*
A: *Yes.*

In compliance with the Americans with Disabilities Act, schools are required to provide students with gluten intolerance and other food allergies a safe and nutritional lunch option. For kids with a 504 plan (see Chapter 18), the school is required to provide lunch and a classroom management plan.

Q: Is it possible to be gluten-intolerant and still serve my country?
A: Yes, but your country may not serve you.

There may not be a free lunch, but there is a gluten-free one. According to the Department of Defense, Army Regulation 40-501 (Standards of Medical Fitness), "intestinal malabsorption syndromes" disqualify one from joining the U.S. Army, Navy, Marine Corps, Air Force, Coast Guard, National Guard, or any other military service requiring a special haircut and a uniform. As a member of the armed forces, you are expected to deploy to some pretty rough places to enforce policy or engage in conflict as necessary. This means that, as part of a rapid deployment force, you're going to have to take along Meals Ready-to-Eat: high-calorie field rations containing a dehydrated entrée, milk shake, crackers or bread, fruit, dessert, and energy bar; utensils; and a heating device. It's not going to be convenient to call the company that produced the meal in your pack when you're in a war zone. If you're in a tank, you're not going to get food you can eat.

You can get gluten-free in a military hospital, but if you're wounded you may have more to worry about than dinner. If you are determined to enlist, you'll lie about your celiac disease or gluten sensitivity, and you may want to read *Gluten-Free in Afghanistan* by Captain B. Donald Andrasik, whose determination to serve, help other soldiers, and generally shake things up is downright heroic.

Q: But what if I'm diagnosed after I join the military?
A: Things get murky.

The armed forces policies toward those with medical conditions vary depending on the mission and the branch of the service. The definition of *fit to deploy* is a relative term, especially as it pertains to celiac disease. Some cases are not well defined and are mild, while others are disabling. An individual may be retained in the military or released to the civilian community.

The most influential factor in the decision to retain is the amount of time served. Just like a corporation, the military will weigh its investment. If you are fresh out of basic training, you can pretty much expect to be jettisoned. If you have rank and have been a productive member of the military for many years, your chances of being kept on are higher. If there is a shortage of personnel in your area and you are considered indispensable, even better. Thanks to Captain Andrasik, whose Afghanistan support group included those with non-celiac gluten sensitivity, things may change.

> **Q: *A gluten-free friend was sentenced to a year in a federal prison for a white-collar crime. Will he be able to get a gluten-free diet?***
> **A: *No, you won't. I mean, no, your friend won't.***

Not even Martha Stewart has enough pull to order gluten-free French toast in a federal prison. Cushy or barbed wired, locked down or wide open, the rules are the same. The Federal Bureau of Prisons tells us the only diets available to prisoners are those eaten for religious purposes, for example, kosher for Jewish prisoners and halal or vegetarian for followers of Islam, or as the prison system calls it, *no flesh.*

Whether it's wheat, gluten, lactose, peanut, tree nut, casein, diabetes, low-cholesterol, or low-salt, it is incumbent upon each inmate to manage his or her special diet by asking to see the ingredient labels, which will be made available, and to self-select the proper food (a quick review of cafeteria scenes in *Orange Is the New Black* proves that this is not as easy as it sounds). Prison is punishment. They don't go out of their way to make it easy. A way around this, I am told, is to contact the prison doctor and he or she will assign a medically necessary diet, which is then put into the computer and reviewed periodically.

If inmates do have bad gluten reactions, they may find they are doing time in a prison hospital, which may not be so bad given they *can* get a gluten-free meal there. Just not in a prison cafeteria. If they are in a position of having to choose a last meal, gluten is the least of their worries.

Jokes aside, given all the other things to worry about, the health and well-being of our prison population doesn't rate much public outrage. Still, captive populations suffer long-term health problems, which may affect recidivism and social behavior. Something to think about.

> **Q: *What happens in nursing homes, homeless shelters, psychiatric wards, and other places where there is captive feeding?***
> **A: *The news is not good for people who cannot insist on a gluten-free diet.***

Sadly, many consumers of such services are not well enough, sane enough, or strong enough to make their wishes known and have no one to advocate for them. The mentally ill are especially vulnerable, and we all have a story of an elderly resident of a nursing home who has been the recipient of a serious error in care. Phone calls to various facilities assured me that all special diets are honored, and I believe most do their best in light of the fact that many of their residents cannot ask for a gluten-free meal. Still, many residents are difficult, have cognitive problems, and are alone and unable to ask for or even remember what they need to eat.

There is no way of knowing what percentage of the homeless population is gluten-intolerant because medical services are usually the first to go on a downward spiral into poverty. Malnutrition combined with malabsorption is a terrible cross to bear.

For many, church and community groups and food charities are often the only sources of food for the needy, homeless, homebound, and chronically ill. Observing my neighborhood church's efforts on this score, food packages are carbohydrate-intensive. A product like VitaMeal, a gluten-free and vegan rice-and-lentil meal in a pouch distributed by international relief organizations all over the world would go a long way to help. With so many professional gluten-free kitchens in business, how hard could it be to develop a nutrient-dense product and make it available to those who do not have the means to cook or look after themselves? As a community, we must come up with ways to take care of the most vulnerable among us. We can dream of a kinder, gentler society.

Q: *My dog's food is loaded with gluten. Poor thing doesn't understand why I wear rubber gloves to feed him. What do I do?*
A. *Could be gluten-free kibble in Fido's future.*

Man and woman's best friend not only eats, he slobbers, drools, licks the hand and the face that feeds him, and fetches your slippers on occasion. What's the point of having a pet if you treat him like a furry nuclear waste dump?

One way to solve the problem is to feed the family pet one of the gluten-free pet foods like Sensible Choice or Nutro. Some owners report that their dogs are healthier and their coats are glossier on this diet, while others complain that the soy-based foods give some breeds more than a bit of a gas problem. If you don't go with gluten-free dog chow, keep food bowls separate from the family utensils and always wash your hands after feeding your pet or cleaning out the dishes. If your gluten-free child loves to feed the family pet, as many toddlers do, it's especially important to teach hand washing the minute the chore is accomplished. The fastest way for gluten to get into a tummy is via fingers that go into mouths after touching Fido's dinner.

Like humans, dogs and cats need cuddling and love. If you can't deliver on your end of the bargain because of gluten fears, don't have a pet in the first place.

Q: *Why do some restaurants use food brought in by customers and some don't?*
A: *Litigation issues, most likely. They are covering their you-know-whats.*

Some restaurants, citing health codes, won't serve food brought in by customers. Many do, so I don't know if this is really a health code violation or a fear of being sued should said customers get sick on the premises. I have to say that the ones who won't work with your food usually have a bigger profile than the mom-and-pop operations that do. It's safe to say that corporate policy and concern over litigation determine the answer. Honestly, I can't argue with it. I'm glad restaurants are concerned with cross-contamination and potential mishaps delivering to the right table. No reason not to get the omelet the way you like it and slip your gluten-free biscuit on the plate beside it. Given that all the rest of the ingredients are gluten-free, you're good to go. Clean, easy, no risk of contamination.

Q: *When I go out to a restaurant, I've heard it's not enough to order a gluten-free meal; it's necessary to ask the kitchen to cook and handle my food in a special way.*
A: *You heard right.*

Cross-contamination rears its ugly head again. Anything can happen on the way to your plate. Your gluten-free salad could be tossed in the same bowl that contained croutons or some other breaded ingredient. Your pasta could be cooked in semolina water, and your burger could be grilled right on top of the last grilled cheese sandwich. Not to mention those rubber gloves kitchen workers wear. If these are not changed for you, the gluten on the gloves goes right into your dinner. And consider the ice cream scoop that's just been in cookie dough when it scoops yours. Many restaurant kitchens are good about this and getting better. But you still have to ask.

A Word About Healing

As you begin the gluten-free diet, you may be running at a nutritional deficit. Before you jump into all the gluten-free goodies out there, think a minute.

Why not kick-start the healing process by eating soothing, easy-to-digest foods during the transition? Like a baby who has just been weaned and learning to eat solid foods for the first time, try one food, then another, adding slowly until you are confident each food agrees with you. Save the gluten-free cupcakes, snicker doodles, and cream doughnuts for when you feel better.

It's not glamorous and it's still a hippie at heart, but with its polish intact, brown rice, full of fiber and nutrients, is a great way to start. Prepared in a pressure cooker the way the macro chefs do it, it is also one of the easiest foods to digest. Mixed with calcium-rich kale that's been sautéed in a bit of toasted sesame oil, it can make for a soothing supper.

Add some beans, cooked well to aid digestion, and you've got a complete protein.

Leftover rice makes a fortifying breakfast porridge with some soy, rice, or almond milk, a little maple or agave syrup, and a few raisins. If you can tolerate soy, miso soup is one of the all-time healing foods, a great antidote to wheat belly. With its mineral-rich wakame, a sea vegetable in the kelp family, protein-rich tofu, and warming broth or dashi, few dishes are as strengthening or as soothing.

Learn to make a traditional dashi or broth instead of using plain spring water (see recipe on page 308). It makes all the difference. Use only gluten-free miso paste. Once you get the hang of it, add 100 percent gluten-free soba noodles for a more substantial soup.

Experiment with other whole, low-fat foods like adzuki beans, a staple in Japan, where they are eaten for their healing properties and high vitamin B_{12}, potassium, and iron content, especially if you've been anemic.

Learn to cook with fresh or dried daikon, a peppery Japanese radish said to aid in the digestion of fats and protein. Sea vegetables are full of protein, calcium, potassium, and iron and are a great way to replace lost or depleted minerals. Look for crisp and salty dulse, sushi nori, and hiziki, traditionally used in pressed salads.

To learn more about other healing whole foods, health seminars, and cooking classes and where to buy the highest-quality, hand-harvested, sun-dried sea vegetables, contact the Kushi Institute, (800) 975-8744, or go to www.kushiinstitute.org.

In the spirit of getting you started on a healthier path, here is a simple vegan bean salad full of protein and anti-oxidants I invented when my husband had heart surgery and all fat, as well as gluten, was banished. Nowadays, I can't make enough of it for everyone. Canned beans are fine as long as they are non-GMO and organic.

BASIC BLACK BEAN SALAD

1 15.5-ounce can black beans, rinsed well and drained
¾ red onion, thinly sliced
1 avocado, chopped
4 small plum tomatoes, pulp removed and chopped
1 yellow bell pepper, seeds removed and chopped
¼ small jalapeño pepper, seeds removed, and chopped into tiny pieces
1 ear of corn, boiled or roasted, cut off the cob (optional)
½ small bunch cilantro, torn or snipped with kitchen shears
Juice of 1 lime

1. Put the black beans, onion, avocado, tomatoes, bell pepper, jalapeño, corn (if using), and cilantro in a large bowl. Drizzle the lime juice over the salad and gently toss.
2. Eat as is. Fold into an omelet. Add a little slivered cooked chicken and wrap it up in a gluten-free tortilla. Serve as a side dish. Easy. Healthy. No gluten.

Okay. Let's go shopping.

5

Marketing 101

Caveat emptor

—PROVERB

- ◆ The Supermarket
- ◆ Natural Food Stores and Organic Markets
- ◆ Farmers' Markets
- ◆ Virtual Markets
- ◆ Don't Forget the Coupons
- ◆ Food Cooperatives and Buying Clubs
- ◆ Bakeries
- ◆ Nothing but the Best for You
  - All-Purpose Gluten-Free Flour Blends, Mixes, and Nut and Specialty Flours
  - Beer and Ale
  - Bread, Cookies, Biscotti, Crackers, and Bread Crumbs
  - Butter and Cheese Alternatives, Egg Replacer, and Spreads
  - Cake Mixes and Piecrust
  - Cakes, Store-bought
  - Cereals and Waffles

  Condiments
  Crackers
  Deli Meats
  Ice Cream, Gelato and Frozen Yogurt, and Dairy-Free Ice Cream
  Miso Paste and Mochi
  Oats
  Pasta and Noodles
  Pizza, Frozen
  Pizza Crust/Mixes/Dough
  Rice, Whole-Grain
  Sauces
  Snacks
  Soups and Broths
  Vanilla and Other Extracts
  Veggie Burgers
  Wraps
  Yogurt

You're new at this, a little confused, and, like everyone else, pressed for time and money. Not to worry: where once gluten-free shopping was a difficult chore requiring an encyclopedic knowledge of arcane ingredients and a magnifying glass, it is now an exciting adventure and much easier than you think. Once you get the hang of it, the hunt yields real rewards.

There are many more shopping venues, too, including the supermarket, which is beginning to yield an impressive gluten-free selection. I'm not a big fan of dough in a can, but I honestly never thought I'd see the Pillsbury Doughboy go gluten-free. Or that Betty Crocker would jump on the bandwagon and offer a line of gluten-free cake and brownie mixes. (Notice that I said gluten-free; I did not say even remotely healthy!) Or that fresh gluten-free ravioli would sit side by side along with the other specialty pastas.

If you're willing to venture beyond your comfort zone, it gets even more exciting. Today's whole foods markets are veritable gold mines of gluten-free. A stroll through a local farmers' market garners gluten-free wonders that are fresh, organic, and artisanal to boot. These community markets are a must for any serious gluten-free citizen committed to eating locally and making a smaller footprint. They are wonderful places to meet your neighbors and chat with the growers about how best to prepare their produce, meat, fish, and poultry. Bakeries and gluten-free shopping sites are a phone call, mouse click, or screen tap away.

Gluten-free choices are now so ubiquitous that the challenge isn't finding safe food; it's finding the best food. Grab your recycled market bag.

It's time for a short course in Marketing 101.

Some Ground Rules

I'm going to assume you know not to shop while hungry. It's too tempting to nosh a little cheesecake at the bakery counter.

No more texting, gabbing, and googling (unless, of course, you have one of the gluten-free shopping smartphone apps on page 117), at least not until you can do this in your sleep.

You need to be alert, laser focused, lest you miss the latest find or fail to notice the knots of gluten-free shoppers comparing notes and discussing the merits of this frozen pizza over that in front of the freezer case. You need to stay on the balls of your feet, ready to grab a bag of Tate's gluten-free chocolate chip cookies before they're all gone!

Do leave the kids at home until you get the hang of this. The management is counting on your grabby little darlings to beg, whine, melt down, do whatever it takes to get you to load up on no-nos.

Don't forget your coupons, store flyer, and frequent shopper card. This new food can be expensive. You want all the rebates, store specials, and two-for-ones you can find.

Do download first. I'm all for exploration and finding something serendipitously, but sometimes you're just too busy. Go to the store Web site and get a list of their gluten-free products.

Don't forget to ask for the aisle-by-aisle organization chart. Many stores have dedicated gluten-free sections for shelved items and frozen, but some still stock gluten-free products according to category.

Let's roll.

The Supermarket

Double coupons, cash back, two-for-one deals, frequent buyer cards, and a growing list of gluten-free products help, but the average American supermarket, a place I once called a toxic waste dump, while ever more gluten aware, is still not the friendliest place for those committed to conscious eating.

Within each store there are notable exceptions—new organic produce sections, prepared food counters offering bento boxes of sushi, barbecued chicken, salads, soups, and entrées ready to take home, and fish caught in the wild as an alternative to the farmed variety. It is possible in some stores to find hormone-free eggs and milk, vegan products, and grain-fed beef and poultry raised in humane conditions.

Despite these welcome advancements, this is still the place where major food processors sell products made with GMOs, additives, stabilizers, fillers, emulsifiers, and preservatives, not to mention excessive fat, sodium, sugar, calories, artificial colors, chemicals, and palm kernel oil. Much of what you will find in boxes, bags, cans, pouches, and single-serving freezer trays have little nutritional value and barely resemble the foods they purport to be. So yes, you will find gluten-free Rice Krispies, Rice Chex, Betty Crocker cake mixes, Bisquick pancake and baking mix, and gluten-free Progresso soups, but don't expect miracles. It's the same stuff, minus the gluten. To make matters worse, regulation is lax and legislation favors the big producers and agri-giants, not the consumer. It's enough to make a cow mad.

Another reason the supermarket isn't the best place to find the healthiest gluten-free products is that within the food industry there are powerful distribution chains vying for the lucrative and all-important shelf position. As the big producers go gluten-free, this is changing, but only to their advantage. Smaller brands like Glutino, Against the Grain Gourmet, and Nature's Path just don't have the clout of a General Mills, ConAgra, and Kraft. Nor do they have the chemicals, additives, and GMO ingredients.

Still, gluten-free companies are making inroads in the supermarket.

Depending on where you live, you may find Amy's gluten-free pizza and frozen entrées, Feel Good Foods Handmade Asian-Style Chicken Dumplings, Van's Gluten-Free Waffles, or kid-friendly Annie's Gluten-Free Rice Shells and Creamy White Cheddar. And yes, there is Pillsbury's new gluten-free dough.

If you're lucky, you may find fresh Via Roma Gluten-Free Five Cheese Ravioli as I did in my local Super Fresh. Even pasta giant Ronzoni is getting in on the act. I live in a state where the Liquor Control Board forbids the selling of alcohol in supermarkets or anywhere but state liquor stores, but you may be surprised to discover Green's ales, Bard's beer, and other gluten-free brews in the wine and spirits aisle near you.

Good sleuthing may unearth Bob's Red Mill cereals, Glutenfreeda instant oatmeal, Pocono Cream of Buckwheat cereal, gluten-free spaghetti from Ronzoni, and a selection of dried pastas and noodles from dedicated gluten-free pasta makers, including fiber- and protein-packed Ancient Harvest Quinoa Pasta.

With the mandatory labeling laws effective next year, many of the products you already love are displaying the gluten-free label. Read the labels anyway. No law is perfect.

SUPERMARKET TRUTHS

Better to buy the ingredients and assemble a meal yourself than to buy one that has already been boxed, bagged, canned, hermetically sealed, or otherwise rendered shelf-stable. It's just as easy to bake or broil a juicy chicken breast with a little garlic and olive oil as it is to warm one that's already cooked, sauced, and maybe not so full of gluten, but loaded with calories and chemicals. Better for the budget, too.

⟜

It pays to clip coupons and use them and to get familiar with the unit price of any given item as well as the package price. When buying gluten-free, you want to be able to compare apples to apples.

⟜

Just as the words *fat-free* scrawled across a package do not mean "sugar-and calorie-free" and *all natural* means pretty much anything in nature, *wheat-free* does not always mean "gluten-free."

✦

It's best to do homework at home. Lighting and other conditions conducive to reading are not exactly ideal in a supermarket aisle and, at peak shopping times, may even be dangerous. Explore store and company Web sites for gluten-free products. The more you know ahead of time, the faster it will go.

✦

Products and conditions vary according to regional tastes and test markets and from store to store. Formulations change without warning, even on a product that has been declared gluten-free. This often happens ahead of new labels. A good example of this is the Boca Burger. One day it was, the next day it wasn't.

✦

A good toll-free number, Web address, or smartphone app is your best friend.

Natural Food Stores and Organic Markets: Gluten-Free Heaven

With rare exceptions, gone are the plum balls and plain brown rice we once associated with the term *health food store*. The new natural and organic markets are slick, modern places still offering exotic items like kudzu and kombu—the former a gluten-free thickener, the latter a kind of seaweed used in soups and stews to make them more digestible, both gluten-free—as well as a vast array of healthy mainstream items.

Gluten-free vegetarians and vegans will find a selection of raw foods, mochi, brown or white rice miso paste, organic vegetables and fruits, every imaginable variety of tofu, nut milks and soy milks and shakes, gluten-free kale chips, dairy-free and gluten-free frozen desserts like Almond Dream and Rice Dream products and Julie's Organic Gluten-Free Ice Cream Sandwich Cookies, and, often, cookbooks and magazines.

These are the places to buy holistic and herbal medicines, gluten-free and cruelty-free cosmetics, environmentally friendly cleaning products, and pressure cookers, heatproof glass mugs, metal bento boxes, and water bottles, with not a scintilla of plastic in the place. Produce is organic and pesticide-free. You won't often find meat, fish, or poultry

Where Can Gluten Hide in a Clear Broth?

This was my beginner's question, too. I have since learned that gluten is a master of disguise. Better to buy Progresso, Healthy Valley, Pacific Foods, or just buy a chicken and make it yourself. Edward and Sons is a safe, good choice for bouillon cubes.

here, only vegetarian and vegan variations thereof, some of which you want to steer clear of. In some stores, you will find cooking demonstrations and classes, as well as organic vegetarian pet food.

Most health food stores have a selection of Japanese essentials such as nori and wakame for making sushi rolls and miso soup, and esoteric items like bonito flakes for miso soup and gomasio, a Japanese sesame seed and salt condiment, as well as gluten-free soba and millet noodles and gluten-free tamari. You can grind your own peanut butter, but I wouldn't advise it: you don't know where the nuts have been. Better to buy jarred peanut, cashew, and almond butters from organic brands like Erewhon or Santa Cruz Organic.

Avoid open bins of grains, seeds, cereals, nuts and nut mixes, tofu, and pickles, too. Always buy the packaged versions with the ingredients or additives clearly listed. Chair massages, food tastings, coffee and teas from self-sustaining farms (not agri-businesses) around the world, fruits and vegetables, cards, flowers, handmade soaps, exotic oils, aluminum-free cookware, colorful handmade brooms from Guatemala, and, yes, a huge inventory of gluten-free, vegan, dairy-free, nut-free, raw, and refined-sugar-free foods are to be found in the new organic, whole, and natural foods markets.

ESSENE MARKET AND CAFÉ

This is one of the finest independently owned whole foods emporiums in the country, and it's a mere two blocks from my home in Philadelphia. I know how lucky I am. People drive hundreds of miles to get to it and not merely for gluten-free food; it is one of the important centers of the macrobiotic cooking movement in the United States.

I take a break from my shopping to sit in their café and enjoy a bowl of brown rice miso soup or a cup of roasted twig tea, feeling virtuous, even with treats like Bakery On Main gluten-free granola, a fresh supply of Crunchmaster roasted vegetable crackers, and my favorite King Soba Noodle Culture gluten-free sweet potato and buckwheat and pumpkin and ginger noodles in my market bag.

I do not keep a macrobiotic kitchen because it is too work-intensive and I am not given to extremes, but that doesn't prevent me from enjoying a soul-satisfying supper already prepared in Essene's kitchen.

Every now and again I spot a newly gluten-free shopper—the bewildered look is a dead giveaway—and offer a tour. Sometimes I find myself being paged—*Attention Jax, gluten-free question in Aisle 3!* I love seeing faces light up when presented with the gluten-free possibilities.

I do what I can. As you will, too. Check out www.essenemarket.com.

SUNSET FOODS

In addition to purveying organic vegetables, flowers, hormone-free beef and poultry, and wine and spirits, this is the Chicago-area headquarters for the best of the best gluten-free brands like Ancient Harvest; Leo's pasta; World Peas; Kinnikinnick bread, buns, and cookies; Local Oven gluten-free, dairy-free baked goods; and baking mixes from Namaste Foods. An entire aisle dedicated to you, dear reader. As we go to press, this gluten-free-friendly market not only offers the best gluten-free products available, it's playing host to a forty-vendor gluten-free fair in Highland Park. Once a family-owned grocery, now a five-store chain in Northbrook, Lake Forest, Libertyville, and Long Grove, Illinois, the vibe is decidedly friendly.

Sunset Foods is a sponsor of the University of Chicago Celiac Disease Center, donating a portion of customer receipts to the program and participating in the center's Gluten-Free Care Package Program by providing baskets of food and resource materials to the newly gluten-free. To find a location near you and learn about their gluten-free event, go to www.sunsetfoods.com.

TRADER JOE'S

With 398 stores as of 2013 and plans for more every day, Trader Joe's no-frills philosophy has taken hold. This is cause for celebration because not only do they carry a great selection of gluten-free items, the freight is kinder and gentler than many of the pricier specialty natural foods stores. The company states that their private label products contain no artificial colors, flavors, preservatives, MSG (monosodium glutamate), or trans fats and are sourced from non-GMO ingredients. Trader Joe's dairy products are made from milk from cows not given the artificial hormone rBST (recombinant bovine somatotropin).

The list of gluten-free products is long and impressive.

Most are Trader Joe's own brand—Gluten-Free French Rolls, Rye-less "Rye" Bread, Gluten-Free Bagels, Toaster Waffles, and those addictive alternatives to Oreos, Joe-Joe's. There are Tortillas, Dairy-Free Cream Cheese Alternative, Black Licorice Scottie Dogs, Salmon Burgers, plain frozen seafood, and Tofu Veggie Burgers.

Other brands include EnviroKidz Organic Gorilla Munch and Panda Puffs cereal, Lärabars, Udi's bagels and breads, and Bob's Red Mill Flaxseed

Marketing Strategy

Find a natural foods store near you. Go to www.greenpeople.org/health-food-stores.htm for a state-by-state directory of independent organic, whole, natural, and health food markets.

Marketing Strategy

As you make discoveries, share your favorites with your non-gluten-free friends, so they know what you like when you come for dinner. Don't overlook store employees. Some products are naturally gluten-free and just plain safe to eat but are not marketed as such. When you find one, pay it forward and ask that it be put on the gluten-free store list.

Meal, not to mention, cut flowers priced as near wholesale as I've ever seen. The trail mixes alone are cause for shopping-cart gridlock, and there is, of course, the most wonderful chocolate in the world—all at amazing prices. This is where you want to stock up. For locations and the complete and updated gluten-free items, see www.traderjoes.com.

WEGMANS FOOD MARKET

Started in Rochester, New York, in 1915 with a pushcart and some fruit, Wegmans has not only become an empire, it is one of the easiest places to do gluten-free. You can sign up for monthly gluten-free e-mails, confer with one of the ten registered dieticians on staff, see videos on gluten-free cooking and baking, download FAQs on gluten-free diets and celiac disease, and link to local support groups and additional resources. Little orange dots on all gluten-free recipes and products guarantee that Wegmans brands and its suppliers have produced these foods without risk of cross-contamination. All gluten-free prepared and deli foods clearly display NO GLUTEN INGREDIENTS. Here, though, the store suggests you ask questions about possible cross-contamination. The downside is that they are pricey.

Still, these people have done everything they can to shorten your learning curve, with a Web site that includes a link to browse gluten-free products and prompts to create a personalized shopping list. With eighty-one stores in Maryland, Massachusetts, New Jersey, New York, Pennsylvania, and Virginia, and more on the drawing board, you may want to make this store your headquarters: www.wegmans.com.

WHOLE FOODS MARKETS

This is where gluten-free is codified, pamphleteered, and elevated to a shopping art form. Ditto for dairy-free. And just recently, all foods containing GMOs have to be labeled or will not be sold at Whole Foods Markets.

Some days, this urban and suburban phenomenon feels like the twenty-first-century answer to the community center where neighbor meets neighbor at the prepared foods counter, and café, where shopping seems to take longer as friends turn up at the sampling tables dotted throughout the store—a danger zone, I must say, for those shy about asking questions before tasting.

The Whole Foods Market in the Time Warner Center at Columbus Circle in New York is the largest of its kind in the country, maybe even the

Marketing Strategy

Don't get more than you paid for. The Environmental Working Group says US-grown raspberries, strawberries, apples, and peaches and Mexican cantaloupe are often contaminated with pesticides. POP, persistent organic pollutants forbidden in organic agriculture, are found in butter, cucumbers and pickles, meat loaf, peanuts, popcorn, radishes, spinach, summer squash, and winter squash. Dinner shouldn't be an E. coli and salmonella scare. Avoid the recall. Go organic.

world. (It's a bit too big to absorb, in my humble opinion, but certainly worth a stop on any gluten-free itinerary.)

In 2013 this community-centric company partnered with Gotham Greens to build America's first commercial rooftop greenhouse in Brooklyn. Whole Foods is also home to GlutenFree Bakehouse products, a line of gluten-free breads, and rolls, cakes, cupcakes, muffins, cookies, and seasonal items like gluten-free stuffing and pumpkin pies created by Chef Lee Tobin when he learned he was one of us. Find them in the freezer case.

The gluten-free product list is vast and ever-changing in response to customer requests and also to reflect regional tastes. For example, you may find a fresh gluten-free baguette in the bakery section of some stores, along with kitchen-made gluten-free pizza, and not in others. Whole Foods is an entrepreneurial corporate structure, so managers differ in what they offer from one store to another. Your job is to ask, Why not *my* Whole Foods?

A quick walk down a Whole Foods Market aisle nets a bigger selection of gluten-free specialty flours, mixes, and blends than you have time to try. This is where you will find Tate's legendary chocolate chip cookies, now gluten-free, and organic gluten-free baby food; Hillary's vegan veggie burgers, free of all common allergens, including gluten; and La Pasta fresh, organic, and small-batch gluten-free cheese, spinach and cheese, and dairy-free crimini and portobello mushroom ravioli. RP's Pasta Company's fresh linguini, fusilli, and fettuccine (plain and spinach) are certified gluten-free and as light and slippery as any artisanal Italian hand-made pasta.

Some stores carry Graeter's ice creams, which are made in small batches, using the French Pot method. All but the flavors that use non-gluten-free mix-ins are gluten-free, and the chocolate chips are huge. There is no better flourless chocolate torte than the one you will find at the bakery counter: no gluten, just butter, sugar, and chocolate.

For gluten-free product lists, news, specials, and free bicycle delivery in some areas, go to www.wholefoodsmarket.com.

Farmers' Markets

This is where we find produce still beaded with moisture, carrots wearing their tops, and giant purple hybrids of broccoli and cauliflower so beautiful we are tempted to paint rather than roast them. Organic farmers and producers with dirt under their fingernails are eager to give us

---

There Are Apps for This!

The Allergy and Gluten Free Diet Tracker app by Fooducate allows you to scan a product barcode by category to see if it contains gluten, peanuts, tree nuts, fish, shellfish, egg, milk, lactose, or soy. There is an option to call the manufacturer for more information. www.food ucate.com.

Is That Gluten Free? Grocery app contains twenty thousand manufacturer-verified gluten-free products from over six hundred companies. Search by category, keyword, brand, or ingredient. $7.99 for iPhone and iPad.

Marketing Strategy

For gluten-free shopping that's easier on the budget, divide your list between staples and commodities found in the supermarket and more expensive specialty items found in organic markets and online shopping sites. If you go the online route, don't forget to factor in the shipping.

the provenance of their bounty. They talk about rain, drought, heat, and cold, the hardness of the winter that shaped this season's crop.

We sense pride here, missing from the way we usually shop. Uniformity matters little, only beauty and freshness. We ask for recipes, sample chocolates and peach jam. We find salted caramel ice cream; organic, gluten-free, and handmade soups; artisanal cheeses, pâtés and sausages; gluten-free cookies, scones, granolas, and breads.

On any given Saturday or Sunday or weekday, we come home with a bag of fresh vegetables and gluten-free goodies, and with instructions for serving or cooking. Our sense of health is renewed, as well as an important American tradition. We return again and again, having forged a connection to the people who grow and make our food. Each spring, we greet our rural friends like the long-lost cousins they are.

I try not to miss a Sunday at my own market at Second and Head House Square where, on those same cobblestones, the good people of the Philadelphia colony came to gossip with their neighbors and buy corn, pumpkins, and fish from the native tribes living alongside them, as well as tea and household goods from English ships at anchor nearby. Today it's a festival of dogs and double strollers, flowers, food trucks, meeting and greeting, and tables overflowing with the best of the farm-to-table movement.

Finding a farmers' market near you is probably the best thing you can do for your health, and for the future of independent farmers, Davids up against Agri-Goliaths. The farm-to-table movement has taken hold and is growing fast, but if we want clean, sustainable food, we have to vote with our wallets.

Crescent City Farmers' Market, New Orleans, Louisiana—Tuesday, Thursday, and Saturday in the Warehouse District. Freshly caught fish and farm-raised meats.

Dane County Farmers' Market, Madison, Wisconsin—More than three hundred growers and vendors. Market days Wednesday and Saturday.

Des Moines Farmers' Market, Des Moines, Iowa—Locally grown produce, artisanal jams, baked goods. Corn high as an elephant's eye. Every Saturday. Downtown Des Moines.

Ferry Plaza Farmers' Market, San Francisco, California—Fresh, local, organic with hard-to-find items like Meyer lemons, Tahitian pomelos, persimmons, mission figs. Added bonus: Just inside the Ferry Building, gluten-free Mariposa Baking company. Saturdays.

Green City Market, Chicago, Illinois—Saturdays all year. Wednesdays in summer and fall. In addition to locally grown produce, Chicago's best chefs show marketgoers how it's done.

Hilo Famous Market, Big Island, Hawaii—Tropical fruits and vegetables not seen in the lower forty-eight. Crafts, artwork, artisanal products, and tropical flowers. With fewer tourists here than on Maui or Oahu, this is a local, authentic taste of Hawaii. Wednesdays and Saturdays.

Portland Farmers' Market, Portland Oregon—Fresh organic food Tuesday through Thursday. Saturday market is the main event. Portland State University.

Santa Monica Farmers' Market, Santa Monica, California—Local, organic produce, herbs, and handmade goods. L.A.'s top chefs shop here on Wednesday.

St. Paul Farmers' Market, St. Paul, Minnesota—Vendors come from no farther than a seventy-five-mile radius. Small-batch honey, hormone-free poultry, artisanal cheeses. Downtown on Saturdays.

Union Square Greenmarket, New York City—Proof farmers' markets can make it anywhere. Locally grown produce, fish, flowers, wines, maple syrup in season, cooking and gardening demonstrations. Monday, Wednesday, Friday, and Saturday.

University District Farmers' Market, Seattle, Washington—Sixty growers, producers, and bakers; Alaska Pacific prawns; Pacific oysters. University Heights Community Center. Saturdays.

Virtual Markets

Not everyone lives in an area surrounded by choices. For easy, one-click shopping, nothing beats online. Trolling for new gluten-free products may even replace eBay as an addiction. Before you submit your order, familiarize yourself with shipping fees and how long you may have to wait for your order. With tight border regulations, this could be expensive *and* time-consuming.

Each site differs, so read the small print regarding spoilage and other reasons for dissatisfaction. If you return something, is there a restocking fee?

Don't buy blind. Better to order a product sampler before you order a carton. Compare prices, deals, and frequent-buyer programs to see which one makes the most sense for you.

Marketing Strategy

Go to www.farmersmarkets .com to find a market near you. When traveling, don't forget to google the nearest farmers' market. Not just for eating well on the road, but for shipping back home. Gluten-free stars often make their first appearances in such places.

If all meets with your approval, load up your shopping cart and hit "Purchase."

For business trips, vacations, or visits to friends and family, send a package ahead of your arrival. Leave behind any leftovers as a hint to your host to reorder for your next visit.

Gift baskets are a great idea, too. These are especially thoughtful for someone new to the diet, or as a way to sample for yourself.

AMAZON

You think books and other products when you think Amazon. But you can save a ton of money on food orders. If you sign up for their Subscribe and Save program, shipping is free and you save at least 5 percent and up to 15 percent on every order. In addition to the top specialty gluten-free brands, find gluten-free vitamins and supplements, Amazing Grass Green Superfood, coconut milk, Miracle Noodles, and commodities like dried beans, grains, and rice. Kosher, vegan, vegetarian, low-carb, non-GMO, fair- and free-trade products are available as well. Books, too, of course, including this one. www.amazon.com/gluten-free

THE GLUTEN-FREE MALL

They call themselves "Your Special Diet Superstore" for good reason. Not only is the selection of foods huge; there are coupons, rewards, bulk specials, books, cleaning products, gluten test kits, gift vouchers, and more. You'll find products for lactose-free and casein-free diets as well. Free shipping. www.celiac.com/glutenfreemall

GLUTEN-FREE SMART STORE

In addition to certified gluten-free products, this relatively new site offers allergy-friendly, organic, non-GMO, and eco-friendly foods and products. There is an emphasis on brands by Allergic Solution and chef Kathy Smart, partners in the site. Brands like Mrs. Glees's baking mixes and Italpasta gluten-free pastas and pasta sauces are also available. www.glutenfree smartstore.com

GLUTEN SOLUTIONS

A trusted name in the gluten-free community, they do gluten-free/dairy-free and gluten-free/raw foods as well as gluten-free. Among the many offerings are Glutino; Betty Crocker; Bisquick; Schär; Bob's Red Mill;

Marketing Strategy

Wouldn't you love to buy fresh bread on the way home? Every day a new gluten-free bakery pops up. We are, happily, faced with an embarrassment of riches. If ever there was a reason to join a gluten-free community, this is it. These people know about it before anybody. And so, too, shall you. Get on the gluten-free grapevine.

Namaste Foods; Authentic Foods dairy-free, soy-free, nut-free baking mix; and Miracle Noodle low-carb gluten-free angel hair and spinach pasta. News, coupons, recipes and special offers. www.glutensolutions.com

GLUTERRA

This gluten-free shopping site with a holistic vibe tells us, "Take care of your body. It's the only place you have to live." In addition to cooking and baking mixes, breads, bagels, snacks, pastas, and noodles, there are baby foods, gifts and gift baskets, books, bath and body products, and hair care and skin care products. A terrific service is a link to gluten-free vegan and vegetarian restaurants in your area, gluten-free community, articles, and food blogs. All purchases go through Amazon's checkout system. www.gluterra.com

Don't Forget the Coupons

BE FREE FOR ME.COM

After being diagnosed with celiac disease, founder Kathleen Reale soon found her new diet took more time and a whole lot more money than she expected. Save, sample, share. www.befreeforme.com

EBATES

This site operates on the travel and hotel site principle. Maximize your savings by checking here first to see if the site from which you are buying offers even more savings through Ebates. www.ebates.com

GLUTEN-FREE SAVER

This site offers daily deals for gluten-free products, including frozen foods, which often include free shipping. Start with daily specials for the best prices. www.glutenfreesaver.com

SWAG BUCKS

This free membership site powered by Google offers "swag bucks" or reward points for downloading its tool bar and using it as your search engine. (Can you say brilliant move, Google?)

Reward points can be redeemed for any number of things, but if you match Swag Bucks certificates to deals and free shipping on Amazon, you've got savings on steroids. www.swagbucks.com

Magazine Clippings

One of many good reasons to subscribe to magazines like *Living Without*, *Gluten-Free Living*, and *Simply Gluten-Free Magazine* are the coupons in the back. Often these are better sources for gluten-free deals than supermarket fliers. Good marketing strategy for everyone concerned.

VITACOST

This site boasts more than one thousand gluten-free and organic products at an average of 30 to 70 percent off. Purchases over $49 qualify for free shipping. E-mail newsletter brings sales and special offers. Share with friends and get an extra $10 coupon when they shop. www.vitacost.com

Go Big or Go Home

In the hunt for good prices on gluten-free items, don't overlook superstores like Target, Walmart, Meijer, and membership bulk buying clubs like Costco, Sam's Club, BJ Wholesale Club, and Loblaws and Hudson's Bay superstores and hypermarkets in Canada. Some are gluten-friendlier than others, but all are jumping on the bandwagon. A great opportunity to save or buy in bulk those items your family loves. Make sure your purchases warrant the club fees. Shop with a list. It's easy to buy too much in these places.

Food Cooperatives and Buying Clubs

If your family is large and goes through food like, as my grandmother used to say, "Grant took Richmond," *and* you want to keep a conscious kitchen, food co-ops are much like the buying clubs above but with natural, organic, sustainable, non-GMO foods. For great prices on organic fruits and vegetables, these places cannot be beat. But don't buy gluten-free grains or flours from bulk bins or from containers that list no provenance or assurance of being milled or processed in a certified gluten-free facility. Unless these can be verified, cross-contamination is almost always the issue.

Marketing Strategy

Sometimes it takes a village. To find a food cooperative or buying club in your area or to learn how to start one with a like-minded gluten-free community interested in clean, non-processed food, go to www.coopdirectory.org.

UNITED BUYING CLUBS

This huge food co-op sells to gluten-free specialty companies as well as to individuals, is presently in thirty-four states, and is served by a purveyor of natural foods, United Natural Foods. The list of gluten-free foods is long, as well as the list of kosher, vegan, vegetarian, and dairy-free foods. You will find organic produce, hormone-free meats, and all manner of locally grown and raised food. For a club near you, visit www.unitedbuyingclubs.com.

Bakeries

Once upon a time, when gluten-free specialty stores were as rare as a rainstorm in the Sahara, I drove one hundred miles to find gluten-free ravioli and lasagna noodles and chocolate brownies. When visiting Los Angeles to autograph copies of my first book, *Against the Grain*, I insisted the event take place at the long-gone Goody's, the first totally gluten-free bakery I'd ever seen. It was difficult to stay focused in the presence of all the gluten-free sweets I could eat.

Every day a new dedicated gluten-free bakery opens its doors in a town or city near you. There are several of these in Center City, Philadelphia, where I live, and that doesn't take into account the surrounding suburbs. There is nothing like getting your daily bread and rolls and bagels fresh from the oven, full of good whole grains and free of gluten and other allergens.

I've listed only a handful here and apologize to those whose reputations have not yet reached my ears. Be assured that they will.

ATLANTA

Dr. Sweet's Cake Emporium—Cakes, cookies, cupcakes, and brownies for any and every intolerance—sweet. www.drsweetscakes.com

BOSTON AREA

Glutenus Minimus—Glorious baked goods, many of which are nut-free and dairy-free; many vegan options. www.glutenusminimus.com

Violette Gluten-Free Bakery—Boasts a totally gluten-free facility and organic and locally sourced ingredients. www.violettegf.com

CHICAGO AREA

Defloured—Amazing baked goods; let it be your first gluten-free experience. www.deflouredbakery.com

Rose's Café and Bakery—On Christmas Eve and in the depths of the great recession, a secret millionaire wrote them a check and saved one of the best gluten-free bakeries on the planet from extinction. www .rosesbakery.com

Sweet Ali's—One of Chicago's most popular gluten-free outposts. www.sweetalis.com

DALLAS

Tu Lu's Gluten-Free Bakery—Gluten-free cupcakes, cookies, muffins, panini, and more; New York City location, too. www.tu-lusbakery.com

EAGAN, MINNESOTA

BitterSweet Gluten Free Bakery—Gluten-free, dairy-free and preservative-free breads and cakes in the Land of Lakes. www.bittersweetgf.com

FORDS, NEW JERSEY

Fallon's Gluten Free Bakeshop—Italian specialty breads and pastries and sweets in a gluten-free and nut-free facility. www.fallonsglutenfreebakeshop.com

LANCASTER, PENNSYLVANIA

Amaranth Gluten Free Bakery—Wonderful dinner and sandwich rolls, cupcakes, and raspberry thumbprint cookies. www.spiceoflifelancaster.com

LOS ANGELES

Breakaway Bakery—Organic, fruit-sweetened goodies free of gluten, wheat, dairy, casein, nuts, soy, and gums, advertised as being made with 400 percent less starch than most gluten-free products. How do they do that? www.breakawaybakery.com

MIAMI/FORT LAUDERDALE

Weezie's Gluten Free Kitchen—What happens when a star chef discovers she's gluten-intolerant? Perfect key lime tarts and gluten-free dining on a whole new level. www.weeziesgfkitchen.com

NEW YORK CITY

BabyCakes NYC—Erin McKenna launched her gluten-free, mostly vegan cupcake empire from this tiny Lower East Side location; shops in L.A. and Disney World. www.babycakesnyc.com

Clementine Bakery—Where Brooklyn goes for exceptional gluten-free treats. Clinton Hill. www.clementinebakery.com

Pip's Place—Upper East Side bakery free of most major allergens. www.pipsplacenyc.com

PHILADELPHIA

Sweet Freedom—Dairy-free, sugar-free, casein-free, gluten-free, lactose-free, corn-free, and nut-free desserts. www.sweetfreedombakery.com

Taffets Bakery and Store—This Italian market gluten-free bakery specializes in amazing bagels, focaccia, biscotti, baguettes, and teff and quinoa breads. Sweets, too. www.taffets.com

PORTLAND, OREGON

Petunia's Pies & Pastries—Jaw-dropping vegan and gluten-free desserts like Bumble-Berry Peach Pie with Hazelnut-Coconut Streusel. www.petuniaspiesandpastries.com

SAN FRANCISCO

Mariposa Baking Company, Ferry Building and Berkeley—Uncommon gluten-free bakery. www.mariposabaking.com

SEATTLE

Flying Apron Bakery—Gluten-free vegan bread, cakes, sweets. www.flyingapron.com

VANCOUVER, BRITISH COLUMBIA

Panne Rizo—This award-winning bakery and café is a must for gluten-free visitors. www.pannerizo.com

WASHINGTON, DC

The Happy Tart—Tarts, cakes, cupcakes, meringues, baguettes, pastries. Classic patisserie, totally gluten-free. www.happytartbakery.com

Hello Cupcake—They do one thing very well. A different flavor gluten-free cupcake every day. www.hellocupcakeonline.com

Nothing but the Best for You

The question I am asked most often is What do you eat? What is your favorite bread? Whose bagels do you swear by? What do you eat for breakfast? What brand of pasta do you serve?

After years of being grateful for any gluten-free crumb, I am much more exacting about the food I eat. You may or may not agree, but for me the idea is to eat consciously and well, not simply to eat gluten-free at all costs. Why eat empty processed foods just because they lack the one ingredient we know will make us sick? Why not get rid of most things that will make us sick?

This is the new way to be gluten-free *and* healthy.

Like more and more Americans, I look for naturally gluten-free and organic foods free of GMOs (although that's hard to do without full disclosure on labels; see Chapter 22, "Food Fights").

I try to eat simply, and as close to home and as green and pesticide-free as possible.

I don't like it, but I pay a little more for organic produce and would rather put my money directly into the pocket of the farmer who comes to market than pay a middleman. Sometimes that is impossible, so the next stop is a store that can assure me their products are pure, organic, and made with actual food instead of taste-enhancing chemicals and high-fructose corn syrup.

I don't eat so many carbohydrates either, and those breads and bagels and cereals I do enjoy, as part of my determination to eat a healthy, whole-grain diet, tend to be less sweet and more nutrient dense and offer far more fiber and protein than some popular brands. My pantry is full of buckwheat, sorghum, and quinoa products and very little white rice flour.

I buy packaged foods like Glutenfreeda oatmeal that have been certified gluten-free by a stricter standard than the FDA and given an identifiable seal. I am more comfortable with those brands.

I am not a vegan, but I am impressed by the variety and taste of products I once wrongly associated with a nuts-and-sprouts mentality. I actually love kale chips and vegan veggie burgers. I prefer Vegenaise to Hellmann's, and I happen to think all kinds of seeds, chia included, are powerhouses of nutrition, either ground or sprinkled whole onto cereal.

I'm not perfect, far from it.

I've cut back on butter, sugar, and chocolate and prefer to buy and bake vegan when I can. I try to use natural sweeteners, coconut cream, nut meals, and nut flours that offer some protein and fiber along with a spectacular taste.

The Whole Foods flourless chocolate torte is a notable example of how the best intentions go awry. So is the Moondance cheesecake. My strategy is to enjoy a slice or two and freeze the rest or make sure friends and family leave with the remainder of the cake.

I've learned that the freezer is my friend. It is so easy to stash small

Buy Certified

While the FDA works out the kinks in the new gluten-free labeling law, which allows companies to *voluntarily* label foods that contain less than 20 parts per million of gluten, these are the seals you can trust. Products tested by these organizations are held to a much higher standard (15 and 10 parts per million) than the government's. Production facilities and their procedures for eliminating cross-contamination are scrutinized and verified as well.

Gluten-Free Certification Organization

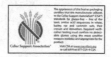

Celiac Support Association

Canadian Celiac Association

National Foundation for Celiac Awareness

portions and to make a loaf of bread or a box of cookies or some other sweet treat last. When I do eat pasta, baby, it better be good.

There is so much gluten-free food out there, and taste is so subjective.

Here's a short list of companies catering not only to the gluten-free diet but also to other food sensitivities. Take your time, experiment, and see what you like; order a sample before plunging in. Play around with some of the new flours here, and try your hand at the recipes in the coming chapters. Homemade isn't as hard as you think. Many of the bakeries listed here ship, and you may find not all artisanal breads and baked goods are more expensive than the commercial varieties. Don't overlook organic, small-batch companies and start-ups offering products both vegan and gluten-free.

I hope you will be pleasantly surprised, as I continue to be.

ALL-PURPOSE GLUTEN-FREE FLOUR BLENDS, MIXES, AND NUT AND SPECIALTY FLOURS

Amazing-Grains: Montina Flour. www.amazinggrains.com
Ancient Harvest: Quinoa Flour and Quinoa. www.quinoa.net
Arrowhead Mills. www.arrowheadmills.com
Authentic Foods Garfava Flour. www.authenticfoods.com

Bisquick. www.bisquick.com
Bob's Red Mill: Chickpea flour and Sorghum flour.
    www.bobsredmill.com
Chēbē Original Cheese Bread Mix. www.chebe.com
Cup4Cup. www.williams-sonoma.com
Dakota Prairie: Organic amaranth flour. www.dakota-prairie.com
Dowd and Rogers Chestnut Flour. www.dowdandrogers.com
Ener-G Foods: Tapioca flour. www.ener-g.com
Gluten Free Mama Coconut Blend or Almond Blend.
    www.glutenfreemama.com
Hodgson Mill. www.hodgsonmill.com
Jules Gluten-Free. www.julesglutenfree.com
King Arthur. www.kingarthurflour.com
Kinnikinnick Foods. www.kinnikinnick.com
Now Foods: Almond flour. www.nowfoods.com
Zócalo Sweet Potato, Peruvian Purple Corn, Amaranth, Mesquite, and
    Kañiwa Flours. www.culinarycollective.com

BEER AND ALE

Bard's Beer. www.bardsbeer.com
Epic Brewing Company Glutenator Gluten-Free Beer.
    www.epicbrewing.com
Green's gluten-free beers—craft-brewed in Belgium.
    www.glutenfreebeers.co.uk
Harvester Pale Ale—Dedicated gluten-free brewery.
    www.harvesterbrewing.com
New Grist Beer. www.newgrist.com
New Planet Beer and New Planet Brown Ale—gluten-free brewery.
    www.newplanetbeer.com
Ramapo Valley beers. www.rvbrewery.com
Woodchuck Draft Hard Cider. www.woodchuck.com

Cheers!

BREAD, COOKIES, BISCOTTI, CRACKERS

Amaranth Gluten Free Bakery—Sandwich Rolls, 4-Seed Bread.
    www.spiceoflifelancaster.com.
Canyon Bakehouse—7-Grain Bread. www.canyonbakehouse.com
Ginny Bakes—Coconut Oatmeal Bliss Cookies. www.ginnybakes.com

Glow Gluten Free—Double Chocolate Chip Cookies.
www.glowglutenfree.com

Katz Gluten Free—Challah, Rugelach, Bagels. www.katzglutenfree.com

Schär's—Heat and Serve Breads, Baguettes, and Rolls. www.schar.com

Taffets Bakery and Store—Teff and Quinoa Bread, *everything* bagels,
baguettes. www.taffets.com

Tate's—Chocolate Chip Cookies. www.tatesbakeshop.com

Udi's Bagels. www.udisglutenfree.com

FOR IMPROMPTU CRUSTS OR CRUMBLES

Health Valley Organic Rice Bran Crackers. www.healthvalley.com.

MI-DEL Ginger Snaps—Soft, gingery, thoroughly satisfying.
www.midelcookies.com.

BREAD CRUMBS

Gillian's Bread Crumbs, Plain and Italian.
www.gilliansfoodsglutenfree.com

Kinnikinnick Panko Style Bread Crumbs. www.kinnikinnick.com

Schär Bread Crumbs. www.schar.com

BUTTER AND CHEESE ALTERNATIVES, EGG REPLACER, AND SPREADS

Crofter's Organic Just Fruit Spreads. www.croftersorganic.com

Daiya Foods—Dairy-free cheese alternative. www.daiyafoods.com

Divine Organics—Nut and seed butters. www.divineorganics.com

Earth Balance. www.earthbalance.com

Ener-G Foods—Egg replacer. www.ener-g.com

Follow Your Heart—Cream cheese. www.followyourheart.com

Once Again Nut Butter. www.onceagainnutbutter.com

Spectrum. www.spectrumorganics.com

CAKE MIXES AND PIECRUST

Ad Hoc/Thomas Keller Cake Mixes. www.williams-sonoma.com

The Adventuresome Kitchen Gluten-Free, Vegan Piecrust.
www.adventuresomekitchen.com

Dowd and Rogers Artisan Baking Mixes. www.dowdandrogers.com

1-2-3 Gluten Free nutrient-fortified, sugar-free baking mixes.
www.123glutenfree.com

Wholesome Chow Vegan, Non-GMO, Organic Baking Mixes.
www.wholesomechow.com

How Many Girl Scouts Does It Take to Bake a Gluten-Free Girl Scout Cookie?

Apparently, more than we imagine. After years of requests and petitions, they are just getting around to test-marketing a chocolate-chip shortbread cookie for booth sales only. Don't even ask about brownies. Shouldn't there be a merit badge for getting this done?

Weird Gluten-Free Fact: World's Biggest Gluten-Free Pizza

Dr. Schär Group, parent company of gluten-free baker Schar USA, baked the world's biggest pizza, using 20,000 pounds of gluten-free flour, 2,500 gallons of water, 10,000 pounds of tomato sauce, and 8,000 pounds of mozzarella cheese, setting a Guinness World Record for any pizza, gluten free or not. It measured 131 feet in diameter, weighed more than 51,000 pounds, and covered nearly one-third of an acre. Some people will do anything for your business.

CAKES, STORE-BOUGHT

Lilly's Bake Shop Gluten-Free Chocolate Roll, Kosher for Passover.
    www.lillysbakeryshop.com
Moondance Cheesecakes with Pecan Shortbread Crust.
    www.moondancedesserts.com
Whole Foods Flourless Chocolate Torte. www.wholefoodsmarket.com

CEREALS AND WAFFLES

Arrowhead Mills Organic Rice and Shine Hot Cereal.
    www.arrowheadmills.com
Bakery On Main Gluten-Free Granola. www.bakeryonmain.com
Bob's Red Mill Mighty Tasty Hot Cereal—Whole-grain brown rice,
    corn, sorghum, and buckwheat. www.bobsredmill.com
Bob's Red Mill Steel Cut Oats. www.bobsredmill.com
Erewhon Supergrains Cereals—Quinoa and Chia Flakes.
    www.erewhonmarket.com
Gluten-Free Oats Rolled Oats. www.glutenfreeoats.com
Glutenfreeda Instant Oatmeal. www.glutenfreeda.com
Nature's Path Mesa Sunrise corn, flax, buckwheat quinoa, and amaranth
    cereal. www.naturespath.com
Van's Gluten-Free Flax Waffles. www.vansfoods.com

CONDIMENTS

Annie's Naturals Organic Honey Mustard. www.annies.com
Hellmann's Mayonnaise. www.hellmanns.com
Maille Original Dijon Mustard. www.maille.us
Vegenaise. www.vegenaise.com

CRACKERS

Crunchmaster Multi-Grain Roasted Vegetable Crackers.
    www.crunchmaster.com
Doctor In The Kitchen Rosemary Flackers. www.drinthekitchen.com
Glutino Table Crackers. www.glutino.com
Mary's Gone Crackers Organic Crackers. www.marysgonecrackers.com

DELI MEATS

Applegate Organic and Natural Meats—No preservatives, antibiotics,
    humanely raised, gluten-free, and casein-free. www.applegate.com
Boar's Head Cold Cuts—Fresh only, and only if the server cleans the
    slicer. www.boarshead.com

ICE CREAM, GELATO, AND FROZEN YOGURT

Graeter's Small-Batch Ice Cream—Most flavors. www.graeters.com

Häagen-Dazs—Extensive list of gluten-free flavors. www.haagendazs.com

Julie's Organic Ice Cream Sandwiches. www.juliesorganic.com

Pinkberry—Franchise frozen yogurt. www.pinkberry.com

Red Mango—Franchise frozen yogurt. www.redmangousa.com

Skinny Cow Ice Cream Bars. www.skinnycow.com

Talenti Gelato—All flavors are gluten-free except caramel cookie
   crunch, which should be obvious. www.talentigelato.com

IF YOU CAN'T EAT ICE CREAM WITHOUT THE CONE

Goldbaum's. www.goldbaums.com

Joy Cones. www.joycone.com

DAIRY-FREE ICE CREAM

Coconut Bliss Ice Cream. www.coconutbliss.com

Purely Decadent Ice Cream. www.turtlemountain.com

MISO PASTE

South River Certified Organic Miso Pastes for authentic Japanese soups
   and sauces—Sweet White, Chickpea, Brown Rice, Azuki Bean and
   Dandelion, Leek and Brown Rice. www.southrivermiso.com

MOCHI

Grainaissance—Traditional Japanese crunchy, chewy, sticky brown rice
   cakes. www.grainaissance.com

OATS

Bob's Red Mill. www.bobsredmill.com

Cream Hill Estates. www.creamhillestates.com

GF Harvest. www.glutenfreeoats.com

Gifts of Nature. www.giftsofnature.net

Glutenfreeda. www.glutenfreedafoods.com

Only Oats. www.avenafoods.com

PASTA AND NOODLES

Ancient Harvest—Dried quinoa pasta. www.quinoa.net

DeLallo—Dried corn and rice and whole-grain brown rice pastas.
   www.delallo.com

GreeNoodle Pasta—Made with ancient Egyptian super vegetable, moroheiya. www.eongoods.com

Jovial Foods—Egg tagliatelle. www.jovialfoods.com

King Soba Noodle Culture—Buckwheat soba, millet and brown rice, pumpkin, ginger, and rice noodles. www.kingsoba.com

La Pasta—Fresh ravioli: spinach and cheese and wild mushroom. www.lapastainc.com

Leo's Gluten Free—Ravioli, fettuccine, rotini, and penne made in a dedicated facility. www.leosglutenfree.com

Lundberg Family Farms—Dried brown rice penne. www.lundberg.com

Pappardelle's Pasta—Non-GMO, artisanal pasta in all the usual shapes and flavors, plus chipotle lime orzo, sweet potato, and chocolate. www.pappardellesonline.com

Quattrobimbi—Le Veneziane dried corn pasta. www.quattrobimbi.com

RP's Pasta Company—Fresh linguini, fettuccini, lasagna sheets. www.rpspasta.com

Thai Kitchen—Stir-fry rice noodles. www.thaikitchen.com

Tinkyada—Dried brown rice spaghetti with rice bran. www.tinkyada.com

Tru Roots Ancient Grain Pasta—Quinoa, amaranth, brown rice, and whole grain corn, made in Italy. www.truroots.com

PIZZA, FROZEN

Against the Grain Gourmet Pizza No GMOs, no preservatives, no stabilizers or flavor enhancers. www.againstthegraingourmet.com

Glutenfreeda Pizza Wraps. www.glutenfreeda.com

Udi's Gluten Free Frozen Pizza. www.udisglutenfree.com

PIZZA CRUSTS/MIXES/DOUGH

Cup4Cup Pizza Crust Mix. www.williams-sonoma.com

Gillian's Foods Pizza Dough. www.gilliansfoodsglutenfree.com

Katz Gluten Free Flat Bread/Personal Pizza Crust. www.katzglutenfree.com

Udi's Pizza Crusts—Two to a pack. www.udisglutenfree.com

RICE, WHOLE-GRAIN

Acquerello Carnaroli Rice. www.williams-sonoma.com

Bob's Red Mill Long Grain Brown Rice. www.bobsredmill.com

Hershey's Shout-Out

Great example of a company that not only provides a clear gluten-free product list, but offers recipes, videos, tips, caveats, and encouragement for gluten-free bakers. www.hersheys.com.

Goya Organic Long-Grain White Rice. www.goya.com

Lotus Foods Organic Forbidden Rice and other Asian specialty rices.
    www.lotusfoods.com

Lundberg Family Farms Basmati, Organic Brown Rice.
    www.lundberg.com

Lundberg Family Farms White Arborio Rice. www.lundberg.com

Organic Texmati Brown Rice and White Rice. www.riceselect.com

Texas Best Brown Jasmine Rice and Jasmine White Rice.
    www.texasbestorganics.com

365 Organic Short Grain Brown Rice. www.wholefoodsmarket.com

SAUCES

A Taste of Thai Fish Sauce. www.atasteofthai.com

Annie's Naturals salad dressings. www.annies.com

Bone Suckin' Sauce—Regular, Hot, Thicker, and Hot Thicker.
    www.bonesuckin.com

Kikkoman Gluten-Free Soy Sauce. www.kikkomanusa.com

Little Soya Individual Soy Sauce Packets—Less sodium, non-GMO.
    www.littlesoya.com

Premier Japan Gluten Free Hoisin Sauce. www.edwardandsons.com

San J Teriyaki Sauce. www.san-J.com

Thai Kitchen Fish, Satay, and Chili Sauces. www.thaikitchen.com

Whidbey Fresh WildeBerryaki Sauce. www.whidbeyfresh.com

The Wizard's Organic Vegan Worcestershire Sauce.
    www.edwardandsons.com

SNACKS

ANDI Bars—Free of gluten, casein, corn, soy, GMOs, artificial flavoring,
    and preservatives. Made by the Autism Network for Dietary
    Intervention. www.autismndi.com

Brad's Raw Kale Chips—No GMOs, vegan, gluten-free, paleo friendly;
    nuts are involved. www.bradsrawchips.com

Glutino pretzels. www.glutino.com

Kind Bars. www.kindsnacks.com

Lärabar. www.larabar.com

Pirate's Booty—Aged White Cheddar popcorn snacks.
    www.piratebrands.com

Ricebliss—Creamy brown rice superfood custard/porridge energy
    snacks. www.ricebliss.com

Sun Cups—Nut-free, gluten-free chocolate cups. www.suncups.com

York Peppermint Patty. www.hersheys.com

SOUPS AND BROTHS

College Inn—Broths. www.collegeinn.com

Imagine Soups—Most are gluten-free and dairy-free.
www.imaginefoods.com

Pacific Free-Range Chicken Broth and Organic Vegetable Broth.
www.pacificfoods.com

Progresso Light—Creamy Mushroom Soup. www.progresso.com

Shelton's Turkey and Chicken Broths. www.sheltons.com

VANILLA AND OTHER EXTRACTS

Flavorganics—Organic, non-GMO, gluten-free extracts. Almond,
anise, orange, chocolate, coconut, coffee, hazelnut, vanilla.
www.flavorganics.com

Nielsen-Massey Pure Extracts—Certified gluten-free, certified kosher
and free of allergens. Madagascar Bourbon vanilla, almond,
chocolate, coffee, lemon, orange, and peppermint extracts, and
orange blossom water and rose water. www.nielsenmassey.com

VEGGIE BURGERS

Hilary's Veggie Burgers—No corn, dairy, gluten, yeast, egg, nut, soy,
gluten, or GMOs. Vegan and toaster ready. www.hilaryseatwell.com

Sol Cuisine's Original Burger—Vegan veggie burger. www.solcuisine.com

WRAPS

Food For Life Brown Rice Tortillas. www.foodforlife.com

La Tortilla Factory Ivory Teff Wraps. www.latortillafactory.com

Mission Corn Tortillas. www.missionfoods.com

YOGURT

Dannon—All yogurts except Activia Breakfast Blends, Activia Parfait,
Activia Fiber, and Danimals Crunchers. www.dannon.com

Fage—Thick Greek yogurt. 0% fat, 2% fat, and total classic. usa.fage.eu

Redwood Hill Farm—Goat kefir, yogurts, lactose-free line, 100 percent
humane. www.redwoodhill.com

So Delicious Coconut Yogurt—Dairy-free. www.sodeliciousdairyfree.com

Part II

What's for Dinner?

Essential Skills

6

The most perfect technique
is that which is not noticed at all.
—PABLO CASALS

Beth Crossman, my first Holt editor and a woman of considerable culinary skills, loved to say that when Bette Hagman, author of the Gluten-Free Gourmet series, was diagnosed with celiac disease, she marched into her kitchen to fix it, but when Jax Lowell was diagnosed a full generation later, she marched right into somebody else's, usually a well-known chef's.

I believed then, and still do, that knowledge of the gluten-free diet, a healthy dose of self-assertion (by this I do not mean arrogant self-entitlement), and a good sense of what the chef is trying to accomplish can net a truly memorable meal. I have acquired some serious kitchen skills since then, but I am smart enough to know that even if you know your way around a saddle of lamb, it takes a whole lot more than that to call yourself a cookbook writer.

If I have learned anything from those generous souls who have allowed me into their kitchens, have contributed to past editions, and have come out en masse for this one, it's this: knowing how to execute basic cooking techniques can give us control over our diets. It can release us from having to slavishly follow a recipe and assume we can't accomplish it just because we are missing one ingredient.

If we know how to sauté or roast any vegetable using simple ingredients like olive oil and garlic, or a few drops of truffle oil, we free ourselves from lists and expectations. We are able to see what foods are the freshest and buy accordingly. We don't fear the winter gulag of root vegetables. If we know that ceviche requires citrus fruits to marinate or "cook" the seafood, we aren't thrown if the market only has lemons instead of limes or the scallops don't look as good as the shrimp. With a solid grounding in technique, we are confident enough to make the substitution. We can wing it.

Knowing how to poach, sauté, roast, coddle, braise, blanch, and properly wash our leafy greens emboldens us to try something new and be much more knowledgeable when shopping for what is fresh and in season. We start to see portions as a taste issue, not a mathematical one. We discover what we love and use more of it. We find ourselves out of one thing, but we have enough know-how to substitute another. We understand the true meaning of *from scratch*.

Even more important, a working knowledge of technique releases us from the unhealthy tyranny of processed, so-called convenience foods. Knowing what we are doing in the kitchen frees us from the ready-made, frozen, packaged, and prefab passing for food these days. Knowing how to get past an artichoke's prickly exterior or dig the meat out of a chestnut is how we develop an appreciation for what is fresh, local, and real. We begin to see our food as cyclical, passing opportunities if you will, not the year-round, pallid offerings of the supermarket.

Even better, we get to know the people who grow our food with care and a minimum of pesticides. We look forward to the spring's first asparagus and to that brief exquisite season of soft-shell crabs that presages sweet summer fruits and tomatoes, and beyond that, the Brussels sprouts, pumpkins, and pears of autumn. When we know how to poach winter fruit, we can wait until summer to try our hands at blueberry pie.

Right now you stand, literally, at a fork in the road. You want to feel your best again. The path you choose is going to make all the difference. One way leads to foods that are naturally gluten-free, protein- and fiber-rich, full of vitamins and energy—whole-grain pastas, breads, and cereals; wild, not farmed, fish; poultry and grain-fed meats raised without hormones and antibiotics; organic vegetables and fruits, nuts and seeds; non-processed cheeses—real food offset by gluten-free treats free of excessive sugar, fat, common allergens, and genetically modified ingredients made by the many small-batch bakeries, kitchens, and companies whose mission it is to deliver more than just gluten-free substitutes. There are no risks on this road; only reward. This is the way to renewed vigor, long life, and a healthy weight.

The other path is an express lane straight to the mega billion dollar market that is gluten-free packaged food: cakes, cookies, brownies, muffins, and pastries the size of hubcaps, all touting the gluten-free label, but full of unhealthy fats and excessive sugar   a trade off, essentially, of one empty food for another.

I looked at the label of a very popular iced chocolate cupcake recently; it weighed in at 440 calories with 21 grams of fat and a whopping 47 grams of sugar. Servings? Three. When was the last time you ate a third of a cupcake?

While subsistence on these products may offer relief from cravings and give us the sense that we have not lost our comfort foods, they doom us to the same chronic problems anyone who lives on this stuff is at risk for developing. Bloating and leaky gut issues aside, I am convinced that this is the source of the disconnect between those who say the gluten-free diet is healthier and those who do not, between those who say it is a way to lose weight and those who say they've packed on the pounds.

Hot Tip

For well-seared steaks and chops, and browned beef, pork, and poultry for stews: Always let meat come to room temperature before pan searing. Otherwise the meat will stew in its own juices. Allow the meat to rest for a few minutes to let the juices settle before slicing and serving.

The difference between these two paths is a working knowledge of what to do with food that does not come in a box, pouch, or bag.

In other words, technique.

The Essential Art of Rice

If there is one gluten-free food you want to do perfectly every time, it's rice. Aim not for the obligatory heap of brown or white rice next to a protein and a vegetable, but for something more aromatic, exotic, spectacular—risotto, pilaf, paella, stir-fried, southern dirty rice, sushi rice, rice cakes, jambalaya, Creole. Learn the differences between rice varieties and which one is right for which recipe. Master the cooking technique for each and there's no end to the dishes you can produce. You may want to put the rice cooker in the next garage sale.

American long-grain Carolina white rice is highly refined, and polished (hull, bran, and germ removed). Experts say it doesn't require washing, although I find that tough to swallow and would do it anyway. The most ubiquitous of grains, you might say this is rice's version of refined white pasta or bread. Pretty, but a little empty. Add wild rice, nuts, or quinoa for interest and extra nutrients.

American long-grain brown rice with its intact nutrient-rich bran and germ layers is a better nutritional deal with a nutty flavor and a chewy bite. Having shed its hippie image, brown rice is quickly replacing white for most main dishes. It's always a good idea to wash brown rice.

Indian basmati is long-grain rice with a nutty fragrance and flavor in both white and brown varieties, and its texture is perfect for absorbing rich sauces. Soak it for half an hour or so before cooking.

Italian risotto rice—arborio, carnaroli, vialone nano—is a creamy-textured, medium-grain rice sometimes considered a short-grain rice because of its ability to absorb far more liquid than the long-grain varieties.

Japanese-style sushi rice is sticky when cooked, but different from the sticky rice used to make sweets like mochi.

Spanish bomba rice is highly absorbable and therefore the perfect choice for paella.

Thai jasmine long-grain rice is slightly flowery and has a soft, pliable texture. It needs to be washed before cooking to remove excess starch. This is a good choice for Asian or Indian dishes.

Boiling

+ Put 1 cup of long-grain white rice and 1½ cups water in a saucepan with a tight-fitting lid. Bring the water to a boil. No peeking under the lid.
+ Reduce the heat to low so as not to scorch the bottom of the pot. Let cook for 20 minutes.
+ Turn off the burner, remove the pan from the heat, and let sit for 5 minutes.

Note: For brown rice, use 1 cup rice and 2 cups water. Simmer on low for 45 minutes. Let stand, covered, for 10 minutes.

Pasta Method

+ Cook 1 cup long-grain brown rice in an abundant amount of water, tasting the rice for doneness just as you would with pasta.
+ Drain.

Steaming

+ This traditional Asian method involves placing a quantity of sticky rice or sushi rice in a fine-mesh rice-steamer basket over boiling water.

Traditional Indian Method

+ Combine 1 cup rice with 1¾ cups water in a 3-quart saucepan.
+ Let soak for 20 minutes.
+ Bring the water and rice to a boil, then cover with a tight-fitting lid, reduce the heat to low, and simmer for 15 minutes. No peeking.
+ Remove the pan from heat and let stand, covered, for 5 to 10 minutes.

Basic Risotto Method

+ Sauté ½ chopped onion in ½ stick butter and olive oil. Add 1 cup rice and stir to coat, until rice is slightly translucent, about 2 minutes.
+ Add about ½ cup of any dry white wine, then add 1 cup warm chicken broth, stirring constantly until the liquid is absorbed, about 4 minutes.
+ Stir in another cup of broth, until it is fully absorbed.
+ Repeat until you have incorporated 3 cups of broth and the rice is creamy.
+ Stir in about 2 tablespoons butter and Parmesan cheese.

✦ Look up all the ways you can make risotto, starting with the Pumpkin Sage Risotto on page 181.

Cutting-Edge Skills

Do you avoid big, impenetrable-looking fruits and vegetables because, well, they seem like too much work and too dangerous to cut? Buying precut is certainly easier and requires less muscle, but it's more expensive, too, and, despite preservatives that make some of us sneeze, or worse, it spoils really, really fast.

HOW TO CUT A PINEAPPLE

1. Lay pineapple on its side and cut off the top and bottom.
2. Stand the pineapple up on its bottom and cut the skin off, following the contours of the fruit.
3. Remove remaining eyes with the tip of a potato peeler.
4. Turn the pineapple on its side and cut into ½-inch-thick slices.
5. Cut out core with a paring knife to make rings.

HOW TO CUT A BUTTERNUT SQUASH

1. Lay the squash on its side and cut ½ inch off each end.
2. Halve the squash just above the bulge where the neck meets the bulb.
3. Remove the tough outer skin with a potato peeler. Spoon out the seeds and stringy membrane.
4. Slice the neck and the bulb and cut into the pieces you need.

Cut to the Chase

You wouldn't shave your face day after day with a dull razor. So why are you dicing vegetables with a dull knife? Invest in a good sharpener or have your knives honed periodically by a professional. They'll make quick work for you. Watch your fingers, though.

HOW TO CUT A PUMPKIN AND GET IT READY FOR COOKING

1. Scrub the outside of the pumpkin with a stiff vegetable brush.
2. Cut the pumpkin in half and spoon out the fibers and seeds with a serrated spoon.
3. Preheat the oven to 350°F.
4. Place the pumpkin halves in an ovenproof dish with enough water to cover the bottom to 1 inch and cover tightly with foil.
5. Bake until the pumpkin is fork tender, about 1 to 1½ hours.
6. Let cool, then scoop out the flesh.
7. Make Spiced Pumpkin Torte (page 232).

REVEREND MICHAEL ALAN'S PERFECT, POSSIBLY PALEO, PUMPKIN PIE

Now that you know how to prepare a fresh pumpkin, artist, master baker, food consultant, and man of the cloth Michael Alan shows us how to use good-for-you flours to bake a much better pumpkin pie than you can buy. Once you've got the hang of it, feel free to play with different fillings. Leave out the sugar, and you've got a healthy template for savory tarts and quiche crusts. You'll need one 10-inch ovenproof pie pan, a rolling pin dusted in gluten-free flour, parchment paper, pie weights or dried beans, and a board, a marble slab, or a big enough section of the kitchen counter to flour and comfortably roll out the dough.

MAKES ONE 10-INCH PIE

1. Blend the flours, sugar, and salt in the bowl of a food processor. Add the butter and coconut oil and pulse until its consistency is that of wet sand.
2. Add the egg and pulse until a dough forms. Turn onto plastic wrap and refrigerate until firm and ready to use.
3. Mix all of the filling ingredients together thoroughly. Refrigerate until ready to use.

To assemble the pie:

1. Preheat the oven to 375°F.
2. Roll the dough out into a 14-inch round and gently place into the pie pan. With a knife or clean kitchen shears, trim off the excess, leaving about a 1/2-inch to 1-inch overhang all around.
3. Crimp the dough and place in the freezer for about 15 minutes.
4. Brush the chilled pie shell with egg wash—one egg whisked with a splash of water. Line the dough with parchment paper and fill the pie shell with weights or dried beans.
5. Par bake for about 20 minutes. Remove the shell and allow it to cool for about an hour, longer if your kitchen is hot or humid.
6. Reduce the oven temperature to 350°F.
7. Fill the cooled pie shell with the pumpkin filling and bake until the center is set, about 40 minutes. Cool on a rack, add whipped cream, and serve.

For the crust:
1/4 cup quinoa flour
1/4 cup chickpea flour
1/4 cup amaranth flour
1/3 cup potato flour
1/3 cup arrowroot flour
1 tablespoon sugar
1/2 teaspoon salt
4 tablespoons (1/2 stick) unsalted cold butter
4 tablespoons cold coconut oil
1 large egg

For the filling:
15 ounces fresh pumpkin, puréed (about 2 cups)
1 large egg
1/2 cup light brown sugar, packed down
1/2 cup honey
1 cup whole, soy, or almond milk
1 teaspoon ground cinnamon
1/2 teaspoon ground ginger
1/4 teaspoon nutmeg, freshly grated
1/4 teaspoon ground allspice
1/4 teaspoon ground cloves
1/2 teaspoon vanilla extract
1/2 teaspoon salt

The Life of Pie

Using ice water and cold butter and oils, and chilling the dough before baking, allows the dough to relax and firms up the fats for a tender, flakier crust. ∗ Partially baking the crust and chilling it before filling keeps the pie from getting soggy. ∗ Egg wash on a chilled crust ensures the filling won't seep into the crust. ∗ Weighing down the crust while it par bakes keeps it from bubbling and warping. ∗ Crimping the edges keeps the filling from leaking and keeps the bottom crust from getting soggy. ∗ Overkneading the dough toughens it. ∗ Wet your hands to knead sticky dough. ∗ Use an oven liner to catch spills, but not a cookie sheet. It will make the bottom crust soggy.

A Word About Vanilla Extract

Hard to find a great baking recipe that does not include vanilla extract. Many gluten-free bakers assume that vanilla and other flavored extracts are pure and natural and gluten free because the alcohol distilling processes renders gluten safe for consumption. (See page 25 for full explanation.) That is true, but not all extracts are equal. Many commercial brands contain additives and list corn syrup as an ingredient and some even contain sulfites. If you are allergic to additives as well as gluten-free, or determined not to consume GMO ingredients, you will do well to read the small print. For our purposes going forward, all recipe ingredient lists assume pure gluten-free vanilla.

The World's First Vegan Egg Yolk

The Vegg is a kind of miracle powder for vegans. No gluten, GMO, cholesterol, or other allergens, and free of animal products. Add water and you've got yourself an egg-free frittata, egg noodles, even vegan hollandaise. A full percent of all sales go to Compassion Over Killing, a nonprofit animal advocacy organization. Get the Vegg online or at natural foods retailers. www.thevegg.com

A Good Egg

Who can't boil an egg? You'd be surprised.

Here's a foolproof way to boil an easy-to-peel, perfect egg. Cage-free and organic should go without saying. Never, under any circumstances, cook an egg that's cracked. Resolve to examine every egg in the box next time.

- Place eggs in a pot and cover with cold water.
- Add a teaspoon of baking soda or salt. Either will keep shells from sticking.
- Bring the water to a rolling boil and cook for about 6 to 10 minutes based on the size of the eggs.
- Remove the pot from the heat and let sit for another 6 to 10 minutes.
- Pour out some water and replace with ice cubes. Let the eggs cool.
- Crack the eggs on the counter and roll the shells between your fingers until you feel them sliding off. Peel the eggs. Refrigerate immediately.

Egg White Sleight of Hand

You'll need two small bowls to play this slippery shell game:

+ Crack an egg in half over one bowl, as clean a crack as you can, no shells.
+ Let the yolk slide back and forth from one shell to another, allowing the white to run into the bowl.
+ Keep transferring the yolk back and forth until all of the white is in the bowl and you're left with a clean yolk.
+ Place the yolk in the second bowl and reserve it for another use.
+ Repeat.

How to Blanch Vegetables

Want bright color and crunchy texture without boiling all the nourishment out of your vegetables? Bring a pot of salted water to a rolling boil. (The salt causes the vegetable to retain vitamins.) Have a bowl of ice water ready next to the sink. Add the vegetables to the boiling water and blanch until crisp tender—about 40 seconds for green beans, snap peas, and other thin vegetables, and about 2 minutes for thicker vegetables like cauliflower, broccoli, and carrots. Drain and immediately plunge into the ice water to shock the cooking process into a sudden halt. Instant crudités.

Deconstructing the Artichoke

You know there's a heart in there somewhere, but where?

+ Remove an inch off the top of the artichoke with a serrated knife. Think flattop haircut.
+ Trim the stem and peel off any withered or black leaves.
+ Snap off the small leaves around the bottom and, with kitchen shears, trim any pointy and sharp edges on the remaining leaves.
+ If you are steaming the artichoke, leave the prickly choke intact. It will pull away easily after cooking.
+ If you are stuffing the artichoke, pry it open and pull out the choke with a melon scoop.

The simplest and best way to eat a whole steamed artichoke is to peel off the leaves, dip them, one at a time, into a good vinaigrette dressing, and scrape off the fleshy part of the leaf with your front teeth (very similar to Oreo cookie–eating technique) and leave the scraped leaf on the side of your plate, working your way to the grand finale—the tender heart.

How to Tell a Ramp from a Leek and Everything in Between

You're at the farmers' market and frankly you're a little confused. You've eaten ramps at restaurants and like their tender leaves and garlicky vibe, but what the heck do they look like, and how do I know I'm not buying scallions or spring onions or leeks?

Think bulbs.

From small to large in the order I just mentioned them:

+ Ramps are tiny with tender leaves and a very small bulb to snip and stir into egg dishes or to grill intact.
+ Scallions are the most familiar, with their green stems and white bulb usually chopped and served raw.
+ A spring onion is a bit bigger and more like an onion, with its purple bulb, but with a mellower flavor.
+ Leeks are the best of both garlic and onion and require a bit of braising before incorporating into recipes.

Aw, Shucks

You've traded fresh organic corn for the frozen GMO variety. You are not bashful about stripping down a bit of the husk to examine the kernels before you toss it in your market bag. You cook it the same day you buy it because you know that's when it's at its sweetest. You've husked each ear and stripped off the silk over newspaper to catch all of the clingy filaments. You've boiled the water and turned it off at its highest roll. You've dropped in the corn, covered the pot, and let it get tender for about twenty minutes. You're a corn connoisseur.

Except when it's time to get the kernels off the cob. No matter how neat you try to be, you end up with kernels all over the floor and counter.

Here's a simple trick.

Place a small bowl, upside down, inside a big bowl, so that it's sitting in the bottom of the big bowl. Stand the shucked ear on top of the upside-down bowl. With a sharp knife, working from top to bottom, cut the kernels off the ear. They'll collect in the large bowl. How easy is that?

Souper Confused

What's the difference between stock, broth, and bouillon? Soup stock is the gold standard for soup making. It is the stuff of bones and meat scraps, leftover vegetables, corncobs, aromatic herbs, and peppercorns, cooked down for hours, strained, and frozen to be used for soup and other recipes. Broth is a commercially available version of homemade stock. Some brands are gluten-free; some are not. Bouillon is dehydrated stock in little cubes or granules. It's intensely salty, full of MSG and other additives. Use when all else fails.

How to Make Spectacularly Simple Non-Processed Vegetable Side Dishes

Who needs limp green beans, overboiled carrots, broccoli, and cauliflower, and frozen side dishes when you've got the fresh, real, and naturally gluten-free thing staring you in the face? If it got any easier to do vegetables and greens, they'd sauté themselves.

Foolproof formula: Sauté pan + olive oil + garlic + greens = really simple, sensational side dish.

Enough with the Spinach!

Get out of your comfort zone with collard greens, bok choy, mustard greens, dandelion greens, kale, beet greens, turnip greens, Swiss chard, and escarole.

How to Roast Vegetables So People Will Actually Want to Eat Them

1. Preheat the oven to 400°F.
2. Scrub, trim, peel, and cut into 2-inch chunks your choice of hard vegetables, such as cauliflower, broccoli, beets, carrots, turnips, sweet potatoes, white potatoes, onions, asparagus, eggplant, zucchini, or celery root.
3. Toss with salt and freshly ground pepper, olive oil or white truffle oil, and dried rosemary.
4. Roast without stirring for about 20 minutes. Then stir or turn vegetables with tongs.
5. Give them another 20 to 45 minutes, depending on the hardness of the vegetables, or until they are golden brown and easily pierced with a fork.
6. Sprinkle with something aromatic, like fresh rosemary or basil.

Old New York Proverb:

A nickel will get you on the subway, but garlic will get you a seat.

What to Do with Vegetables Once You've Roasted Them (Besides Parking Them Next to a Protein)

1. Broiled open-faced roasted vegetable sandwich with fresh mozzarella on gluten-free baguette.
2. Roasted vegetables and cheese panini on gluten-free quinoa bread.
3. Chilled roasted vegetable salad with sun-dried tomatoes and greens.
4. Vegetable turkey hash: Add chopped chicken or turkey to the vegetables, melt a little butter in a pan, mash it all down, and cook on one side until it's brown and crisp, then flip and do the other. Finish by frying an egg on top.

Braising

A slow-cooking method, the slower the better, by which meats are dusted with a bit of all-purpose gluten-free flour, seared or browned in fat or oil, and then simmered on a very low heat in a small amount of liquid, usually wine, until tender and falling off the bone. This is usually done in a deep skillet or Dutch oven with plenty of room for the juices to accumulate and create a richly flavored sauce. Classic examples are Greek braised leg of lamb, osso buco or braised veal shanks, and brisket. No need to go for the expensive cuts. You could cook a shoe this way, and it would taste good.

Wilting Greens

After sautéing garlic or onion or mushrooms in a bit of butter or olive oil, toss in the greens of your choice, cover the pan, and wait about 2 minutes. The greens will be nicely wilted. Stir to coat the greens with the sauce. Or let your soup do the wilting. Toss in the greens at the final stage. Cover and wait for about 2 minutes. Stir. Same principle as going out on a damp day and feeling, well, wilted.

The Art of Stir-Fry

Always start with hot oil. Use a pan with high, sloping sides. Always cut vegetables and meats the same size. Start with foods that take the longest and cook in descending order, the fastest last. Sauté in quick succession, pushing the cooked foods out along the sides of the pan as you do the next batch. Experiment with gluten-free fish sauce, hoisin sauce, or teriyaki sauce.

5. Fold into an omelet with cheese.
6. Toss with pasta and a little pesto sauce.

The Art of Goi Cuon (Vietnamese Rice Wrapper or Spring Roll)

These lovely paper-thin, gluten-free rice wraps found in Asian markets are well worth getting the hang of handling. Make sure you buy Vietnamese rice paper rather than the thicker Chinese version, which can tear more easily.

+ Fill a bowl with warm water mixed with a little sugar and cider vinegar and soak the wraps for 4 to 5 seconds, until they are pliable but not falling apart.
+ Pluck them out, lay them flat, and keep them separate to prevent sticking.
+ Fill, but not overly, with bits of peeled cooked shrimp, or slivers of chicken or pork, or rice vermicelli, bits of lettuce, radish, bean sprout, mint, or cilantro.
+ Fold one corner over the filling, then both ends (think gift wrap), and roll, brushing a little water over the end that isn't folded to seal. Cover with a clean dish towel to prevent drying out.

How to Choose a Nice Piece of Safe, Eco-Friendly Fish

You know you should load up on your omega-3s and eat fish twice a week, but what about all the mercury and PCBs (polychlorinated biphenyls) and other pollutants floating around out there? What to do besides buying tired old tilapia? *U.S. News and World Report* says it's important to think small, sustainable, and wild. Consider buying farmed fish, too, as long as it's from US farmers using aquaculture techniques that don't pollute or allow farmed fish to escape into the wild. Some high-omega-3 suggestions:

+ Wild-caught Pacific sardines
+ Wild-caught Alaska salmon
+ Wild-caught anchovies
+ U.S.-farmed rainbow trout
+ U.S.-farmed or wild-caught striped bass
+ U.S.-farmed barramundi (a.k.a. Asian sea bass)
+ Wild-caught Arctic char
+ Wild-caught Pacific halibut

At the Fish Counter

Never buy a fish that has been color-enhanced.
Never buy a fish whose eyes are cloudy.
Never buy a fish that smells, well, fishy.

~ A Good Rule: Fish, like guests,
keeps for two days! ~

Poachers Welcome

Many a jaw-dropping and naturally gluten-free dessert is overlooked because we've gotten it into our heads that poaching fruit is hard to do.
This couldn't be further from the truth.

Basic Poached Fresh Fruits

1. Choose firm pears, apricots, plums, or peaches.
2. Combine water or white wine or red wine or orange juice and/or lemon juice with sugar, honey, agave syrup, or maple syrup.
3. Add vanilla, cinnamon stick, cloves, fresh ginger, lavender, rosemary, thyme, cardamom, or star anise.
4. Add the fruit and bring to a boil. Reduce the heat and simmer uncovered until the fruit begins to soften, anywhere from 10 to 25 minutes, depending on the fruit and its size.

Does It Pass the Smell Test?

If you've ruined whipped cream with a fishy or onion-scented spatula, you know what I mean when I say you need to smell your utensils, cutting boards, salad bowls, and coffee and spice grinders before you use them. Sniff out the culprits that can ruin a nice dinner.

5. With a slotted spoon, transfer the fruit to a platter, cutting the bottoms, if necessary, to make them stand up.

6. Cook the poaching liquid until it's reduced by half to two-thirds. Pour the syrup over fruit and serve with ice cream, whipped cream, fresh mint, or a few caramels or chocolates.

Basic Sweet Reduction for Dried Fruits

1. Combine 1 cup juice, or wine, or calvados, or balsamic vinegar and up to 8 tablespoons honey, sugar, agave syrup, or maple syrup.

2. Add rosemary and/or thyme and/or lavender and/or spices like cinnamon stick, nutmeg, cloves, and vanilla.

3. Add dried prunes, mission figs, apricots, apples, cranberries, and/or cherries.

4. Boil the mixture until syrupy and reduced by half.

5. Chill. Serve over ice cream, sponge cake (see recipe, page 153), with sweetened cream or yogurt and slivers of toasted almonds.

What to Do with Fresh Figs

1. Eat whole or chop into yogurt or cereal.

2. Mash with a bit of honey and spread on a sandwich.

3. Roast with a little olive oil, quartered, so they open like flowers. Heat a little cream and honey for a minute, then drizzle over the fruit. Add mint. Sprinkle with pine nuts or pistachios.

4. Quarter, stuff with goat cheese, and roast. Drizzle with honey and mint or basil.

5. Poach using the method above (see page 149) in red wine and fresh herbs.

6. Split and roast with honey. Serve with crème fraîche.

7. Cut an X three-quarters of the way through the figs from the top and stuff with Saint André or Brie. Sprinkle with thyme. Roast for 5 minutes.

Stinky Cheese Trick They'll Thank You For

If you are able to eat soy, combine a scant ounce of pungent, oozy, gorgeous cheese like Époisses, Pont l'Évêque, or Taleggio with an entire package of silken tofu. Mix well and refrigerate overnight, letting the chameleon of foods absorb the flavor of the cheese. It will taste creamy and sinful, but isn't. No need to use the T word.

A CLASSIC SALADE NIÇOISE

If you can pull off a classic Niçoise (pronounced "nee-SWAZ") made with fresh green beans and French potato salad, you've got the perfect unprocessed lunch or dinner, a tribute to fresh ingredients and simple technique. A far cry from the overly dressed, trumped-up, seared tuna and otherwise limp concoctions found on all but a few menus, this one was inspired by the doyenne of French cuisine, Julia Child herself. This simplified version was adapted from her much-used tutorial, *Mastering the Art of French Cooking*, and has been in my arsenal for as long as I have known how to boil water. With a few items from the farmers' market, this essential salad comes straight from the pantry.

SERVES 6 TO 8

1. To prepare the green beans: In a large pot, add the salt to 6 quarts of water and bring to a boil.
2. Drop in the beans, cover, and return to a boil. Uncover the pot and boil the beans gently for 3 to 4 minutes, or until they are tender and still have a slight crunch. Drain.
3. Plunge the beans into a bowl of ice water to stop the cooking. Drain, pat dry, and let cool in the refrigerator.
4. To make the potato salad: While the green beans are cooling, put the potatoes into a steamer basket in a large saucepan with a few inches of water. Bring the water to a boil. Reduce the heat, cover, and let the potatoes steam until fully cooked, about 20 minutes. Peel and slice the potatoes, approximately 1/4- to 1/2-inch thick. Set aside.
5. In a large bowl, blend together the wine, water, shallots, olive oil, salt, and pepper. Very gently toss the potatoes with the dressing. Set aside to cool.
6. To make the dressing: In a screw-top jar, place the mustard, shallot, lemon juice, salt, and pepper. Pour in the olive oil and shake. Add more salt and pepper, if necessary.
7. To arrange the salad: To avoid an overly dressed salad, toss only the Boston lettuce leaves with the dressing and arrange on a platter or on individual dinner plates. Spoon the potato salad into center and arrange boiled eggs, anchovies, tomatoes, beans, and tuna into a pleasing design. Scatter with the capers, black olives, and parsley. Serve with a gluten-free baguette.

For the green beans:
1½ teaspoons salt
1½ pounds crisp green beans, strings removed and ends snapped off

For the potato salad:
1½ pounds small red potatoes, gently scrubbed
1/3 cup dry white wine
1/3 cup water
1 tablespoon shallots, minced
3 tablespoons extra-virgin olive oil
Salt and freshly ground black pepper to taste

For the dressing:
½ tablespoon Dijon mustard
½ tablespoon shallot, finely minced
1 tablespoon freshly squeezed lemon juice
Salt and freshly ground black pepper to taste
½ cup extra-virgin olive oil

For the salad:
1 head of Boston lettuce, leaves snapped, washed, and dried
6 large eggs, hard-boiled and quartered
1 2-ounce can oil-packed anchovy fillets
3 to 4 ripe tomatoes, quartered
2 5-ounce cans light, oil-packed chunk tuna
2 tablespoons capers
10 black, brine-packed Niçoise olives
½ cup fresh parsley, chopped
Salt

The Icing on the Carrot Cake

Ditch the canned frosting. Forget the high-fructose corn syrup, additives, and trans fats. Okay, there's butter and sugar, but hey, this is carrot cake. Or come to think of it, red velvet. Sometimes all you have to do is read the package.

ESSENTIAL CREAM CHEESE FROSTING

---

1 8-ounce package Philadelphia cream cheese, softened
¼ cup (½ stick) unsalted butter, softened
½ tablespoon vanilla extract
1 16-ounce package confectioners' sugar, sifted

ENOUGH TO ICE TWO 8- OR 9-INCH LAYERS

1. In the large bowl of an electric mixer, beat the cream cheese, butter, and vanilla on medium speed until well blended.
2. Add the sugar gradually, beating after each addition, until well blended.
3. Slather the frosting on cooled red velvet, carrot, or spice cake. Lick fingers. Repeat.

AFFOGATO: TEMPEST IN A COFFEE CUP

I first tasted this amazingly simple and totally satisfying dessert at Chez Panisse and was determined to duplicate it at home. It's nothing more than ice cream in a coffee cup, any flavor you choose (I am partial to the double wallop of coffee ice cream), splashed with finely chopped chocolate, or rum or espresso, or a little of each. If you've got a pint of ice cream and a chocolate bar hidden away, you've got skills.

1. Put any flavor ice cream or gelato you like into a coffee cup.
2. Sprinkle with chocolate bits.
3. Splash with a little liquor or dark rum.
4. Pour espresso over the top.

The Best Way to Zest

The grated zest of thick-skinned citrus fruits—like oranges, lemons, and limes—imparts a rich flavor to many recipes. Before you get out the Microplane, scrub the fruit vigorously with a wire brush to remove any pesticide residue that may linger on the skin.

A SIMPLE SPONGE CAKE FOR YOUR REPERTOIRE

A sponge cake is just that, a blank, eminently infusible canvas for all the fabulous gluten-free desserts you can think of. No need to rely on the less than ideal store-bought variety, which may be full of the sorts of things you've sworn off. This Victoria sponge comes with permission from Nigella Lawson's *How to Eat: The Pleasures and Principles of Good Food*, as part of Nigella Lawson's Proper English Trifle, on page 240. Cornstarch gives it a feathery lightness and it can be blended in a food processor to dispense with the bother of all the creaming most cakes require. Let the butter get very soft or it won't blend well. Always use organic eggs. Substitute soy or almond milk for whole milk if necessary.

MAKES TWO 8-INCH LAYERS

1. Preheat oven to 350°F. Butter two 8-inch round pans.
2. Put all the ingredients, except milk, into a food processor and process to mix. When everything is well mixed, process while pouring the milk through the funnel. You want a batter of a soft, dropping consistency. Add more milk if necessary.
3. Pour the batter into the prepared pans and bake for about 25 minutes. When ready, the tops should spring back when pressed and a cake tester or fine skewer should come out clean.
4. Let the cakes stand in their pans for a minute or so and then turn them onto a wire rack to cool. Sandwich together with cream, jam, crushed fresh raspberries, or whatever you like. Sprinkle with superfine sugar. Or reserve, plain, for any number of desserts.

1 cup (2 sticks) very soft unsalted butter, plus more to butter the pans
1½ cups all-purpose gluten-free flour
¼ cup cornstarch
1 cup plus 2 tablespoons superfine sugar
2 teaspoons baking powder
1½ teaspoons vanilla extract or zest of ½ lemon or orange, depending on the flavor you want
4 large eggs
2 tablespoons milk, plus more if needed

Now what?

+ Use for English trifle.
+ Soak in orange liqueur or brandy and top with poached fruits.
+ Soak in coffee and rum and top with ice cream, mascarpone, and chocolate curls.
+ Spread with one layer of jam, then another of jam and beaten cream. Roll. Freeze. Sprinkle with confectioners' sugar. Slice.
+ Fill with pears, plums, apricots, fresh figs, peaches, blueberries, strawberries, or raspberries macerated with sugar.

Macerate

To make soft or to break down, usually by soaking. Sprinkling a bit of sugar over fresh berries, peaches, apricots, and pears draws out the liquid and softens the fruit to use as fillings or to top gluten-free French toast, ice cream, and other frozen desserts.

Rising to the Occasion

Everybody's got to have one spectacular culinary magic trick. Soufflés may sound fancy and they do impress the pants off people, but they are really simple to pull off with ingredients you've most likely already got on hand.

Follow these hard-and-fast rules and you can't go wrong:

+ Always handle egg whites gently. Imagine you are mixing clouds.
+ As tempting as it may be, never open the oven to check on the soufflé.
+ A soufflé waits for no one. The second it comes out of the oven, take it, triumphant, to the table.

CLASSIC CHEESE SOUFFLÉ

Here are two classics—cheese soufflé and chocolate soufflé—one savory, one sweet, rendered gluten-free by Shola Olunloyo, globe-hopping chef and StudioKitchen master teacher. In the bargain, you get to learn how to make a gluten-free béchamel sauce. Potato starch creates the spectacular effect. As with all uncomplicated foods, buy the best ingredients you can find.

SERVES 8

8 8-ounce ramekins
Nonstick cooking spray or melted butter
Gluten-free flour for dusting ramekins
¼ cup (½ stick) unsalted butter
3 tablespoons potato starch
2 cups half-and-half
Salt, freshly ground black pepper, and ground nutmeg to taste
2 large egg yolks
Fresh thyme to taste
4 ounces (1 cup) Gruyère cheese, grated, plus extra to sprinkle over the soufflés
5 large egg whites

1. Preheat oven to 375°F. Spray the ramekins with nonstick cooking spray or brush with melted butter and coat with gluten-free flour, coating the bottom and sides evenly. Refrigerate to chill and set.
2. To prepare the béchamel sauce, in a medium saucepan, melt the butter over low heat. Add the potato starch and whisk until well blended. Add all of the half-and-half at once and whisk to blend. Raise the heat to medium and whisk frequently, paying particular attention to scraping the bottom of the pan so that it doesn't burn.
3. When the mixture thickens, reduce the heat to low and season with salt, pepper, and nutmeg to taste. Remove from the heat and pass the mixture through a fine strainer to remove any lumps. Cool over a bowl of ice. When cool, whisk the egg yolks, thyme to taste, and cheese into the sauce. (Béchamel can be made a day ahead and refrigerated.)
4. In the bowl of a stand mixer or with a handheld electric whisk, whisk the egg whites until they form firm peaks. Fold the whites into the

béchamel and cheese mixture, a third at a time, with a rubber spatula. Fold gently until well combined, without losing too much volume on the egg whites.

5. Spoon the combined batter into ramekins to just below the rim. Sprinkle the tops with the additional cheese. (Soufflés can be chilled in the refrigerator for about 1 hour or baked immediately.) Bake for 15 to 20 minutes, until the tops are puffed and golden. Serve immediately. Take a bow.

DARK CHOCOLATE SOUFFLÉ

SERVES 8

1. Preheat oven to 375°F. Brush the ramekins with the melted butter and coat with cocoa powder (foil ramekins should be well coated). Chill in the refrigerator.

2. In a large bowl or double boiler, melt the chocolate and the remaining 8 tablespoons butter together over simmering water. Stir together with a rubber spatula until smooth. Let the mixture cool slightly.

3. In the bowl of a mixer, whisk the eggs, sugar, and vanilla at high speed until tripled in volume. Fold one-third of the egg/sugar mixture into the chocolate/butter mixture. Add the rice flour. Fold in the rest of the egg/sugar mixture carefully.

4. Fill the ramekins to just below the rim. Soufflés can be kept in the refrigerator at this point for up to 24 hours.

5. Bake for 12 to 15 minutes, or until the soufflés have risen and are slightly liquid in the middle. Make an entrance. Serve straight from the ramekins.

8 8-ounce ramekins, ceramic or foil
½ cup (1 stick) unsalted butter, plus melted unsalted butter for coating the ramekins
Cocoa powder for dusting the ramekins
½ pound semisweet chocolate, chopped into small chunks
5 large eggs
½ cup sugar
1 teaspoon vanilla extract
3 tablespoons rice flour, sifted

Learn to Make a Healthy Loaf of Bread

Not because there aren't wonderful gluten-free bakery loaves to be gotten in half the time. There are.

Not because you can't pick up a commercial loaf or a mix that's decent. You can.

Not because you have the time, which sometimes you don't.

But because there is nothing more satisfying than sitting in a fragrant kitchen, slicing into a still-warm loaf, and knowing you have produced something alive and irresistible.

You'll want to ask yourself, If I can do this, what else can I do?

SWEET POTATO ROSEMARY BREAD

You don't have to be gluten-free to love this nourishing, protein-rich, and fiber-rich essential loaf. Sweet potato gives it its earthy color, maple syrup its sweetness, and rosemary its rich Tuscan aroma. With thanks to Jennifer Katzinger and Flying Apron Bakery. Reprinted with permission from *Flying Apron's Gluten-Free and Vegan Baking Book* (Sasquatch Books).

MAKES 1 LOAF

3½ cups brown rice flour, plus more for dusting the work surface
1 cup garbanzo bean flour
¼ cup flax meal
½ tablespoon dried rosemary
¾ teaspoon sea salt
¾ teaspoon xanthan gum
¼ cup extra-virgin olive oil
¼ cup maple syrup
1 cup lukewarm water (94°F)
½ tablespoon cake yeast
1 cup puréed sweet potatoes or yams

1. Preheat the oven to 300°F. Lightly oil a baking pan or pizza stone. Dust your work surface liberally with brown rice flour.
2. In a large bowl, combine the brown rice flour, garbanzo bean flour, flax meal, rosemary, salt, and xanthan gum. In the bowl of a standing mixer fitted with a dough hook, combine the olive oil, maple syrup, water, and yeast. As soon as the yeast is activated (the mixture will look cloudy and bubbles should form on the surface, about 3 to 5 minutes), turn the mixer on low speed.
3. Add the flour mixture and sweet potatoes alternately, a little at a time, until just incorporated, being careful not to overmix. (Note: You can mix the dough by hand. Simply add the flour mixture and sweet potatoes alternately to the oil mixture and mix until just incorporated.)
4. Once all of the ingredients are incorporated, remove the dough from the bowl and quickly and gently knead it three or four times on your floured surface. Shape the dough into a 12-inch-long loaf.
5. Moving quickly, place the loaf on the prepared baking pan or pizza stone. Lightly slash the loaf along the length of the top; this will allow excess air to escape so that the bread does not crack.
6. Bake until a knife inserted deep into the center of the loaf comes out clean, about 2 hours 5 minutes.
7. Let cool.

CHICKPEA SOCCA

Who says bread must be made of flour? In Mediterranean seacoast towns like Nice and Naples, where borders blur, little chickpea crepes called socca abound. Street vendors wrap them around anchovies, black olive tapenade, hard-boiled eggs, and saucisson. A thin batter will make a crispier socca, a thick one results in a soft chickpea bread to butter or to dip into a pool of rosemary- or basil-scented olive oil. Bryan Sikora, owner of La Fia in Wilmington, Delaware, first made these for me. Now they're a house staple, full of protein and a regular in the breadbasket.

MAKES 20

1. In a medium bowl, mix the chickpea flour, water, olive oil, and salt. Pour the batter into a hot crepe pan, tilting to coat pan in an even layer of batter.
2. Cook on one side until golden brown. (For thicker crepes, you may have to flip and cook on the other side.)
3. Remove the socca from the pan and set aside to crisp in a warm place (near the pilot light or in a warm oven that has been turned off).
4. Repeat until all of the batter is used.

1 cup chickpea flour
1 cup water
¼ cup olive oil
1 tablespoon salt

The Art of Bread Crumbs

Of course you can buy gluten-free bread crumbs, but this is something more wholesome and maybe a bit more frugal. It is so much easier to produce and far better than those bags of sawdust. Crab cakes, anyone?

1. Cut the crust off a loaf of slightly stale, but still somewhat pliable, gluten-free bread. Cut the bread into chunks and crumb them in the bowl of a food processor.
2. Spread the crumbs onto a plate and let them dry out a bit more.
3. Pop them into a ziplock bag and store in the freezer. Use them straight out of the bag. No need to defrost.
4. For superfine crumbs, leave the bread out to get really, really dry before crumbing.

Learn More

ESSENTIAL READING

Cook with Jamie: My Guide to Making You a Better Cook by Jamie Oliver
(Hyperion)

Flying Apron's Gluten-Free and Vegan Baking Book by Jennifer Katzinger
(Sasquatch Books)

How to Cook Everything: The Basics by Mark Bittman (Wiley)

In the Green Kitchen: Techniques to Learn by Heart by Alice Waters
(Clarkson Potter)

Risotto: Delicious Recipes for Italy's Classic Rice Dish by Maxine Clark
(Ryland Peters & Small)

Seductions of Rice by Jeffrey Alford (Artisan)

Shola Olunloyo Studio Kitchen—Blog, tastes, menus.
www.studiokitchen.com.

*Stir-Frying to the Sky's Edge: The Ultimate Guide to Mastery, with
Authentic Recipes and Stories* by Grace Young (Simon and Schuster)

*Vegetable Literacy: Cooking and Gardening with Twelve Families from the
Edible Plant Kingdom* by Deborah Madison (Ten Speed Press)

The Way to Cook by Julia Child (Knopf)

SAFE SEAFOOD

Wallet- and purse-size cards for ordering and buying safe seafood.
www.seafoodwatch.com

ESSENTIAL EQUIPMENT

Chefs Catalog. www.chefscatalog.com

Kitchen Krafts. www.kitchenkrafts.com

Sur La Table. www.surlatable.com

Williams-Sonoma. www.williams-sonoma.com

Cooking with the Stars

'Tis an ill cook who cannot lick his own fingers.
—SHAKESPEARE, *ROMEO AND JULIET*

- ◆ Alice Waters: *Moroccan Braised Eggplant*
- ◆ Traci Des Jardins: *Grilled Corn and Squash Salad with Chipotle Crema, Lime Vinaigrette, and Cotija Cheese*
- ◆ Thomas Keller: *Bouchon Bakery Gluten-Free Brioche Rolls*
- ◆ Rick Bayless: *Quesadillas Asadas • Essential Chopped Tomato-Serrano Salsa*
- ◆ Molly O'Neill: *Corn and Lobster Pie in a Chili-Polenta Crust*
- ◆ Aimee Olexy: *A Trio of Savory Sides: Cauliflower with Fontina Mornay, Nutmeg, and Bread Crumbs • Pan-Roasted Mushrooms Galore with Fine Herbs and Shallots with Coriander Vinaigrette • Raw Radish and Cucumber Salad, Pine Nuts, Feta, Mint, and Sauvignon Blanc Vinaigrette*
- ◆ Katy Sparks: *Buckwheat Crepes Gratin with Cauliflower, Chanterelles, and Cave-Aged Gruyère*
- ◆ Steve DiFillippo: *Gluten-Free Gnocchi with Wild Mushrooms, Garlic, and White Truffle Oil*
- ◆ Kristine Kidd: *Arctic Char with Kumquat Gremolata, Roasted Fennel, and Potatoes*
- ◆ Marcie Turney: *Crispy Squash Blossoms Barbuzzo*
- ◆ Bobby Flay: *Saffron Risotto Cakes with Shrimp, Red Chili Oil, and Chive Oil*
- ◆ Michael Cole: *Beau Monde Cider-Brined Berkshire Pork Chops with Pumpkin Sage Risotto, Grilled Pear, Soubise Purée, and Smoked Balsamic Reduction*

My kitchen apron says SEPARATE THE WHEAT FROM THE CHEF! This is not something I wear to keep food from splattering all over the front of me, even though I am not the neatest cook in the world. I do it to entertain, to elicit questions, and to show everybody what it means to go through life *against the grain*. I wear it to put the world on notice that this kitchen is a gluten-free zone and this chef (I use the term loosely) can produce a meal everyone will enjoy without so much as a whiff of wheat or gluten. With its little pin, CELIACS DO IT GLUTEN-FREE, a gift from Elaine Monarch, visionary and founder of the Celiac Disease Foundation, my apron is a way of folding a little humor in with the egg whites as I wield my non-contaminated whisk.

These talismans are delicious proof that we can find joy and inspiration by not seeing the gluten-free diet as the end of something but rather as the beginning of a new and healthier relationship with food. A culinary adventure, actually. They remind me again and again of how generous professional chefs can be, creative souls who have made it their business to nourish us with their ideas and their deep-hearted love of good food.

When *Against the Grain* first debuted, most chefs had no idea what gluten was, much less how to cook gluten-free. Still, they took up the challenge. Life is too short for crustless pizza, mock apple pie, and rolls that taste like hockey pucks and fool no one. Who can forget Molly O'Neill's glorious Corn and Lobster Pie in a Chili-Polenta Crust (page 167), reprised here for this special edition? Or Alex Cormier's Bananas Financier, an exquisite almond torte with caramelized fruit and John Rivera Sedlar's Sweet Corn Soufflé with Passion Fruit and Chocolate Sauce? These miracles from that first book still appear in my kitchen when there is ample time.

This time around there is very little need for explanation. Special diets are a way of life in professional kitchens. They are a challenge to a chef's very nature. As often as not, we discover chefs who eat gluten-free themselves or have a gluten-free family member or good friend in need of something wonderful to eat. Necessity is still the mother of invention and nurtures the impulse of every chef I have had the pleasure of knowing.

As home cooks and as diners we, too, have become more sophisticated, more familiar with exotic foods and cooking techniques. Thanks to the Food Network, and the explosion of cooking shows, cookbooks, and magazines that have given birth to new culinary stars, our appetite for new recipes has never been more voracious. If you can't enjoy a meal at your own table, where can you?

I am amazed and honored by the stature of the chefs assembled here, the generosity represented on these pages, and the range of mouthwatering choices, many of them vegetarian. If you had any doubt, these good and gifted souls will prove once and for all that there has never been a better time to be gluten-free.

Read, learn, shop, chop, simmer, cook, lick your fingers, and share the results with those you cherish. Be glad you are that special.

With apologies to the Bard, *Ah, what foods these morsels be.*

Alice Waters

Icon, owner of the legendary Chez Panisse, food activist and visionary, founder of the Edible Schoolyard Project, Alice Waters is a tireless teacher and advocate for sustainability, as well as lobbyist in chief and muse for the first White House organic garden. Perhaps more than anyone in our time, she is responsible for revolutionizing the way we eat, cook, and think about food. Her deceptively simple dishes are the focus of a lifelong passion for flavor and reverence for locally produced, seasonal foods. The *New York Times* says she has "singlehandedly changed the American palate." I don't doubt it.

MOROCCAN BRAISED EGGPLANT

Reminiscent of a ratatouille, this gorgeous braised eggplant with its smoky North African heat is from *The Art of Simple Food II*. There is no greater argument for eating simply and buying only the freshest organic produce than this naturally gluten-free and vegan dish. As the flavors merge and layer, this tastes even better the next day. Double it for a crowd and serve over steamed basmati rice.

1 medium onion, peeled
½ large bunch of fresh cilantro
1 tablespoon extra virgin olive oil
1-inch piece of fresh ginger, peeled and minced
Large pinch of saffron
¼ teaspoon cayenne pepper
1 teaspoon cumin seeds, crushed
Salt to taste
4 Japanese eggplants, trimmed and cut into 1½-inch chunks
3 medium tomatoes, cored and cut into 1½-inch chunks
3 medium summer squash, cut into 1½-inch chunks (optional)

SERVES 4

1. Grate the onion on the coarse holes of a box grater.
2. Trim off the stem ends of the cilantro and cut the leaves away from the stems and set aside. Cut the stems finely.
3. In a 2-quart heavy-bottomed pot, heat the oil over medium heat. Add the grated onion and cook for 3 minutes. Stir in the cilantro stems, ginger, saffron, cayenne, cumin seeds, and salt and cook for 5 minutes.

4. Stir in eggplant, tomatoes, and, if you like, the summer squash. Reduce the heat to low and continue cooking uncovered at a simmer until the vegetables are soft, about 15 to 20 minutes. Check for salt and add more, if necessary.

5. Add half the chopped cilantro leaves to the vegetables and cook for 2 minutes.

6. Serve garnished with the rest of the chopped cilantro.

Traci Des Jardins

No matter that she has worked in some of the most acclaimed kitchens in Los Angeles, France, and New York, is a two-time James Beard Award–winner, founded the wildly successful San Francisco restaurants Jardinière, Acme Chophouse, and Mijita Cocina Mexicana and is one of the top female chefs in the country, Traci Des Jardins has never forgotten her roots on her family's farm in the San Joaquin Valley. With the same passion she brings to her food, this deeply committed chef and activist champions and works with hunger-relief organizations like Share Our Strength, Citymeals-on-Wheels, and her own charity, La Cocina. In the land of plenty, is there anything more important than making sure everyone eats?

GRILLED CORN AND SQUASH SALAD WITH CHIPOTLE CREMA, LIME VINAIGRETTE, AND COTIJA CHEESE

If ever there was a reason to go to the farmers' market, this vegetarian salad of bright and complex flavors is it. Relying on the freshest produce possible, it is the perfect foil for grilled vegetables, meat, and fish. Chipotle in adobo or chipotle purée and Cotija cheese can be found in Mexican markets. For the grated radish, try using a mandoline for the prettiest results.

SERVES 8

1. Brush the corn and toss the squash with 2 tablespoons of olive oil and season with salt and pepper. Grill over medium high until lightly browned.

2. In a mixing bowl, whisk together half of the lime juice, the extra-virgin olive oil, and salt and pepper.

3. Purée the chipotle in a mortar and pestle or in the bowl of a blender and add the crème fraîche. Add the remaining lime juice and a little water if necessary to bring to the consistency of cream.

4. In a mixing bowl, combine the squash and corn; add half of the lime vinaigrette, toss, and season with salt and pepper.

5. On each plate, or one long platter, spread the chipotle crema to form a thin layer. Place the squash-corn mixture in the middle. Toss the purslane and radishes in the remaining lime vinaigrette and place the leaves over the top. Top with Cotija cheese.

8 ears of corn, shucked and cut from the cob
4 assorted squash, zucchini, sunburst, yellow, and crookneck, sliced into ⅛-inch-thick pieces
2 tablespoons olive oil
Salt and freshly ground black pepper to taste
Freshly squeezed juice of 2 limes
¼ cup extra-virgin olive oil
1 chipotle in adobo or 1 tablespoon chipotle purée
¼ cup crème fraîche or sour cream
2 cups purslane
½ cup shaved radishes
1 ounce (¼ cup) grated Cotija cheese

Thomas Keller

Chef-proprietor of the legendary French Laundry, Per Se, Ad Hoc, Bouchon Bistro, and Bouchon Bakery, and author of visually stunning cookbooks (*The French Laundry Cookbook, Bouchon, Under Pressure: Cooking Sous Vide, Ad Hoc at Home,* and *Bouchon Bakery*), Thomas Keller is the only American chef who holds multiple and simultaneous three stars from the notoriously snooty Michelin Guide and has been accorded so many honors and awards, it would be impossible to list them all here. During an unforgettable and once-in-a-lifetime anniversary dinner at The French Laundry, I was served this gluten-free brioche the likes of which I thought I'd never taste again.

BOUCHON BAKERY GLUTEN-FREE BRIOCHE ROLLS

Using Chef Keller's Cup4Cup all-purpose gluten-free baking mix, these come via *Bouchon Bakery* by Thomas Keller and Sebastien Rouxel, executive pastry chef for the Thomas Keller Restaurant Group, twice declared to be one of the "Top Ten Best Pastry Chefs in America" by *Pastry Art and Design* magazine. You'll need egg wash, Maldon salt for sprinkling (found in specialty stores and fancy markets), and a 12-cup muffin pan prepared with nonstick spray. Gather yourself and breathe; they are easier than you think. Serve with rosemary-scented olive oil for a special dinner party, sliced as a mini sandwich, or spread with butter and French raspberry jam anytime you wish to transform an ordinary morning into something exquisite.

2 teaspoons instant yeast

1 tablespoon plus 2 teaspoons granulated sugar

¾ cup plus 2 tablespoons plus 1¾ teaspoons warm water (at 75°F)

3¾ cups plus 1 tablespoon Cup4Cup baking blend

2 tablespoons plus ¾ teaspoon kosher salt

½ cup plus 2 tablespoons eggs

1½ tablespoons egg yolks

¼ cup honey

7 tablespoons unsalted butter, melted and cooled

Egg wash (see recipe below)

1 tablespoon Maldon salt for sprinkling

MAKES 12 BRIOCHE ROLLS

1. In a small bowl, combine the yeast and sugar. Stir in the warm water, and set the bowl in a warm spot to proof (rise) for about 10 minutes, or until the yeast mixture is foaming and bubbly.

2. Meanwhile, in the bowl of a stand mixer fitted with the paddle attachment, combine the Cup4Cup and salt. Separately, in a medium bowl, whisk together the eggs, yolks, honey, butter, and proofed yeast mixture.

3. Turn the mixer to low speed and slowly add the egg mixture. Increase the speed to medium and mix the dough for 10 minutes. It will be very silky and not as stiff as regular bread dough.

4. Scrape down the sides of the bowl, cover with plastic wrap, and set the bowl in a warm spot until the dough has about doubled in size, about 1 hour.

5. Using a rubber spatula, deflate the dough, turning it over a few times in the bowl. Scrape down the sides of the bowl, cover the bowl tightly with plastic wrap, and refrigerate for 2 hours.

6. Spray the muffin pan with nonstick spray. Spoon ⅓ cup of the dough into each cup. Brush the tops of the rolls with egg wash, sprinkle with the Maldon salt, and set in a warm spot to proof uncovered for about 40 minutes, until they rise (but are not doubled) and spread slightly.

7. Preheat the oven to 350°F. Bake the rolls for 15 to 17 minutes, until the tops are a golden brown and a wooden skewer inserted in the center of a roll comes out clean.

8. Transfer to a wire rack and cool completely.

Egg Wash

1. Break 1 or more eggs, as needed, into a small bowl and whip with a fork or small whisk to combine the white(s) and yolk(s) well.

2. Strain through a fine mesh strainer before using.

Rick Bayless

There is no greater authority on Mexican cooking than Rick Bayless. This star chef and owner of Frontera Grill, Topolobampo, Xoco, Frontera Fresco, and Tortas Frontera has made a career of interpreting the depth and timeless flavors of old Mexico. These crusty griddle-baked quesadillas are from his Julia Child Cookbook Award–winning cookbook *Rick Bayless's Mexican Kitchen* and serve as a wonderful introduction to a country that is as near to heaven as the gluten avoidant can come. With thanks.

QUESADILLAS ASADAS

You can make quesadillas with ready-made corn tortillas, but the difference is worth the trouble of making them yourself. With peppery roasted poblano rajas, these cheesy, chewy stuffed tortillas are a marvel of texture, spice, and heat made by a master. Once you get the hang of laying down a thin circle of dough onto the griddle, spreading on the filling, and folding it over to bake until crusty, you may want to invest in a tortilla press.

MAKES 12 QUESADILLAS, SERVING 4 TO 6

1. Roast the chilies directly over a gas flame or 4 inches below a very hot broiler until blackened on all sides, about 5 minutes over the open flame, about 10 minutes under the broiler. Cover with a kitchen towel and let stand 5 minutes. Peel, pull out the stem and seed pod, then rinse briefly to remove any bits of skin and seeds. Slice into ¼-inch strips.

2. In an 8- or 9-inch skillet, heat the vegetable oil over medium to medium-high heat, then add the onion and cook, stirring frequently, until nicely browned but still a little crunchy, about 5 minutes. Add the garlic and oregano, toss a minute longer, then stir in the chilies and heat through. Taste and season with salt.

NOTE: Rajas can be made 2 days ahead; cover and refrigerate.

1. Cut two squares of medium-heavy plastic (a garbage bag works well) to cover the plates of your tortilla press. If necessary, knead a few more drops of water into the masa to give it the consistency of soft cookie dough, then roll it into 12 balls. Cover the dough with plastic. Divide the cheese into 12 equal portions, and cover with plastic.

2. Turn on the oven to the lowest setting. Heat a large griddle or heavy skillet over medium heat. Use the tortilla press to press out the dough one by one between the two sheets of plastic. Peel off the top sheet, then flip the uncovered side of the tortilla onto your hand (the top of the tortilla should align with your index finger, and your fingers should be slightly spread to give support).

3. Carefully peel off the plastic. Then, with a gentle, swift motion, lay the tortilla on the hot griddle. Evenly sprinkle on a portion of the cheese, leaving a ½-inch border all around so that the cheese doesn't run out onto the griddle, then lay a portion of the rajas down the center. When the tortilla comes free from the griddle (it will take about 20 seconds),

For 2 cups roasted poblano rajas:

1 pound fresh poblano chilies (6 medium-large)
1 tablespoon vegetable or olive oil
1 large white onion, cut into ¼-inch-thick slices
3 cloves garlic, finely chopped
1 teaspoon dried oregano, preferably Mexican
½ teaspoon salt or to taste

For the quesadillas:

1 pound (2 cups) fresh masa for tortillas or 1¾ cups masa harina mixed with 1 cup plus 2 tablespoons hot water
1½ cups shredded Mexican Chihuahua cheese or other melting cheese such as brick cheddar or Monterey Jack

use a spatula to fold it in half, and gently press the edges together, more or less sealing them.

4. Move the quesadilla to the side to continue baking as you begin the next one. Continue making and folding quesadillas, letting them bake on the griddle until crispy/crunchy and nicely browned (the masa on the inside will still be a little soft), 2 to 3 minutes in all.

5. Keep finished quesadillas warm on a rack set on a baking pan in the oven. When all are made, line them up on a warm serving platter or wooden board or a basket lined with a napkin, and serve with salsa below.

Essential Chopped Tomato-Serrano Salsa

For the salsa:

12 ounces ripe tomatoes (2 medium-small round tomatoes or 4 or 5 plum tomatoes)

Fresh serrano chilies to taste (roughly 3 to 5, or more if you like it spicy)

12 large sprigs of fresh cilantro

1 large clove garlic, very finely chopped

1 small white onion

1½ teaspoons freshly squeezed lime juice

¼ teaspoon salt or to taste

1. Core the tomatoes, then cut them in half and squeeze out the seeds if you wish (this will give the sauce a less rustic appearance). Finely dice the flesh by slicing it into ¼-inch-thick pieces, then cutting each slice into small dice. Scoop into a medium bowl.

2. Cut the chilies in half lengthwise (wear gloves if your hands are sensitive) and scrape out the seeds if you wish (this will make the salsa a little less spicy). Chop the chilies as finely as you can, then add them to the tomatoes.

3. Carefully bunch up the cilantro sprigs and, with a sharp knife, slice them ¹⁄₁₆-inch thick, stems and all, working from the leafy end toward the stems. Scoop into the tomato mixture, along with the garlic.

4. Finely dice the onion with a knife, scoop it into a small strainer, and then rinse it under cold water. Shake to remove any excess water and add to the tomato mixture.

5. Taste and season with lime juice and salt. Let stand a few minutes for the flavors to meld.

Molly O'Neill

I moved away from Manhattan years ago, but my Sundays still belong to the *New York Times*. There is nothing I like better than the slow, ritual unfolding of the paper, sipping tea, nibbling a gluten-free muffin, reading, clipping, circling, lazing my way through the *Book Review* and the *Magazine*. I still miss that final sweet moment reserved for Molly O'Neill's weekly rhapsody on food. I console myself with her gorgeous book, *One Big Table: A Portrait of American Cooking*, and her delicious memoir, *Mostly True*.

CORN AND LOBSTER PIE IN A CHILI-POLENTA CRUST

This, from *Play It by Ear* by Molly O'Neill, is not one of those meal-on-the-table-in-an-hour deals. It is not inexpensive. It requires the husking and cooking of fresh corn, the steaming of lobsters, and the coddling of a custard in something the French call a bain-marie, a method of resting one pot in another filled with water and cooking in the oven. Nice, but not necessary, would be a sunny kitchen with a porch overlooking an August sea, waves of Puccini in the background. Short of that, the act of creating such a beautiful dinner as this will transport the cook, as it has me, to this perfect summer place in the heart. With gratitude to the *New York Times*.

SERVES 6

To make the polenta:

1. In a medium saucepan, bring the water to a boil over high heat.
2. Stir together the cornmeal, chili powder, and salt and pepper. Whisking constantly, add the cornmeal mixture to the water in a slow, steady stream.
3. Switch to a wooden spoon, reduce the heat slightly, and cook, stirring constantly, until the mixture is very thick, about 25 minutes.
4. Spray a 9-inch pie plate with the olive oil spray and spoon the polenta into it. Place a large sheet of plastic wrap over the polenta and press it out with your hands so that the polenta covers the bottom and the sides of the pie plate evenly. Remove the plastic and set the dish aside.

For the polenta:
2¾ cups water
⅔ cup yellow cornmeal
1 teaspoon chili powder
¾ teaspoon salt
Freshly ground black pepper
  to taste
Olive oil spray (non-alcohol)

To make the custard:

1. Preheat oven to 350°F.
2. Wrap the garlic in aluminum foil and roast it in the oven until soft, about 45 minutes.
3. Reduce the temperature to 325°F.
4. Peel the garlic and place it in a large mixing bowl, and whisk to purée it. Add the eggs and whisk lightly. Add the milk, salt, and pepper, and whisk just until well combined. Stir in the corn.
5. Pour the mixture into the polenta shell. Place the pie plate in a large roasting pan and fill the pan with enough hot water to come halfway up the sides of the pie plate. Bake until the custard is set, about 1 hour.

For the custard:
3 large cloves garlic, unpeeled
2 large eggs
1 cup milk
1 teaspoon salt
Freshly ground black pepper
  to taste
Kernels from 2 large ears of
  corn (about 2 cups)

For the lobster mix:

Kernels from 1 large ear of corn (about 1 cup)

2 lobsters, steamed, tail and claw meat removed and diced into ½-inch cubes

1 red bell pepper and 1 yellow bell pepper, stemmed, cored, de-ribbed, and diced into ¼-inch cubes

1 jalapeño pepper, seeded and minced

1 tablespoon chopped fresh cilantro

2 scallions (white and green parts), chopped

1 tablespoon freshly squeezed lime juice

½ teaspoon salt, plus more to taste

Freshly ground black pepper to taste

To make the lobster mix:

1. Toss together the corn, lobster, bell peppers, jalapeño, cilantro, and scallions.

2. Add the lime juice, salt, and pepper. Taste and adjust seasoning, if needed.

3. Spoon the mixture evenly over the custard. Cut the pie into wedges and serve immediately.

Aimee Olexy

Owner, muse, and genius behind award-winning Talula's Garden and Talula's Daily on Washington Square in Philadelphia, as well as Talula's Table in Kennett Square, and pioneer of the Philly BYOB movement with the wildly popular Django, Aimee Olexy is one of the brightest stars in the farm-to-table firmament. She is also one of the country's most respected experts on artisan cheeses (see her spectacular Seven Sinful Cheeses on page 226). Steeped in big-city style and a passion for fresh, local, organic fruits and vegetables, Olexy's knowledge of and reverence for the care farmers and ranchers put into the foods they produce is the inspiration that shapes her menus.

A TRIO OF SAVORY SIDES

These sublime side dishes rely on the finest farmers' market produce you can find. Serve one or two for a casual lunch or all three as the main event. Piment d'Espelette, a dried pepper found in the south of France and similar to paprika, can be found in specialty stores. To sweat shallots, cook them in butter while keeping them white. For the cauliflower, try a mix of cheddar, purple, or green Romanesco varieties. Use different varieties of mushrooms and cucumbers. In order to duplicate Olexy's precise measurements, I would recommend using an inexpensive kitchen scale, rather than trying to convert to cups or tablespoons.

Cauliflower with Fontina Mornay, Nutmeg, and Bread Crumbs

SERVES 4

1. Bring a large pot of well-salted water to a boil and blanch the cauliflower until not quite tender, about 3 to 4 minutes. Set aside.

2. In a tall pot, melt the butter over medium heat. Add shallots, salt lightly, and sweat slightly. Once the shallots have begun cooking, add the flour and stir constantly with a wooden spoon until the flour-butter mixture is golden brown, taking care to cook the flour evenly and not allowing it to stick or burn.

3. Add the milk, slowly stirring with a whisk. As the milk warms, the flour will begin to thicken. Continue stirring frequently to prevent sticking. Keep a close eye on the mixture. When the sauce reaches a creamy texture, taste to make sure the flour is cooked completely. If grainy, cook a bit longer.

4. Remove the sauce from the heat and whisk in the Fontina, Piave Vecchio, and nutmeg. Season with salt and pepper to taste.

5. Stir in the cauliflower florets and mix thoroughly. Add the bread crumbs and mix again.

6. Serve immediately.

Pan-Roasted Mushrooms Galore with Fine Herbs and Shallots with Coriander Vinaigrette

SERVES 4

1. Clean the mushrooms and slice them into uniform pieces, keeping each variety separate.

2. Heat up a large pan over medium-high heat and add a little olive oil. Add oil as needed to ensure the end result is not greasy. Allow the oil to get hot enough to slightly smoke.

3. Add the mushrooms, starting with the maitake and trumpet, allowing them to brown slightly as you roll them or toss them around in the pan. Next add the oyster mushrooms, allowing them to brown evenly and adding more oil as needed, cooking until any moisture released by the mushrooms dries.

4. Add the shiitake and crimini mushrooms, along with oil, if needed. Brown them and cook their juices down to concentrate the flavor.

5. Add the shallots. At this point, the mushrooms should have a nice color. Season with salt and pepper, moving quickly to keep the shallots from burning.

For the cauliflower gratin:

3 heads of cauliflower—cheddar, purple, or Romanesco cauliflower, broken into bite-size florets

6 tablespoons (¾ stick) unsalted butter, cubed

3 shallots, minced

Salt to taste

3 ounces gluten-free all-purpose flour

1 quart cold whole milk

4 ounces Fontina Val d'Aosta, grated

2 ounces Piave Vecchio or Parmesan, grated

¼ teaspoon fresh nutmeg, finely grated

Freshly ground black pepper to taste

2 cups gluten-free bread crumbs or gluten-free panko crumbs

For the mushrooms:

Olive oil for cooking the mushrooms

10 ounces maitake mushrooms

6 ounces king trumpet mushrooms

2 ounces oyster mushrooms

6 ounces shiitake mushrooms

6 ounces crimini mushrooms

2 tablespoons shallots, minced

Salt and freshly ground black pepper

2 tablespoons fresh parsley, chopped

1 tablespoon fresh chives, minced

Dash of sherry vinegar or freshly squeezed lemon juice (optional)

For the coriander vinaigrette:

1 ounce garlic, minced
3 ounces shallots, minced
1 ounce fresh ginger, minced
1 cup sauvignon blanc vinegar
2 cups blended oil such as canola or avocado–olive oil blend
3 teaspoons coriander seeds, toasted and finely ground
1 teaspoon piment d'Espellette, or paprika if not available
1 tablespoon honey
½ cup extra-virgin olive oil
Salt and freshly ground pepper to taste

For the sauvignon blanc vinaigrette:

1 ounce garlic, minced
3 ounces shallots, minced
1 ounce fresh ginger, minced
1 cup sauvignon blanc vinegar
1 tablespoon honey
½ cup extra-virgin olive oil
Salt and freshly ground black pepper to taste

For the cucumber salad:

12 medium cucumbers, peeled and seeded
8 ounces Greek feta cheese
3 ounces fresh mint, torn into small pieces
15 radishes, sliced thin on a mandolin
4 ounces pine nuts, lightly toasted and crumbled

6. Once seasoned, add the parsley, chives, and a dash of sherry vinegar or a fresh squeeze of lemon.
7. Toss with Coriander Vinaigrette and serve immediately (recipe follows).

1. Mince the garlic, shallots, and ginger and mix them together in a small bowl. Add the vinegar to "cook" and season lightly with salt.
2. In a small saucepan, warm the blended oil gently over low heat. Add the coriander and piment d'Espelette, turn off the heat, and allow the mixture to steep as it cools down.
3. Once the oil is cool and the aromatics have been softened by the vinegar, add the honey to the oil and whisk until it is dissolved. In a stream, add the infused oil to the garlic-shallot-ginger-vinegar mixture and finish with the extra-virgin olive oil.
4. Season with salt and pepper to taste and set aside to toss with mushrooms.

Raw Radish and Cucumber Salad, Pine Nuts, Feta, Mint, and Sauvignon Blanc Vinaigrette

SERVES 4

Mix all ingredients well and reserve to dress the salad.

1. Cut the cucumbers into bite-size chunks, making jagged shapes for texture. Move the cucumbers to a serving bowl and dress evenly with the reserved vinaigrette. Let the cucumbers marinate for 10 minutes.
2. Mix the feta cheese into the cucumbers and the vinaigrette. If the cucumbers look dry, add more vinaigrette.
3. Just before serving, add mint and radishes, so they retain their crunch and bright color, and add crumbled pine nuts.

Note: Talula's Garden holds the nuts for last in case of allergy.

Katy Sparks

Her cookbook isn't called *Sparks in the Kitchen* for nothing. By the time this book goes to press, this culinary dynamo and veteran of Quilted Giraffe, Bolo, Mesa Grill, and Brooklyn's Union Market will have transformed New York's legendary Tavern on the Green into the prettiest table in town. Cozy and casual, perched on the western edge of Central Park, a meal here might be what it's like to dine inside a Rousseau painting. We couldn't imagine a more perfect backdrop for Sparks's thoroughly modern American simplicity and farm-to-table sensibility.

BUCKWHEAT CREPES GRATIN WITH CAULIFLOWER, CHANTERELLES, AND CAVE-AGED GRUYÈRE

The beauty of this latticed dish is in its assembly. No need for last-minute crepe making, always dicey when there's an audience. Crepes can be made a day ahead. Serve it as a hearty winter supper for four or as a side with something simple and roasted.

SERVES 6 TO 8 AS A SIDE DISH

To make the crepes:

1. In a medium bowl, place the flour. Whisk in the eggs, butter, milk, water, and salt.
2. Heat a 10-inch nonstick skillet over medium-high heat; brush the pan with the remaining melted butter.
3. Add ¼ cup of the batter to the skillet; tilt to coat the bottom. Cook the crepe, adjusting the heat to prevent burning, until golden on the bottom, 35 to 40 seconds. Using spatula, turn crepe over; cook 30 seconds. Transfer the crepe to a plate.
4. Repeat with the remaining batter, stacking the crepes between sheets of plastic wrap. The crepes can be made 1 day ahead. Cover and chill.
5. Remove the crepes from the refrigerator, cut into thin strips, and reserve.

To make the chanterelles:

1. Clean the mushrooms and slice them.
2. In a 10-inch sauté pan, heat the butter over medium heat, until foaming. Add the sliced mushrooms and the shallot and sauté until tender, about 2 minutes. Add the thyme, tarragon, and cream.
3. Season with salt and pepper and remove the pan from heat. Set aside.

To make the cauliflower:

1. Preheat the oven to 450°F.
2. Cut the cauliflower into small florets. Roast it uncovered in a 9×11-inch casserole dish with the cherry tomatoes, garlic, coriander, and lemon zest, and drizzled with olive oil, until the cauliflower is tender and a little browned, about 20 minutes. Season with salt and pepper and set aside.

To make the gratin:

1. Preheat oven to 400°F.
2. Butter a 9×11-inch gratin dish.

For the crepes:
1¼ cups gluten-free buckwheat flour
3 large eggs
¼ cup (½ stick) melted unsalted butter, plus additional for the skillet
¾ cup milk
1¼ cups water, or more as needed
¼ teaspoon sea salt

For the chanterelles:
¾ pound fresh chanterelles
1 tablespoon unsalted butter
1 shallot, minced
1 teaspoon fresh thyme, minced
1 teaspoon fresh tarragon, minced
¼ cup heavy cream
Sea salt and freshly ground black pepper to taste

For the cauliflower:
½ head of cauliflower
8 to 10 small whole cherry tomatoes
2 cloves garlic, minced
½ teaspoon crushed coriander seeds
½ teaspoon freshly grated lemon zest
1 tablespoon olive oil
Sea salt and freshly ground black pepper to taste

For the gratin:
Unsalted butter for greasing the gratin dish
½ cup heavy cream
6 ounces (1½ cups) grated cave-aged Gruyère

3. Add the cream and half of the Gruyère to the bowl with the crepes and toss to combine. Pour the mixture into the prepared gratin dish. Sprinkle the remaining Gruyère over the top of the crepes.

4. Bake uncovered until heated through and the cheese on top has browned, about 20 minutes. Serve hot.

Steve DiFillippo

Restaurant Hall of Famer, impresario of Davio's restaurants in Boston, Atlanta, and Philadelphia, and author of the bestselling business memoir, *It's All About the Guest*, Steve DiFillippo proves exceptional Italian food is a slam dunk on a gluten-free diet. Specializing in Northern Italian and regional classics handed down through his family, then giving them a modern edge, Chef DiFillippo doesn't just adapt to special diets, he takes them to a whole new level. If this is how the father of a daughter with celiac disease shows his love, we're all for it.

GLUTEN-FREE GNOCCHI WITH WILD MUSHROOMS, GARLIC, AND WHITE TRUFFLE OIL

Old World meets four-star. Handmade gnocchi made in the traditional way is the perfect foil for the woodsy depth of fresh, wild mushrooms and truffle oil. As with all simple dishes, this one relies on the best crimini, porcini, shiitake, portobello, or chanterelle mushrooms you can find. If you've never used highly flavored truffle oil, a little goes a long way. Enough for a spectacular dinner party.

For the gnocchi:
2 pounds (or about 3 large) Idaho potatoes, scrubbed and boiled in their skins until tender
2 ounces (½ cup) Parmesan cheese, finely grated
1 large egg
1 teaspoon salt
Freshly ground black pepper to taste
2 to 3 cups rice flour, plus more to flour the work surface and a rimmed baking sheet
Salted water for cooking gnocchi
Olive oil, to coat second rimmed baking sheet

MAKES APPROXIMATELY 4 DOZEN

1. Allow the cooked potatoes to cool slightly, then carefully peel while holding the potatoes with a kitchen mitt.

2. While still hot, purée the potatoes through a ricer or food mill into a large mixing bowl and allow the potatoes to cool completely before proceeding.

3. Add the Parmesan, egg, salt, and pepper to the potatoes and mix well.

4. Gradually add enough rice flour to form a smooth, slightly sticky dough. (You may not need all of the rice flour. It should stick to itself, but not to your hands. Avoid making it too dry.) Briefly knead the dough to incorporate the flour, being careful not to overwork the dough.

5. Bring a large pot of salted water to a rolling boil.

6. Cut the dough into 10 equal pieces and place 1 piece on a lightly floured work surface. Roll the piece into a long rope, about ½ inch in diameter, flouring lightly if needed. Cut the rope into ½ inch cubes. Repeat with each piece of dough, setting the formed gnocchi on a floured rimmed baking sheet.

7. Immediately add the gnocchi to the boiling water and continue cooking for 2 to 3 minutes, until they have risen to the top. Remove the cooked gnocchi with a slotted spoon or skimmer. Set aside on a rimmed baking sheet coated lightly with olive oil to prevent sticking while preparing the sauce.

1. Place a sauté pan over medium heat. When hot, add the olive oil and garlic. Brown slightly.

2. Add the wild mushrooms and toss well.

3. Cook the mushrooms for about 5 minutes or until slightly brown, tossing often.

4. Season to taste with salt and pepper. Add the truffle oil. Toss well.

5. Toss the mushrooms with the gnocchi and garnish with parsley and shaved Parmesan.

For the wild mushrooms, garlic, and white truffle oil:

3 tablespoons olive oil
3 cloves garlic, thinly sliced
1-pound mix of wild mushrooms, including portobollo, shiitake, and cremini
Salt and freshly ground black pepper to taste
Splash of white truffle oil
Chopped fresh flat-leaf parsley for garnish
Shaved parmesan cheese for garnish

Kristine Kidd

Former food editor of *Bon Appétit*, author of *Weeknight Gluten Free*, and newest star in the gluten-free galaxy, Kristine Kidd is truly one of us. When her childhood gluten sensitivity roared back as celiac disease, this virtuoso of wholesome ingredients and intense flavors set out to prove the most memorable meals are not the most difficult or complicated and are naturally gluten-free. Her simple approach relies not on makeovers and substitutions, but on experiment, peak freshness, and seasonal produce at the height of perfection. With thanks to Kristine and a warm welcome to the family.

ARCTIC CHAR WITH KUMQUAT GREMOLATA, ROASTED FENNEL, AND POTATOES

The simplest dishes are the ones we come back to again and again, and this Arctic char—with its delicate and sweet flavor roasted with fennel, potatoes, and the sweet-tartness of kumquats—is a one-dish wonder. If Arctic char is not available, wild salmon or trout fillets will do nicely, but some fish markets and Whole Foods Market locations will order char for you with a day's notice. Always remember that the safest and most environmentally correct seafood is wild, not farm raised or color enhanced. Look for fresh kumquats in season.

SERVES 2

3 tablespoons olive oil, plus more to dab on the fish and more to coat the rimmed baking sheets (if not using olive oil spray)

2 tablespoons plus 1 teaspoon fennel seeds

1¼ to 1⅓ pounds Yukon gold or russet potatoes

2 small fennel bulbs, tops trimmed

Coarse kosher salt and freshly ground black pepper to taste

3 6-ounce fillets of Arctic char, wild salmon, or trout

8 kumquats

¼ cup chopped fresh flat-leaf Italian parsley

1 small shallot, finely chopped

For the potatoes:

1. Place one rack in the lower third and another in the center of the oven. Preheat oven to 400°F. Spray 1 large rimmed baking sheet and one small rimmed baking sheet with olive oil spray or brush the baking sheets with olive oil.

2. In a small, dry skillet, stir the fennel seeds over medium-high heat until fragrant, about 2 minutes. Transfer the fennel seeds to a mortar or spice mill and grind coarsely.

3. Cut the potatoes in half lengthwise, then cut each piece lengthwise again into 4 wedges that measure about ¾ inch at the widest part. Place the potatoes in a large bowl.

4. Halve the fennel bulbs lengthwise, then cut them into wedges that measure about ½ inch at the widest part. Place the fennel pieces in the bowl with the potatoes.

5. Add 3 tablespoons olive oil, 2 tablespoons toasted fennel seeds, and salt and pepper to the potatoes and toss to coat. Spread the potato-fennel mixture on the large rimmed baking sheet. Place the sheet on the center rack in the oven and roast until the vegetables are beginning to brown on the bottom and are almost tender, about 35 minutes.

For fish and gremolata:

1. Arrange the fish fillets skin-side down on the small rimmed baking sheet. Sprinkle the fish with the remaining 2 teaspoons of toasted fennel seeds, coarse kosher salt, and pepper.

2. Dip a pastry brush in the remaining olive oil, and dab over the fish.
3. Halve the kumquats lengthwise, then thinly slice them lengthwise (it is easier to slice the cut side of the fruit than the skin side), discarding the seeds. Cut the slices finely crosswise, forming chopped kumquats. Sprinkle one-half of the chopped kumquats over the fish.
4. Place the remaining kumquats in a small bowl. Mix in the parsley and shallot for the gremolata.
5. After the vegetables have roasted for 35 minutes, place the fish on the lower oven rack. Roast the fish and vegetables until the fish is just springy to the touch and opaque in the center and the vegetables are brown on the bottom and tender, about 10 minutes.
6. Transfer the fish and vegetables to plates, sprinkle with the gremolata, and serve.

Marcie Turney

I like to call star chef Marcie Turney and her partner, business wizard Valerie Safran, the Empresses of 13th Street. Thanks to their vision and chutzpah, a block that was once the epicenter of crime, check-cashing joints, and porn parlors is now the beating heart of Philadelphia's Midtown Village food scene. With Verde, Open House, Marcie Blaine Artisanal Chocolates, Grocery, and six wildly popular restaurants, among them Barbuzzo, Jamonera, Little Nonna's, and the newly opened Lolita, all of them with Marcie at the helm, these two have not only raised the culinary bar, they have reclaimed an entire neighborhood. Love and thanks to this gifted, creative, and apparently tireless pair.

CRISPY SQUASH BLOSSOMS BARBUZZO

Otherwise known as fleur de courgette or zucchini flower, the delicate texture of squash blossoms takes well to frying. Look for them in farmers' markets and good grocery stores, or grow them yourself in the garden. The combination of fresh buffalo mozzarella, pickled farm tomatoes, and charred corn salad make for an unforgettable lunch or appetizer. Leftover pickled farm tomatoes are wonderful with fish, pork, or grilled steak.

SERVES 4

For the squash blossoms:
4-ounce ball of fresh buffalo mozzarella, cut into 8 blossom-size pieces
¼ teaspoon kosher salt
8 squash blossoms, wiped clean with a tea towel

For the pickled farm tomatoes:
1 quart small mixed farm tomatoes, halved
½ cup white balsamic vinegar
2 tablespoons (packed) brown sugar
1 teaspoon salt
¾ cup extra-virgin olive oil
1 clove garlic, minced
1 teaspoon fresh ginger, minced
½ teaspoon yellow mustard seeds
½ teaspoon freshly ground black pepper
½ teaspoon turmeric
½ teaspoon cumin seeds, toasted and ground

For the charred corn salad:
3 ears fresh corn, shucked and silk removed with a damp tea towel
1 jalapeño pepper, stem and seeds removed, finely diced
3 tablespoons red onion, diced finely

To prepare the squash blossoms:
1. Season the mozzarella pieces with the salt.
2. Carefully open each squash blossom enough to tuck a piece of mozzarella inside. Gently pinch the tips of the squash blossoms together. Refrigerate.

To pickle the tomatoes:
1. Put the tomatoes in a medium-sized, non-reactive bowl, either glass or stainless steel.
2. In a medium saucepan, add the vinegar, brown sugar, and salt. Stir to dissolve and bring to a boil.
3. In a small sauté pan, warm the olive oil over low heat. Add the garlic, ginger, mustard seeds, pepper, turmeric, and cumin seeds and cook until fragrant, about 2 minutes, stirring frequently with a wooden spoon.
4. Pour the hot oil mixture into the vinegar mixture and stir. Pour this over the tomatoes and allow to come to room temperature. Set aside.

To make the corn salad:
1. Place the ears of corn on an outdoor or indoor grill and roll with tongs until slightly charred in spots, approximately 3 minutes. Remove them and let cool.
2. In a large bowl, hold the ears of corn upright one at a time and, using a knife, cut the kernels from the cobs. The bowl will capture the kernels. Dispose of the cobs or reserve them for vegetable stock.
3. Add the jalapeño, onion, scallion, mint, cilantro, garlic, lime zest, lime juice, and olive oil to the corn kernels and set aside.

1. Heat the canola oil until it reaches 375°F on a deep-fry thermometer.
2. While the oil is heating, put the rice flour, salt, paprika if using, and pepper in a medium bowl and whisk to combine. Slowly add the seltzer while whisking to prevent any lumps. Add the egg whites and whisk the mixture for 30 seconds.
3. Hold a stuffed squash blossom by the stem and dip it into the batter, making sure to coat it completely. Place the blossom in heated oil and repeat with the others. Do not crowd the pan. The blossoms should not touch each other.
4. Fry for 1 to 2 minutes, turning often, until golden and crispy. Transfer the blossoms to to a paper towel–lined tray. Season with salt and pepper.
5. To serve, place on each plate ¼ cup of the pickled farm tomatoes. Place 2 fried squash blossoms on top, and finish with 3 tablespoons of the charred corn salad. Drizzle each plate with good-quality olive oil.

1 scallion (white and green parts), sliced thinly
1 tablespoon fresh mint leaves, stacked and sliced into thin strips
1 tablespoon fresh cilantro leaves, stacked and sliced into thin strips
1 clove garlic, grated on a Microplane
Zest and freshly squeezed juice of 1 lime
2 tablespoons extra-virgin olive oil

For the squash blossom batter:
Canola oil, enough for 2 inches on the bottom of a deep pot
10 ounces (about 1¼ cups) rice flour
¼ teaspoon kosher salt, plus more to season the squash blossoms
¼ teaspoon smoked Spanish paprika (optional)
Pinch of freshly ground black pepper, plus more to season the squash blossoms
8 ounces seltzer
2 large egg whites

Bobby Flay

No doubt about it. Bobby Flay is a culinary rock star. This James Beard Award–winning chef, *Boy Meets Grill* Food Network darling, Iron Chef, and bestselling author is the mastermind behind Bar Americain, Mesa Grill, Bobby Flay Steak, and Bobby's Burger Palace and has been a huge influence on the way we cook and eat.

SAFFRON RISOTTO CAKES WITH SHRIMP, RED CHILI OIL, AND CHIVE OIL

Tapas, or small plates, are a *pasión* of Spaniards who love to dine late and prefer sophisticated grazing to a heavy meal. These savory risotto cakes can just as easily be served as a spectacular first course or a light lunch. Use arborio rice and look for chiles de arbol in specialty stores or the international section of markets.

MAKES 24 TAPAS

4½ cups (or more) low-sodium, gluten-free chicken broth
⅛ teaspoon crumbled saffron threads
2 tablespoons olive oil
1½ cups chopped onion
1½ cups arborio rice
½ cup dry white wine
Salt and freshly ground black pepper to taste
Nonstick vegetable oil spray
1 cup white rice flour, plus more for dredging the risotto cakes
¾ cup canola oil
24 large uncooked shrimp, peeled, deveined, and butterflied

1. Combine the broth and saffron in a medium saucepan, and bring to a boil. Remove the saucepan from the heat and cover it to keep warm.
2. In another medium saucepan, heat the olive oil over medium heat. Add the onion and sauté until tender, about 6 minutes. Add the rice and stir for 1 minute. Add the wine and stir until absorbed, about 1 minute. Add ½ cup of the saffron broth and stir until absorbed, about 4 minutes. Continue adding broth, ½ cup at a time and stirring frequently, until the rice is just tender, allowing each addition to be absorbed before adding more, about 20 minutes total. Season with salt and pepper.
3. Spray a rimmed baking sheet with nonstick spray. Spread the risotto on the prepared sheet, forming an irregular 13×9-inch rectangle. Cover the risotto with plastic wrap and refrigerate until cold and firm, about 2 hours. (This can be made 1 day ahead. Keep chilled.)
4. Preheat the oven to 300°F.
5. In a medium bowl, place the rice flour and season with salt and pepper. Using a 2-inch-diameter cookie cutter, cut out 24 rounds from the risotto. Dredge the risotto cakes in rice flour and place them on a clean rimmed baking sheet.
6. In a large nonstick skillet, heat ¼ cup canola oil over medium heat. Working in batches, add the risotto cakes to the skillet and cook until golden brown, about 2 minutes per side. Transfer the risotto cakes to another baking sheet and place them in the oven to keep warm.
7. Sprinkle the shrimp with salt and pepper. In another large skillet, heat the remaining 2 tablespoons of canola oil over high heat. Add the shrimp and sauté until just opaque in the center, about 2 minutes per side.
8. Top each risotto cake with 1 shrimp. Drizzle the shrimp with Red Chili Oil and Chive Oil (recipes follow) and serve.

Red Chili Oil

MAKES ⅓ CUP

1. In a small bowl, place the chilies. Add enough hot water to cover. Let stand until chilies soften slightly, about 1 hour. Drain.
2. Coarsely chop the chilies. In the bowl of a blender, combine the chiles and olive oil and blend until smooth.
3. Season to taste with salt and pepper.
4. Cover and refrigerate. Bring to room temperature before using. Will keep for 3 days.

4 chilies de arbol
½ cup olive oil
Salt and freshly ground black pepper to taste

Chive Oil

MAKES ½ CUP

1. In the bowl of a blender, blend the olive oil and chives until smooth. Strain into a small bowl. Discard the solids left in the strainer.
2. Season to taste with salt and pepper.
3. Cover the chive oil and refrigerate. Bring it to room temperature before using. Will keep for 3 days.

½ cup olive oil
⅓ cup chopped fresh chives
Salt and freshly ground black pepper to taste

Michael Cole

There is nothing more thrilling than discovering a rising star. The fact that this one has risen just steps away from my front door is even more remarkable. This self-taught chef, art school graduate, and most recently executive chef of Philadelphia's Crêperie Beau Monde, is the genuine article. I have long enjoyed his complex salads and smoky soups, as well as his gluten-free adaptations the waitstaff like to call Jax Specials. Now he has upped his game and shown us what miracles can come from a chef's curiosity and an artist's aesthetic. Maybe he'll be the first to master both.

BEAU MONDE CIDER-BRINED BERKSHIRE PORK CHOPS WITH PUMPKIN SAGE RISOTTO, GRILLED PEAR, SOUBISE PURÉE, AND SMOKED BALSAMIC REDUCTION

This remarkable dish takes some time, but it is not particularly difficult. I can't think of anything more spectacular for an autumn dinner party followed by a sliver of Reverend Michael's Apple and Fig Crisp (page 221) or poached winter fruit and cheese. Make sure you leave enough time for the pork chops to marinate in the apple cider brine, preferably overnight. The sauces can be made ahead of time, held warm or gently reheated and stirred occasionally while making the risotto and pork. The balsamic reduction is best at room temperature. Begin the risotto 10 to 15 minutes before you start cooking the pork, so both are ready at the same time.

SERVES 4

For the brine:

2 sprigs of fresh rosemary, chopped
4 Berkshire pork chops, trimmed of excessive fat
1 cup water
1 cup apple cider
½ cup salt
¼ cup (packed) dark brown sugar
¼ cup sherry vinegar
2 bay leaves
10 black peppercorns (Szechuan peppercorns if available)
1 teaspoon red pepper flakes

For the soubise purée:

¼ cup (½ stick) unsalted butter
2 medium white onions, chopped
4 cloves garlic, chopped
4 sprigs of fresh thyme leaves, stripped
¼ teaspoon grated fresh nutmeg
¼ cup dry white wine
½ cup heavy cream
½ cup cooked white jasmine rice
Salt and freshly ground pepper to taste

To brine the pork chops:

1. Rub the rosemary into the pork chops. Set aside.
2. In a medium saucepan, combine the water, apple cider, salt, brown sugar, vinegar, bay leaves, black peppercorns, and red pepper flakes. Bring the ingredients to a simmer over medium heat and stir until the brown sugar and salt are dissolved. Remove the pan from heat and let cool.
3. Put the pork in a plastic ziplock bag with the cooled brine and fasten securely. Refrigerate at least 4 hours, preferably overnight.

To prepare the soubise purée:

1. In a medium saucepan, melt the butter over medium heat. Add the onion and garlic and cook until soft, about 5 to 10 minutes. Stir in the thyme and nutmeg and cook for about 1 minute, until aromatic. Add the wine and simmer until the liquid reduces by half, about 20 to 25 minutes.
2. Remove the mixture from the heat and place it in the bowl of a food processor. Process until smooth, while slowly adding the cream.
3. Return the mixture to the saucepan and bring to a simmer over low heat. Add the rice and simmer over medium heat until thickened, about 10 minutes. Strain through a fine mesh sieve. Add salt and pepper. Keep warm, or set aside for reheating.

To make the balsamic reduction:

1. In a small saucepan, bring the balsamic vinegar, sherry vinegar, apple cider vinegar, honey, basil, and shallot to a boil. Reduce the heat to low and simmer until the liquid is reduced by three-quarters and is syrupy, about 20 to 25 minutes.
2. Strain the reduction through a sieve. Let it cool to room temperature.

To make the risotto:

1. Preheat the oven to 350°F.
2. Place the pumpkin halves cut-side down on a lightly oiled rimmed baking sheet. Bake until the pumpkin is tender, or until it is easily pierced with a fork, about 1 hour.
3. Let the pumpkin cool and scrape out all of the flesh. In the bowl of a food processor, place the pumpkin flesh and pulse until slightly creamy. Set aside.
4. In a medium saucepan, melt 2 tablespoons butter over medium heat. Add the shallots and garlic and sauté for about 10 minutes, until the shallots are transparent. Mix in the rice and sage and continue cooking until the rice is slightly translucent. Add the wine and sherry.
5. Reduce the heat and gently simmer until all of the liquid is absorbed. Add a 6 to 8-ounce ladle of broth and simmer until it is also absorbed. Stir often.
6. Repeat this process until the rice is al dente, about 20 minutes, stirring constantly and adding more broth if necessary.
7. Stir in the remaining 2 tablespoons of butter, the Parmesan, pumpkin, salt, and pepper until well incorporated.
8. Serve immediately.

To make the pork chops:

1. Preheat oven to 400°F.
2. In a large oven-proof sauté pan place the olive oil. Heat the oil over medium-high heat.
3. Remove the pork chops from the brine and pat dry with paper towels. Sear both sides until browned.
4. Put the sauté pan in the oven and cook until medium-rare, 6 to 8 minutes.

Assembly:

1. Slice the pears in half and remove the cores. Slice the pear halves vertically, but keep them intact.

For the smoked balsamic reduction:
1 cup balsamic vinegar
¼ cup sherry vinegar
¼ cup apple cider vinegar
¼ cup honey
6 fresh basil leaves
1 shallot, chopped
2 teaspoons smoked paprika (hot or sweet, depending on your preference)

For the pumpkin sage risotto:
1 small pumpkin, halved and seeds removed
Oil for coating the rimmed baking sheet
¼ cup (½ stick) unsalted butter
3 shallots, minced
2 cloves garlic, minced
1½ cups arborio rice
10 fresh sage leaves, chopped
½ cup dry white wine
½ cup sherry
3 cups gluten-free chicken or vegetable broth, heated
½ cup grated Parmesan cheese
Salt and freshly ground black pepper to taste

For cooking the pork chops:
2 tablespoons olive oil
2 pears
Unsalted butter to grease the sauté pan, if using

2. Place the cut sides down either on a grill or in a lightly buttered sauté pan over medium heat for a few minutes.
3. Divide the risotto among four plates, place a pork chop on each one, and spoon the soubise over all.
4. Drizzle the reduction on each plate and garnish with ½ cooked pear, fanned and placed on top of the pork chop.

Learn More

The Art of Simple Food: Notes, Lessons, and Recipes from a Delicious Revolution and *The Art of Simple Food II* by Alice Waters (Clarkson Potter)

Bobby Flay's Mesa Grill Cookbook by Bobby Flay, Stephanie Banyas, and Sally Jackson (Clarkson Potter)

Bobby Flay's Throwdown! (based on the Food Network show *Throwdown*) by Bobby Flay, Stephanie Banyas, and Miriam Garron (Clarkson Potter)

Bouchon Bakery by Thomas Keller and Sebastien Rouxel (Artisan)

The Essential Thomas Keller: The French Laundry Cookbook and Ad Hoc at Home by Thomas Keller (Artisan)

It's All About the Guest by Steve DiFillippo, a memoir with recipes (Lyons Press)

One Big Table by Molly O'Neill (Simon and Schuster)

Sparks in the Kitchen by Katy Sparks (Knopf)

Thomas Keller Baking Mixes. www.williams-sonoma.com

Weeknight Gluten Free by Kristine Kidd (Williams-Sonoma)

A Baker's Dozen

Pat-a-cake, pat-a-cake, baker's man,
Bake me a cake as fast as you can;
Pat it and prick it, and mark it with a B,
Put it in the oven for baby and me.

—NURSERY RHYME

- Flying Apron Bakery, Seattle: *Fresh Strawberry and Blueberry Fruit Tart*
- Risotteria, New York City: *Bleecker Street Breadsticks*
- Helmut Newcake, Paris: *Dark Chocolate Fondant with Ginger and Raspberry Coeur*
- Zix Cookies, Sonoma, California: *Glenn Minervini-Zick's Raspberry Almond Ravioli Cookie*
- Nigella Lawson: *Cinnamon Almond Cake*
- Gwyneth Paltrow and Julia Turshen: *Sweet Potato and Five-Spice Muffins*
- Pure Fare, Philadelphia: *French Toast Pineapple Upside-Down Cake*
- BabyCakes NYC: *Meyer Lemon and Bing Cherry Cupcakes with Vanilla Frosting*
- Kelli and Peter Bronski: *Almond Pâte-à-Choux Florentines*
- Tate's Bake Shop, Southampton, New York: *Kathleen King's Gluten-Free Chocolate Crinkles*
- Christina Pirello: *Chocolate-Glazed Coconut Macaroons*
- Taffets Bakery, Philadelphia: *Mediterranean Focaccia*
- Miglet's Cupcake Shop, Danville, California: *Vanilla Salted Caramel Cake with Vanilla Buttercream*

If you're like me, there's nothing more exciting than discovering the perfect gluten-free muffin or slice of carrot cake made in small batches by one of the many artisanal bakers popping up around the country. I'm not talking about weekend bakers or talented amateurs like myself; these are top-notch pastry chefs and bread makers who have dedicated themselves to raising the bar for gluten-free baked goods. The best of them shun trans fats, high-fructose corn syrup, preservatives, and excessive sugar, working their wonders with fresh ingredients and new combinations of flours, textures, and flavors, and many of them take into account vegan and lactose-free diets. They are not substituting, or doing the quick makeover; they are inventing an altogether new language for gluten-free indulgences.

On a recent Sunday morning, I was strolling around my favorite farm-to-city market, greeting neighbors and enjoying the community vibe, when I spotted a table piled high with gluten-free oatmeal cakes that were a cross between a scone and a cookie, chewy inside, brown and crisp at the edges. What was I here to buy? I couldn't remember, so divine were these confections. In San Francisco, on the way to lunch at the very gluten-free-friendly Slanted Door in the Ferry Building, I came upon the Mariposa Bakery kiosk and a gluten-free coffee cake I'm still dreaming about. Munching to my heart's desire, I floated the idea of moving west. In the deliciousness of that moment, it seemed like the only sensible thing to do.

Stepping for the first time into the tiny Lower East Side shop at the heart of what is now the BabyCakes empire was a thrill equal to my inaugural visit to Risotteria across town in Greenwich Village, where I was given a warm rosemary breadstick to nibble on while waiting for one of the best gluten-free pizzas on the planet. During an unexpected cupcake encounter in Northbrook, Illinois, I managed to beat a pack of indecisive toddlers and their overcaffeinated parents to the counter before the goodies were all gone. It wasn't pretty, but these were caramel cupcakes the likes of which I'd never tasted. Some may feel that knowing about these places beforehand and planning an itinerary around them is the way to go, but for me there is no pleasure more acute than the moment presenting itself.

Many bakeries will ship anywhere in the United States and sometimes farther afield. But mail order can be dicey and shipping costs prohibitive when you don't know enough about the baker you're ordering from. There is a dizzying array of baking books, but which one to invest in? You don't want a shelf full of expensive duds.

The following is a sampler of recipes from the best of the best baking today and some from those who will soon be. Browse their books, stop in when you're in their towns and cities, and look for them in gourmet groceries and farmers' markets. And always, always keep your eyes open for the new kid on the block. Every week, it seems, there's someone worth noticing.

Herewith a little taste.

Flying Apron Bakery, Seattle

Flying Apron's founder, Jennifer Katzinger, set out to prove that gluten-free vegan can be sweet, sublime, and as sinfully rich as any creamy concoction. She has more than succeeded with gluten-free, dairy-free cakes, pastries, and breads as good as any found in a French patisserie. I dare say, they're even better for their lack of common allergens. How is it possible to make a classic fruit tart without dairy? The answer is this stunner from *Gluten-Free and Vegan Holidays* by Jennifer Katzinger. With thanks.

FRESH STRAWBERRY AND BLUEBERRY FRUIT TART

Master this marvel of crust and custard and who needs dinner? Sorghum flour gives the crust its tender flake, and raw cashew butter is the secret to its creamy heart. Apricot jam lends the tart a spectacular glaze. Use the sweetest and freshest organic strawberries and blueberries you can find.

MAKES ONE 9-INCH TART

1. Preheat the oven to 350°F.
2. In the bowl of a stand mixer fitted with a paddle attachment, add all of the crust ingredients and mix until they are just combined; the dough will look like little pearls.
3. Using your hands, press the crumbly dough into a 9-inch tart pan with a removable bottom. (Do not use a rolling pin.) The crust will be very thin; the base should be the thinnest, with the sides a bit more substantial.
4. Bake for about 15 minutes, or until golden. Remove from the oven. If the sides have slumped during baking, push them gently back into place while the crust is still warm. Let cool.

For the crust:
⅓ cup coconut oil
1 cup sorghum flour
¼ teaspoon sea salt
½ teaspoon vanilla extract
1 tablespoon maple syrup

For the custard:
½ cup raw cashew butter
1 tablespoon maple syrup
Zest of 1 medium orange
  (about 2 tablespoons)
Freshly squeezed juice of ½
  medium lemon (about 1½
  tablespoons)
1 teaspoon vanilla extract
Pinch of salt

For the topping:
2 cups strawberries
1 cup blueberries
1 tablespoon apricot jam
1 tablespoon water

5. While the crust is cooling, combine all of the custard ingredients in the cleaned stand mixer bowl fitted with the paddle attachment. Whip on high speed until thick and creamy. You may need to scrape the bowl with your spatula a few times between beatings to ensure that all of the ingredients have been thoroughly incorporated.

6. To make the topping, rinse the strawberries and blueberries and pat them dry. Create a flat base on each strawberry by cutting off the stem.

7. In a small saucepan over low heat, combine the apricot jam and water. Heat until a thin syrup forms and just starts to bubble.

8. To assemble the tart, spoon the custard into the crust and gently spread with a spatula to cover evenly. Arrange the strawberries, cut-side down, and blueberries atop the custard.

9. With a small pastry brush, gently brush the apricot glaze onto the berries. Remove the rim of the tart pan but keep the base in place to easily transfer the tart to a serving platter. Serve immediately or chill, lightly covered, up to 2 days in the refrigerator.

Risotteria, New York City

There is always a crowd waiting for a table outside Joseph Pace's tiny West Village café that seats twenty and takes no reservations. Mostly they come for the risotti—arborio or vialone or carnaroli—in dozens of varieties. And they bus, train, drive, and fly in from all over the country for gluten-free panini and pizza, thin-crust or Sicilian, saving enough room for something sweet from the bakery. There is a collective sigh as the breadsticks are placed on the table. Warm and yeasty, inexplicably soft *and* crunchy, salty and scented with rosemary, these gluten-free marvels are positive proof that heaven resides on Bleecker Street.

BLEECKER STREET BREADSTICKS

Serendipity so often plays a part in how good things come to us. This breadstick recipe first appeared quite some time ago in the *New York Times* and, to put it as delicately as possible, did not quite work. California baker Jane Oswaks, whose notes I'd saved and had only recently rediscovered in time to include them here, adapted, perfected, and generously shared the recipe with us. The first time you taste them, you'll have to remind yourself to breathe. It takes a village to bake a breadstick this good. With thanks to all.

MAKES 12 TO 18 BREADSTICKS

1. Preheat oven to 425°F.
2. Combine the yeast, sugar, and warm water and let sit until frothy.
3. In the medium bowl of a stand mixer fitted with standard mixers (not a dough hook), combine the rice flour, tapioca starch, dry milk powder, xanthan gum, gelatin powder, sea salt, and herbes de Provence. Mix on low speed to blend.
4. Add the proofed yeast mixture to the dry ingredients. Add the olive oil and vinegar. Raise the speed to high and beat for 6 minutes. (The dough will stay very soft and should not pull off the sides of the bowl. If necessary, add water, 1 tablespoon at a time, until the dough does not resist beaters.)
5. Liberally spray or oil a rimmed baking sheet and set aside.
6. Put the dough into a large pastry bag with a plain round ½-inch tip, and pipe 12 to 18 breadsticks about 8 inches long, leaving 2 inches in between. Spray or brush the tops of the breadsticks liberally with oil, and salt generously with sea salt.
7. Bake the breadsticks for 10 minutes, turn them, and spray or brush them again with oil. Continue to bake until golden brown, about 10 minutes more. Serve warm.

1¼ teaspoon active dry yeast
½ teaspoon sugar
1 cup warm water
1½ cups organic brown rice flour
1 cup tapioca starch
2 tablespoons nonfat dry milk powder
1 tablespoon xanthan gum
1 teaspoon unflavored gelatin powder
½ teaspoon sea salt
1 tablespoon dried herbes de Provence
3 tablespoons extra-virgin olive oil
3 tablespoons cider vinegar
Nonstick spray or vegetable oil for greasing the rimmed baking sheet and breadsticks
Fleur de sel or other flaky sea salt to salt the breadsticks

Helmut Newcake, Paris

As if you need another reason to book a trip to Paris. In an old loft nestled in the rue Bichat in the 10th arrondissement near Canal St. Martin is a tiny patisserie and café named after photographer Helmut Newton. It is here that Le Nôtre–trained pastry chef and celiac Marie Tagliaferro and her husband François created the first truly authentic gluten-free pastries in Paris. Here you'll find all the classics—éclairs, religieuses, canelés, mille-feuilles, Madame de Fontenays, les petits gâteaux, tartes, marrons glacés, and bûches de Noël—all of them flaky, sublime, and unforgettable. These are the delights we dream about, brave time zones for. My thanks to Marie and François for making their American debut on these pages.

DARK CHOCOLATE FONDANT WITH GINGER
AND RASPBERRY COEUR

These tiny cakes with their molten raspberry hearts are surprisingly easy to make for such a dramatic and romantic dessert. Rather than converting and getting mixed up in the differences between weight and volume, I suggest a simple, inexpensive kitchen scale to measure out grams and assure the authenticity of this divine French creation. You will need small round or heart-shaped bottomless stainless-steel tins, 2¾ inches in diameter and 2 inches high. Buy the best raspberries and chocolate you can afford, at least 70% cacao. Serve warm with their hearts still melting.

MAKES 6 TO 8 CAKES, DEPENDING ON THE SIZE OF THE TIN

190g dark chocolate, chopped
180g unsalted butter, plus more for greasing the rimmed baking sheet and the stainless steel tins
90g cornstarch or gluten-free baking mix without buckwheat
200g sugar
Pinch of salt
7 large eggs
20g crystallized ginger, thinly sliced
125g fresh raspberries

1. In a microwave oven or over a double boiler, melt the chocolate and butter together. Do not mix until the butter is totally liquid. Let cool slightly.
2. Place the cornstarch and sugar and pinch of salt in a medium bowl. Set aside.
3. Stir the chocolate and butter with a spatula until smooth and shiny. (Note: Do not use a whisk; you want to avoid adding air into the mixture.) Set aside.
4. Beat the eggs in another bowl.
5. Gradually pour the eggs into the cornstarch-sugar mixture to avoid lumps.
6. Add the chocolate-butter mixture. Add the ginger and mix.
7. Let cool in refrigerator for 5 hours. (Note: The batter can be made a day ahead.)

Baking and assembly:
1. Preheat oven to 400°F. Butter a large rimmed baking sheet and butter each tin.
2. Cut squares of parchment paper, slightly larger than the molds, and butter each square. Place two squares under each tin.
3. Spoon an even layer of batter, about ½-inch thick, into each mold. Add 3 raspberries and top with a second layer of batter.
4. Bake for 10 to 12 minutes. If you use frozen berries, baking may take a bit longer, 12 to 14 minutes. Watch carefully and insert a toothpick into the cake's center; the cakes will be flowing slightly.

5. Cool 2 minutes and gently turn out of the molds without damaging the sides of the cake.
6. Serve warm and melted with a dollop of caramel ice cream.
7. Pretend you are in Paris.

Zix Cookies, Sonoma, California

I met Glenn Minervini-Zick, a.k.a. the Sonoma Dough Man, in the most unexpected way. My husband and I had just driven up from San Francisco to the small town of Sebastopol to meet our friend Jane for lunch. We arrived at the restaurant first, a bit wobbly from the hairpin turns on the coast highway, and as I got my bearings, I noticed a display of gorgeous cookies and asked if any were gluten-free.

"There *were*," said the baker, "but someone bought them all this morning."

Then, taking a second look, he asked, "Are you Jax?"

"Yes," I said, dumbfounded.

"Jane bought them all for you, but don't tell her I told you and ruin the surprise."

Of course, we told. She waved Glenn over for a proper introduction and a good laugh. Oh, the joys of asking questions of strangers.

When he is not fly-fishing, experimenting with gluten-free flours indigenous to other cultures, teaching techniques to culinary arts students, working on his bake books, or chatting up strangers, GM-Z is wowing them at regional fairs, professional food shows, and Sonoma's Santa Rosa Farmers' Market.

GLENN MINERVINI-ZICK'S RASPBERRY ALMOND RAVIOLI COOKIE

This sweet hybrid of ravioli and pastry gets its rustic sensibility from millet flour and an almond paste that is coarser than commercial varieties. Glenn uses his own raspberry jam, but you can use any high-quality preserves. Pre-blanched almonds are available in specialty markets but can be pricey. See the recipe for Blanched Almonds on page 192. It's best to prepare the dough the day before baking to ensure the proper consistency. Glenn uses Bob's Red Mill or Arrowhead Mills Organic for the flours and Spectrum Organic for the shortening.

For the most tender, flaky shell, all ingredients should be cold before starting the mixing process.

1¼ cups millet flour
½ cup tapioca flour
¾ cup white rice flour, plus more as necessary for dusting countertop or baking slab
¼ cup granulated sugar, plus more for sprinkling on top of the cookies.
1 teaspoon salt
1 teaspoon xanthan gum
10 tablespoons cold unsalted butter
6 tablespoons cold organic, all-vegetable shortening
2 tablespoons cold water
1⅔ cups almonds, blanched
1¼ cups confectioners' sugar
1 cup raspberry jam
1 teaspoon almond extract
1 large egg, separated
Splash of milk

MAKES APPROXIMATELY 30 COOKIES

For the ravioli shell:

1. In the bowl of a food processor, using the blade attachment, briefly mix the flours, granulated sugar, salt, and xanthan gum on the pulse setting.
2. Cut the butter into ½-inch cubes and chop the shortening into small pieces.
3. Add the shortening to the dry ingredients and pulse the food processor until the shortening is chopped into pieces the size of fine shavings and they are well mixed into the dry ingredients, approximately 30 to 60 seconds.
4. Add the butter and pulse again in 10- to 15-second intervals until the mixture resembles coarse crumbs with no larger pieces remaining. Resist the urge to overmix the dough, which will reduce its flakiness.
5. Transfer the dough to the bowl of a standing mixer with a paddle attachment.
6. Turn the mixer on at low speed, and immediately begin to add the water a little at a time.
7. Continue mixing until the dough begins to form a ball. If the dough is wet or sticky, add a little more rice flour to the dough and mix in.
8. Take the dough to a dry, gluten-free floured countertop or baking slab.
9. Divide the dough into 2 equal pieces, form into balls, and wrap with plastic wrap.
10. Flatten the balls slightly with the palm of your hand. Refrigerate for at least 1 hour or overnight. The dough is easier to work with when cold.

For the filling:

1. Place the almonds and half the confectioners' sugar into the bowl of a food processor fitted with a blade attachment. Process the almonds until they are finely ground, periodically stopping the food processor to scrape the sides and bottom of the bowl.
2. After about 2 minutes, add the remaining confectioners' sugar and

continue to process until the almonds will not grind any finer. This process may take up to 5 minutes.

3. Transfer the almond mix to the bowl of a stand mixer with a paddle attachment. Add the raspberry jam and almond extract and mix thoroughly.

4. Transfer the raspberry-almond filling to a covered bowl and chill.

For the ravioli construction:

1. Remove the dough disks from the refrigerator one at a time to keep them cold.

2. On a countertop dusted with gluten-free flour, dust the top of the disk and roll out the dough to ⅛-inch thick as follows: Roll the dough starting from the middle of the disk heading away from you. Give the disk a quarter turn and repeat, rolling the dough away from you. Continue turning the dough and rolling until the disk is ⅛-inch thick.

3. Cut an even number of circles with a 3-inch cookie cutter. Half will be tops and half will be bottoms. Separate the circles from the scraps. Set aside the scraps to use later.

4. Whisk the egg white and brush over the circles.

5. With a spoon or ½-ounce (1 tablespoon) cookie scoop, add approximately 2 teaspoons of filling in the center of the bottom circles. Flatten slightly with a damp finger or two.

6. For each cookie, spoon ¼ teaspoon raspberry jam on top of the filling.

7. With a small metal spatula or flat knife, pick up a top circle and flip it over onto each of the bottoms. The egg wash on the top circle will now be touching the mix. The side of the ravioli showing will be dry.

8. Using a 2½-inch circle ravioli stamp, press down on the circle to seal the ravioli. Work quickly so that the egg wash seals the ravioli well. The ravioli stamp seals the edges.

9. Transfer the ravioli to the freezer. Repeat this process for the remaining dough ball.

For baking:

1. Preheat oven to 375°F.

2. While the oven is heating, place the frozen ravioli, no closer than 1 inch apart, on a parchment paper–covered cookie sheet to allow them to defrost a bit before they go into the oven.

3. In a small bowl, combine the egg yolk and milk. Brush the tops of the ravioli with egg yolk–milk wash. Sprinkle granulated sugar over the wash and, with a small, sharp knife, cut a slit in the top of the ravioli.

4. Bake for 12 to 15 minutes, until just golden brown. Remove the cookies to wire racks and cool. If a bit of filling leaks out of the sides of the ravioli, wait until the cookie cools, then carefully cut away the excess. These cookies are best eaten within 7 to 10 days. Store in an air-tight container.

Blanched Almonds
Make these well ahead and store remainder in an air-tight container for other uses.

1. Submerge whole raw almonds in boiling water. Bring the water back to boil and continue boiling for 5 minutes.

2. Drain the almonds into a sieve and pour cold water over them. Let them stand and cool for at least 15 minutes.

3. The skins will now be loose. Peel the skins off the almonds and place them on a cookie sheet to air-dry for a couple of hours or overnight. At this point they can be incorporated into the recipe.

Nigella Lawson

How many chefs can claim a smartphone app? As a young girl, domestic goddess, celebrity, bestselling author of eight cookbooks, Food Network star, and contributor to the *Oxford Companion to Italian Literature*, British-born Nigella Lawson found her way to Florence and learned how to cook like an Italian. Now she shows us how to bake like one with her trademark light touch and faithfulness to simple ingredients. Deceptively plain, but with a restrained richness, redolent of marzipan, meltingly damp, cinnamon scented, and naturally *senza glutine*, this cake represents what Nigella does best. From *Nigellissima: Easy Italian-Inspired Recipes* by Nigella Lawson with permission. *Mille grazie.*

CINNAMON ALMOND CAKE

A grating of clementine zest, ground cinnamon, and a dusting of confectioners' sugar gives this simple and elegant cake a decidedly wintry look, but it can be made all year round and is especially wonderful with summer's freshest raspberries. Nigella tells us to use olive oil labeled mild and light rather than a more robust extra-virgin olive oil and to use free-range pasteurized egg whites out of a carton to spare ourselves having eight leftover yolks "gazing reproachfully at us from the refrigerator."

SERVES 8 TO 12

8 egg whites
¾ cup superfine sugar
Few drops of almond extract
Zest of 1 clementine or
    ½ orange
½ cup mild and light olive oil,
    plus more for greasing the
    pan
½ cup almond meal (flour)
1 teaspoon baking powder
1 cup sliced almonds
1 teaspoon ground cinnamon
Approximately 2 teaspoons
    confectioners' sugar, for
    decorating the cake

1. Preheat the oven to 350°F. Grease a 9-inch springform cake pan with olive oil and line the base with parchment paper.

2. In a large clean, grease-free bowl, whisk the egg whites until they are opaque and start to hold their shape, then slowly add the sugar, whisking until it's all incorporated and the mixture is thick and shiny.

3. Add the almond extract and the clementine or orange zest. Then, in about three batches, alternately whisk the olive oil and the almond meal until they are both smoothly incorporated into the meringue.

4. Pour the mixture into the prepared pan, then mix together the sliced almonds and cinnamon and sprinkle them over the top of the cake.

5. Bake for 30 to 40 minutes (start checking at 30 minutes), by which time the top should have risen and set, the almonds become golden, and a cake tester should come out clean, barring the odd almond crumb.

6. Remove from the oven and let the cake cool, in its pan, on a wire rack. Once it is no longer hot, spring open the sides of the pan, but don't try to remove the cake from the base until completely cooled.

7. When you are ready to serve, push the confectioners' sugar through a small strainer and over the cake to create a snowy effect, and take to the table.

Gwyneth Paltrow

How does an Oscar-winning actor, busy mother, and author of the *New York Times* bestselling cookbook *My Father's Daughter*, commute between homes in New York and London, blog about food, travel, fashion, and wellness, globe hop with Mario Batali, and still manage to look gorgeous and glowing with health? Those clear eyes and sylph's body we all envy came at a price. When the stress of overwork, life, and responsibility took its toll, leaving her anemic and depleted, her doctor suggested she eat only organic, mostly vegan, and give up coffee, alcohol, dairy, sugar, shellfish, gluten, soy, and anything processed. She shows us here that transformations don't have to be boring or bland, but as rich and satisfying as the foods we once craved. From *It's All Good* with thanks to Gwyneth Paltrow and Julia Turshen.

SWEET POTATO AND FIVE-SPICE MUFFINS

Who says vegan can't hold its own in the barrage of butter and sugar of conventional baking? The secret to these tender, slightly spicy, slightly sweet muffins is sweet potatoes, olive oil, and almond milk. Paltrow and Turshen use Thomas Keller's Cup4Cup flour blend, but also recommend Bob's Red Mill All-Purpose Baking Flour. Serve with a good, rough-cut English marmalade and organic blueberries.

MAKES 1 DOZEN MUFFINS

1 large sweet potato
½ cup extra-virgin olive oil
½ cup unsweetened almond milk
⅔ cup good-quality maple syrup or xylitol (a natural sweetener made from fruit and vegetable fibers), plus 2 tablespoons for brushing the muffins.
1 teaspoon vanilla extract
2 cups gluten-free flour mix (if the blend doesn't include xanthan gum, add 1 teaspoon)
2 teaspoons baking powder
2 teaspoons baking soda
1½ tablespoons Chinese five-spice powder
½ teaspoon fine sea salt

1. Preheat the oven to 400°F.
2. Prick the sweet potato a few times with a paring knife or a fork. Bake until soft (when a paring knife can cut through with zero resistance), about 1 hour. Set the sweet potato aside until it's completely cool.
3. Peel the sweet potato, discard the skin, and mash the flesh in a large mixing bowl with a fork.
4. Whisk the olive oil, almond milk, maple syrup, and vanilla into the sweet potato. In a separate large bowl, whisk together the flour mix, baking powder, baking soda, five-spice powder, and salt. Fold the dry ingredients into the wet ingredients.
5. Line a 12-cup muffin tin with paper liners and evenly distribute the muffin batter among the cups.
6. Bake for 20 to 25 minutes, or until a toothpick comes out clean, brushing the tops with the extra maple syrup during the last 5 minutes of baking. Let the muffins cool before serving.

Pure Fare, Philadelphia

Kriti Sehgal hated how she felt after eating out—bloated, stuffed, foggy. Why do restaurants have to serve so much fat and sugar, and a simple snack or a sandwich have to be loaded with fat and high-fructose corn syrup? Does good food always have to be a guilty pleasure? Kriti's answer was Agno Grill, a new kind of restaurant minus the post dinner remorse, and Pure Fare, an oasis of organic, local, gluten-free and dairy-free, vegetarian, and vegan delights so satisfying, she's had to take the overflow to two more locations. Who says you can't have your cake and feel good, too?

FRENCH TOAST PINEAPPLE UPSIDE-DOWN CAKE

You'll want a cast-iron or sturdy ovenproof skillet to bake this inventive and kind of retro, bready, cakey teatime/brunch-time indulgence from Pure Fare executive chef Sarah Ginn. Maple syrup and coconut oil more than make up for the absence of dairy and refined sugar. If possible, use fresh pineapple and whole-grain sandwich bread. If the bread's unavailable, make your own or buy it from the bakery, or buy the highest-quality commercial brand you can find. Many thanks to Sarah for this creative take on the upside-down cake.

SERVES 8

½ cup extra-virgin coconut oil, plus 2 tablespoons for preparing the skillet
6 large eggs
¾ cup maple syrup
½ teaspoon ground cinnamon
¼ teaspoon ground ginger
1 teaspoon salt
2 teaspoons vanilla extract
8 slices gluten-free sandwich bread, cut into ½-inch cubes
½ pineapple, cut into small pieces

1. Preheat the oven to 375°F. Grease a medium oven-proof skillet with 2 tablespoons coconut oil.
2. In a medium bowl, mix the eggs, maple syrup, cinnamon, ginger, salt, and vanilla. Add the bread cubes and mix well. Use your clean hands to massage the eggs into the bread and to break apart larger pieces of bread. You want the mixture to be chunky.
3. Add three-quarters of the pineapple and mix well.
4. Transfer the mixture to the prepared skillet and bake for 30 to 35 minutes, until the top is golden brown and the cake is firm. Let cool before slicing and serving.
5. Garnish with remainder of fresh pineapple.

BabyCakes NYC

In a world of reckless desserts overflowing with ever more flour, sugar, and buttercream, Erin McKenna is the queen of the conscious cupcake, presiding over an empire that began in a Lower East Side outpost no bigger than a postage stamp and now stretches from West Hollywood to Disneyland. Winner of Best Cupcake award from *New York* magazine (notice I didn't say best vegan or gluten-free cupcake), author, and veteran of the Food Network and Martha Stewart television, McKenna proves food sensitivity is no match for her brand of baked bliss. Reprinted with permission from *BabyCakes: Vegan, (Mostly) Gluten-Free, and (Mostly) Sugar-Free Recipes from New York's Most Talked-About Bakery* by Erin McKenna (Clarkson Potter).

MEYER LEMON AND BING CHERRY CUPCAKES WITH VANILLA FROSTING

Erin McKenna likes to say the still-life aesthetic of this cupcake is its own reward, and swears on her highlights its taste surpasses its beauty. She warns us to avoid overchopping the cherries and to try for a nice, thick lemon zest for an added texture that pairs neatly with the creamy frosting. Oh, baby.

1¾ cups agave nectar
Grated zest and freshly squeezed juice of 6 Meyer lemons
24 fresh Bing cherries, pitted and diced
2 teaspoons salt
½ cup garbanzo–fava bean flour
1½ cups brown rice flour
1 cup potato starch
½ cup arrowroot
1 tablespoon plus 1 teaspoon baking powder
½ teaspoon baking soda
1½ teaspoons xanthan gum
¾ cup coconut oil
¾ cup homemade applesauce or store-bought unsweetened applesauce
1 tablespoon vanilla extract
1 tablespoon pure lemon extract
⅔ cup hot water

MAKES 2 DOZEN CUPCAKES

1. In a small saucepan, whisk together the agave nectar, lemon zest, and lemon juice. Cook over medium heat until the mixture boils. Reduce the heat and continue to simmer for 10 minutes. Set aside.

2. Place half the cherries in a small mixing bowl and add ¼ cup of the lemon-infused agave nectar and ½ teaspoon of the salt.

3. Preheat oven to 325°F. Line two standard 12-cup muffin tins with paper liners.

4. In a medium bowl, whisk together the flours, potato starch, arrowroot, baking powder, baking soda, xanthan gum, and remaining 1½ teaspoons of salt. Add the lemon-agave nectar mixture, coconut oil, applesauce, and vanilla and lemon extracts to the dry ingredients. Mix until completely combined. Add the hot water and stir the batter until smooth.

5. Scoop ¼ cup batter into each prepared baking cup. Spoon 1 teaspoon prepared cherries onto the center of each cupcake, then top with

another 1 tablespoon of batter. Bake the cupcakes on the center rack for 24 minutes, rotating the tins 180 degrees after 12 minutes. The finished cupcakes will bounce back slightly when pressed, and a toothpick inserted into the center will come out clean.

6. Let the cupcakes stand in the tins for 20 minutes, then transfer them to a rack and cool completely. Using a plastic spatula, gently fold the remaining chopped cherries into the frosting (recipe below). With a frosting knife, liberally apply the vanilla frosting to the top of the cooled cupcakes. Store the cupcakes in an airtight container in the refrigerator for up to 3 days.

Vanilla Frosting

This thick and creamy frosting also doubles as a whipped topping, and left unrefrigerated, it becomes a vanilla sauce to serve with fruit, shortcakes, corn breads, and muffins. If you want to steer clear of soy, replace the liquid and powdered soy with rice milk varieties of both in equal measure, but be advised that the result will taste slightly sweeter. If you want the full frosting effect, factor in a full 6 hours for it to chill and set.

ENOUGH FROSTING FOR 24 CUPCAKES

1½ cups unsweetened soy milk
¾ cup dry soy milk powder
1 tablespoon coconut flour
¼ cup agave nectar
1 tablespoon vanilla extract
1½ cups coconut oil
2 tablespoons fresh lemon juice

1. In the bowl of a blender or food processor, combine the soy milk, soy powder, coconut flour, agave nectar, and vanilla. Blend the ingredients for 2 minutes. With the machine running, slowly add the coconut oil and lemon juice, alternating between the two until both are fully incorporated.

2. Pour the mixture into an airtight container and refrigerate for 6 hours or for up to 1 month. (If you plan to use it as a sauce, store the mixture at room temperature for up to 1 week.)

Kelli and Peter Bronski

You'd expect sacrificial nuts and seeds from greyhound-lean Peter Bronski, endurance athlete, ultra-marathoner, and author of *The Gluten-Free Edge: A Nutrition and Training Gide for Peak Athletic Performance and an Active Gluten-Free Life*. But add Kelli, lifelong baker and cook, Cornell-trained food industry veteran with a decade of experience at New York's fabled Waldorf Astoria Hotel, and you've got swoon-worthy French pastry from the most dynamic duo cooking, teaching, blogging, and baking today. With thanks to the Bronskis, and reprinted with permission from *Artisanal*

Gluten-Free Cooking by Kelli and Peter Bronski, this is incontrovertible evidence that gluten-free is not the end of anything, but just the beginning.

ALMOND PÂTE-À-CHOUX FLORENTINES

These ethereal almond pastries are the stuff of Parisian patisseries, café au lait, and languorous afternoons reading *Le Figaro*. Relax and take a deep breath. Loosen up the wrists. This kinder, gentler pâte-à-choux dough is surprisingly easy to master and will add to your legend.

MAKES 12 PASTRIES

For the pâte-à-choux pastry dough:

1¼ cups water, approximately
½ cup (1 stick) salted butter
1 teaspoon granulated sugar
1 teaspoon salt
1½ cups Artisan Gluten-Free Flour Blend (see recipe below)
4 eggs

1. In a saucepan, add the water, butter, sugar, and salt. Bring to a boil. Then remove from the heat, add the flour all at once, and stir vigorously until it forms a dough ball and pulls away from the sides of the pan.
2. Transfer the dough to the bowl of a stand mixer and beat with the paddle attachment at low speed until it cools to be just warm to the touch, about 5 minutes.
3. With the mixer at medium speed, add the eggs one at a time and beat until they are completely incorporated and the dough is smooth.

For the almond Florentines:

1 batch of prepared pâte-à-choux pastry
Baking spray for greasing the rimmed baking sheet
2 tablespoons cornstarch
¼ cup sugar
2 egg yolks
1 cup milk
1 tablespoon salted butter
½ teaspoon pure almond extract
4 ounces gluten-free almond paste (½ can Solo brand)
12 whole shelled almonds

1. Preheat the oven to 375°F.
2. Transfer the pâte-à-choux dough to a pastry bag fitted with a large star tip. On a lightly oiled baking sheet, pipe the dough to form 2½-inch-diameter circles. Then pipe a second circle within each larger circle, filling the center. Finally, pipe a second layer of dough on top of the outer circle.
3. Bake for 20 to 25 minutes, until golden brown. Let cool on the baking sheet.

For the almond pastry cream:

1. In a small bowl, mix the cornstarch and sugar. Whisk in the egg yolks, beating until light in color.
2. In a saucepan, bring the milk to a boil over high heat, then remove the pan from the heat.
3. To temper the egg yolk mixture with the heated milk: slowly pour

about half of the milk into the egg mixture while whisking vigorously, then pour the egg mixture into the saucepan with the rest of the milk, still whisking vigorously.

4. Bring the mixture to a boil, whisking constantly for 1 minute. Remove from the heat and stir in the butter and almond extract.

5. While the pastry cream is still warm, stir in the almond paste, whisking to incorporate until smooth. Refrigerate until cool.

To assemble:

1. Transfer the pastry cream to a pastry bag fitted with a star tip.
2. Pipe a rosette in the center of each pastry.
3. Top each pastry with a whole almond.

The Bronskis' Artisan Gluten-Free Flour Blend
Combine all of the ingredients and store in an airtight container in the refrigerator.

1 ¼ cups brown rice flour
¾ cup sorghum flour
⅔ cup cornstarch
¼ cup potato starch
1 tablespoon plus 1 teaspoon potato flour
1 teaspoon xanthan gum

Tate's Bake Shop, Southampton, New York

Kathleen King knows her cookies. She started baking them as a child, selling them from a fold-out card table at her family's farm stand. Pretty soon, she couldn't keep up with demand, left her mother's kitchen, opened a bakery, and named it for her father, Tate King. The rest, as they say, is Hamptons history. On visits back to Long Island, Tate's Bake Shop was a place I avoided for fear of fainting with longing. A few years ago, a friend convinced me to go in, made me close my eyes, and led me to the gluten-free chocolate chip cookies the whole country is raving about. Thin, crisp, *and* chewy—unforgettable.

KATHLEEN KING'S GLUTEN-FREE CHOCOLATE CRINKLES

Kathleen created these soft, cakey cookies for Colleen Seiler, Tate's wheat-intolerant assistant retail manager, so she'd have something wonderful to snack on at work. If this is an employee retention program, sign me up. Chocolate, cocoa, and espresso powder give these mini marvels their richness, while coconut flour and ground almonds add to their lightness.

MAKES ABOUT 7 DOZEN COOKIES

½ cup (1 stick) salted butter, cut into 8 pieces

4 ounces unsweetened chocolate, finely chopped

2 teaspoons vanilla extract

1 teaspoon instant espresso powder

1¼ cups almond flour or finely ground slivered almonds

½ cup potato starch

½ cup white or brown rice flour

¼ cup coconut flour

¼ cup natural or Dutch-processed cocoa powder

2 teaspoons baking powder

1½ cups plus ⅓ cup granulated sugar

4 large eggs, at room temperature

1 cup semisweet chocolate chips

1 cup confectioners' sugar

1. In a small saucepan, melt the butter over medium heat. Remove the pan from the heat, add the unsweetened chocolate, and let stand for 2 minutes to soften. Whisk until the chocolate is melted and smooth. Whisk in the vanilla and espresso powder. Let the mixture cool until tepid.

2. In a medium bowl, whisk together the almond flour, potato starch, rice flour, coconut flour, cocoa powder, and baking powder.

3. In a large bowl, beat 1½ cups of the granulated sugar and the eggs with an electric mixer set on high speed until the mixture is pale yellow and thick, about 3 minutes. Beat in the tepid chocolate mixture. Using a wooden spoon, gradually stir in the almond flour mixture. Stir in the chocolate chips. Cover the bowl with plastic wrap and refrigerate until the dough is chilled enough to handle easily, about 2 hours.

4. Position the oven racks in the top third and center of the oven and preheat oven to 350°F. Line two large, rimmed baking sheets with parchment paper or silicon baking mats.

5. Using about 1 tablespoon for each, roll the dough into balls. Put the remaining ⅓ cup of granulated sugar and the confectioners' sugar into two separate bowls. Roll each ball first in the granulated sugar, then in confectioners' sugar, and place the balls 3 inches apart on the prepared baking sheets. Bake just until the edges of the cookies are firm and the tops are cracked, about 10 minutes. The cookies should be soft and cakey; do not overbake. Let the cookies cool on the pans for 5 minutes. Transfer the cookies to a wire cooling rack and let cool completely.

6. Repeat with the remaining dough balls, using cooled baking sheets.

Christina Pirello

Star of the new show *Christina: America's Healthy Cooking Teacher*, this Emmy Award–winning whole foods chef understands the power of healing food more than most. At the age of twenty-six, gravely ill and with little chance of recovery, she embarked on a diet based on whole and unprocessed foods and proved it's possible to save your own life and eat happily ever after. Thirty years later, this red-haired dynamo is teaching us to do the same. Reprinted with permission from *Glow: A Prescription for Radiant Health and Beauty* by Christina Pirello (HP Trade). With thanks and great affection for setting me on a healthier path.

CHOCOLATE-GLAZED COCONUT MACAROONS

There is nothing quite like the paradox of macaroons—rich and decadent, yet decidedly light. And therein lies the art. If these gluten-free and dairy-free vegan delights were easier to make, they would make themselves. Herewith, a coconut lover's dream.

MAKES ABOUT 3 DOZEN MACAROONS

1. Preheat the oven to 400°F. Line two rimmed baking sheets with parchment paper.
2. Combine the coconut, coconut flour, baking powder, salt, syrup, almond extract, and almond milk. Mix well and add up to 1 cup of almond meal to create a sticky batter. Set aside so that the coconut gets saturated, about 5 minutes. You should have a thick batter, but it will not be very cohesive.
3. Drop the dough by teaspoons onto the prepared baking sheets, forming peaked cookies with your fingers. Bake until the coconut begins to brown, 18 to 20 minutes. Transfer the cookies to a wire rack to cool.

2½ cups unsweetened, shredded coconut
⅓ cup coconut flour
½ teaspoon baking powder
Pinch of sea salt
⅓ cup brown rice syrup
½ teaspoon almond or vanilla extract
⅔ to 1 cup unsweetened almond milk
Up to 1 cup almond meal

1. Place the chocolate in a heat-resistant bowl.
2. In a small saucepan, combine the almond milk and rice syrup and bring to a boil over high heat. As soon as the milk mixture comes to a rolling boil, pour it over the chocolate and whisk to form a smooth, satiny ganache.
3. Slip a piece of parchment paper under the wire rack to catch any drips. Moving in a zigzag direction, use a fork coated in the chocolate to drizzle the cookies with the chocolate glaze. Allow the cookies to stand for a few minutes to set the glaze.

For the chocolate glaze:
½ cup chopped nondairy dark chocolate
2 to 3 tablespoons unsweetened organic almond milk or soy milk
2 teaspoons gluten-free brown rice syrup

Taffets Bakery, Philadelphia

Blink and you've missed Omer and Natasha Taffet's tiny shop in South Philly's bustling Italian Market, where they devote themselves to raising the bar for gluten-free baked goods. There are sweets, of course—decadent brownies and exceptional biscotti. But bread is the heart of this place and these people know their stuff. Their baguette, one of the most difficult textural combinations to render gluten-free, is the real deal, crusty outside, soft and yeasty inside. I recently served it to a chef friend and watched as he tore off a hunk, dipped it into my Fish Stew (page 227), and never raised an eyebrow. There are bagels, too, teff and quinoa loaves, and, thanks to this generous pair, a thyme-, rosemary-, and garlic-studded focaccia to try at home.

TAFFETS MEDITERRANEAN FOCACCIA

This is Omer Taffet's homage to the fresh flavors of his childhood in Tel Aviv. Serve it as a starter with briny olives, feta, fresh basil, and summer tomatoes from the garden. Make it a savory foundation for winter's deeper spices, sun-dried tomatoes, robust cheeses, and vegetables. Spread it with roasted garlic or pesto and serve it with a salad. This recipe calls for dried herbs, but fresh, local, or homegrown herbs are even better. Taffet uses Bob's Red Mill flours, but you can substitute your favorite brand.

Olive oil for greasing the rimmed baking sheet and brushing the focaccia before baking
1½ cups millet flour
1½ cups brown rice flour
2 cups tapioca flour
1 tablespoon xanthan gum
1 tablespoon salt, plus more to sprinkle on the focaccia before baking
1 teaspoon dried basil
1 teaspoon dried thyme
1 teaspoon dried rosemary
¼ cup instant yeast
5 large egg whites
1 tablespoon honey
2 teaspoons vinegar
2⅜ cups water

SERVES 4

1. Preheat oven to 350°F. Spray olive oil on a 13 by 18-inch rimmed baking sheet.
2. In a large bowl, combine the millet flour, brown rice flour, tapioca flour, xanthan gum, salt, basil, thyme, rosemary and instant yeast prepared according to package directions. Add egg whites, honey, vinegar, and water and blend well.
3. Pour the batter onto the prepared baking sheet and spread evenly to the corners. Place near the stove or on a warm windowsill in the kitchen and let rise for 15 to 30 minutes, or until the batter doubles in size.
4. Brush with oil and sprinkle with salt. Bake for about 35 minutes, or until golden brown and a toothpick through the middle comes out clean.

Miglet's Cupcake Shop, Danville, California

It's not often that a world-class baker begins her career at a summer camp. Katie Taylor, founder of Miglet's and maker of the most beautiful wedding cakes in the world, started out as a volunteer for the Taylor Family Foundation gluten-free summer camp. The kids raved about the treats she baked for them, giving the young Katie the confidence to strike out on her own. Now the faithful flock to Danville for her pastries, cakes, brownies, breads and savory quiches, macaroni and cheese, chicken potpies (see Old-Fashioned Chicken Potpie, page 216), and, of course, cupcakes, created in a kitchen totally free of gluten. Rumor has it alarms are set all over town for Katie's Early Bird Delights. Alas Miglet's doesn't ship, but it supplies many area bakeries, including Mariposa in Berkeley and San Francisco. Moving to California is not out of the question.

VANILLA SALTED CARAMEL CAKE WITH VANILLA BUTTERCREAM

This vanilla salted caramel wedding extravaganza may just be worth getting married for. Add a garden, champagne, a few close friends, and some candied violets for the top of the cake. Eat happily ever after.

MAKES TWO 9-INCH LAYERS

1. Preheat oven to 325°F. Grease and flour two 9-inch pans.
2. In the bowl of an electric mixer, cream the sugar and egg yolks until light and fluffy, about 2 minutes. In a small saucepan, melt the shortening and butter together over low heat and add half to the mixture. Mix, then add the rest.
3. In a small bowl, combine the buttermilk and vanilla and set aside. In a larger bowl, sift together soda, salt, and xanthan gum. In the bowl of a standing mixer, with the mixer on low speed, alternate adding small amounts of the buttermilk and the sifted ingredients until well incorporated.
4. In a separate bowl, beat the egg whites until stiff and then gently fold them into the batter. Pour the batter into prepared cake pans, making sure the batter is evenly divided, and place in the oven for 30 to 35 minutes, until golden brown and a tester comes out clean when inserted in the middle of the cake.
5. Let the cakes cool in the pans for no more than 8 minutes before turning them onto a wire rack to finish cooling.

½ cup organic palm shortening, plus more for greasing the cake pans
2 cups all-purpose gluten-free flour, such as Cup4Cup, plus extra for dusting the cake pans
2 cups sugar
5 large eggs, separated, at room temperature
½ cup (1 stick) unsalted butter
1 cup buttermilk
1 teaspoon vanilla extract
1 teaspoon baking soda
½ teaspoon salt
If your all-purpose gluten-free flour does not contain xanthan gum, add ¾ teaspoon

Vanilla Buttercream

1. In the bowl of a standing mixer, cream the butter while slowly adding the milk and vanilla. Beat for 4 minutes.
2. Sift the sugar and add on low speed to the mixture, 1 cup at a time. Scrape the edges and bottom of the bowl and continue mixing until well incorporated. Set aside.

1 pound (2 sticks) unsalted butter, at room temperature
¼ cup milk
1 tablespoon vanilla extract
7 cups confectioners' sugar

2 cups sugar
2 tablespoons corn syrup
Water, enough to saturate
¾ cup heavy cream
2 tablespoons unsalted butter
1 teaspoon sea salt
1 tablespoon vanilla extract

Salted Caramel Filling

1. In a small saucepan, mix the sugar and corn syrup together with enough water to saturate the mixture. Place over medium to high heat and boil until the mixture reaches a deep amber color or reaches 350°F on a candy thermometer.
2. Remove from the heat immediately. Slowly whisk in the cream, butter, sea salt, and vanilla. Set aside until completely cooled.

Assembly:

1. If the cakes have formed peaks on top, cut them off with a serrated knife so that they are level.
2. Place one layer on a serving plate. Frost an even layer of vanilla buttercream onto the cake and place it in the refrigerator for 5 minutes to set. This is important because it will allow the frosting to set up before pouring the caramel over it.
3. Remove the layer from the refrigerator. Pour the caramel on top until it oozes a bit down the sides of the cake. Place the second layer on top and put the cake back in the refrigerator for 5 minutes. Remove it from the refrigerator. Frost the top of the cake with vanilla buttercream and drizzle the cake with the rest of the caramel. Serve at room temperature.

Learn More

Artisanal Gluten-Free Cooking and *Artisanal Gluten-Free Cupcakes* by Kelli and Peter Bronski (The Experiment). www.noglutennoproblem.blogspot.com

BabyCakes: Vegan, (Mostly) Gluten-Free, and (Mostly) Sugar-Free Recipes from New York's Most Talked-About Bakery by Erin McKenna (Clarkson Potter) and *BabyCakes Covers the Classics: Gluten-Free Vegan Recipes from Donuts to Snickerdoodles* by Erin McKenna and Tara Donne (Clarkson Potter). www.babycakesnyc.com

Flying Apron Bakery, Seattle, Washington, www.flyingapron.com, *Flying Apron's Gluten-Free and Vegan Baking Book* and *Gluten-Free and Vegan Holidays* by Jennifer Katzinger (Sasquatch Books)

Helmut Newcake, Paris. www.helmutnewcake.com

It's All Good by Gwyneth Paltrow with Julia Turshen (Grand Central)

Miglet's Bakery, Danville, California. www.migletsgf.com

Glenn Minervini-Zick—Books forthcoming: *A Cookie Baker's Touch, Gluten-Free and Gluten-Full Artisanal Cookies* and *Traditional Bakers of Ecuador*. www.zixcookies.wordpress.com

Nigellissima: Easy Italian-Inspired Recipes by Nigella Lawson (Clarkson Potter). www.foodnetwork.com/nigella

Pure Fare, Philadelphia. www.purefare.com and Agno Grill. www.agnogrill.com

Risotteria, New York City. www.risotteria.com

Taffets Bakery, Philadelphia. www.taffets.com

The Talk—Food Network

Tate's Bake Shop, Southampton, New York. www.tatesbakeshop.com. *Baking for Friends* by Kathleen King (Tate's Bake Shop)

This Crazy Vegan Life, Cooking the Whole Foods Way and *Glow: A Prescription for Radiant Health and Beauty* by Christina Pirello (HP Trade). www.christinacooks.com. *Christina: America's Healthy Cooking Teacher*, www.createtv.com

9

You Gotta Have It

Jonesing/vb: to have a strong need, desire
or craving for something.
—URBAN DICTIONARY

◆ Caroline Winge-Bogar: *Grown-Up Macaroni and Cheese*
◆ Glenn Minervini-Zick: *Pizza Just Like Mamma Makes (or Wishes She Could)*
◆ Eileen Plato: *Judy's Cafe Oh, Mama! Meatloaf*
◆ Kelli and Peter Bronski: *Chicken Tikka Masala*
◆ Jilly Lagasse and Jessie Lagasse Swanson: *French Onion Soup with Gruyère-Smothered Crostini • Jilly and Jessie's Spiced Carrot Cake with Sweet Mascarpone Frosting*
◆ Katie Taylor: *Old-Fashioned Chicken Potpie*
◆ Kevin Smith: *Mexican Lasagna*
◆ Lynn Jamison: *Mother of All Tortes*
◆ Reverend Michael Alan: *Apple and Fig Crisp*
◆ Lowell Family: *Vegetarian Pad Thai*

No matter how pure you are, how consciously you eat, or how scrupulously you avoid fat and calories, sugar and carbs, the day will come when you absolutely must eat something that satisfies physical hunger *and* feeds the soul. Usually that food is bound up with the sense memory of family, friends, falling in love, the need to be comforted and cosseted against life's rough edges, or a sudden longing for long-gone and pre-gluten-free pleasures. You will resist, because most likely what you are jonesing for isn't the healthiest or the lowest-calorie choice. You may have something else instead, but no amount of eating around this craving will suffice. It won't let go until you give in.

When I was growing up my father often brought us homemade ice cream from a neighborhood ice cream parlor: a quart of intense black raspberry and coffee with a hint of butterscotch packed down hard in a cardboard carton. Even now, those two flavors conjure glinting spoons; my mother's voice, low and house warm; my father's satisfied smile; my grandmother's sly look as she offered me the rest of hers.

Every now and then I sit down at a local ice cream store (pre-vetted for gluten-freeness) and order two scoops, coffee on top, black raspberry on the bottom, just the way my father brought it home. One taste and I am a small girl again, circled, safe.

Nothing else will do.

Herewith are some recipes (and some amazing packaged treats, too) for nursery foods, comfort foods, simple foods, and splurges that summon the particular tastes of the stories of our lives and, in so doing, take us to a new level of nourishment. I do not advocate living on foods like these, but I wholeheartedly embrace them for those times when, well, *you gotta have it*. Lost and now found again, sweet or savory, these pleasures are still as potent without the gluten.

Mac Attack

Forget the fat. Forgo the mea culpa. You don't do this often, so enjoy it. This decidedly grown-up version of the ultimate comfort food combines Brie, Muenster, and provolone, and once you get the hang of it, you can experiment with other variations like sharp cheddar, Emmentaler, and Gruyère. The trick is coming up with combinations that work well together and will not overwhelm each other. Cheese is the star here, so splurge a little; nothing processed, please. Let out your waistband and succumb to gooey, cheesy goodness.

GROWN-UP MACARONI AND CHEESE

No additive-addled supper-in-a-box here. From Caroline Winge-Bogar, a Culinary Institute of America–trained chef with a genius for updating classics, this savory macaroni and cheese is what soothing tastes like on a very sophisticated tongue. With a simple salad, it can be a humble family meal, or it can be an elegant and unexpected side at a dinner party. Then again, you could just eat it out of a bowl in your pajamas.

SERVES 4

½ cup (1 stick) unsalted butter, plus more to butter the baking dish

10-ounce box elbow macaroni

2 tablespoons cornstarch

1½ cups milk

1½ cups half-and-half

4 ounces (1 cup) Brie, cut into medium dice

2 ounces (½ cup) Muenster, cut into medium dice

2 ounces (½ cup) provolone, cut into medium dice

2 large egg yolks

½ teaspoon salt

½ teaspoon coarsely ground black pepper

2 slices gluten-free bread chopped in the bowl of a food processor, or packaged gluten-free bread crumbs (optional)

1. Preheat oven to 350°F. Butter well a large Pyrex baking dish.
2. Cook the pasta al dente according to the package directions, taking care not to overcook.
3. In a small bowl, combine the cornstarch with 2 tablespoons of the milk and stir until well blended. In a large saucepan, combine the rest of the milk, the half-and-half, and the butter and bring to a boil, watching carefully to avoid boiling over. Add the cornstarch mixture and continue boiling until thickened, about 1 minute.
4. Reduce the heat to medium low and add the cheeses. Stir until the sauce is smooth. Remove from the heat and quickly stir in the yolks, one at a time, stirring constantly. Season with the salt and pepper.
5. Pour the cheese over the cooked pasta and transfer to the prepared baking dish. Top with the bread crumbs, if desired. Bake for about 25 minutes, until the top is lightly browned and bubbly.

Gotta-Have-Pizza Pizza

There are some pretty good gluten-free frozen pizzas these days, most notably the offerings from Against the Grain Gourmet. There are wonderful restaurant pizzas, too, for a night out with family and friends. But sometimes you just want something homemade. This one reminds me of the pies left on our cottage doorstep when I was a child, still warm and covered with a kitchen towel, our Italian neighbor's way of thanking my parents for some kindness or another. Those were the best, crusty on the edges, soft at the center, scented with basil and gorgeous homegrown tomatoes, melting with good cheeses and a bit of meatball or sweet Italian sausage to eat on a summer porch.

PIZZA JUST LIKE MAMA MAKES (OR WISHES SHE COULD)

This comes from master baker Glenn Minervini-Zick (see page 189 for his Raspberry Almond Ravioli Cookie), who is proving one treat at a time that gluten-free isn't a substitute for anything. The folks at the Sonoma County Community College baking program apparently think so, too. They tasted two pizzas with the same toppings, one gluten-free, the other wheat, with care taken to avoid cross-contamination, of course. The bake master's pizzas won hands down. Once you get the hang of the dough, experiment with toppings. Fresh vegetables, meatballs, sweet Italian sausage, pitted olives (maybe a little Greek feta), grilled artichokes, zucchini, roasted peppers, pesto: the sky's the limit. This recipe is guaranteed to make your modern kitchen fragrant with memories of slower times. The crust can be made and frozen and toppings added. Talk about thinking outside the box.

MAKES TWO 10-INCH PIZZAS

1. In a large mixing bowl, put the rice flour. In a 2-cup measuring cup, combine 1 cup warm water, the yeast, the olive oil, and the honey. Add liquids to the rice flour and mix with a wooden spoon. Then add the remaining ¾ cup of warm water and stir until well blended.

2. Cover bowl with plastic wrap and let sit in warm location for 2 to 3 hours, or until the volume doubles.

3. In a large bowl, combine the millet, sorghum, and tapioca flours, the potato starch, and the salt. Mix well with a whisk. Add to the wet rice flour mix and stir until well blended.

4. Transfer the dough to the bowl of a standing mixer. Using the dough hook attachment, mix the dough until it is very smooth, 2 to 3 minutes. Or you can transfer the dough to a floured countertop (use a mix of rice and tapioca flours for flouring the countertop surface) and

For the dough:
1 cup rice flour, plus more to dust the countertop (optional)
1¾ cups warm water
1 tablespoon or one package active dry yeast
4 tablespoons olive oil
1 tablespoon honey
1 cup millet flour
½ cup sorghum flour
1 cup tapioca flour, plus more to dust the countertop (optional)
½ cup potato starch
2 teaspoons kosher salt, plus more for sprinkling on the pizza
Olive oil, for oiling the baking sheets and brushing on the pizzas

For the topping:
5 medium ripe tomatoes, chopped into small dice (note: if the tomatoes are out of season, substitute good-quality organic canned diced tomatoes)
6 ounces (1½ cups) mozzarella cheese, grated
3 ounces (¾ cup) Parmigiano Reggiano cheese, grated
1 tablespoon garlic finely chopped
¼ cup fresh basil, chiffonade or finely sliced, chopped, or torn
Freshly ground black pepper

knead by hand for 5 minutes. The dough will be soft and sticky and a little tough to work with, but messiness is part of the magic.

5. After the dough is smooth and a bit stretchy from kneading, put it back in the bowl to rest while you preheat the oven to 500°F.

6. Lightly oil 2 baking sheets. Divide the dough into 5 pieces. For each piece, place the dough on the baking sheet and spread out with your fingers and palms. The dough will shrink a bit as you push it out. Let the dough relax from time to time, but keep pushing it until the dough is very thin, about ¼-inch thick or less. (Note: With baking sheets you will have one 10-inch circular pizza per sheet. Small pizzas are easier to work with and bake faster.) Repeat this process for the remaining 3 dough pieces.

7. Brush the pizza dough with olive oil and sprinkle with salt. Bake for 4 to 5 minutes. Partially baked pizza will have a bit of color on top but will not be golden brown. If the crust sticks to the baking sheet, loosen it with a metal spatula.

8. Remove the pizzas from the oven and sprinkle with topping—the tomatoes, mozzarella, Parmigiano-Romano, garlic, and basil—on each pizza. Sprinkle with salt and pepper and put back in the oven for an additional 6 to 8 minutes.

9. Peek at the underside of the pizza as the cheese becomes golden brown to ensure that the bottom of the pizza is also golden brown. Resist the urge to take the pizza out of the oven too soon. Bake a minute longer to ensure that the crust is done.

Option: You can complete the recipe through Step 6, bake the pizza crusts, and freeze them plain for up to 1 month. When you've gotta have it, add the toppings and bake for 4 to 6 minutes at 500°F.

Judy's Cafe Meat Loaf

Once upon a time there was a place where everyone knew your name and you could eat at the bar if you were on your own and wanted a quick supper and a little dishing with the neighbors. You could go to Judy's in your pajamas if you felt like it, and in that part of town this wasn't such an outlandish idea. Bill, the maître d', art expert, and resident raconteur, regaled the regulars with tales of lost treasures and museum misadventures. The chef once parked my car. Eileen Plato, ringmaster, owner, and baker of apple pies and towering layer cakes, was the soul and spirit of the place. She understood what foods we were jonesing for.

Mix Master

Thomas Keller, one of America's most celebrated chefs, owner of The French Laundry, Bouchon, Ad Hoc, and Per Se, and with several Michelin stars under his toque, has taken gluten-free baking mixes to the next level. His Ad Hoc Gluten-Free Waffle and Pancake Mix is a new reason to make brunch and his Bouchon Bakery Gluten-Free Chocolate Chunk Cookie Mix, made with Callebaut chocolate chips and Nielsen-Massey vanilla, and Gluten-Free Carrot and Corn Muffin Mixes can make an afternoon treat into a special occasion. Pricey, but it's not as if you are doing this every day. Exclusively at Williams-Sonoma. www.williams-sonoma.com

There is something gentrified and expensive on that corner now, small plates served with greens resembling cocktail hats and with a waiting list longer than both my arms. Thanks to Eileen, who has kept this recipe a state secret until now, the meat loaf lives on.

OH, MAMA! MEAT LOAF

I am told that the inspiration for this classic Italian polpettone came from Elizabeth David's classic cookbook, *Italian Food*. Many iterations and fine tunings came later, including this one, which calls for gluten-free bread crumbs. This is a meat loaf to tweet about. You'll need plastic wrap for molding and shaping, a small pastry brush, and the best ground pork, veal, and beef you can find. This recipe will yield three small loaves, enough for a hungry crowd and game day meat loaf sandwiches. Or you can freeze half for the next time you've gotta have it. The only way to serve it is with potatoes mashed with garlic, butter, salt, pepper, and plenty of cream. (Okay, light cream.) You've got your whole life to eat like a Spartan.

SERVES 6 TO 8 WITH LEFTOVERS

1. Preheat the oven to 375°F.
2. In a large bowl and using protective gloves, hand mix the meats thoroughly.
3. In another bowl, whisk together eggs, garlic, shallots, tomato paste, Worcestershire sauce, salt, and pepper. Add the wet mix to the meat mix and blend thoroughly. Add enough bread crumbs to bind the mixture. Shape the meat into 3 loaves.
4. In another bowl, mix the spinach, bell pepper, and 1 cup of Parmesan. In a separate, smaller bowl, put the provolone.

Assembly:

1. Line a rimmed baking sheet with parchment paper. Set aside.
2. Spread a large piece of plastic wrap on your work surface. Place 1 loaf in the middle and flatten it. Cover with another piece of wrap and roll out into a uniform rectangle.
3. Remove the top sheet of plastic wrap and spread one-third of the spinach mix down the center of the loaf. Top with a third of the provolone. Roll the loaf up on the long side toward the middle, starting on the side

1 pound each of pork, veal, and beef, ground together
3 whole large eggs plus 1 large egg white for glazing
6 cloves garlic, finely chopped
3 large shallots, finely chopped
1/3 cup tomato paste
1½ tablespoons Worcestershire sauce
2 teaspoons kosher salt
2 teaspoons freshly ground black pepper
½ to 1 cup gluten-free bread crumbs, enough to bind the loaves
½ 6-ounce bag of spinach, stemmed and chopped
1 large red bell pepper, finely diced
½ to ¾ cup grated Parmesan cheese
1 ounce (¼ cup) provolone cheese, diced, or more to taste

closest to you. Repeat the roll toward you from the other side. Seal lengthwise and tuck in the ends. Note: To ensure that the loaf does not burst open while in the oven, seal the seams tightly using your fingers and plastic wrap.

4. Keeping the loaf in plastic, transfer it to the prepared baking sheet. Then flip it open, bottom to top. Discard the plastic wrap. Repeat with the remaining loaves.

5. Brush the loaves with lightly beaten egg white.

6. Bake for 35 to 40 minutes, until the loaves are a little oozy and give slightly when pushed with your finger.

Subcontinental Comfort

When Kelli and Peter Bronski are not creating world-class gluten-free pâte-à-choux pastry for their Almond Florentines (page 198), these passionate artisanal cooks love nothing more than adapting traditional Indian cuisine like this classic chicken dish from the Tandoori Grill in Boulder, Colorado. The result is a rich tomato cream sauce enlivened by layers of spice and a touch of sweetness from caramelized onions. From *Artisanal Gluten-Free Cooking* with many thanks to Kelli and Peter Bronski.

Tate's Bake Shop Gluten-Free Chocolate Chip Cookies

Crispy, chewy, buttery, rich, but not overly so. You need to get up early—these crave-worthy cookies fly off the shelf at Whole Foods and other specialty stores faster than regular Tate's. A total of 80 calories a pop, 4 grams fat, 9 carbs. How do they do that? www.tatesbakeshop.com

---

KELLI AND PETER BRONSKI'S CHICKEN TIKKA MASALA

3 boneless, skinless chicken breasts, cubed
Salt
3 tablespoons olive oil
1 tablespoon butter
1 medium onion, sliced
1 large garlic clove, minced
1 tablespoon fresh ginger, minced
½ teaspoon cayenne pepper (optional)
2 teaspoons ground cumin
2 teaspoons paprika
1 teaspoon garam masala
1½ cups diced tomatoes or 1 14.5-ounce can no-salt-added diced tomatoes
1 cup heavy cream
½ cup gluten-free chicken broth
⅓ cup fresh cilantro, chopped

Paired with steamed basmati or jasmine rice and Garlic Naan (page 302) to mop up all of the sauce and the savory bits, this is as far from ghee-laden takeout as Minneapolis is from Mumbai.

SERVES 4

1. Season the chicken with salt. Heat a bit of olive oil (about 1 to 2 tablespoons) in a large skillet over medium-high heat. Sauté the chicken until cooked. Remove from the pan and set aside.

2. In the same skillet, over medium heat, melt the butter and the additional tablespoon of olive oil. Add the onion, garlic, and ginger and sauté until very soft, about 10 minutes.

3. Add the cayenne, if using, cumin, paprika, and garam masala and stir to combine. Cook for an additional minute.

4. Add the tomatoes, heavy cream, and chicken broth. Using a hand-

held immersion blender, or a traditional blender, purée until smooth.

5. Simmer uncovered for 10 minutes. Add the chicken and simmer for an additional 10 to 20 minutes. (Simmering longer will yield a richer, more flavorful and thicker sauce, but be careful, as simmering for too long may cause the sauce to separate.)

6. Add the fresh cilantro just before serving. Serve over rice.

Jilly Lagasse and Jessie Lagasse Swanson's French Onion Soup with Gruyère-Smothered Crostini

Imagine having Emeril as a father: spoon-fed and cosseted in his kitchen, wrapped in the bigness of a chef's heart; all of your growing pains eased with good Louisiana comfort food, maybe a beignet for being a good girl. Then BAM! You're gluten-free and all that breaded southern comfort is a thing of the past. But you are the apples that have not fallen far from the tree and you have learned from the master. You yearn for the onion soup–soaked crostini of your childhood and you transform that yearning into something warming and buttery, cheesy and satisfying for a bitter winter's night.

OH, DADDY! ONION SOUP

The sisters suggest using a premade gluten-free baguette like the ones made by Against the Grain Gourmet. If you are lucky to have a gluten-free bakery near you, all the better. This recipe brings out the flavor of red onions, but any type you prefer will work just as well. Tying the sprigs of herbs together with some butcher's twine will make it a lot easier to fish out the parsley and thyme when the soup is done. With many thanks to Jilly and Jessie, reprinted with permission from *The Gluten-Free Table* (Grand Central).

2 tablespoons olive oil
3 pounds red onions, thinly sliced (about 10 cups)
Salt
4 sprigs of fresh thyme
2 sprigs of fresh parsley
4 cups gluten-free chicken stock
4 cups gluten-free beef stock
½ cup dry red wine
1 bay leaf
1 tablespoon balsamic vinegar
Freshly ground black pepper to taste
1 gluten-free baguette, cut into ½- to ¾-inch slices
8 ounces (about 2 cups) Gruyère cheese, grated
Finely sliced green onions, for garnish (optional)

SERVES 6

1. In an 8-quart nonstick stockpot, heat the olive oil over medium-high heat for 1 to 2 minutes, just to get the oil warm.

2. Add the onions and ½ teaspoon salt. Stir so that the oil coats all of the onions.

3. Cook for 30 to 40 minutes over medium heat, stirring the onions often. The onions will become caramelized and brownish and begin to form a syrupy crust on the bottom of the pan.

4. Meanwhile, with butcher's twine, gently tie the stems of the thyme and parsley together to form a mini herb bouquet. Set aside.

5. Once the onions are fully caramelized, stir in the chicken stock, beef stock, wine, thyme-and-parsley bouquet, and bay leaf. Loosen the browned crust on the pan's bottom with a wooden spoon and stir until those bits become incorporated into the liquid.

6. Bring the soup to a simmer and cook for another 20 to 30 minutes to meld all of the flavors.

7. Preheat the oven to broil.

8. Remove the soup from the heat. Stir in the balsamic vinegar and add salt and black pepper as desired. Remove the herbs, including the bay leaf.

9. Ladle about 1 cup of soup into each of 6 ovenproof soup bowls and place on a baking sheet.

10. Top the soup in each bowl with 1 to 2 slices of the baguette and sprinkle the bread with approximately ⅓ cup cheese.

11. Broil the soup until the cheese is bubbly and browned, 3 to 5 minutes, depending on your oven.

12. Remove the soup bowls from the oven and garnish with green onions, if desired. Let cool for several minutes and serve.

Big Fat Pretend-It's-Your-Birthday Carrot Cake

Sometimes you just want cake, sweet, moist, airy, and iced to within an inch of its life. It can't be a cupcake or a brownie or even a cookie. It's got to be the real deal, like your mother made or, in this case, your father. This is the stuff of bake sales, birthdays, covered-dish suppers with a spare for the family, the kind of cake you can press a fork into and lift every last crumb. You know you should substitute applesauce and agave syrup for butter and cane sugar. But we are talking craving here, the kind that grabs you by the lapels and won't let go until you've had at least two slices before you freeze the rest and try to forget it behind the gluten-free flax waffles.

JILLY AND JESSIE'S SPICED CARROT CAKE WITH SWEET MASCARPONE FROSTING

I like to think this is how Emeril got them to eat their carrots. More delicate than the layer cakes of long ago, and more grown-up, this is the one that will take you back to that sweet burnt air of birthday candles and big wishes. For an even more spectacular effect, garnish with grated carrot and chopped pecans. From *The Gluten-Free Table* with thanks to Jilly Lagasse and Jessie Lagasse Swanson.

SERVES 8 TO 10

1. Preheat the oven to 350°F. Grease and flour two 9-inch cake pans.
2. In a large bowl, cream the butter and brown sugar until light and fluffy, using either a handheld or stand electric mixer. Add the eggs and vanilla and beat until creamy.
3. In a separate bowl, sift together the flour blend, baking powder, cinnamon, and salt. Stir in the almond meal/flour. Gently fold the dry ingredients into the butter mixture and blend until it becomes thick.
4. Add 1½ cups of the carrots, ⅔ cup of the walnuts, if using, and the milk and mix well.
5. Spoon the batter into the prepared cake pans, dividing evenly. Bake for 35 to 40 minutes, or until a toothpick inserted in one of the layers comes out clean. Allow the layers to cool fully in the pans before trying to invert them onto a cake plate.
6. While the layers are cooling, make the frosting. In a medium bowl, using a handheld or stand mixer, combine the mascarpone, confectioners' sugar, and ¼ cup of the remaining walnuts, mixing until thoroughly incorporated. The consistency should be fluffy. Set aside.
7. Carefully invert one of the cake layers onto a serving plate or cake stand and frost the top with a small amount of the frosting. You'll need a thin layer to act like a glue to hold the next layer on.
8. Carefully invert the second cake layer on top of the frosted layer. Generously cover the cake on the top and sides with the remaining frosting. Decorate with the remaining ½ cup grated carrot and any remaining nuts.
9. Store the cake in the refrigerator until serving time.

12 tablespoons (1½ sticks) unsalted butter, softened to room temperature, plus more to grease the cake pans

1½ cups all-purpose gluten-free flour blend (Arrowhead Mills was used here), plus more to dust the cake pans

1½ cups (packed) soft light brown sugar

6 large eggs

1 teaspoon all-natural vanilla extract

1 heaping tablespoon plus 1 heaping teaspoon baking powder

½ teaspoon ground cinnamon

1 teaspoon salt

½ cup almond meal/flour

2 cups finely grated carrots (about 2 large carrots, peeled)

1 cup walnuts or pecans (about 4 ounces), roughly chopped (optional)

2 tablespoons milk, any % fat you prefer

2 14-ounce containers good-quality mascarpone cheese, softened to room temperature

½ cup confectioners' sugar

Julie's Gluten-Free Organic Ice Cream Sandwiches

I don't know about you, but my idea of heaven is a Carvel Flying Saucer on a hot summer night—vanilla ice cream, chocolate cookie a little bit soggy, a little bit crisp. Made with Glutenfreeda gluten-free organic cookies, these are lightweights at 200 calories a pop, certified organic, no chemical additives, no GMOs. Lemon cookie, too. Four slightly Flying Saucer–ish sandwiches in a round can. www.juliesorganic.com.

Oh, My Potpie

Katie Taylor, founder of Miglet's Cupcake Shop, is barely out of her twenties, and yet this wunderkind understands the need for something that evokes simpler times both savory and comforting. The allure of this old-fashioned combination of pie and chicken stew never fades. Maybe it's because our lives move so fast and are so stressful, and these little wonders are so hearty and unfussy. This one takes me back to my own nana's kitchen, scent of sage and butter, steam escaping from an X carved into a golden crust, the anticipation of waiting for it to cool enough to eat.

OLD-FASHIONED CHICKEN POTPIE

Katie's gluten-free variation on the classic is redolent of thyme and cream, carrots and onion, and she relies on a good gluten-free flour blend; she recommends Cup4Cup. This recipe makes one 9-inch pie to serve in separate bowls. While the pie is baking, toss field greens dressed with vinaigrette. Open a bottle of wine and let it breathe. You, too.

For the dough:

4½ cups all-purpose gluten-free flour blend, plus more for dusting the pastry board
½ cup sweet rice flour
¼ cup sugar
2 teaspoons xanthan gum
1 teaspoon salt
1¼ cups (2½ sticks) cold unsalted butter, cut into cubes
4 large eggs
2 to 3 tablespoons water

SERVES 4

1. Preheat oven to 350°F.
2. In the large bowl of a standing mixer, sift together the flours, sugar, xanthan gum, and salt. Add the butter and mix on low speed until the pieces of butter are the size of peas or smaller. Add the eggs and mix until combined. Slowly add water until the dough comes together.

3. Roll out the dough on a pastry board dusted with gluten-free flour. Cut 2 rounds, using your favorite 9-inch pie pan as a guide. Use one dough round for the bottom crust and reserve the other for the top crust.

4. Press the pie dough into the pan and par bake your pie shell for 10 minutes.

1. In a large saucepan, heat olive oil over medium heat. Add the onion and cook until softened, about 4 minutes.

2. Add the butter and flour and cook for 1 to 2 minutes, whisking continuously. Slowly add the stock and whisk out any lumps.

3. Add the carrots, peas, corn, and chicken and cook until the filling has thickened, about 5 minutes. Add the thyme.

4. Fill the pie shell and place the second crust on top. Gently pinch the edges of the pie to create a seal.

5. In a small bowl, whisk the egg and cream together and generously brush the top of the pie with the mixture. Cut an X shape into the top crust and bake for 30 to 40 minutes, or until the top of the pie is golden brown and bubbling.

6. Let the potpie rest for 10 minutes before serving.

For the chicken filling:
1 tablespoon olive oil
1 medium yellow onion, chopped
¼ cup (½ stick) unsalted butter
¼ cup plus 2 tablespoons all-purpose gluten-free flour blend
2½ cups low-sodium gluten-free chicken stock
1 large carrot, peeled, diced and blanched
4 ounces (about ½ cup) frozen peas
4 ounces (about ½ cup) frozen corn
4 to 5 ounces (about ⅔ cup) chicken, fully cooked and diced, preferably chicken thigh
1½ teaspoon fresh thyme, minced
1 large egg
1 tablespoon heavy cream

Hilary's Eat Well—the World's Best Veggie Burger

Who says cravings can't be healthy? These crunchy and delicious patties from Local Burger founder Hilary Brown can be prepared the conventional way or popped into the toaster: no gluten, corn, yeast, dairy, egg, GMO, soy, or nuts, 200 vegan calories, and a whopping 4 grams of fiber. Among the healthy and planet-friendly ingredients are coconut oil, spinach, sweet potato, and apple cider vinegar. I like mine slathered with guacamole, sliced tomato, and lettuce on a big, soft, gluten-free roll. www.hilaryseatwell.com.

I Want Tacos! Enchiladas! Pizza!

You're craving something spicy, but you yearn for the texture and gooeyness of something cheesy. You want tomatoes, cheese, chicken, and beef and something crispy, too. A little jalapeño would be nice. You want it all before you have a meltdown. Richly textured, creamy, and crisp, redolent of oregano, chopped chilies, and cream—Mexico City meets Palermo in a casserole dish.

MEXICAN LASAGNA

Here is Kevin Smith's masterpiece of international indulgence adapted from *The Frog Commissary Cookbook*. At my house we call this richly filling and supremely satisfying concoction the Pearl Harbor of lasagnas because just when you think you have room for another piece, you're sunk. Make it for supper and divide up leftovers into single microwavable portions and freeze. Save it for one of those days when putting on your shoes is too much work.

SERVES 8

For the chicken layer:
1½ cups gluten-free chicken stock
2 teaspoons crushed coriander seeds
6 bay leaves
1 pound boneless, skinless chicken breasts, cut into 1-inch strips
¼ teaspoon salt
½ teaspoon freshly ground black pepper

For the beef layer:
¾ pound ground beef
1½ teaspoons ground coriander
⅛ teaspoon ground cloves
¼ teaspoon freshly ground black pepper
½ teaspoon dried oregano
½ teaspoon ground cumin
1 teaspoon minced garlic
¾ teaspoon salt
2 tablespoons minced roasted jalapeño peppers or ¼ teaspoon crushed red pepper flakes
2 tablespoons balsamic or red wine vinegar

For the onion mixture:
2 tablespoons olive oil
3 cups yellow onions, thinly sliced
½ teaspoon salt
2 4-ounce cans mild green chilies, chopped

To make the chicken layer:
1. In a deep skillet, combine the stock, coriander seeds, and bay leaves over high heat and bring to a boil. Reduce the heat to very low and simmer for 5 minutes. Add the chicken, cover, raise the heat to high and bring back to a boil. Reduce the heat to very low and cook for 7 to 10 minutes more, or until the chicken is just done.
2. Pour the contents of the skillet into a sieve set over a bowl to catch the broth. Let the chicken cool.
3. Return the broth to the pan and reduce the liquid to ½ cup over medium heat. Set aside.
4. Remove any bay leaves and seeds from the chicken and cut the meat into ½-inch pieces. Combine the chicken with the reduced broth and the salt and pepper. Set aside.

To make the beef layer:
1. In a large skillet, combine the beef, coriander, cloves, pepper, oregano, cumin, garlic, salt, jalapeño, and vinegar. Cover and cook over medium heat until the beef loses its pink color and all the vinegar has evaporated, about 8 to 10 minutes.
2. Set aside.

To make the onion mixture:
1. In a 9-inch skillet, heat the olive oil over medium heat. Add the onions, salt, and chilies. Cook for about 10 minutes, stirring frequently.
2. Set aside.

To make the tomato sauce:

1. Preheat oven to 475°F. Line a rimmed baking sheet with aluminum foil.
2. Put the tomatoes stem side down in a single layer on the prepared baking sheet. Bake for 25 to 30 minutes, or until the skins are lightly charred.
3. In a blender or in the bowl of a food processor, purée the tomatoes, skins, stems, and all, and then put them through a sieve.
4. In a large skillet, heat the olive oil over medium heat. Add the garlic and sauté for about 15 seconds. Add the puréed tomatoes, sugar, salt, and pepper. Cook, stirring occasionally, for 10 to 15 minutes, until the mixture has thickened. Set aside.

For the tomato sauce:
4 pounds ripe tomatoes
2 tablespoons olive oil
1 tablespoon garlic, minced
2 tablespoons sugar
1¾ teaspoons salt
½ teaspoon freshly ground black pepper

Assembly:

1. Preheat the oven to 350°F. Lightly oil a 9 by 13 by 2-inch baking dish. Put down a layer of 6 tostadas.
2. Mix the chicken with half of the onion mixture and 1 cup tomato sauce. Spread the mixture over the tostados. Drizzle with 1 cup of crème fraîche. Sprinkle l cup of the cheese on top.
3. Lay down 6 more tostadas, pressing and flattening down the layer below.
4. Combine the beef with the remaining onions and 1 cup tomato sauce. Spread this over the tostados. Top with 1 cup crème fraîche and 1 cup cheese.
5. Lay down the last 6 tostados and the remaining cheese.
6. Set the pan on a rimmed baking sheet and bake for 35 to 40 minutes, until golden and bubbly. Let the lasagna rest for 15 minutes before serving. Garnish with coriander and sliced black olives.

18 5-inch gluten-free tostados (corn tortillas fried until crisp in ½ inch corn oil and well drained)
3 cups crème fraîche
1 pound (4 cups) cheddar cheese, grated
1 tablespoon fresh cilantro or parsley, minced
Handful of pitted black olives, sliced

The Chocolate-Butter-Sugar Jones

You've had a rough week. Forget messing around with flour. You want the richest torte you can find. You don't care how many calories. This is an emergency. If you don't feed this craving, you'll do something bad like eat toothache-sweet frosting straight out of the Betty Crocker can. You swear you'll only eat a sliver and freeze the rest. But you know you can't be trusted. Bet you can round up some friends whose weeks have been as bad as yours.

MOTHER OF ALL TORTES

Lynn Jamison, owner of the long-gone and much-missed Jamison's Bakery, calls this tribute to the major food groups—chocolate, butter, sugar, and cream—Queen Mother Cake. This is a moist cake, not quite molten, but quite wet after baking. To avoid collapse, let it cool completely in the pan before turning it out onto a cake plate, if you can bear to wait that long.

MAKES TWO 9-INCH LAYERS

Butter and gluten-free all-purpose flour for preparing the pans
12 ounces bittersweet chocolate
¾ pound (3 sticks) unsalted butter
1½ cups sugar
½ teaspoon salt
12 large eggs, separated
Pinch of cream of tartar
¾ pound (about ½ cup) almonds, finely ground

1. Preheat the oven to 300°F. Generously butter 2 round 9-inch cake pans and dust them well with flour.
2. In the top of a double boiler, melt the chocolate over low heat. Set aside and let cool.
3. In a large bowl, cream the butter, sugar, and salt together. In a separate bowl, gently whisk the egg yolks. Add the whisked yolks to the creamed butter and sugar, mixing thoroughly. Add the cooled chocolate and fold in.
4. In a small chilled bowl, place the reserved egg whites. Add the cream of tartar to the egg whites and whip into soft peaks. Using a spatula gently fold the egg whites into the chocolate mixture, then gently fold in the almonds, one-third at a time.
5. Pour the batter into the prepared pans and bake for about 40 minutes, or until a sharp knife inserted comes out almost clean. Cool thoroughly before removing the cake from the pans.

Chocolate Glaze

1½ cups heavy cream
6 ounces bittersweet chocolate, chopped into small pieces
1 cup sliced, un-blanched almonds

1. In a small saucepan, heat the cream over medium heat to scalding, until bubbles appear around the outside edge of the liquid. Remove from the heat and mix in the chocolate until it's melted. Stir until thick.
2. Let cool. Pour over the cake and chill thoroughly before serving.
3. While the cake is chilling, preheat the oven to 350°F. Sprinkle the sliced almonds on a rimmed baking sheet and toast for 7 minutes, watching carefully to make sure they don't burn.
4. Just before serving, sprinkle the almonds all over the top.

The Air Is Crisp and Full of Apples

On one level, a crisp is nothing more than something wonderful to do with the baskets of apples we can't resist overbuying. On a deeper one, it's that first hunkering down we do before winter sets in for real. We lay a fire in the hearth, and in a kitchen redolent of fruit and spices, we dispense with the formality of crust. We are hungry for the simplest of family comforts, crumbled pie, fruit, and ice cream in a bowl.

REVEREND MICHAEL ALAN'S APPLE AND FIG CRISP

Gone are leaden chunks of dough and runny, overly sweet apples. This beautiful crisp is as full of protein and fiber as it is honeyed figs, raisins, seeds, almonds, and apples. In the hands of an artist, food consultant, and man of the cloth, this American classic is gotta-have-it-new again.

SERVES 6 TO 8

1. Preheat oven to 375°F. Butter a 9 by 13-inch baking dish.
2. In a large mixing bowl, add all of the ingredients for the filling and mix well. Pour the mixture into the prepared baking dish.
3. In a separate mixing bowl, add the flours, oats, brown sugar, and salt. With a fork, cut the butter into the flour mixture until it has the texture of wet sand. Stir in the almonds, sunflower seeds, and pumpkin seeds. Cover the filling with the topping in an even layer and bake for 40 to 45 minutes, or until the juices are bubbling.
4. Serve warm with ice cream, whipped cream, or thick yogurt.

For the filling:
3 pounds apples, cored and cut into ½-inch slices
½ cup golden raisins
1 pint fresh figs, quartered
2 tablespoons honey
1 lemon, zest and freshly squeezed juice
1 tablespoon fresh ginger, grated
1 tablespoon ground cinnamon
½ teaspoon ground nutmeg
½ teaspoon ground cardamom
¼ teaspoon ground cloves
1 tablespoon arrowroot powder
¼ tablespoon salt

For the topping:
¼ cup brown rice flour
¼ cup quinoa flour
⅓ cup gluten-free oats
½ cup (packed) dark brown sugar
½ teaspoon salt
½ cup (1 stick) cold, unsalted butter cut into cubes, plus more to butter the baking dish
½ cup sliced almonds
¼ cup sunflower seeds
¼ cup pumpkin seeds

La Pasta Fresh Ravioli

Silky pillows of gluten-free pasta, two minutes from pot to table. Tucked inside, fluffy ricotta cheese, spinach and cheese, or vegetarian wild mushrooms. No going back to the frozen hockey pucks of old. Look for it at Whole Foods Markets and other whole foods stores where they refrigerate the pasta. Holy Ravioli!

Dying for Thai

Nothing beats the calming, frankly sedative effect of the rice noodle. A little sweet, a little spicy, crunchy and comforting, and naturally gluten-free, Pad Thai satisfies on every level. In Thailand, it's the national craving, made in as many versions as there are street vendors and restaurants. Not high-fat takeout here. This is food to get comfortable with, eat with chopsticks from a bowl cupped in your hand.

VEGETARIAN PAD THAI

You can get fancy with hard-to-find tamarind paste, shrimp, chicken, bean curd, and lots of bells and whistles, but I've stuck with this simple classic adapted from a yellowed recipe clipped from *Vegetarian Times* and with a little help from Whole Foods chef Lee Tobin. If you prefer more protein, briefly stir-fry fish, poultry, or tofu in peanut oil, then add the sauce and noodles. For authenticity, and better absorption of the sauce, use the dried, flat-sided rice noodles called sen lek, found in Asian markets.

SERVES 6

2 quarts plus 3 tablespoons water

8 to 10 ounces dried rice noodles

¼ cup rice vinegar

3 tablespoons tomato paste

2 tablespoons (packed) brown sugar

2 tablespoons gluten-free fish sauce

2 tablespoons peanut oil

2 cloves garlic, finely minced

1 fresh green chili, seeded and finely minced

2 large eggs

½ cup fresh cilantro, snipped

1 cup bean sprouts

1 lime, cut in wedges

½ cup unsalted peanuts, coarsely chopped

6 scallions (white and green parts), sliced

1. In a large saucepan, bring 2 quarts water to a boil over high heat. Then remove from the heat. Soak the rice noodles in the hot water for 20 minutes. Drain and set aside.
2. In a small bowl, blend the rice vinegar, tomato paste, the remaining 3 tablespoons of water, the brown sugar, and the fish sauce.
3. In a large skillet or stir-fry pan, heat the peanut oil over medium heat. Add the garlic and chili and stir-fry for 3 minutes.
4. Make a well in the center of the pan and crack eggs into it, cooking until the eggs are mostly set. Scramble the eggs quickly into the sauce. Add the fresh cilantro and stir in noodles, mixing thoroughly with the sauce. Remove from the heat.
5. Garnish each bowl or plate with lime wedges, chopped peanuts, and scallion slices.

Learn More

Kelli and Peter Bronski—books and recipes.
    www.noglutennoproblem.blogspot.com
The Gluten-Free Table by Jilly Lagasse and Jessie Lagasse Swanson (Grand
    Central)
Miglet's Gluten-Free Potpies. www.migletsgf.com

10

Gather

We should look for someone to eat and drink with
before looking for something to eat and drink.
— EPICURUS

- ◆ The Deep Pleasures of Sharing a Table
- ◆ Just Dessert: *Aimee Olexy's Seven Sinful Cheeses and Brandied Sour Cherries*
- ◆ An Autumn Supper: *Lowell Family Fish Stew with Scallops, Halibut, and Shrimp*
- ◆ A Dublin Tea: *Rebecca Bunting's Irish Soda Bread* and *Lemon-Blueberry Scones*
- ◆ In an Artist's Studio: *Anna Jurinich's Chocolate-Dipped Brandy-Soaked Raisin Almond Biscotti, Chocolate Brandy-Glazed Walnut Cake*, and *Spiced Pumpkin Torte*
- ◆ A Thanksgiving Feast: *Mary Capone's Apple Cider–Brined Roast Turkey, Apple Cider–Bourbon Gravy*, and *Pear Ginger Cranberry Relish*
- ◆ A Birthday Party: *Jennifer Katzinger's Banana Split Cake*
- ◆ A Hanukkah Celebration: *Lisa Stander-Horel's Sweet Potato, Pumpkin, and Sage Latkes* and *Harvest Tzimmes*
- ◆ A Dickens Christmas: *Nigella Lawson's Proper English Trifle*
- ◆ A Gathering of Gifts: *Lowell Family Incredibly Rich Date Nut Loaf, Walnut Cherry Chocolate Bark, Tarragon Mustard*, and *Jules Shepard's Cranberry Chutney*
- ◆ Entertaining Cookbooks and Web sites

I remember a sunset gathering on a beach, three achingly young couples sipping wine and nibbling cheese while mosquitoes dove and the ocean gently rolled, sand cooling beneath us as we talked ourselves into the people we would become.

The salty brine of a certain kind of olive can summon it all again. So potent is the sense memory of food shared with others. We look into the faces of those gathered with us and think Yes, I belong here. This is my tribe. We gather around festive holiday tables, on quiet summer porches, at kitchen tables for plainspoken suppers with family. We understand that this shared connection is the narrative thread that runs through the stories of our lives.

Remember the time she made us a gluten-free dinner and tried to poison us! How the family laughed when I served that first, really awful, post-gluten peach cobbler loaded down with enough brown rice flour to sink the *Bismarck. Wasn't that the Christmas she roasted a goose and almost burned down the house? Do you remember that Seder where everyone was so old, poor Uncle Mort had to ask the questions?* We can almost taste the sweet and sour of that night. The Thanksgiving we almost lost my husband, I made corn bread stuffing and homemade cranberry sauce, hoping somehow it would change everything. Years later, those foods evoke the image of my usually voluble father standing to say grace, unable to speak.

We break bread together, even if that bread is gluten-free, and we understand we are better off together than alone. *That was the worst wedding I'd ever been to, but I met your father that night.*

My friend Gingy Beckerman wrote a book called *Love, Loss, and What I Wore.* It could just as well have been *Love, Loss, and What I Ate.*

The most unforgettable times are those that seem small: a spontaneous meal cooked with friends; a table set in the garden; a gathering of two—heads tilted toward each other, the rest of the world a held breath. Never has ice cream tasted so sweet or felt as conspiratorial.

We gather just for the fun of it. Any excuse will do. We picked too much corn at the farmers' market. We made two pies. We've been housebound too long. We couldn't sleep and made enough chili for a crowd. We cobble together a lunch when friends show up unexpectedly. We host a neighborhood potluck. We plan a dinner party with great attention for the one newly gluten-free and sow the seeds of reciprocity.

With careful attention and from faded bits of paper, we prepare the dishes handed down from one generation to the next. We open our great-grandmother's *Joy of Cooking* and read her notes in the margins. We gather for weddings and birthday celebrations, to warm a house and to ease the sorrow of others. When we gather, we give generously of our time and our affection. We draw the circle close and warm ourselves in the light of one another.

Just Dessert

There is something to be said for simple gatherings. We are busy, we are overcommitted; sit-down dinners with all the bells and whistles are daunting and impossible for some, especially for those with small children. Why not ask friends to join you for a decadent dessert after dinner when the kids are safely tucked away? As in all simple things, the idea is to make it count.

SEVEN SINFUL CHEESES AND BRANDIED SOUR CHERRIES

No run-of-the-mill cheese plate, this. This is an ooh-and-aah deal from Aimee Olexy, epicure and owner of Talula's Table, Talula's Daily, and Talula's Garden, her inspired collaboration with Stephen Starr, restaurants the *New York Times* called "spiritual retreats." At the heart of it all is her passionate love affair with fromage, about which she has an encyclopedic knowledge.

It should go without saying that these cheeses are the stars, all of them buttery, creamy, rich, runny, boozy, sublime, and downright sensual with their drizzle of brandied cherries. They are to sliver, savor, experience, and, yes, lick off your fingers. Olexy gives us nine that live together gorgeously. Choose your favorite seven or go for the whole plate. Shop for them in a first-rate cheese shop. Sample. Let the flavors bloom. Take your time. A good sparkling wine like Gruet Rose, with hints of strawberry, raspberry, and cherry, would be perfect. Decorate plates with bits of Walnut-Cherry Chocolate Bark (page 242).

BUY ENOUGH TO SERVE 6 TO 8

- ✦ Harbison from Cellars at Jasper Hill, Vermont—Earthy, oozy, mildly pungent cow's milk
- ✦ Green Hill from Sweet Grass Dairy, Georgia—Buttery, runny cow's milk

- Dancing Fern from Sequatchie Cove Farms, Tennessee—Pungent, oozy, washed rind cow's milk
- Cocoa Cardona from Carr Valley Cheese Company, Wisconsin—Firm, sweet, slightly nutty goat's milk with notes of cocoa
- Époisses from Époisses, France—Very runny, pungent cow's milk
- Kunik from Nettle Meadow Farm, New York—Creamy, bright-tasting mixture of cow's and goat's milk
- Délice de Bourgogne from Burgundy, France—Very rich, creamy, and runny cow's milk
- Mt. Tam from Cowgirl Creamery, California—Oozy, luscious cow's milk
- Rogue River Blue from Rogue Creamery, Oregon—Wrapped with brandy-soaked fig leaves, boozy, creamy, raw cow's milk

Boozy Cherries

1. In a large saucepan, heat the water and sugar over medium heat and whisk until the sugar is dissolved.
2. Let the mixture cool to room temperature. Stir in the brandy. Add the cherries and let them marinate for at least 2 hours.
3. Keep the cherries in the liquid and stir before serving.

¼ cup water
¼ cup sugar
½ cup brandy
2 cups sour cherries, pitted

An Autumn Supper

If you're like me, you're not in love with last-minute pyrotechnics, especially when your kitchen is wide open to an audience, as mine is. I like easy dinner parties, beautifully choreographed, but deceptively simple and based on the freshest ingredients I can find. This saffron-scented fish stew is a miracle of advanced planning and always seems more flamboyant than it is.

FISH STEW WITH SCALLOPS, HALIBUT, AND SHRIMP

Buy the fish the morning of the dinner. Don't be afraid to substitute cod for halibut if one looks better than the other. The sauce, scented with a little cumin, saffron, and just a pinch of hot pepper, can be made at your leisure and set aside until the fish is ready to be cooked in it. For the roasted peppers, buy the Italian kind swimming in olive oil and spices; it makes for a deeper flavor than roasting your own over an open flame, and it's worth the extra expense. Fresh corn in season is always preferable and, if you have time, roast it before adding it to the stew. Frozen is fine, but make sure it's organic and non-GMO. Don't forget a gluten-free baguette or two to mop up the wonderful sauce. Make basmati rice ahead of time and keep it tightly sealed in a 250°F oven.

Start with a salad of field greens, oranges, beets, and goat cheese and finish with poached figs, prunes, and apricots in calvados over ice cream.

SERVES 8

3 tablespoons olive oil
2 cups yellow onion, chopped
4 celery stalks, chopped
6 cloves garlic, minced
2 teaspoons dried thyme
3 bay leaves
½ teaspoon crushed red pepper flakes
1 teaspoon ground cumin
2 or 3 saffron threads
1 cup vermouth
2 28-ounce cans diced fire-roasted tomatoes
¾ cup roasted red bell peppers, chopped
2 cups gluten-free chicken or vegetable broth
1 cup fresh corn kernels
1 pound raw medium shrimp, peeled, deveined, tails on
1 pound Pacific halibut or cod, cut into bite-size pieces
1 pound sea scallops
½ cup fresh parsley, chopped
Salt and freshly ground black pepper to taste

1. In a large soup pot, heat the olive oil over medium-high heat. Add the onion, celery, and garlic and sauté until the vegetables are soft, 5 to 7 minutes. Add the thyme, bay leaves, red pepper flakes, cumin, and saffron and stir to coat. Stir and cook until the thyme is fragrant, about 2 minutes.

2. Add the vermouth, reduce the heat to medium low and simmer, about 2 minutes.

3. Add tomatoes, bell peppers, broth, and corn. Raise the heat to high and bring to boil. Reduce the heat and simmer for about 5 minutes.

4. At this point, set aside. When you are ready to serve the stew, bring the soup to simmer over medium heat and carefully add shrimp, halibut, and scallops and simmer, watching carefully, until shrimp are pink and the fish is opaque and cooked through, about 7 minutes. Note: If the scallops are large, put them into the broth before the halibut and shrimp.

5. Remove the soup pot from the heat and stir in the parsley, reserving a bit for each guest's bowl. Add salt and freshly ground pepper to taste.

6. Into each bowl, place a little basmati rice. Place a portion of fish on top of the rice. Spoon a generous amount of broth over the top. Garnish with fresh parsley.

7. Separate the fish from the sauce to store leftovers. Add the fish to the reheated sauce, which will warm it. Otherwise, the fish will get rubbery.

A Dublin Tea

Before the coffee shop, that hectic hive of connectivity and hissing espresso machines, there was tea, a quiet hour or so in the afternoon to gather in the garden or in front of a fire for a bit of conversation over something sweet and fortifying. This one comes courtesy of Rebecca Bunting, award-winning goldsmith, cooking teacher, and gluten-free baker, Irish right down to the roots of her bright red hair. Like all Dublin teas, this one requires Irish soda bread, scones, butter, and jam, fresh berries and cream, a proper pot, and a lovely jasmine, Darjeeling, or Irish breakfast tea.

IRISH SODA BREAD

This is basically one dough for two breads, so it's a whole lot easier than it may look. The effect is spectacular, authentic, unhurried, from another time. No texting @ teatime.

MAKES 1 LOAF

1. Preheat oven to 375°F (350°F for a convection oven). Grease a 9-inch pie pan with vegetable oil spray.
2. In the bowl of a food processor, mix the all-purpose flour, tapioca flour, baking soda, baking powder, xanthan gum, salt, and sugar. Add the butter chunks and process until the mixture resembles coarse cornmeal.
3. Pour the mixture into a large mixing bowl and add the caraway seeds, buttermilk, and raisins, stirring with a wooden spoon until all is incorporated.
4. Turn the mixture onto a kneading surface dusted with cornstarch, and lightly knead the dough into a ball, adding only as much cornstarch as needed to keep it from sticking.
5. Place the dough in the prepared pie pan and flatten slightly. Cut a cross in the top with a greased knife.
6. Bake until loaf is well browned, 45 to 50 minutes. Cool completely on a wire rack before slicing.

Vegetable oil spray, for greasing the pan
2¾ cups all-purpose gluten-free flour mix
6 tablespoons tapioca flour
2 teaspoons baking soda
1 tablespoon baking powder
1½ tablespoons xanthan gum
¾ teaspoon salt
4 tablespoons sugar
6 tablespoons (¾ stick) cold unsalted butter, cut into chunks
1 tablespoon caraway seeds
1½ cups buttermilk
1½ cups golden raisins
Cornstarch for kneading

LEMON-BLUEBERRY SCONES

These can be cut into 3-inch rounds or into the more classic wedge shape. The secret to these slightly lower-calorie confections is low-fat vanilla yogurt instead of cream and a mixture of fresh and dried blueberries. As with all thick-skinned fruit, buy organic lemons to avoid any chemical residue in the zest.

¼ cup (½ stick) unsalted cold butter, cut into chunks, plus extra for greasing baking sheet

1¾ cups gluten-free all-purpose flour mix

¼ cup tapioca flour

1¼ teaspoon baking soda

2 teaspoons baking powder

1 teaspoon xanthan gum

¼ teaspoon salt

¼ cup sugar

1 cup low-fat organic vanilla yogurt

⅓ cup fresh blueberries, slightly chopped

⅓ cup dried blueberries

1 teaspoon lemon zest

Cornstarch for rolling out the dough

MAKES 8 LARGE SCONES

1. Preheat oven to 350°F. Grease a baking sheet.
2. In the bowl of a food processor, measure out flour mix, tapioca flour, baking soda, baking powder, xanthan gum, salt, and sugar. Add the chunks of butter and process until the butter is cut into the dry ingredients and the mixture resembles the texture of cornmeal.
3. Transfer the dough to a mixing bowl. Add the yogurt, fresh blueberries, dried blueberries, and lemon zest and stir with a mixing spoon to form a stiff dough. Turn onto a kneading surface that has been dusted with cornstarch, sprinkling more on top. Briefly knead the dough and form it into a ball.
4. Roll or pat out the dough to about 1-inch thick. Cut the dough into triangles or rounds. Place on the prepared baking sheet and bake until lightly browned, 15 to 20 minutes. Cool the scones on a wire rack.

In an Artist's Studio

On a meandering tine of Long Island's north fork, amid vineyards and horse farms, Croatian artist Anna Jurinich paints haunting images of innocence and warnings, secrets and survival, and, always, transcendent grace. On a crisp fall afternoon, the surrounding fields full of ripe pumpkins, she and her Italian husband, inventor Giampaolo Fallai, greeted friends to celebrate her new studio. On the walls a mysterious Madonna wearing dozens of tiny buttons, another veiled and furtive, jagged landscapes blooming with chrysalises. On the long table, Giampaolo's wine, rugged as the Adriatic coast, Brandy-Soaked Raisin Almond Biscotti, Spiced Pumpkin Torte, and a walnut cake that survived the diaspora. All the senses well fed.

CHOCOLATE-DIPPED BRANDY-SOAKED RAISIN ALMOND BISCOTTI

Soaking the raisins in a bit of brandy makes these moister than the typical biscotti, which is why they taste even better the next day. Make sure the brandy you use contains no gluten ingredients. For a more baked cookie, after slicing, separate them with your hands, then slip them into the oven for another five minutes. Gold Medal gluten-free flour did the trick, but you can substitute your favorite all-purpose gluten-free flour. Depending on how you cut them, this recipe yields quite a few cookies—plenty to serve for a party and to give as gifts.

MAKES APPROXIMATELY 4 DOZEN BISCOTTI

1. Preheat oven to 350°F. Grease a 10×15-inch rimmed baking sheet with cooking spray or a light coating of butter.
2. In a small bowl, combine the brandy and raisins and allow to soak for a few minutes. Set aside.
3. In a large bowl, mix the sugar, flour, eggs, brandied raisins (a little liquid left in raisins is fine), salt, vanilla, and almonds. Mix well, until the dough looks creamy. Pour dough onto the baking sheet and spread with a wooden spoon in an even layer, about ¾-inch thick.
4. Bake until slightly browned, about 18 minutes. Let cool for a few minutes and cut into 1-inch sticks vertically from top to bottom, and then cut the sticks in half horizontally.
5. When cooled, coat with chocolate.

1. Over a double boiler, melt the butter and chocolate with the milk.
2. Dip half the biscotti in the melted chocolate. Place the biscotti on waxed paper to cool. Repeat.
3. Store the biscotti in an airtight container.

Cooking spray or butter to grease the baking sheet
¼ cup brandy
1 cup dark raisins
1 cup sugar
1 cup all-purpose gluten-free flour
3 large eggs
Pinch of salt
1 tablespoon vanilla extract
1 cup almonds, chopped

For chocolate coating:
1 tablespoon unsalted butter
10 ounces dark chocolate pieces
4 tablespoons milk

CHOCOLATE BRANDY-GLAZED WALNUT CAKE

A wealthy German family for whom she worked as a young girl gave the recipe for this naturally gluten-free cake to the artist's mother. It is most likely from the period before World War I when Croatia was part of the Austro-Hungarian Empire. Using no flour, only ground walnuts, the nuts give it a dark chocolatey color and moist texture. It's best to grind the walnuts by hand to avoid the oiliness that can accompany machine-ground nut meals. Using a combination of ground almonds and walnuts works as well for this cake.

MAKES ONE 9-INCH CAKE

1. Preheat oven to 350°F. Butter the bottom and sides of a 9-inch springform cake pan and dust with gluten-free flour.
2. In a large bowl, mix the sugar with the egg yolks and cream well with

Butter, to grease the springform pan
Gluten-free flour to dust the springform pan
7 ounces sugar (about ¾ cup)
8 medium or large eggs, separated
7 ounces ground walnuts (about ¾ cup)
1 tablespoon vanilla extract

an eggbeater until pale in color, about 10 minutes. Add the ground nuts and mix well. Add the vanilla.

3. In a separate bowl, beat the egg whites until stiff and, with a circular motion, gently so as not to deflate the meringue, blend into the yolk mixture, starting with about a third of the mixture. When that is well incorporated, add the rest.

4. Pour the batter into the prepared pan and bake for 45 minutes, taking care not to open the oven door as this will cause the meringue to fall.

5. At the 45-minute mark, open the oven door gently and insert a fine knife in the middle of the cake. If the knife comes out clean, it's done. If not, reduce the oven temperature to 250°F and bake for another 5 minutes.

6. Let the cake cool for about 5 minutes. With a knife, very gently loosen the cake from the pan.

For glazing the cake:
⅓ cup water
⅓ cup gluten-free brandy
1 tablespoon unsalted butter
10 ounces dark chocolate
  pieces
4 tablespoons milk

1. In a cup, mix the water and brandy and brush generously over the top and sides of the cake.

2. Over a double boiler, melt the butter and chocolate with the milk.

3. With a spatula, spread the melted chocolate on the top and sides of cake to seal in the brandy.

SPICED PUMPKIN TORTE

An artist makes art of everything beautiful, in this case the pumpkins outside the studio door. The secret to this rich Umbrian flourless cake is fresh pumpkin, peeled, scraped, and slow-cooked in milk and raisins soaked overnight in rum. Pumpkins are always time-consuming and take a bit of muscle (see Chapter 6, "Essential Skills"), but well worth the effort, especially if you prepare it the day before the party.

If you want the pleasure of freshly roasted pumpkin seeds, wash them quickly and pat dry after scooping them out of the pumpkin. Slowly roast in a 250°F oven for 1 to 2 hours, checking on them every now and then.

MAKES ONE 10-INCH BUNDT CAKE

1. Preheat the oven to 350°F. Liberally butter a 10-inch bundt pan, then cover the sides and bottom with bread crumbs, pressing slightly.

2. Peel the pumpkins and remove the seeds. Then cut the pumpkins into melon-like wedges.

3. In the bowl of a food processor, or with a hand grater, grate the pumpkin into long strips.

4. In a large saucepan, mix the grated pumpkin with the milk and cook, covered, over medium heat, until tender, about 45 minutes.

5. In a colander, allow the cooked pumpkin to thoroughly drain and cool, about 2 hours. Toss from time to time to keep the liquids draining, until most of the liquid is gone.

6. In a small bowl, combine the raisins and rum. Soak the raisins in the rum for 5 to 6 hours or overnight.

7. In a large bowl, place the raisins and cooked pumpkin. Add the vanilla, salt, sugar, lemon zest, and eggs. Mix until the ingredients are well incorporated. Pour the batter into the prepared pan.

8. Bake on the center rack until the top of the cake is golden brown, about 1 hour 45 minutes, or until a cake tester inserted in the center comes out clean.

9. If the cake is not quite done, reduce the oven temperature to 250°F and allow the cake to bake another 10 to 15 minutes.

10. Let the cake cool completely before turning it out onto a serving plate. When cake is well cooled, dust with confectioners' sugar.

Butter for greasing the bundt pan
Gluten-free bread crumbs, enough to coat the sides and bottom of the bundt pan
2 small pumpkins (about 2½ to 3 pounds after peeling, coring, and scraping out the seeds)
2 cups milk, enough to cover the pumpkin
1 cup raisins
Rum, enough to soak the raisins
1 cup granulated sugar
1 teaspoon vanilla extract
Pinch of salt
1 teaspoon lemon zest
4 large eggs, beaten
Confectioners' sugar, for dusting the cake

A Thanksgiving Feast

If this is your first gluten-free Thanksgiving, rejoice. Magazines like *Living Without* are required reading for holiday entertaining. With recipes from top chefs and luscious photography, it's easy to plan a feast fit for the most food-obsessed guest, so good even Uncle Arthur will never suspect the whole thing is gluten-free.

Chef Mary Capone, author of *The Gluten-Free Italian Cookbook: Classic Cuisine from the Italian Countryside* and founder of Bella Gluten-Free, gives us an unforgettable harvest gathering with Apple Cider–Brined Roast Turkey with Apple Cider–Bourbon Gravy and Pear Ginger Cranberry relish. Add some cornbread sage stuffing, Pumpkin Sage Risotto (page 180), and Reverend Michael Alan's Apple and Fig Crisp (page 221). Look into the faces of those assembled (even the brother your father loved best) and count your blessings.

APPLE CIDER–BRINED ROAST TURKEY

Brining a turkey ensures a juicy, tender bird, and apple cider imbues it with a wonderful flavor. Like marinating, brining is an overnight process. Make sure the turkey is completely thawed before placing it in the brine mixture. For an even moister turkey breast, roast your turkey unstuffed.

SERVES 16–20

For the apple cider brine:
8 cups apple cider
8 cups cold water
1 cup kosher salt
⅔ cup (packed) brown sugar
1 tablespoon whole peppercorns, crushed in mortar and pestle
4 bay leaves
4 sprigs of fresh parsley
4 sprigs of fresh sage
4 sprigs of fresh thyme

For the turkey:
1 16- to 20-pound turkey, rinsed and patted dry
Salt
2 teaspoons freshly ground black pepper, plus more to season the turkey cavities
¼ cup (½ stick) unsalted butter or dairy-free alternative, softened
1 tablespoon apple cider
Zest of 1 lemon, carefully scrubbed to remove residue
1 teaspoon fresh thyme, stemmed
2 tablespoons all-purpose gluten-free flour
2 cups gluten-free, dairy-free turkey or chicken broth, plus more as needed

1. To make the apple cider brine, in a large stockpot, place the apple cider, water, salt, brown sugar, peppercorns, bay leaves, parsley, sage, and thyme. Bring the mixture to a boil over medium heat, stirring until the sugar and salt are dissolved. Let cool.

2. To make the turkey, remove the giblets and neck from the turkey. Trim any excess fat at the neck area. Rinse the turkey thoroughly inside and out and pat dry. Place the turkey inside a double-lined oven bag (1 oven bag placed inside another to prevent leaking) and put the bagged turkey in a large stockpot or roasting pan. Add the brine to the bag and tie it securely with twist ties to prevent leaking. Refrigerate the turkey for 12 to 24 hours.

3. Remove turkey from the brining liquid and rinse thoroughly. Pat it dry. Salt and pepper the inside cavities of the bird. Set aside, letting the turkey return to room temperature.

4. Preheat oven to 425°F.

5. In the bowl of a food processor or in a small bowl, mix together the butter, apple cider, lemon zest, pepper, and thyme to make a coarse paste. Slide one hand between the skin and meat of the turkey breast and lift gently. Spread several tablespoons of the herb paste under the skin. Spread the remaining paste over the outside of the thighs, drumsticks, and the back of the bird. Sprinkle flour over the entire bird. This helps to brown the skin. Tuck the wings under.

6. Place the turkey, breast-side down, on the rack of a large roasting pan. Add 2 cups broth. Place the turkey in the preheated oven and cook uncovered for 45 minutes. (This sears the outside of the turkey, keeping the juices in the breast meat.)

7. Remove the bird from the oven. Reduce the oven temperature to 325°F Turn the turkey, breast-side up, on the roasting rack. Insert a meat thermometer into the thickest part of the thigh and tent the bird loosely with foil. Return the turkey to the preheated oven and baste every 30 minutes. Add more broth, if necessary.

8. Remove the turkey from the oven when the temperature registers 165°F to 170°F on the thermometer. Transfer the bird to a platter and tent with foil. Let it rest for 30 minutes before carving.

Apple Cider–Bourbon Gravy

1. In a small skillet, melt the butter over medium heat. Add the flour blend and whisk. Cook the mixture for 3 to 5 minutes, until the roux is light brown and well combined. Set aside.

2. In a medium saucepan, combine the broth, pan drippings, and apple cider. Bring to a gentle boil over medium heat. (If you don't have 2 cups of pan drippings, supplement with additional broth equal to 2 cups.)

3. Add the roux, 1 tablespoon at time, whisking constantly. Simmer over low heat until the gravy reduces to about 4 cups, about 10 minutes.

Note: To judge the consistency of your gravy, allow 1 to 2 minutes of whisking between each addition of roux before adding more. The gravy is ready when it has reduced to about 4 cups and is thick enough to coat the back of a spoon. If the gravy becomes too thick, add more drippings or broth. If it's too thin, continue to reduce or add additional roux.

4. Add the bourbon. Season with salt and pepper to taste and continue to simmer, about 3 minutes.

5. Serve with the turkey and Pear Ginger Cranberry Relish (recipe follows).

Mary's All-Purpose Flour Blend

1. Mix together the rice flours, potato starch, and tapioca flour.
2. Store in a tightly covered container in the refrigerator.

Pear Ginger Cranberry Relish

MAKES 2 CUPS

1. In a medium saucepan, mix together the cranberries, brown sugar, water, lemon zest, pears, ginger, cinnamon, allspice, and salt.

2. Heat, uncovered, over medium-low heat. Simmer until mixture thickens, about 20 to 30 minutes.

3. Refrigerate at least 1 hour before serving to heighten the flavors.

¼ cup (½ stick) unsalted butter or dairy-free butter alternative

¼ cup Mary's All-Purpose Gluten-Free Flour Blend (recipe follows)

2 cups gluten-free, dairy-free turkey or chicken broth, plus more if needed

2 cups turkey pan drippings

2 cups apple cider

2 tablespoons bourbon

Salt and freshly ground black pepper to taste

For the flour blend:

2 cups brown rice flour

2 cups white rice flour

1⅓ cups potato starch

⅔ cup tapioca flour

For the relish:

1 10-ounce package fresh or frozen cranberries

⅓ cup (packed) light brown sugar or honey

1⅔ cups water

1 tablespoon lemon or lime zest, washed of any residue and finely grated

2 pears, cored and cubed

1 teaspoon fresh ginger, finely grated, or ¼ teaspoon ground ginger

2 cinnamon sticks

¼ teaspoon allspice

¼ teaspoon salt

A Birthday Party

They say the origin of the birthday cake came from the ancient Greeks who, in order to please Artemis, goddess of the moon, baked round honey cakes and decorated them with lit candles so she could see their glowing offerings. The Germans and Romans lit candles to ward off evil spirits. Adding another for good luck is a little extra insurance. Making a secret wish and blowing all of the candles out in one breath is one way of whistling in the dark. We are all fragile as flames. When we lift our eyes up from the waxy smoke into the warm circle of those celebrating the flesh-and-blood fact of us, it is a joy both primal and unparalleled. Besides, who doesn't look good in candlelight?

BANANA SPLIT CAKE

No toothache-sweet sheet cake here. This luscious vegan cake is from Jennifer Katzinger, founder of the fabled Flying Apron Bakery in Seattle, created to celebrate her little girl's first birthday. Gooey and rich and ever so candle worthy, this dark chocolate concoction with its secret heart of pecans and dates is something that would send Artemis herself over the moon. From *Gluten-Free and Vegan Holidays* by Jennifer Katzinger (Sasquatch Books) with thanks.

MAKES ONE 9-INCH 2-LAYER CAKE

1. Begin by starting the filling. In a large saucepan, place the dates and water over low heat and simmer for about 1 hour, stirring occasionally, until the dates are quite soft. Be sure that the liquid does not completely evaporate.
2. While the dates cook, begin making the frosting. In a double boiler or using a metal bowl set over a saucepan of simmering water, melt the chocolate with the coconut oil. When all of the chocolate has melted, whisk in the water, vanilla, and salt. Refrigerate the frosting for 1 hour, taking it out and whisking occasionally.
3. Preheat the oven to 350°F. Lightly grease two 9-inch cake pans.
4. In a large mixing bowl or the bowl of a stand mixer fitted with the paddle attachment, combine the canola oil, coconut milk, vanilla, maple syrup, and bananas.

For the filling:
1 pound pitted dates, coarsely chopped
1½ cups water
2 cups lightly toasted pecan halves, plus another 10 pecan halves for decorating the cake
Pinch of salt

For the frosting:
5½ ounces dark baking chocolate (72% cacao), finely chopped
⅓ cup coconut oil
½ cup water
1 teaspoon vanilla extract
Pinch of salt

For the cake:
½ cup canola or extra-virgin olive oil, plus more for greasing the cake pans
1 cup canned unsweetened coconut milk
2 teaspoons vanilla extract
1 cup maple syrup
1 medium banana, mashed
2½ cups brown rice flour
1½ teaspoons baking soda
1 teaspoon sea salt

5. In a separate bowl, combine the brown rice flour, baking soda, and salt. Gradually incorporate the dry ingredients into the wet ingredients, mixing thoroughly. Divide the batter equally between the 2 prepared cake pans.

6. Bake for 30 minutes, or until the cakes spring back when you press the center with your finger and a toothpick inserted into the middle comes out clean. Allow the cakes to cool completely before removing them from the pans and assembling.

7. While the cakes cook, drain the dates. In the bowl of a food processor, place the dates and pulse them until they have a smooth consistency. Transfer the date paste to a separate bowl, clean the food processor, and add the pecans and salt. Pulse until a creamy nut butter forms.

8. To assemble, place 1 cake layer on a platter and, using a spatula or butter knife, spread the pecan butter on it. Atop the pecan butter, spread about 1 cup of the date paste. Place the second layer atop the first and spread the remaining date paste on it. Spread the chocolate frosting over the date filling, covering the sides of the cake as well. (Note: If the frosting has become too solid after refrigeration, try spreading it with a heated knife, or heat the frosting slightly and whip in a stand mixer until it is spreadable.)

9. Arrange the pecan halves in a circle on top of the cake.

10. Make a wish. Blow out the candles.

A Hanukkah Celebration

The children are opening presents, running around looking for chocolate coins, and, of course, the door is left open to friends whose families are too far away. The menorah is glowing on the sideboard and good smells are wafting out of the kitchen. In all of the business and preparation, there is a sense of peace that you've all made it through another year. You light the final candle, say the prayer you know as well as your child's face, and whisper your own. *Thank you for everyone gathered here.*

SWEET POTATO, PUMPKIN, AND SAGE LATKES

These gluten-free latkes are baked and crisp, infused with pumpkin and sage, and can be made egg-free as well. Of course, you don't have to tell the family any of that. With thanks to Lisa Stander-Horel, creator of the popular blog *Gluten Free Canteen*, baker, and author of *Nosh on This: Gluten-Free Baking from a Jewish-American Kitchen* (The Experiment), you can bend tradition and start a new one the whole *mishpocheh* will love.

MAKES 24 SMALL LATKES

1 teaspoon high-heat vegetable oil, such as sunflower oil

1 large sweet potato (1½ pounds)

2 extra-large eggs

¼ cup organic pumpkin purée

2 tablespoons olive oil

2 tablespoons all-purpose gluten-free flour

2 teaspoons baking powder

½ to 1 teaspoon kosher salt, to taste

freshly ground black pepper to taste

2 tablespoons fresh sage, coarsely chopped, plus extra for garnish

1 scallion (white and green parts), coarsely chopped

1. Preheat the oven to 400°F. Line 2 baking sheets with parchment paper. Grease the parchment with the vegetable oil. (Because the oven is very hot, make sure that the oil is labeled high-heat.)
2. Using a box grater or a food processor, grate the sweet potato. Wring the grated sweet potato in a clean dish towel to remove excess moisture. Place the sweet potato in a large bowl.
3. In a small bowl, whisk together the eggs, pumpkin purée, olive oil, flour, baking powder, salt to taste, and pepper. Add the egg mixture to the grated sweet potato and mix until blended. Stir in the sage and scallion.
4. Scoop the mixture in 2-tablespoon amounts and place them on the prepared baking sheets, 10 to 12 scoops to a sheet. Flatten the latkes slightly with wet fingers.
5. Place the latkes in the oven and bake for 5 minutes. Then reduce the oven temperature to 375°F and bake for 15 minutes more. Flip the latkes over, rotate the baking sheets in the oven, and bake for 15 minutes more, or until both sides are lightly browned and the latkes are puffy.
6. Let the latkes cool on the pans for a few minutes. Serve warm.

For egg-free latkes:

1. Combine 2 tablespoons flax meal or ground chia seeds with 6 tablespoons warm, unsweetened applesauce.
2. Let sit for 5 minutes to thicken. Add this mixture to replace the 2 eggs in Step 3, above.

HARVEST TZIMMES

Translated literally, *tzimmes* means "a big deal." And when it comes to Jewish holiday food, it wouldn't be Hanukkah without this big deal stew. This one, made of winter vegetables and fresh or dried fruit, is for the vegetarians at the table. Vegans, too, if you substitute agave syrup for the honey. As with all stews, tzimmes flavors are even better the next day and need only to be reheated in a 300°F oven for 30 to 45 minutes.

SERVES 14 TO 16

1. Preheat the oven to 325°F. Grease a 5-quart Dutch oven (with a lid that seals tightly) with nonstick spray.
2. Cube the sweet potato, red potatoes, carrots, and apples into 2-inch pieces and place them in the bottom of the Dutch oven. Add the shallots, figs, apricots, prunes, raisins, cranberries, broth, orange zest, orange juice, brown sugar, olive oil, honey, cinnamon, salt, pepper, and garlic. Stir the ingredients until well blended.
3. Cover, place in the oven, and bake for 1½ to 2 hours, until soft but not mushy. When fully baked, scoop the tzimmes gently into a serving bowl to avoid breaking up the ingredients. Serve with brisket, latkes, and roasted chicken.

Nonstick spray to grease the Dutch oven
1 large sweet potato (1½ pounds)
3 to 4 large red potatoes
4 to 6 medium carrots
2 large apples, any variety
1 medium shallot, finely diced
10 dried figs, cut in half
½ cup dried apricots, cut in half
½ cup pitted prunes
⅓ cup raisins
¼ cup dried cranberries or ½ cup fresh cranberries
1 cup gluten-free vegetable broth
Zest of 1 orange
¼ cup freshly squeezed orange juice
2 tablespoons (packed) light brown sugar
2 tablespoons olive oil
2 tablespoons honey
1 teaspoon ground cinnamon
1 teaspoon kosher salt
¼ teaspoon freshly ground black pepper
3 cloves garlic, smashed

A Dickens Christmas

Well, maybe not *absolutely* Dickens because you really don't want to roast a goose and have the whole house smelling of rendered goose fat. But yes, a lighted tree, a little eggnog, a good Leicestershire cheese and spiced pecans for starters, maybe a nice standing rib roast, with Brussels sprouts roasted in truffle oil, and Yorkshire pudding, gluten-free, of course, and a simple salad of greens, pears, and walnuts.

For the inevitable photo op, and the priceless memory of Grandma and the kids in ridiculous paper hats, set each place with Christmas crackers stuffed with toys and silly English riddles to read aloud at the table. Don't even think about trying to pull off a gluten-free plum pudding; it's just not worth it. Herewith, British down to its roots, from the domestic goddess herself, a rich Christmas trifle Dickens would have loved.

NIGELLA LAWSON'S PROPER ENGLISH TRIFLE

When Nigella says "proper," she means lots of jam, lots of custard, and lots of cream. She uses sponge cake soaked in orange liqueur instead of the traditional sherry (see recipe on page 153). She advises us to bring out our best and biggest crystal bowl—the quantities below will fill a bowl of 10-cup capacity or a 9 by 13-inch rectangular dish. You can use a store-bought cake, something porous to soak up the booze. In a pinch, a gluten-free pound cake will do. With thanks, reprinted with permission from *How to Eat* by Nigella Lawson (Hougton Mifflin Harcourt).

2½ cups light cream half-and-half

Zest and freshly squeezed juice of 1 orange

½ cup Grand Marnier

¼ cup Marsala wine

1 8-inch sponge cake (for recipe, see A Simple Sponge Cake for Your Repertoire, page 153)

10 heaping teaspoons best-quality raspberry or boysenberry jam

2 pints ripe raspberries

8 large egg yolks

1 cup superfine sugar, or more if needed

2 cups heavy cream

½ cup slivered almonds

1 orange

SERVES 8 TO 10

1. Pour the light cream or half-and-half into a wide, heavy-bottomed saucepan, add the orange zest—reserving the juice separately for a moment—and bring just to a boil over medium heat. Remove the pot from heat and set aside for the orange flavor to infuse.

2. In a separate small bowl, mix together the Grand Marnier, Marsala wine, and the reserved orange juice. Pour half of it into a shallow soup bowl, keeping the rest for replenishing halfway through.

3. Split the sponge cake horizontally. Make little sandwiches of the sponge and dunk each one, first one side, then the other, into the booze in the bowl. Arrange the alcohol-saturated slices at the bottom of the trifle bowl. When the bottom of the bowl is covered, top with the jam and raspberries and put in the refrigerator to settle.

4. Bring the orange-zested half-and-half back to the boil, while you whisk together the egg yolks and ½ cup sugar in a bowl large enough to accommodate the cream. When the yolks and sugar are thick and frothy, pour the about-to-bubble cream into them, whisking as you do so. Wash out the saucepan, dry it well, and return to it the custard mixture, making sure you disentangle every whisk-attached string of orange zest.

5. Fill your sink with enough cold water to come about halfway up the custard pan. Over medium to low heat, cook the custard, stirring all the time with a wooden spoon or spatula. With so many egg yolks, the custard should take hardly any time to thicken (and it will continue to thicken as it cools), about 7 minutes. If it looks as if it might be about to boil or break, quickly plunge the pan into the sink of cold water, beating furiously until the danger is averted.

6. When the custard has cooked and thickened, take the pan over to the sink of cold water and beat robustly, but calmly, for a minute or so.

When it's smooth and cooled, strain it over the fruit-topped sponge and put the bowl back in the refrigerator for 24 hours.

7. Not long before serving, whip the heavy cream until thick and, with a spatula, smear it generously over the top of the custard. Put it back in the refrigerator. Toast the slivered almonds by tossing them in a hot, dry frying pan for a couple of minutes, and remove them to a plate until cool.

8. Squeeze the orange and pour the juice into a measuring cup. Measure out an equal quantity of sugar, usually about ½ cup. Pour the orange juice into a small saucepan and stir in the sugar to help it caramelize. Bring to a boil over medium high heat and let bubble until you have a thick, but still runny, caramel. If you let it boil too much until you have toffee, it's not the end of the world, but you're aiming for a dense, syrupy, sticky caramel.

9. Remove from the heat when cooled slightly and dribble it over the whipped cream; you may find this easier to do teaspoon by teaspoon. You can do this an hour or so before you want to eat it. Scatter the toasted almonds over the top before serving.

A Gathering of Gifts

We arrive with small boxes, repurposed cookie tins, and old-fashioned glass jars. Inside, nestled in tissue, wrapped in ribbon, are gifts of food, made by hand. So much better than a flashy last-minute purchase at a pricey gourmet market, these are presents you'll be remembered for and may even be expected to repeat year after year. Here, some sweets and savories for a holiday table, to tuck into a suitcase for a weekend hostess, for whenever we gather for absolutely no reason at all.

INCREDIBLY RICH DATE NUT LOAF

Christmas Eve was always a big deal at our house. Friends gathered to help us trim the tree, sip eggnog, and enjoy a buffet supper while Bing Crosby, Willie Nelson, and Handel's *Messiah* gave us all a rosy glow. At the end of the evening, these dense and rich loaves waited in a basket by the door, a thank-you for being part our beloved tradition. The whole deal is a bit more restrained these days, but the definitive date nut loaves live on.

The original recipe for this dark spiced cake came from one of Craig

Claiborne's *New York Times* columns and has been rendered gluten-free over the years, not that anyone has ever noticed. Buy whole dates, not pieces, because these are often dusted with flour to keep them from sticking together. Make several loaves—you are going to want to keep one for yourself.

MAKES 1 LOAF

½ cup (1 stick) unsalted butter, plus more for buttering the loaf pan
1 cup sifted all-purpose gluten-free flour, plus extra for dusting the loaf pan
1 cup dates, pitted and diced
¾ cup dark seedless raisins
¼ cup golden raisins
1 teaspoon baking soda
1 cup boiling water
1 cup sugar
1 teaspoon vanilla extract
1 large egg
1 teaspoon ground allspice
1 teaspoon ground ginger
1 teaspoon ground cinnamon
¾ cup walnuts, chopped

1. Preheat the oven to 350°F. Butter a loaf pan and cut waxed paper to fit the bottom. Butter again and dust with flour.
2. In mixing bowl, place dates and raisins. Dissolve the baking soda with the boiling water and pour over the fruit. Set aside.
3. In a large mixing bowl or using an electric mixer, cream the butter and sugar together. Beat in the vanilla, egg, and spices. Add the flour and mix well. Add the nuts.
4. Pour the batter into the loaf pan and bake until a knife comes out clean, approximately 60 to 70 minutes.
5. Let cool for 5 minutes and turn onto a wire rack.
6. Gift wrap or serve with whipped cream laced with a bit of rum or top with pumpkin or salted caramel ice cream.

WALNUT CHERRY CHOCOLATE BARK

This salty sweet treat couldn't be easier. Arrive with a box of this and you'll be invited back. Sprinkle bits of it in unexpected places—the cheese plate, with jasmine tea or espresso, or as garnish on a simple dish of ice cream. I like to set it out as an intermezzo for guests to nibble on while I'm organizing dessert. Make as much or as little as you like. Experiment with interesting combinations of nuts and dried fruits, such as white chocolate with cranberries or blueberries and lavender.

1. Line a baking sheet with parchment paper.
2. In a double boiler, melt 12 ounces of high-quality dark or milk chocolate, stirring until the chocolate is smooth.
3. Add to the chocolate mixture chopped walnuts, dried cherries, and a bit of sea salt, pressing them slightly.
4. Spread the mixture on the prepared baking sheet and let cool for several hours.
5. Coarsely chop and place in layers between pieces of waxed paper in a pretty tin. Add a ribbon.

TARRAGON MUSTARD

James Beard once said, "I believe that if ever I had to practice cannibalism, I might manage if there were enough tarragon around." That's how strongly some of us feel about tarragon. Pair a pretty jar of this piquant mustard with another of the small pickled gherkins the French call cornichons. If you are feeling really generous, add a slice of vegetable pâté. For your favorite paleo, go with the full-fat goose liver version.

MAKES ENOUGH FOR SEVERAL SMALL JARS AND ONE FOR YOU

1. In a small mixing bowl put the dry mustard and add the vinegar. Do not mix. Cover and let stand in the refrigerator overnight.
2. In a double boiler, put the mustard and vinegar and mix over hot water. Add the eggs one at a time, whisking constantly, until thoroughly blended.
3. Add the sugar, butter, and salt and cook gently over hot water for 5 minutes, taking care not to overcook, otherwise the eggs will curdle.
4. Pour the mustard into small, tightly sealed glass jars and refrigerate.

1 4-ounce can Coleman's dry mustard
1 cup tarragon vinegar
6 large eggs
¾ cup sugar
½ cup (1 stick) unsalted butter
1 teaspoon salt

CRANBERRY CHUTNEY

Wrap this dazzling red chutney in a small glass jar, tie with a red ribbon, and you may as well be handing out garnets. This tangy version is courtesy of Jules Shepard, owner of Jules Gluten Free mixes and activist-baker who rocked the one-ton, thirteen-foot cake (see Chapter 22, "Food Fights") that helped sweet-talk the FDA into finalizing the gluten-free label.

MAKES ABOUT 7 CUPS

1. Preheat the oven to 400°F. Place the butter in a 9 × 13-inch baking dish and melt it in the preheating oven.
2. In a large bowl, place apple cubes. Add the raisins, pecans (if not tolerated, use the sunflower seeds), orange pieces, brown sugar, cider, lemon juice, ginger, and cloves. Stir to combine well.
3. Pour the mixture into the melted butter in the hot baking dish, spreading it in an even layer.
4. Place the mixture in the oven and bake for 1 hour uncovered, stirring every 15 minutes.

3 tablespoons unsalted butter or dairy-free alternative
3 Gala or Fuji apples, peeled and cut into ¾-inch cubes
½ cup raisins
½ cup pecans, chopped, or sunflower seeds
½ orange, peeled and chopped
¾ cup (packed) light brown sugar
½ cup apple cider
2 tablespoons freshly squeezed lemon juice
1 teaspoon ground ginger
¼ teaspoon ground cloves
2½ cups fresh cranberries

5. Stir cranberries into the baked mixture and cook for an additional 20 minutes, or until the cranberries soften and the chutney thickens.

6. Save a little for yourself and pour the rest into a chunky glass jar with a tight-fitting lid. Store in the refrigerator until it's time to wrap. Take beribboned to the gathering with 10 ounces of good dark chocolate.

Learn More

How to Eat: The Pleasures and Principles of Good Food by Nigella Lawson (Houghton Mifflin Harcourt)

Nosh on This: Gluten-Free Baking from a Jewish-American Kitchen by Lisa Stander-Horel (The Experiment)

Gluten-Free and Vegan Holidays by Jennifer Katzinger (Sasquatch Books)

WEB SITES

Aimee Olexy, www.talulasgarden.com

Bella Gluten Free mixes by Mary Capone, www.bellaglutenfree.com

Jules Shepard—Jules Gluten Free, www.julesglutenfree.com

Anna Jurinich paintings, www.annajurinich.com

Part III

You Need to Get Out More

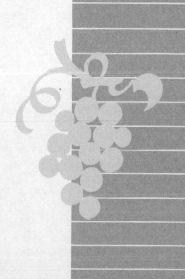

11

The Rules of Engagement

My method is to take the utmost trouble
to find the right thing to say, and then to say it
with the utmost levity.

—GEORGE BERNARD SHAW,
ANSWERS TO NINE QUESTIONS

We're new at this. It's normal not to want to leave the safety of our kitchens.

We need to learn the rules and, in some cases, nurse our wounds. We have to figure out what works for us and what doesn't, what we like and what we don't.

After much experiment and trial and error, we have acquired some skills. We have learned to shop and cook for our families and friends who will tell us the truth if our attempts at gluten-free dishes are worthy of a second helping or if we need to go back to the drawing board. Every day, we get better at this. We slowly build our confidence. We can't eat over the sink forever. It's time to leave the nest.

Whether we are gluten-free by choice or by necessity, what sets us apart also brings us together. To be out in the world and to break bread, so to speak, with others is to receive not only sustenance but also nourishment for the spirit. There is a collective easing over good food and a glass of wine. We look around a friend's table and see a husband who cannot tolerate dairy, a wife whose heart literally relies on a light touch with the saltshaker. There is the diabetic friend, the vegan, the mother of a toddler who risks anaphylaxis at the mere mention of PB and J.

We are not alone.

Given the high profile of the gluten-free diet, we are more likely than not to be the recipients of special dishes and desserts made or brought just for us. There is nothing sweeter than hearing the hostess whisper *gluten-free* as a special dinner roll, gently warmed, makes its way down the table to us.

When we leave the safety of our circle and eat with colleagues or acquaintances who are not yet friends, we may feel a little more precarious. How do we present ourselves? How much talk will we allow about our particular issues? In a culture that is often obsessed with its dietary habits, it's tough to know when enough is enough.

I am reminded of a dinner party many years ago, when someone asked my husband, who had just endured brain surgery, if this was indeed true. All conversation stopped. Spoons hung in midair. Understanding that the wrong answer could cause the party to devolve into a depressing conversation, my husband paused, gave all gathered a wicked look, and said, with perfect timing, "Yes, I've just had one installed."

The room exhaled. We exchanged the look between husband and wife that says, "Well done."

Someone, I believe it may have been Miss Manners, said, "Etiquette is what you do for other people to make yourself feel better." Certainly, knowing what to do in any given situation involves a great deal of empathy. No doubt most social sins are committed not out of malice, ignorance, dimwittedness, or thwarted toilet training, but out of an inability to intuit the moment, how to save it, how to change it, how to avoid the misguided belief that everyone around us will be fascinated by the minutiae of our suffering.

When Abraham Lincoln's butler dropped the Thanksgiving turkey in full view of the distinguished guests, he spared the poor man.

"Why don't we just serve the other one?" the president said.

King George I was said to have lifted his finger bowl to his lips in imitation of his guest, a chieftain from an African tribe, showing all the snickering lords and ladies to be the snobs they really were, thus proving: the greater the man, the greater his courtesy.

Good manners always include, never exclude.

And so my husband saved that evening, not because he's the world's greatest wit but because he knew that as soon as the question was asked, the evening needed saving.

A diet as restrictive as ours is not without its social cost, but I find that the harder I work at helping others become comfortable with my restrictions, the more comfortable they, in turn, attempt to make me. The old saws were never truer: *To be loved, one must love. To receive one must give. To have a friend, be a friend.* I might add: *To be well hosted, host often and well.*

It's time to resume your social life. How do you do that without needlessly obsessing or having an outright panic attack? How can you make sure your presence at the dinner table doesn't cause an allergic reaction all its own? Here are a few simple rules of engagement.

Rule No. 1

For a small dinner, always, always let your host
know about your diet ahead of time.

You may think you don't want to create extra work or be any trouble. The truth is, it's rude not to explain your diet when you RSVP. Send a quick e-mail or text: *I'm gluten-free now. Are you sure you still want me to come?*☺ This will open a conversation in which you can answer the inevitable questions, educate the host about what you can and cannot eat, offer to bring your own crackers or roll or something for everyone to share, and to be reassured that you are more than welcome.

In these days of vegan/paleo/vegetarian/dairy-free/sugar-free/nut-free/casein-free/gluten-free, the host may ask about dietary restrictions before you even have a chance to say a word. Can you imagine anything worse than finding out too late that one of your guests can't eat what you've taken the trouble to prepare? You owe it to your friend, sister-in-law, and next-door neighbor to say something. A dinner party is a gift. Do not let it sit unopened.

Rule No. 2

Never arrive empty-handed.

Leave the wine and flowers to others. After consulting with the host, arrive with a platter of gluten-free canapés, or with a box of gluten-free chocolates or fancy cookies or chocolate-covered strawberries, something sinful that will complement the meal your host has carefully orchestrated. If there is a vegetarian or dairy-free or lactose-free friend in attendance, make sure your offering is suitable for them, too. Aren't consideration and generosity at the heart of being a good guest? Not to mention, you are showing them how it's done, guaranteeing your thoughtfulness will be reciprocated on another occasion. A kind of edible pay-it-forward. If the party is large and chairs are not involved, do bring something for yourself and others, but put yours on a separate plate to ensure that it retains its purity. Depending on the crowd and the formality of the occasion, eat it discreetly or not.

Rule No. 3

Never arrive hungry.

This is going to be a great party or event and you know you will overdo it, so you haven't eaten all day in anticipation of the evening's feast. This is like grocery shopping on an empty stomach—a recipe for disaster. Unless you know what's on the menu and there are some safe and good options for you, eat before you leave the house. You don't have to tuck away several courses; just eat enough to arrive pleasantly full and absolutely impervious to the temptation of gobbling something full of gluten.

Thinking fish was a food I could eat, I once arrived at a traditional Italian Christmas Eve Feast of the Seven Fishes dinner positively ravenous, only to discover that absolutely everything was battered and fried. I did what any polite person would do. I kept my mouth shut and, with the skill of a sidewalk con artist, I pushed food around on my plate. When no one was looking, I slid it all onto my husband's (see Rule No. 10, "Master the art of plate and switch"). Fortunately, dinner was served buffet-style, so I was not in the glare of attention. My dinner that night consisted of chocolate Santas and many cups of espresso. I was up until New Year's. When I got home, I ate everything in the refrigerator, including the baking soda and the spare batteries.

When I thanked our friends for hosting us, I apologized for my shifty behavior and told them why. They've treated me to the gluten-free version of that annual feast ever since.

So yes, do eat before you go out. You'll seem serene, in control, and svelte in your new outfit, focused on catching up with friends rather than chowing down at the buffet.

Do leave a little room for surprises. As more and more party planners are getting the gluten-free memo and are accommodating special diets, chances are there will be something naughty *and* safe.

Rule No. 4

The caterer is not your personal chef.

At large dinners, lunches, and brunches that are catered in someone's home, it is perfectly acceptable to walk into the kitchen and ask the caterer questions about what is being served. It is also possible to negotiate a separate pot of water for pasta or a new bowl and tongs for your salad. (It helps if you know your friend's kitchen and can locate the required pot or utensils.)

But if you've alerted the host to your special diet, this may be unnecessary. You may find that there is a special plate for you. Or you may discover the waitperson passing hors d'oeuvres has identified you and is pointing out what's safe for you on the tray. I was at a party recently where there were lovely spring rolls. I longed to taste one but was afraid to.

"Go ahead," said a voice behind me, "they're rice wrappers and there's no gluten in the filling."

Admittedly, this is rare. When it happens, revel in it.

If you've forgotten to alert your host, by all means ask the caterer to steer you in the right direction. Helping you is a great way to foster word of mouth and get more business. They certainly don't want you to get sick and mention their company's name. Don't overlook the servers at the buffet. They know what's in every dish, including those ingredients not obvious to the naked eye.

Be sensitive to the caterer's responsibilities before asking your questions. The moment before twenty individual chocolate soufflés exit the oven is not an ideal one. It is not polite, nor is it attractive, to ruin everyone else's dessert just because you can't eat it.

When you thank your host, don't forget to mention how accommodating the caterer was and how well you ate. Chances are the response will be, *Why didn't you tell me?*

Rule No. 5

Never sleep in a restaurant or eat in a hotel.

Professional lunches, charity events, mega bar mitzvahs, weddings, prayer breakfasts; room dividers; radish roses everywhere. These are mass feeding events for hundreds of people and should not be mistaken for anything else.

Before you call the catering or banquet office and attempt to negotiate a gluten-free meal, think about what you're missing—probably not much. There are spectacular exceptions, and there is much advance word of mouth about those, but most of the time the food in these big catering establishments isn't so hot in both the literal *and* the figurative sense. You have to ask yourself if you really want to eat a plate of pallid chicken or vegetables because that's what gluten-free is going to be.

Eat before you go and you will not only get through this thing unscathed, you may actually have a great time in the absence of worrying about food. The trick is doing it without calling attention to yourself.

Rule No. 6

Never bother a bride.

Sometimes the polite thing to do is nothing at all.

While it's perfectly acceptable to phone the bride's parents to ask what is being served and what you can bring to a small reception at home or in a club or restaurant, resist the urge to discuss your diet with the bride. Anybody but.

If a large wedding is planned, and you are not in the wedding party, the best strategy is avoiding her altogether in the weeks leading up to the big day. Even if she is a brilliant neurosurgeon or an astrophysicist, most likely she will be temporarily insane, worrying about whether or not she can get into her dress, arguing the finer points of the seating plan, ushers, flowers, and music, and practicing the art of drifting on a cloud of tulle. Anything you say about food will seem hopelessly selfish and ill timed.

Put in a word with the family or, if they are too overwhelmed, call the caterer if you must, but in these days of specialized eating, there may just be a gluten-free option. If not, eat first and nibble carefully at the reception—unless, of course, the bride is gluten-free, which, happily, is becoming more and more the case. Then it's a piece of cake.

Rule No. 7

Never take potluck when you can
eat from your own pot.

At potlucks, picnics, barbecues, church suppers, and other forms of covered-dish affairs, there are just too many cooks and too many ways to get glutened. Even if the author of said covered dish tells you it's gluten-free, you wonder about the pot she cooked it in or the many ways a non-gluten-free cook can unwittingly contaminate food. On my refreshingly friendly city block, we have such a potluck twice a year at the winter and summer solstices. The neighbors gather, some of them exceptional, and, in one or two cases, highly competitive cooks, and they present a gorgeous array of hot foods, cheeses, pâtés, and such.

This is my foolproof method: I make a gluten-free dish big enough to share, put some on my plate before any stray gluten gets inadvertently mingled, and eat only that. If I don't have time to cook, I buy shrimp and dipping sauce or strawberries coated in chocolate or a big basket of gluten-free cookies or a box of gluten-free fudge. No matter what I bring, that is all I eat. I take back the pan, platter, or bowl and wash it in extra-hot water.

Rule No. 8

Never, under penalty of death-by-pasta,
answer the question, "What happens
when you have gluten?"

In this case, it is not a sin to tell a lie. If *trust me you don't want to know* isn't enough to change the subject and avert a round-table discussion of your gastrointestinal tract, make something up. When you are asked what symptoms you get when you eat gluten, tell them you are overcome with the urge to fondle fresh rolls. Tell them you cannot control your compulsion to lick plates. Make up a story about turning into a cereal killer. Tell them anything but the truth, which will put a real kibosh on the evening. No amount of coaxing or encouragement should delude you into thinking people really want to hear about it. Even if they think they do, they don't. By all means, be kind to the person who is considering the diet and really needs a straight answer, but offer to explain another time. Give him your e-mail address or suggest you meet her for coffee one morning. Then move on with a snappy *Speaking of pasta, how was your trip to Italy?* Or *These dumplings remind me of the twins. How are those darling girls?*

You never know. You may run into a baker interested in developing a gluten-free tart or the government person in charge of food labeling, or, as I did once, the inventor of Beano. Still, while the conversation may be fascinating to the two of you, it's best to continue it somewhere less public.

Rule No. 9

Never take a bite to be polite.

You are sitting at a table with friends. Someone is swooning over the home-made meatballs, which you know are full of bread crumbs. The cook is basking in the compliments, telling everyone they came to America with her Sicilian great-grandmother. She glances around at people's plates and her eyes rest on yours. It's piled high with the gluten-free pasta she's prepared in a special pot just for you, not a meatball in sight.

You can't hurt her feelings, can you? After all, she's already made an effort on your behalf. What's the harm if you take a teensy bite?

If you are a celiac, there's plenty of harm in a small taste. If you are gluten-intolerant, you are in for a day or two of feeling truly lousy, which may start the instant you swallow, in which case your friend will feel even worse. If you are voluntarily avoiding gluten and you don't mind a little mild bloating, you will create the impression that the gluten-free diet is one that can be dipped in or out of at will and that you are not someone to be taken seriously.

You could say you pigged out on the spaghetti and have no room. But that wouldn't strike the right note in this situation. You are cornered. Own up. Tell her you knew how much making those meatballs for everyone meant to her and that you didn't have the heart to tell her you couldn't have them. Promise you'll let her know the next time. And apologize.

Rule No. 10

Master the art of plate and switch.

This party trick, which works very well at buffets, involves a quick hand, a willing partner—your date, perhaps, someone who likes a good ruse.

Here's how it goes:

If you find yourself stuck with a whopping big dose of gluten, all you have to do is look for your accomplice, hand over your plate, and try again.

Don't try this at a sit-down dinner, where there is too much scrutiny, unless you are a sleight-of-hand artist. Otherwise you'll end up red faced with food in your lap. If there's no one to play switcheroo with you and another guest comments on your full plate, you could fess up, provided you're in the mood for a conversation about gluten. Otherwise you could just say you made it for someone else and you'll be getting yours shortly. Then without fanfare, slip it into the kitchen or hand it to a waitperson to take away.

Never deconstruct a canapé with your fingers or otherwise scrape off a cracker's topping. Throw it away and start over. If disposing of said inedible canapé has you stumped, think about how creative you were at getting rid of Brussels sprouts when you were a kid. Remember that you are not regarded with as much suspicion as you were then and that no one but your dry cleaner will ever see the insides of your pockets.

Rule No. 11

> Never mistake a business breakfast,
> lunch, or dinner for a meal.

Business has it own etiquette or, to be more accurate, non-etiquette. Alas, to be brash and rude is sometimes considered dynamic, powerful, and plugged-in in corporate circles.

Would you leave your cell phone on the table and take a call at a friend's house? I don't think so. If the answer is yes, you have bigger problems than business etiquette.

A business meal disguises itself as a social occasion, but it is anything but. It is an opportunity to score a point or two, win a client, impress the boss, get the job, and, for some—you know who you are—edge out and otherwise damn your competition with faint praise. To have a condition, special diet, intolerance, or, God forbid, anything with the word *disease* in it is to be perceived as weak. It is not something you bring up unless you work for a food company and you are the idea person in charge of marketing new gluten-free products.

Be polite, charming, and entertaining and make the required small talk before you get down to brass tacks and keep the conversation professional. If it's a breakfast, eat a hearty one at home—amaranth cereal, English muffin, jam, and gluten-free pancakes—and, thus fortified, narrow your eyes, square your shoulders, and order a fruit salad or a small glass of orange juice with your coffee. If it's lunch, grab something near the office before you arrive at the restaurant. Ditto for dinner.

With downsizing, outsourcing, and working weekends with no overtime pay, it's a wonder anybody has time to eat, much less eat safely. I'm not suggesting that everyone you work with is a cutthroat out for your job, and certainly many lifetime friendships have been known to bloom among coworkers, but in the shrinking ranks of today's job market, it's wise to be known for something other than your intolerance to certain foods. Eat first; bond later.

Rule No. 12

Don't expect the gang at work to remember your diet.

Why do companies tell their employees they're family?

Does your family resent you when you get a promotion? Do they fire you? Does your family give you a raise that doesn't even cover carfare? Or not give you one at all? Most companies foster camaraderie, and a family-*like* atmosphere; in our economically challenged times, it's good to feel part of something, that you are all in it together—even if you're just griping about the boss. You may even spend more time with these people than you do with your actual family, but at the end of the day, they are as far from kin as it gets. They do not have to take you in when you have no place to go. And they do not have to remember you are gluten-free.

Ask the bartender at the office hangout to stash a bag of gluten-free pretzels and a few bottles of beer or ale when it's time to blow off the week with your coworkers. Make a study of take-out places near the office that offer gluten-free options. Keep their menus in your desk, and when you find yourself working late or through lunch with colleagues, pass them out and offer to be the designated order taker. You'll be thought of as a team player.

Again, do your research. Identify the pizza place within delivery distance and order enough—gluten-free and regular—for everyone. Many of these restaurant pizzas are really good, so make sure yours is labeled clearly. One pizzeria in Philadelphia tells me that more and more offices are ordering the gluten-free versions of their thin-slice pizza. Secure your slices before they're gone.

Clearly label anything that must go into a shared office kitchen. Be cute. Be funny. Be firm. Long hours and lots of stress make pilferers of us all.

For morale-boosting events designed to make you forget that you haven't had a raise in five years, such as picnics on the boss's lawn or taking over an entire bowling alley, eat first. If your spouse is invited, do the *plate and switch*. If you are alone and desperate, slide your plate over to the empty place next to you. If you get caught, say your throat closes up at these things. He or she will nod knowingly. Don't even think about eating at the annual office party. It's much more fun to see who is flirting with whom and how much your rival is putting away at the bar.

Rule No. 13

> It's perfectly fine to carry your own food
> where other food is served or sold.

Except when it isn't.

Recently I tucked a gluten-free blueberry muffin into my purse and went to the movies. As I happily nibbled my treat and read reviews of upcoming films, the usher rushed over, glaring at me as if I'd brought in an entire colony of bed bugs.

"That's not our muffin," he said, shining an accusatory flashlight on the goods. You'll have to get rid of it or leave the theater."

"I'd love to have one of your muffins," I explained, foolishly thinking common sense would prevail, "but I can't. This one is gluten-free."

Hoping to placate him, I showed him my bottle of prohibitively expensive movie water. "I bought *this*."

He wasn't buying any of it. Either I get rid of it or leave. I refused to budge. Would he Taser me and call the police? Would they put me in plastic handcuffs and cup my head as I ducked into the squad car? I never found out because people around me rose up like an angry mob and threatened to walk out en masse if I couldn't sit there and finish my muffin.

"Leave her alone!" they shouted. "She's gluten-free!"

Okay, maybe don't bring your own food to movie theaters with mean ushers.

But restaurants, diners, snack bars, athletic stadiums, Greyhound buses, airplanes, trains, trolley cars, sidewalk cafés, bistros, and malls are perfectly fine as long as you do it with as little fanfare as you can muster and as politely as possible.

I often buy a biscotti or a cupcake from my favorite gluten-free bakery and walk a block to a friendly café where I order a cappuccino and eat my treat. Most people don't mind. If you do it where you are known, you may be offered a plate and a knife.

If you call ahead, it is perfectly acceptable to hand your bread to a waiter and ask that it be returned to you in the form of French toast, eggs Benedict, Reuben sandwich, or a double cheeseburger as long as you make sure the grill is clean and there is no other gluten involved in the preparation. Again, do this where you are known or ask the questions in a respectful way, and be very, very grateful so that they remember you the next time.

At a local bistro run by a chef whose wife is gluten-free, I order plain gluten-free onion soup, and give them a thick slice of my gluten-free baguette. They slather on the Gruyère, throw it under the broiler, and I've got a crusty cheesy bowl of comfort.

Under no circumstances eat the middle of a premade sandwich or switch the bread for your own because it is almost certainly contaminated with unseen gluten. But it *is* absolutely acceptable to order a sandwich with no bread or roll and transfer it to the bread you carried in with you and kept on a plate on the table. Again, do this after you have been assured that the filling is gluten-free and that it has been prepared on a clean board with a clean knife and assembled by a kitchen worker who has put on a fresh pair of rubber gloves to do it.

Rule No. 14

> A good gluten-free guest arrives
> with a suitcase of food.

But don't expect to be waited on hand and foot.

Just because you have a problem with gluten doesn't mean you can't operate a toaster oven or microwave, or put on your own pot of fresh water for your pasta. Just as you make your bed, squeeze the toothpaste from the bottom, and do not leave muddy footprints on the rug, you shouldn't expect your hosts to race around looking for a gluten-free market to better serve you.

Don't squirrel away your food and refuse to share. Pack enough for everybody. People will be curious and want to try. Make gluten-free oatmeal in the morning. Make everybody a starter course of fresh ravioli. As you are showing them how it's done, they will be learning how to do it for you next time. And there will be a next time because you are the perfect guest.

Rule No. 15

It is acceptable to use your fingers
when all else fails.

Despite your best efforts, should an offending crumb or a stray crouton find its way into your mouth, screaming and spitting it onto your plate is not a good move. Cover your mouth with your napkin, neatly remove the offending food (this is also known as *The Fishbone Maneuver*), and put the food into the napkin. Place the napkin in your lap until you can dispose of it discreetly. Finish with a nice big gulp of water to rinse any gluten particles out of your mouth.

The idea is to attract as little attention to yourself in the process as you possibly can. If you don't think you can pull this off, pretend to drop something, then duck under the table to empty your mouth in private. If you can complete this maneuver without laughing, you're doing well, which will take your mind off the fact that you've just been glutened.

Rule No. 16

Give as good as you get.

Reciprocity.

For my money, this is the most important skill in a friendship. It involves an equal share of receiving and giving, knowing when another's needs trump yours and when they don't. Can you imagine anything worse for a vegetarian than hearing ad nauseam about your friend's new gluten-free diet, only to be treated to cheeseburgers when the plate is on the other table?

Receiving special treatment requires giving the same. When your favorite vegetarian surprises you with gluten-free choices, even when she's serving dinner for twelve, it is your ironclad responsibility to create a veg-etarian feast for her. When someone checks at a restaurant for you before making a reservation, you do the same. Never invite people to your house without first asking what they can and cannot, and in some cases do not want to, eat.

If the person who is most generous is a happy omnivore, not challenged in any way by diet, and couldn't care less what she eats, you are bound by the laws of friendship and love to reciprocate in any way you can think of. Find out which foods are her favorites and cook them when she comes. If she's a picky eater who could take or leave an éclair, keep looking until you find something else that will show the full measure of your appreciation. Not every time, not tit for tat. When she least expects it. When it's clear you didn't have to, but did anyway.

Rule No. 17

Never forget to say thank you.

It's amazing how few people say thank you or write or call the host the next day. Not even for engagement, wedding, and baby presents. We are seeing the demise of the thank-you note. Don't get me started.

In my book, cooking something special for someone is the ultimate demonstration of love. The party hostess who made her miniature quiches gluten-free because she knew you were coming, the weekend hostess who ordered your favorite gluten-free bagels so you could enjoy her nova and cream cheese brunch along with everyone else, the sister who baked you scones.

It is absolutely unacceptable to accept these gifts—and make no mistake; they are gifts—without conveying your gratitude in some meaningful way. An immediate thank-you is a given, sincere and heartfelt. Beyond that a call, text, e-mail, card, flowers, or even a gift is in order. It all depends on the magnitude of the kindness and the extent of your gratitude. I love sending vintage food postcards, such as retro diners and drive-in burger stands, old toasters, Lucille Ball with her Veg-O-Matic. When someone makes or buys a treat for me, I flip through my collection and send the one that most fits the occasion. After a while, matching the postcard to the kindness becomes a game. You'll be surprised at how much food you can find on postcards.

A person who says thank you is always welcome. Simple as that.

Bottom Line

The gluten-free diet, or any diet for that matter, doesn't excuse you from applying the basic rules of courtesy and social conduct—but you knew that. In fact, it requires that you learn some new ones. Tact and diplomacy, empathy, kindness, a good sense of humor, and the ability to shake off disappointments will serve you well. If you miss a meal, you've got another one coming in about four hours.

When in doubt, smile.

Learn More

Emily Post's Etiquette by Peggy Post, Anna Post, Lizzie Post, and Daniel Post Senning (William Morrow)

A Gentleman at the Table by John Bridges and Bryan Curtis (Thomas Nelson)

Tiffany's Table Manners for Teenagers, fiftieth-anniversary edition by Walter Hoving (Random House)

12

Dining Out with No Reservations

You can get anything you want at Alice's Restaurant.

—Arlo Guthrie

The very idea of eating in public is terrifying to anyone new to the gluten-free diet. You feel surrounded by buffalo wings, fried mozzarella, panko, and panini. Brunch with its muffins and pancakes and brioche and sweet rolls breeds a special kind of anxiety. What if your mimosa has come in contact with a croissant on the way in from the bar? What if the French fries are beer-battered? What if they're plunged into the same oil as the onion rings? How are you going to explain your needs to the waiter who, in turn, must explain it to the chef? You worry something will be lost in the translation. Add to this the crash and clatter and the decibel level in the average restaurant kitchen and you wonder if you'll get through dinner alive.

"The woman at table twenty can't have gluten."

"What?"

"No gluten."

"*Vladimir Putin*???"

"No gluten!"

It's enough to make you want to stay home and curl up with a nice safe bowl of cereal.

Welcome to the gluten-free restaurant renaissance.

From multistar establishments to fast food and everything in between, the food industry has become savvy to special diets and common allergies, including gluten-free. You know there's something going on when market analysts on CNBC are discussing the gluten-free boom and its impact on the food industry and on the economy in general.

There's never been a better time to leave your reservations at home and go out. In fact, it is not unusual to find a chef who is not only gluten-free-friendly but who has personal experience with the diet as well.

Word of mouth travels fast, especially when there are smartphone apps to find you a place to eat. Or you can click onto one of the trustworthy gluten-free restaurant registries listed at the end of this chapter.

Still.

There's the dicey-looking diner or the pub near the office, the little bistro that just opened up in the neighborhood, and the four-star tapas bar run by that new chef everybody is buzzing is about. These places may not be on a safe list, but that doesn't mean they are not safe; it just may mean they're not on a list yet. Or they have no idea that there is such a registry. Or your app may not have caught up. Or any number of reasons that have nothing to do with you. Go anyway. You could be disappointed.

Nothing in life can confer immunity from that. On the other hand, you might be pleasantly surprised, which is more likely. If not, you've got three hundred and sixty-four more opportunities to succeed, not counting breakfast, lunch, and snacks. So what if one or two places don't get it or don't want to?

Job number one was getting the gluten-free diet down cold. Now it's time to add a working knowledge of menu terms, negotiating and diplomatic skills, and an appetite for planning ahead. Before you know it, chefs will be eating out of your hand.

Familiarity Breeds Content

The key to dining out well—not to be confused with frequenting places where food is prepared according to corporate formula, something I will talk about a bit later—is educating and cultivating a relationship with the person who prepares your meal. If you do it right, you will have a friend who takes professional pride in pleasing you. Go to one of the sites listed at the end of this chapter and choose a few local restaurants with gluten-free menus. Go there often, often enough for them to know exactly what you need, what you don't like, and, even better, what you do.

Bear in mind—special treatment doesn't have to be expensive treatment. While it is always nice to have in reserve a special restaurant that knows how to cook for you, you don't have to spend more to get more. Whether it's a modest family restaurant or the little café or deli around the corner, the key word is habit.

My neighbors often order the Jax Special at our local bistro, which specializes in crepes, something I would love to order but cannot for obvious reasons. The Jax Special is nothing more than an egg white omelet folded around the crepe filling of my choice—these days it's cheddar cheese, spinach, and andouille sausage (theirs, not everyone's is gluten-free). If I haven't arrived with a hunk of my gluten-free baguette, which I often do, they may surprise me with a Parmesan crisp. Over time, we have established exactly which fillings and sauces are safe for me and which are verboten. The chef's wife is gluten-free so he knows how to keep my food from touching anybody else's.

We go there once a week, and these days even more (writing a book doesn't leave much time to cook). I've gone so far as to supply a gluten-free flour blend to substitute for the crepe batter, but due to cross-contamination concerns, this hasn't been feasible. Yet. In the meantime, the Jax Special is so good, everyone wants one. A lobbying effort is under way to get it on the menu. And you thought you couldn't change the world!

Download Dinner

It's rare to find a restaurant without a menu posted on their Web site, making it a simple matter to choose the place that may be possible for you. The menu won't answer all of your questions, but it will eliminate some places and, depending on your understanding of menu terms and various cuisines, you will be well ahead of the game.

You'll still have questions but, armed with an idea of what you might like to order and what you may have to supply if you go, things will go a lot more smoothly. Besides, it's always easier to negotiate with someone whose work you are familiar with.

Make Requests and Reservations Well Ahead of Time

You can't sashay into a restaurant on a Saturday night with no advance warning and expect to get a safe, gluten-free meal. That's just asking for trouble.

If up to now you've always let someone else make the reservations, you need to step up to the plate and make them yourself. Why? Because whoever makes the calls, calls the shots.

If possible, make the reservation in person. Afternoon or mid-morning is usually best; this is when the kitchen is prepping for dinner or getting organized for lunch. Ask to speak to the chef or to the manager and go over your menu concerns. Ask about dishes that are dusted with flour, contain soy sauce, use bread crumbs or croutons, or involve a marinade or soup stock that contains gluten. Chances are, they'll know exactly what you need.

If a dish has to be adapted, or special arrangements made, don't ask them to do it on a Saturday night, at least until they've gotten to know you better. If this is a one-time-only visit, this is not the time to let them know.

Don't be insulted if you are asked to wait. Anything can happen in a professional kitchen. You don't want to find yourself explaining your diet restrictions to a chef whose dishwasher just quit or is nervous about a visit from a restaurant critic. Offer to call, e-mail, or come back at a better time.

If you're lucky, a chef may just pop out of the kitchen at the right moment and, before you know it, you're both planning your supper. Serendipity? The chef may think so.

First Impressions Count

Start off on your best foot. Be deferential to the chef's greater skill and remember that this is a request, not a confrontation. Asking for help always trumps making demands. Never be defensive. The idea is to appeal to the creative artist as well as to the businessperson, especially if this is a special-occasion restaurant and you don't want an anniversary, birthday, or an important date ruined.

Do mention the rave review you read in the local newspaper, the gluten-free friend who recommended the place highly, and how much you want to eat here. A little flattery will get you everywhere. Try to resist dictating the menu. The idea is for the chef to know the parameters so that he or she can improvise. If the meal doesn't work for the chef, it's not going to work for you. The restaurant knows you're not coming back if all it can offer you are plain vegetables and a boring piece of protein.

Be Clear, Concise, Specific

I need to be gluten-free is a good start. But it isn't enough.

If it's an Italian restaurant, you may want to ask if you can provide your own pasta or ravioli but that it's important for them to cook it in a clean pot of fresh water. Ask about the various sauces and which one is the safest to choose; often Bolognese or other meat sauces are thickened with flour. If the restaurant is known for its vegetarian dishes, you should ask about seitan and other glutenous wheat proteins in their meatless dishes. If it's a Middle Eastern restaurant, you must ask where the cous cous may be lurking. On Chinese and Japanese menus, soy sauce, miso soup, and tempura are issues.

Explain why it's important to clean off the grill before cooking your food and to switch tongs before tossing your salad.

Don't overlook the bar. If you are dairy-free or have a nut allergy, some mixed drinks may contain cream or milk and nut flavorings.

If you are not comfortable explaining what gluten-free is to a chef who may not be fluent in English, use the language cards in Chapter 14.

Go with Your Gut

We all know the kiss-off when we get one. If you are getting a bad vibe from the restaurant, anything at all that tells you they are not taking you seriously or do not understand your request, walk away. You owe them nothing and they could end up making you miserable. There are more restaurants than you have time to try. Keep on stepping.

You're Not Just Doing It for Yourself

On a visit to the restaurant Terra in St. Helena, California, I asked the chef if he would do his haricots verts tempura with rice flour. After comparing the flavor and texture of my green beans to his usual wheat flour version, he realized that rice flour made for a lighter, slightly sweeter, and much more interesting tempura batter. Not only did I negotiate a wonderful meal for myself, I left behind a great dish for other gluten-free diners to discover. I know. I came back again and ordered it.

Just because I've designed them for travel doesn't mean they don't work at home.

Whatever you do, keep it simple.

Timing Is Everything

If the restaurant agrees to use a special ingredient, by all means supply cooking instructions. For example, gluten-free dried pastas usually take longer to cook than regular. Fresh gluten-free pastas and ravioli are ready in two to three minutes. You don't want to hold up everybody's dinner waiting for yours to cook. Ditto for that baguette you want transformed into buttery garlic bread. You need to give it to them when you sit down, so they can run it under the grill when the rest of your table gets theirs.

Leave Your Card

Perhaps you have a business card you can scrawl GLUTEN-FREE across. You can also make a copy of the English Gluten-Intolerance Dining Card in Chapter 14 and leave it behind for reference. Most likely they will make a note of it and put it in your customer profile for future reference. Don't forget to write your name and number on it if they have any questions. At minimum, ask the staff to put "gluten-free" next to your name on the reservation. This way, when you arrive for dinner, they've got a heads-up that you will have questions and requirements.

Trust Exercise

In one of my regular restaurants, I am given a special menu with little hearts drawn by the chef next to items that are safe for me. I am steered gently to selections that not only take into account my needs but my food preferences as well. Small pleasures arrive unbidden—a gluten-free roll scented with rosemary, a soft chickpea socca pancake to dip in olive oil, a spectacular goat cheesecake with lemon curd and nut crust.

My trust in the chef didn't happen overnight. It evolved over time the way a friendship does, with mutual appreciation and a genuine desire to please. When he moved on to his next restaurant and to his next wife, as it turned out, I went right along with him—all in the name of a great cheesecake. Find some relationship material of your own.

Your Compliments to the Chef

There is nothing more satisfying during a long, bruising night behind a hot stove than the sight of a happy and well-satisfied customer. If the meal has been truly extraordinary, by all means, take pen to paper, text, or e-mail when you get home. Leave a rave review on the restaurant Web site. Tweet or blog about it. Post for other gluten-free diners.

At minimum, do the quick after-dinner pop in. *Quick* is the operative word here. Never spend more than a few minutes thanking a chef unless it's the end of the night and he or she has come out of the kitchen. If the kitchen is too small or chaotic to pop into, tap on the glass or stand at the door and blow a kiss, tip a hat, place a hand over your heart, press palms together in *Namaste*. Give a thumbs-up or simply touch your fingers to your lips in the universal gesture of gustatory bliss. Draw a heart on a napkin, or write "I am yours forever!" on a Post-it and stick it on your clean plate. Do anything but leave the restaurant without conveying your compliments to the chef.

There's Always One Bad Apple

For the rare chef who gives you a bad time, there are dozens more who will not disappoint. When a new and much heralded pizza restaurant opened near my home, I stopped in to say hello to the owner and to ask if there would be any gluten-free options on the menu because I had celiac disease and lived just around the corner.

"My daughter's got that."

"So you do," I said, thinking this was my lucky day.

He scowled.

"That's not pizza."

What could I say? If this guy wasn't interested in feeding his daughter, I didn't stand much of a chance. Mine was not to convince, only to convey there's plenty of other pizza out there. I didn't need his.

Sometimes the problem is not with the chef but with the manager or receptionist. Remember my tale of the greeter who told me her gluten-free guests loved their whole-wheat pasta in response to *Do you have any gluten-free options?*

Educate or keep walking? It's up to you to decide.

Sometimes a manager or receptionist or one of the waitstaff will take it upon himself or herself to present their "back-of-the-house" rules to

Rumors Abound

It has come to my attention that certain stratospherically expensive restaurants couldn't care less about special diets and sometimes lie to customers about the safety of their meals. These rumors are unsubstantiated but troubling just the same. I called one such place but forgot to say I was Donald Trump's personal assistant. They said they were booked until 2025. What would The Donald do? I think he'd make a little building out of his potatoes Anna, so he'd know they were the same ones that went back to the kitchen. Then he'd say, *You're fired!*

you. This happens more and more these days, with the emphasis shifting away from customer service toward corporate compliance. Any conversation with a waiter that starts with *"We can't . . ."* should be a red flag to call the manager. Or go elsewhere.

A Word About Waiters

Waiting tables is one of the most exhausting, stressful, poorly paid, footsore, and often thankless jobs on the planet. The majority of waiters are hardworking people, often students and artists, actors, musicians, and writers, many with multiple jobs who honestly want to make your experience a good one.

As hardworking as they are, just because a good waiter knows to serve from the left and can bone a whole fish and operate a complicated corkscrew doesn't mean he or she has any understanding of the gluten-free diet. A good way to get the waiter in your corner is to warn him that some extra trips to the kitchen on your behalf may be necessary. You hope he or she doesn't mind. It's hard to resent extra work you can plan for.

Empathy. There's nothing like it for getting what you want.

Some Tips

+ As soon as you arrive, let your waiter know you have made special arrangements. If you have had an earlier conversation with the chef, now is the time to ask that your arrival be announced to the kitchen.

+ If you have brought some of your own food to fill in—a dinner roll or a portion of pasta—hand it over when you sit down and explain that the kitchen is expecting it.

+ If you have not previously explained your requirements, do so now.

+ Say that you're going to need help ordering and that it may be necessary to ask the chef some important questions. Language like, "I'm on a strict gluten-free diet and really need your help" is far more effective than rude demands, suspicion, or hostility.

+ Avoid phrases like "I'd better not get any gluten." Given the stories about what really goes on in a restaurant kitchen, a waiter with a grudge might see to it you get a whole lot more than crumbs in your food.

+ If a mistake is made, do not scream *CONTAMINATION* at the top of your voice, unless you want to be hosed down by someone in a hazmat suit.

✦ Better to say, *I know you meant well, but there can't be a cookie touching my ice cream. Would you mind bringing me a fresh dish?*

No one is plotting to keep you sick. Waiters are people who make honest mistakes. If the restaurant is worthy of it, give them a chance to make it up to you. Times are tough. The last thing a restaurant wants to do is encourage a gluten reaction.

Get Past No with the What-If Scenario

✦ What if the chef used cornmeal, or ground nuts (if you are not allergic to them), to dust the soft-shell crabs, coat the flounder, or thicken the sauce?
✦ What if the chef put this sauce on my pasta instead of that one?
✦ What if the chef pan-seared my lamb chops in a clean pan instead of using the grill?
✦ What if I ordered the dish without the orzo?
✦ What if the chef put the polenta from that dish on the chicken I'm considering?
✦ What if I asked for a side dish of risotto instead of pasta with my steak?
   If no still means no, dine elsewhere.

GRATUITIES

Despite what you may have heard about four-star restaurant waiters who earn more than some surgeons, the average restaurant server earns a meager salary supplemented by tips, so their reasons for encouraging you to enjoy yourself are not entirely altruistic. Extra service deserves extra consideration. If you have been given special treatment, you should find it in your heart to dig deep and leave a fair and generous tip.

I'm not talking lavish or excessive here. If you budget for a dinner out, factor in the tip. Spending more than you planned is easy in a good restaurant, but stiffing the waiter is not the solution. It is one of the worst restaurant sins, and it all but guarantees a really bad experience next time. Can you say *gratuitous violence*?

THE RUDE (AND OTHERWISE DIFFICULT) WAITER

Okay. You're the most solicitous customer ever born, but this is not a perfect world. You will occasionally run into trouble. This is inevitable, so you may as well be prepared. You know the type. Arched eyebrows, condescending tone, bored expression, points with his or her pinkie as he or she recites the pedigree of every item on your plate.

My friend Jim and I ran into one of these when Jim asked for catsup for his omelet. The waiter's eyebrow shot to his hairline, a look of disgust on his face.

"The chef doesn't believe in catsup."

Jim is good at skewering people like this, but he let it pass. I wondered if he'd heard the man.

After clearing our plates, the waiter returned to set down our coffee cups, along with a pitcher of half-and-half and a bowl of pink and yellow sugar packets.

"Tell me," Jim said, "what is the chef's position on Sweet'N Low?

The waiter is tapping his foot and letting his attention stray to another table as you ask about the ingredients in a particular dish you are thinking of ordering. You sense he hasn't heard a word. Your inedible dinner confirms it. When you ask that the food be taken back, you get an eye roll and a look of undisguised annoyance.

"It's only a little flour," he says with a bored shrug.

Good manners and reason have failed to make an impression.

Even if you probably can't, you have my permission to say, "I'll only sue you a little."

If confrontation isn't your thing, leaving is probably best. But don't forget to make sure the offending item is removed from your check. Paying for bad treatment is adding insult to injury.

In the dark days when few knew what gluten was, much less how to render a meal free of it, it was almost impossible to get a safe meal in a restaurant. It was easy to get snarky with people who refused us special attention. I'm glad to say that those days are over. Today you're more likely to find restaurant staff who will ask if you have celiac disease when you say you have a severe reaction to gluten. You may be surprised when the waiter says, "My sister does, too."

So, too, are the chances good that your chef has more than a passing acquaintance with gluten-free cooking and baking because more and more culinary schools are making these courses mandatory. This doesn't mean that you should abdicate responsibility for the safety of your meal. But it does mean that it is not necessary to walk into every restaurant with a chip on your shoulder.

The Menu: A Crash Course

A few years ago, after a conference at the National Institutes of Health, I joined four of the top women in the gluten-free world at a Washington, DC, restaurant specializing in Asian fusion cuisine. The chef understood that we weren't just gluten-free; we were experts on the subject—in other words, a tough audience. Eager to be written up by the magazine editor at the table, he assured us we did not have to order from the menu; he would feed us safely and royally (he *really* wanted to get into the magazine). Who could resist an offer like that?

A gorgeous miso soup arrived. It was silky smooth, faintly smoky, and unlike any miso soup we'd experienced. We tucked into it like children. At one point, the waiter came to the table and I said I'd never tasted such an exquisite miso soup. What kind was it? I was expecting to hear white or brown rice miso, or some combination thereof. With a great deal of pride, the waiter said a mixture of hatcho and barley miso.

It took a second to sink in.

Barley?!

It wasn't the first time any of us had been accidentally glutened and we accepted our separate fates—five people with five different reactions—with equanimity. We would survive. No one got mad. Actually, we felt sorry for the chef, whose knees were bleeding from so much bowing and scraping and begging our forgiveness. We forgave him, of course, and he, in turn, apologized by making us a gluten-free molten chocolate cake.

We all like to think of ourselves as well informed, sophisticated, and worldly, even if we are not. Two at the table that night were chefs, one of them the magazine's food editor, and nobody knew that the soup was too good to be true.

In hopes of decreasing the odds of an accidental glutening, I've designed the following glossary to help you sharpen your knowledge of cooking techniques commonly and not so commonly found on restaurant menus.

Roux and Other Flour Sources

According to *Larousse Gastronomique*, a roux is not a cheek color but a mixture of flour and a fatty substance, most commonly butter, which is cooked and used as a thickening element for sauces and soups, most notably gumbos and bisques. A roux can be white, blond, or brown, depending on how it is prepared. No matter what color, it is to be avoided by anyone on a gluten-free diet.

Many popular French sauces are based on this technique. Most are not gluten-free unless the chef specifically tells you the roux has been omitted or has been prepared with gluten-free flour. Many modern chefs have omitted this classic and artery-clogging step in the name of enlightened cuisine, and they rely on vegetable reductions for the intensity of their sauces.

That said, you'll never go wrong asking for specific ingredients whenever you see the following sauces listed on the menu:

Africaine	Cardinal	Moutarde
Albert	Chateaubriand	Nantua
Alboni	Chaud-froid (brown	Provençal
Allemande	sauce)	Ravigote
Américaine	Chasseur	Robert
Anglaise	Diable	Soubise
Béarnaise	Hunter	Suprême
Béchamel	Lyonnaise	Velouté
Beurre	Madeira	Véronique
Bigarade	Maître d'hôtel	And plain old American
Bordelaise	Mornay	White Sauce
Bourguignonne		

BREADS AND CAKES

To paraphrase the famously politically incorrect Marie Antoinette, Let you not eat (unless you know it has been rendered gluten-free):

baba	galette	pain anglais
baguette	gâteau	panettone
beignet	genoise	pannequet
brioche	gnocchi	pâté
bûche de Noël	gougère	pavé
charlotte	kugelhopf	petits fours
crepe	kulich	pierogi
croissant	macaroon	praline
croquette	mazarin	profiterole
croustade	napoleon	quenelle
éclair	neapolitan	quiche
fritters	nougatine	roti
galantine	pain	roulé

savarin

St. Honoré

strudel

tarte

terrine

torte

vacherin

vol-au-vent

zuppa inglese

and, yes, cake

WHEAT PASTA BY ANY OTHER NAME IS JUST AS DANGEROUS

bucatini

capelli d'angelo (angel hair)

cannelloni

cappellacci

cappelletti

conchiglie

fettuccine

fusilli

garganelli

lasagna

maccheroncini

maltagliati

orecchiette

pappardelle

penne

pizzoccheri

quadrucci

ravioli

raviolini

rigatoni

spaghetti

spaghettini

stricheti

tagliatelle

tagliolini

tonnarelli

tortelli

tortellini

tortelloni

vermicelli

ziti

Not to mention, noodles:

Chinese yellow noodle

orzo

soba (many brands are not 100% buckwheat)

somen

udon

A Handy Glossary of Menu Terms and Techniques

Familiarize yourself with the following culinary terms and techniques. Not only will you be smarter about what contains gluten, what doesn't, and what may or may not, but your knowledge will be as impressive as your confidence.

SAFE IN ANY LANGUAGE

Acarajé: Brazilian black-eyed pea fritters made with pure chickpea flour

Dal: The gluten-free lentil purée of India

Edamame: Japanese soybeans boiled in the pod

Fagioli: Italian for beans

Finocchio: Not a puppet with a penchant for stretching the truth, but the Italian word for fennel, a green related to the licorice-like anise, but milder. As are all vegetables in their natural state, finocchio is gluten-free.

Flageolet: French for dried beans

Frittata: A flat Italian omelet that is dryer than its French cousin and is never folded. It can be filled with almost anything except flour, which is never used in a frittata.

Fungee: Also called coo coo, and made with pure cornmeal, this is the Caribbean's answer to polenta.

Gravlax: Swedish marinated salmon

Masa harina: Finely ground Mexican corn flour. Perfectly safe.

Meringue: A dessert made with egg whites and sugar. No fat. No flour.

Raita: The cool cucumber, yogurt, and watercress sauce from India. Dip your papadum, but not your naan.

Seviche: Raw shrimp, scallops, lobster, or other fish marinated in fresh limes and hot chilis for at least six hours. Gluten-free.

Tandoori: A mildly spiced style of cooking meats, vegetables, or fish that's been marinated in lemon, garlic, and ginger and cooked in a hot tandoor, or Indian oven.

Zabaglione: A frothy Italian dessert made with whipped egg yolks, sugar, Marsala wine, and, some say, clouds. Have this with an almond cookie for a totally gluten-free dessert.

USUALLY SAFE, BUT ASK ANYWAY:

Cellophane noodle: The flat rice noodle of Shanghai, a.k.a. bean thread, mung bean noodle, glass noodle.

Dosa: The rolled, usually gluten-free pancake of India. Do ask before ordering.

Enchilada: A Mexican dish made with fish, chicken, or beef, sauced and rolled in a corn tortilla served with melted cheese and sour cream. Freshly made enchiladas are almost always gluten-free. In chain or fast-food restaurants, the tortilla is often wheat and bears no resemblance to the real thing. The sauce is often thickened with flour.

Flan: Creamy Spanish caramel custard; in French it's called crème caramel. Ask first.

Macaroon: A dessert cookie made of almond paste, sugar, and egg whites. Many commercial macaroons contain a small amount of flour. Others do not. Ask.

Pakoras: Spicy Indian vegetable fritters that may contain gluten. Ask.

Polenta: A white or yellow, fine-grained or coarse cornmeal that is stirred until it reaches a creamy consistency. Mixed with butter and cheese, it is sometimes allowed to harden, then fried and served as an entrée or an accompaniment. This Northern Italian specialty is wheat-free and gluten-free unless the chef gets fancy and mixes in another grain. Safe 99 percent of the time. Ask.

Posole: Mexican corn stew studded with bits of pork. Ask if it has been thickened with flour.

Risotto: Considered the pasta of Venice, this Italian classic is made with broth or water or wine and a short-grain creamy rice called arborio. There are hundreds of varieties of this rich, satisfying dish—vegetable, cheese, mushroom, shellfish, and meat—and unless the chef has decided to gild a lily, it is always gluten free.

Socca: Mediterranean pancake made with chickpea flour. Always ask if anything else has been added.

Torte: A flourless cake usually made with finely ground almonds or chestnuts. Some modern chefs mix in a tiny bit of cake flour, but most don't. Ask, or risk missing out on one of the all-time classic desserts.

ABSOLUTELY NOT

Albondigas: Mexican fried meat cakes that usually contain wheat flour.

Américaine: A tomato sauce once based on lobster coral but now commonly thickened with the more plentiful wheat flour.

Arlésienne: A dish or garnish composed of fried eggplants and fried onion rings dredged in wheat flour.

Au gratin: Translation: floury cheese sauce and bread crumbs.

Battered: A technique of dipping food in flour, egg, and milk, then into bread crumbs.

Beef Wellington: This dish is always served *en croute* or in a wheat pastry crust that has been slathered with pâté. Forget it.

Beignet: A dessert fritter made with wheat flour popular in Louisiana and restaurants specializing in Cajun cuisine.

Bisque: A thick soup or purée commonly thickened with wheat flour.

Blanquette: A veal or chicken ragout or stew based on a white roux.

Bouchée: Any bite-size puff pastry that is filled with sweet or savory ingredients as a dessert or hors d'oeuvre.

Bourguignonne: A stew containing Burgundy wine and roux.

Cordon Bleu: Meat, usually veal or chicken, wrapped around cheese and ham, then breaded and fried.

Couscous: A North African specialty usually made of crushed durum wheat or millet flour, chickpeas, or rice, and steamed with spices and lamb, mutton, or chicken.

Crépinette: A small, fat sausage encased in bread crumbs.

Croque Monsieur: A grilled sandwich, usually ham and Gruyère cheese.

Croquette: A small roll of mashed potatoes, meat, or fish, encased in bread crumbs and fried.

Crouton: A small, buttered cube of dried bread usually served in salads and soups, often invisible until it ends up in your mouth.

En croute: Anything wrapped and baked in pastry.

Escabeche: A Spanish dish consisting of floured and fried smelts, mackerels, whiting, and red mullets.

Filo: Sometimes spelled phyllo, this is paper-thin Greek pastry dough.

Focaccia: You don't care how it's made. It's bread.

Fricassée: Stew consisting of flour-thickened white sauce and cut-up poultry.

Fritter: Anything battered and fried, usually apples, corn, or potatoes.

Fritto misto: A traditional Italian dish of foods fried in flour and egg batter.

Gnocchi: Italian potato dumplings, which always contain a small amount of flour.

Goulash: A roux-based Hungarian stew flavored with paprika.

Matelote: Any fish stew made with red or white wine and thickened with flour.

Meunière: Usually fillet of sole in a mixture of butter and flour.

Milanaise or **Milanese:** An Italian method of preparation usually involving veal or chicken cutlets dipped in egg and bread crumbs mixed with cheese and fried in butter or olive oil.

Moussaka: A thick Greek eggplant casserole that is thickened with a flour-based béchamel sauce.

Navarin: A ragout or stew of mutton or lamb that has been thickened with roux.

Panini: An Italian grilled sandwich.

Panko: Japanese bread crumbs.

Pasticcio: Any dish that is a mixture of meat, vegetables, or pasta and bound by eggs, béchamel sauce, and topped with breadcrumbs.

Polonaise: A popular method of preparing cauliflower involving bread crumbs.

Quiche: A savory tart bound with eggs, cream, Gruyère, and, alas, pastry crust.

Scaloppini: Veal or chicken scallops, pounded flat, floured, and sauced.

Semolina: A fancy name for wheat flour.

Soufflé: Any sweet or savory dish that consists of puréed ingredients, thickened with egg yolks and stiffly beaten egg whites carefully folded in and baked, frozen, or refrigerated in a high-sided soufflé dish. If the baked version did not contain a tiny bit of flour, it could not rise to such dizzying culinary heights, but frozen soufflés most likely do not contain flour. Ask if it does, or risk missing out on the mother of all French desserts.

Spelt: A form of wheat considered more digestible than the standard. But not for you.

Stroganoff: A ragout of beef containing sour cream, thickened with a dark roux, and most commonly served over egg noodles.

Tagine: A North African stew served with couscous.

Tempura: Japanese battered fish or vegetables and, often, dessert.

Let's Review the Rules of Order

+ Download gluten-free dinner menus.
+ Discuss. Don't dictate.
+ Be clear, be concise; keep it simple.
+ Order uncomplicated grilled or broiled dishes and pass on sauces, soups, marinades, stews, and fried platters.
+ Use the gluten-free dining cards in Chapter 14.
+ Never allow another person (even someone who loves you) to explain your diet.
+ Become a regular. Familiarity breeds content.
+ Always give advance warning when asking for special treatment at peak times.
+ Give cooking instructions for foods supplied to the chef.
+ Show your appreciation often and well.
+ Never discuss your requirements unless you have undivided attention.
+ Never pretend you understand a menu term or method of preparation if you don't.
+ Never pay for what you can't eat. Send it back and tell the waiter why.
+ Be prepared to leave any establishment in which you are denied the attention and consideration you request and deserve.
+ Make sure what you return doesn't come right back. Give your dinner identifying marks.
+ Never accept anyone's best guess, however sincere.
+ Go with your gut. Ignore it at your peril. There's always another restaurant.
+ Without exception, the more you do this, the easier it gets.

Eating High on the Food Chain

Chain restaurants are another story altogether.

All aspects of the chain dining experience are standardized, formularized, and franchised. Many of these places are "eating theme parks" right down to the tablecloths, waitstaff uniforms, and clowns at the front door whose very greeting is lifted from a big fat operating manual. There is not a lot of room for improvisation.

This is very good news for the gluten-free. With so many of these places making the effort to conform to strict certification standards for gluten and other common allergens, you have a much better chance of finding that what's safe for you at one location is safe in all of the others. If there was ever a good argument for sameness, this is it.

That said, although many chain restaurants are making serious attempts to slim down their menus, the average serving in these places pack a fat, calorie, and sugar wallop. Gluten-free or not, they still have a long way to go in terms of healthy eating.

Don't take my word for it. In a recent study reported by ABCNews .com, University of Toronto researchers analyzed the nutritional information of food ordered at nineteen large sit-down restaurant chains and discovered that the average meal contained a belt-busting 1,128 calories—56 percent of the average daily 2,000-calorie intake recommended by the FDA for a healthy adult. Lunch packed an average 1,000 calories, and breakfast came in at a hefty 1,228.

According to Mary Scourboutakos, one of the study's authors, it doesn't stop there. Average sodium levels contained 151 percent of the recommended daily salt intake, 89 percent of daily fat, and 60 percent of daily cholesterol.

The news isn't better at independent and small chains. According to a *JAMA* (*Journal of the American Medical Association*) internal medicine study performed by researchers at Tufts University in Boston, forty items from nine of the most common food categories purchased at independent and small-chain restaurants weighed in at an average 1,327 calories, 17 percent more than similar menu items at larger chains. Nearly 10 percent contained more than a day's worth of calories, and a few packed nearly two days' worth. Both research groups found that the average rack of ribs with all the trimmings weighed in at between 1,850 and 3,500 calories. Bottom line: Given that 40 percent of meals are now eaten out of the home, this is a big problem. On the bright side, ordering a meal with no sauce or bread crumbs or any gluten-containing foods can reduce the average calories you are consuming at these places.

What does a gluten-free citizen do?

It's in everyone's interest to lobby for better food choices and more reasonable restaurant portions and for more FDA oversight in terms of calories, fat, sodium, sugar, and the worst of the worst, high-fructose corn syrup. See Chapter 23 for ways to be more involved. In the meantime, look for chain restaurants that offer low-calorie alternatives as well as gluten-free menus. Choose the ones that list the nutritional contents of each dish.

Eat more consciously, even if it means taking a food carrier to work and zapping it in the microwave. Eat two appetizers instead of a main dish. Order the healthiest meal you can find and take half home. Divide and conquer: Ask that your meal be boxed before you take the first forkful. Otherwise, one bite leads to another. Before you know it, you've eaten enough calories for a family of four. And aren't we gluten-free because we're sick of feeling sick?

ASIAN BOX

This California newcomer with locations in Palo Alto, Mountain View, San Francisco, Burbank, and Los Angeles bills itself as the first gluten-free, fast-casual, all-natural chain and caters to the Silicon Valley tech crowd. The vibe is Asian street food by a chef/owner trained in the upscale San Francisco kitchens of The Slanted Door and Out the Door. Kids' menu, some gluten-free wine and beers, and gluten-free condiments, marinades, and sauces. www.asianbox.com

AUSTIN GRILL

Offering gluten-free tacos, enchiladas, grilled entrées, toasted coconut and cinnamon ice cream, this Tex-Mex–style chain in the Washington Beltway area is careful to point out that, while they make every effort to avoid cross-contamination, their kitchens are not gluten-free, so there is always the possibility. www.austingrill.com

BJ'S RESTAURANT AND BREWHOUSE

Here you will find soups, big salads, giant stuffed potatoes, and gluten-free thin crust pizza topped with anything you want except meatballs, which contain bread crumbs. What goes with pizza? A nice cold Redbridge gluten-free beer or gluten-free hard cider. The restaurants offer information on other allergens and recommend that you alert your server when you sit down. www.bjsbrewhouse.com

BONEFISH GRILL

Mostly fish with meat, too. These folks do not post the specifics of their gluten-free menu on their site. They are careful to remind us that gluten-free doesn't mean fat-free or healthy. We are asked to consult an "angler" or waiter for the details. www.bonefishgrill.com.

CALIFORNIA PIZZA KITCHEN

After a failed attempt at offering gluten-free pizza, this East Coast chain has gotten it right: mushroom, pepperoni sausage, margherita, original BBQ chicken, and pepperoni. Offerings vary from restaurant to restaurant. www.californiapizzakitchen.com

CARRABBA'S ITALIAN GRILL

Omelet Alert

Some chain restaurants, most notably IHOP, add pancake batter to their omelets to make them fluffier. Unless you, too, want to puff up in ways you hadn't counted on, always ask that yours be made with *eggs only* in a *clean* omelet pan.

One of the first chains to be certified by the Gluten Intolerance Group (GIG), this folksy Italian chain tells us up front they do not have a dedicated grill for gluten-free items, nor are they equipped to offer advice on the diet, nor are they responsible for any misinterpretations on the part of their customers. Disclaimers aside, they take gluten-free diners seriously and offer a long list of options on a separate gluten-free menu. www.carrabas.com

CHEESEBURGER IN PARADISE

Owned by singer Jimmy Buffet, this casual burger restaurant started in Florida (where else?) and is currently in sixteen states. You can order a cheeseburger on a gluten-free bun with a side of gluten-free fries and wash it down with a root beer float. This chain develops its menu and addresses cross-contamination prevention with the assistance of the Gluten Intolerance Group. www.cheeseburgerinparadise.com

CHEVY'S FRESH MEX

This is casual Mexican with forty locations. A search did not turn up a gluten-free menu per se, but there are many safe items to choose from and they suggest calling ahead for a gluten-free, un-cross-contaminated dining experience. For example, they offer gluten-free tortillas, but if you do not give them advance notice that you need an oil change, you will find that they are fried in the same cooker with everybody else's. Children's menus are available as well. www.chevys.com

CHILI'S

This huge national and international chain serves up more caveats than real options. Furthermore, they pass the buck to their food suppliers, claiming that they can't guarantee the absence of allergens in the food. There are a couple of gluten-free options, but only by process of elimination. In the widening universe of options, who needs a chilly reception? www.chilis.com

LEGAL SEA FOODS

These people have been doing it right for many years. You can order gluten-free croutons in your salad, ask that a gluten-free roll be served with your calamari fried in chickpea flour, or request that they use gluten-free bread crumbs on baked fish. The children's menu offers fish sticks (catsup movers, as parents like to say) fried in chickpea flour. www.legalseafoods.com

THE OLD SPAGHETTI FACTORY

Gluten-free pasta. Why else would you go? Enjoy it with marinara, meat, clam, mushroom, cheese, browned butter, and Alfredo sauces. www.oldspaghettifactory.com

OUTBACK STEAKHOUSE

This Aussie-inspired chain has spread across the country faster than you can say, "Put another shrimp on the barbie." In 2012 Zagat gave them Best Steak in the national restaurant chain survey. In addition to selections under 600 calories, they offer an extensive gluten-free menu for adults and for kids, with a warning about what you should *not* order, that is, Aussie fries, mustard vinaigrette, and blue cheese dressings, as well as what's safe to enjoy. www.outback.com

P.F. CHANG'S CHINA BISTRO

Within an extensive gluten-free menu there are welcome warnings for spicy dishes, and items are marked vegetarian as well. Special orders are served on plates bearing the P.F. Chang's logo to avoid mishaps and ensure they are delivered to the right table. Clever. They ask that you alert the server to food allergies before placing an order and not to use the soy sauce on the table but to request the gluten-free version. They are well-known for their lettuce wraps with gluten-free filling. www.pfchangs.com

SEASONS 52 FRESH GRILL

This place is a refreshing change from the typical belly-buster menu. The emphasis here is on fresh and seasonally rotating ingredients with dinner choices advertised as being less than 475 calories per item. Mind you, they don't say per plate. There is a gluten-free menu, as well as lactose-free, low-sodium, garlic-free, vegetarian, and vegan menus, and they all come with the usual disclaimers. www.seasons52.com

TED'S MONTANA GRILL

That's Ted as in Ted Turner. The extensive gluten-free menu includes salmon, Angus beef, bison, and gluten-free French fries. There are big-sky portions for those of us who don't have a ranch in Montana. A field day for the gluten-free paleo, this chain took Best Gluten-Free Restaurant Chain in the 2012 Gluten-Free Readers' Choice Awards. www.tedsmontanagrill.com

UNO'S CHICAGO GRILL

Sorry, no gluten-free Chicago deep dish, but thin crust comes in a choice of pepperoni, cheese and tomato, and veggie topping to wash down with Woodchuck gluten-free cider. There are many other gluten-free options as well: steaks, burgers, salads, and an ice cream sundae. Thin crust pizzas are not available in Chicago at Pizzeria Uno or Pizzeria Due. Odd they would not make this available in their namesake city. www.unos.com

Fast-Food Nation

You left the house without tucking a Kind protein bar in your purse and now you're at the mall. Your stomach is growling so loudly, you can't hear the one-hour-sale announcements on Chia Pets. It doesn't help to think about the belly fat you're losing. Before you know it, you've wandered into the food court and are surrounded by pizza, wraps, smoothies, panini, gooey soups, greasy french fries, and potatoes stuffed with things nature never intended. If you choose carefully, you won't get glutened. Unless you order a green salad and iced tea, you won't get healthy either.

But you will get fed.

Believe it or not, in the *JAMA* and Canadian studies quoted earlier, chain restaurants weighed in heavier on average in calories, fat, sugar, and sodium than fast-food chains. Before you break out the mariachi band, understand that this is tantamount to choosing between huge and humongous.

No matter what the spin masters say, it's hard to get a healthy fast-food meal. As Mark Bittman said in his *New York Times* column, "When McDonald's took down the pictures of soda with Happy Meals on the menu boards, it didn't mean you'll be asked whether your kid prefers milk, water, or juice. No. McDonald's will actively discourage the drinking of soda (likely its most profitable item and among the least healthy items in the American diet) only when it's forced to."

Some Fast-Food Tips

+ Always try to eat something before going shopping. Ditto for long drives on roads with nothing but fast-food signs.
+ Fill a baggie with protein-packed mixed nuts, or nuts and raisins and other dried fruits, or stick a banana or an apple in your purse or in the car, or maybe a gluten-free muffin or a gluten-free energy bar. Try not to get crumbs all over the place.
+ If you've remembered to bring two slices of gluten-free bread, head for the nearest deli or sandwich counter and ask them to make a plain roast turkey or roast beef sandwich, Boar's Head brand, if possible. Make sure the meat has not been marinated and that the server wipes the slicer, changes his or her gloves, and uses a clean knife to cut your sandwich.
+ Forget food court toasters. Gluten-free breads no longer need to be toasted to taste good. You don't want to put yours in something full of other people's crumbs.
+ If it's a panini you're hungry for, make sure gloves are changed and the grill is scraped clean before your bread is put on. Ditto for a clean knife. Say no to added sauces or "special ingredients."
+ Carry a gluten-free wrap and ask for a roll-up. Same rules as above. Condiments are usually in individual packets. Read the label or know which brand is gluten-free before you squeeze.
+ Order a cold cut platter with plain lettuce and sliced tomatoes in lieu of a sandwich. Again, ask what kind of cold cuts they are using. Roll up, squirt on mustard. Repeat.

- ✦ If you're really desperate, buy a big box of plain, unbuttered popcorn, and avoid any flavored varieties.
- ✦ Forget salad bars, not only for reasons of gluten contamination but also for basic hygiene. Put down that olive—you never know where it's been.
- ✦ Smoothies are dicey as well, what with all the mix-ins. If you can see a list of ingredients and can coerce the teenager behind the counter to wash out the blender, be my guest.
- ✦ Forget fast-food hamburgers. Do you really want to eat a gray, stripped-down, generic meat patty of dubious provenance?
- ✦ A nice jolt of Starbucks coffee is an option, or chai with a little piece of pure chocolate to fight the four o'clock slump. Avoid the blended drinks that cannot be verified and ask for the gluten-free list before you order anything.
- ✦ When all else fails, think ice cream and frozen yogurt. While this is not the most slimming of choices, it may well be the safest. Tell yourself you're having dessert for lunch.

I Scream, You Scream

Most ice-cream chains offer many gluten-free choices. The obvious culprits are any flavors with the word *dough*, *cookie*, *pie*, *cheesecake*, *cupcake*, *brownie*, or any other kind of cake in the name. But there's more to safety than avoiding cookie dough and blueberry cheesecake.

Get a cup, not a cone, unless you've brought your own. Ask the server to scoop your ice cream out of a fresh container with fresh gloves and a clean scoop.

Avoid toppings. Fresh fruit and M&M's may seem like safe choices, but most likely they have been cross-contaminated by malted milk balls, cookie crumbs, or some other fly-by topping.

If you're an ice cream lover like me, do your homework first. Makes things go faster in the store when the sugar slump hits. Understand that you are asking for a lot and tip accordingly. Here are a few of the bigger chains and where they come down on the issue.

BEN & JERRY'S

There's no gluten-free list, but they will call out any ingredients containing wheat, flour, barley, oats, rye, or malt on the package label. This is great in the grocery store, but there are no labels in their dipping stores.

Go to their Web site and find an ingredient list for every flavor they make. Or ask store manager for it. www.benandjerrys.com

CARVEL

These folks do offer a gluten-free list on their Web site. Click on Nutritional Information, go to Frequently Asked Questions, scroll down to Gluten, and you'll find lots of choices. If you are a fan of the ice cream cake, they are happy to make your special order without chocolate crunchies (not gluten-free) and substitute something like fudge (gluten-free). www.carvel.com

DAIRY QUEEN

This allergy-savvy company recommends that you speak to a manager about your intolerance or sensitivity. They tell us that the Blizzard mixing machine is used to blend *all* drinks, both gluten-free and not. To reduce the risk of cross-contamination, they suggest you ask the crew to thoroughly clean it before making your order. Easy-to-navigate Web site. Go to Nutrition and click on their Gluten Sensitive Guide. www.dairyqueen.com

HÄAGEN-DAZS

They do not have a gluten-free list per se, but they do have an extensive list of ingredients by flavor. The company cautions us to avoid flavors using cookie crumbs, cake dough, or otherwise dubious ingredients and suggests we ask for the ingredient list. I must say my local store is always forthcoming when I have gluten questions. www.haagendazs.com

THE LITE CHOICE

No gluten, artificial additives, corn syrup, hormones, or preservatives and kosher to boot. There are eighty soft-serve flavors blended in any combination. Watch the hard-packed varieties and ask for the ingredient list. Gluten-free waffle and sugar cones, too. Pass up the toppings. Shops are in Manhattan, Long Island, Queens, New Jersey shore towns, Philadelphia, and Montreal, with more to come. www.thelitechoice.com

RED MANGO

According to the company, most Red Mango frozen yogurt flavors are certified gluten-free by the Gluten-Free Certification Organization at a standard of less than 10 parts per million of gluten. Bear in mind that the new standardized FDA labeling mandate sets the limit at 20 parts per million. The exception is those flavors containing soy, which are clearly

Sugar or Waffle?

There is nothing like an ice cream cone for licking the afternoon slump. If you are a waffle cone person, no one will ever convince you to switch to sugar. And vice versa. Hand one of these over at your local ice cream parlor or dip straight out of the carton at home. Edward & Sons gluten-free sugar cones and Let's Do Sprinklez in confetti, carnival, or chocolate. www.edwardandsons.com

Barkat waffle cones—gluten-free, milk-free, egg-free, and vegetarian. www.glutenfreemall.com

marked. The company further states that their yogurts are kosher and contain good bacteria called Super Biotics, which may reduce lactose intolerance. As always, watch the toppings. www.redmangousa.com

Have It Your Way: The Big Three and Some Upstarts

BURGER KING

This chain provides a list for their "gluten sensitive guests," which includes burgers, but no buns. Lots and lots of disclaimers about cross-contamination and their reliance on different suppliers. There are asterisks on French fries, tacos, and the sausage patty, which point to a warning that these items may be fried with gluten. www.burgerking.com

CHICK-FIL-A

Many gluten-free choices are here, including grilled items and gluten-free chicken nuggets for the kids. They state very clearly that they do not have a gluten-free prep area but that their procedures have been written to avoid cross-contamination. www.chick-fil-a.com

CHIPOTLE MEXICAN GRILL

This hybrid of fast-food and restaurant fare really understands the issue of gluten intolerance and sensitivity, as well as other food allergies. Their Web site states that their food contains no peanuts, tree nuts, shellfish, wheat, and gluten (except for the flour tortillas), soy, and milk (except for the cheese dishes) and that if you are extremely sensitive, you should ask them to change their gloves. They tell us it's possible that any of the corn dishes may have commingled with unsafe grains before arriving in their kitchens. They clearly get that some of us, especially those who are exquisitely sensitive, need to make informed decisions. www.chipotle.com

IN-N-OUT BURGER

Fans of this place (lots of us in the gluten-free community) are, well, fanatical. The food is fresh and the menu is ultra simple—burgers, cheeseburgers, fries, shakes, and sodas. Nothing battered or floured or otherwise clogged up with gluten. Everything is gluten-free but the buns. *Protein style* on the "secret menu" means that the burgers or cheeseburgers are wrapped in lettuce leaves. This place is a field day for the gluten-free paleo. Downside: the chain is small, with restaurants in California, Nevada, Arizona, Texas, and Utah. www.innoutburger.com

McDONALD'S

There is no gluten-free list but instead a long and cumbersome list of ingredients you can download. At the end of each item, common allergens—milk, egg, wheat, soy—are listed in bold type. Nowhere do we find the word *gluten*. There's a big flap in the gluten-free community over their French fries. The oil they use contains wheat derivatives, but management maintains that the fries themselves contain no gluten detectable by a test that can measure up to 3 parts per million. Cross-contamination in the fryer is the issue here. If you really must go, study your options carefully. Full disclosure: I don't eat McDonald's fries. www.mcdonalds.com

WENDY'S

There is a rather extensive number of menu items to choose from here, and they are clearly listed on their Web site, which also includes an explanation of what the gluten-free diet is. There are three miles of disclaimers: lots of blah, blah, blah in mice type encouraging you to consult with your physician and consider cross-contamination issues. Read it anyway. www.wendys.com

A Final Word

Whether it's fast, slow, or somewhere in between, the restaurants listed in this chapter are but a few links in a vast nationwide food chain. Remember to check in from time to time as menus change to reflect the tastes of the times. Let's hope they get healthier. As you develop your own gluten-free-friendly favorites, pin, post, and join the chat. Word of mouth travels fast. These Web sites and search apps will reignite your appetite for eating out.

Gluten-Free Restaurant Awareness Program (GFRAP).
    www.glutenfreerestaurants.org
www.allergyeats.com—This free smartphone app for iPhone or Android
    gives feedback on restaurant accommodations and lets you search
    by selecting the top ten allergens, including gluten.
www.findmeglutenfree.com—free iPhone app lets you browse gluten-free
    options by locations or browse popular chains.
Urban Spoon. www.urbanspoon.com
Yelp. www.yelp.com

Nice Buns

If you're going to bring your own, may I suggest Udi's hamburger or hot dog buns. In the frozen case at Whole Foods and other gluten-free groceries. For fresh, stay-soft buns with sesame seeds and a kaiser roll vibe, go to www.amaranthbakery.com.

13

The Melting Pot

The world is your rice noodle.

—JAX PETERS LOWELL,
AGAINST THE GRAIN

One of the benefits of the shrinking global neighborhood and the *celebritizing* of world cuisine is an immediate connection to what is outside of our comfort zones. Cultures transcend borders, and cuisines that were once remote and exotic are as close as the nearest city or town. We gobble up food blogs, tune in to *The Chew,* and indulge in the new culinary voyeurism with *Anthony Bourdain Parts Unknown.* Our mouths water vicariously.

If you've never been an adventurous eater and avoid ethnic foods, now is the time to break out of your shell. If you are willing to look beyond the borders of standard American fare, and explore new cuisines with a healthy curiosity and an open heart, the world's kitchen opens to you. I'm not talking about stingray sushi or piranha steaks, but traditional cuisines that rely on naturally gluten-free staple crops far friendlier than our own. You'll discover there's no going back. When you learn more about each country's cuisine, its singular tastes, and its techniques, the world is not only your oyster. It is your risotto, your rice wrapper, and your rice noodle.

Bye-bye American pie. Hello Pad Thai.

Following my own diagnosis and period of adjustment during which I resisted the urge to embark on a one-woman hunger strike, a wise friend took me to dinner at a local Indian restaurant. I'm not a fan of overly hot curries, especially the hair-curling vindaloo variety, so after checking the temperature of the kitchen, I was assured that gluten intolerance was common in the chef's native Mumbai, and I discovered heaven right here on earth. That night I enjoyed a lamb dish called biryani, made with saffron and fragrant basmati rice, and served with two traditional sauces—a lentil or yellow split pea purée called dal and a cool cucumber, yogurt, and watercress sauce called raita. My host waved away a basket of traditional Indian breads and ordered papadam, a peppery crisp made with lentil flour.

Armed with some basics, eating globally should be an excellent adventure.

A Note of Caution

As with everything you buy or order, you must always ask how a food is prepared and what's in it before you consume it. The following suggestions are merely guidelines, but they should go a long way toward helping you negotiate an unfamiliar menu and decide which dishes to investigate further. In or out, eating ethnic is the gluten-free way to go.

Afghan Cuisine

Once upon a time, few of us could say with certainty where on the map Afghanistan was exactly. Sadly, that is no longer the case. This magnificent mountainous country has fallen to endless war and the worst kind of devastation—all the more reason for us to find and patronize purveyors of

Afghan cuisine. Unlike its neighbors, India and Pakistan, where chefs fight the fiery climate with more heat in their curries, Afghanistan's cooking is subtle and cool, like the temperatures at the country's higher elevations.

Exotic spices and flavors predominate—cardamom, saffron, orange peel, rose water, yogurt, and mint. Lamb and yogurt feature strongly, but dishes are surprisingly mild despite their intricate seasonings.

Skip the appetizers, which are usually turnovers, dumplings, and deep-fried pastries, and move right along to the main course. Not all restaurants use the same ingredients, so remember to ask before you consider the following dishes.

Kabuli-palaw is a gorgeous combination of lamb, rice, carrots, raisins, almonds, and pistachios in a spiced tomato sauce.

Norenge-palaw is a sweeter version of this dish with the addition of cardamom and orange peel soaked in rose water.

Badenjan-chalaw combines lamb and eggplant, and facilliya-chalaw is a mixture of green beans and lamb.

Kabobs of chicken or lamb or ground beef are usually marinated in yogurt, spices, garlic, and lemon before cooking. In this land where meat is not as plentiful or as available as it is here, vegetables make much of Afghan cuisine a vegetarian's dream.

Buranee badenjan is sautéed eggplant with meat sauce and yogurt.

Sabzi is puréed spinach with onions, and buranee kadu is sautéed pumpkin with meat sauce and yogurt.

Afghan desserts tend to be sticky, sweet, and off-limits for the gluten-free, but firnee, a silky Afghan pudding sprinkled with pistachios and almonds, is usually thickened with cornstarch. Ask before ordering.

An Afghan meal is typically finished off with green tea or chai, a traditional tea. You haven't come this far for a cup of coffee.

African Cuisine

In Swahili, *karamu* is the word for "feast." Unusual flavors come together in Africa because of the vast differences in climate, temperatures, and confluence of cultures. North African cuisine, featuring couscous, is heavily grain-based and therefore difficult for those avoiding gluten.

However, Ethiopian teff is the smallest grain in the world and it's gluten-free. Papaya and chili soup is a South African specialty mixing two unexpected flavors. Traditionally, cornstarch is used as a thickener.

Tanzanian fruit and cashew salad with rum cream is worth searching for, and so is the beef and plantain cake from Kenya called matoke. Not a real cake, this is a casserole of highly spiced pieces of beef that have been folded into a plantain and spinach purée, then baked and garnished with shredded coconut.

Cachupa is a vegetable stew of kale, corn, lima, and kidney beans, bananas, name (white yam), and calabaza (acorn squash), among other exotic ingredients from the Cape Verde Islands off the coast of West Africa. This traditional dish often contains chorizo (Spanish sausage), and it's important to find out how the sausage is made before ordering.

Beware of bobotie, a curried beef casserole from South Africa that contains bread crumbs. Yassa is a spicy marinated chicken in onion sauce from Senegal and may be served over rice or couscous. Before ordering, find out. Doro wett is an Ethiopian chicken stew that should not be made with any wheat or gluten. It is typically served over injera, a flat bread made of teff, which is safe to eat only if it is made with no other flour. If there's any doubt, order this over rice and explain why (use the Swahili Gluten Intolerance Dining Card on page 331) so as not to be perceived as rude or unconcerned about tradition.

Angolan shrimp are marinated in a spicy mixture that may turn up on the menu as pilli-pilli or peri-peri. There should be no gluten ingredients in any of these versions, but ask anyway. Tiebou dienne are Senegalese fish fillets stuffed with rice. If prepared properly, they should not contain bread crumbs. Pass up kotokyim, the crab gratin from Ghana. Like gratins everywhere, this one contains bread crumbs.

Drink a cup of strong coffee or soothing mint tea. Then make a *tamsbi la tutaonama*, a statement in Swahili, or just say thank you and pay your bill.

ETHIOPIAN INJERA

The flat, spongy, and slightly sour teff bread of Ethiopia called injera signifies the bonds of loyalty and friendship and is traditionally eaten with the fingers, a piece at a time torn off and wrapped around a mouthful of food. This recipe comes courtesy of Yeworkwoha "Workeye" Ephrem, owner of Ghenet Restaurant in Brooklyn, New York, and uses gluten-free teff flour from The Teff Company in Caldwell, Idaho, which, when mixed with other gluten-free flours, makes a fiber-rich American loaf as well. It's great for dipping and is a change of pace from pizzas and open-faced sandwiches.

MAKES APPROXIMATELY 15 INJERA

2 tablespoons yeast
1½ pounds teff flour
6½ cups warm water

1. Dissolve the yeast according to the package instructions. In a large bowl, combine the yeast, teff flour, and water and mix until smooth. Cover with plastic wrap and let sit in a warm place for 3 days. Yes, 3 days!
2. On the third day, throw away the water that has risen to the top.
3. Add a small amount of fresh warm water until the dough is a little thinner than pancake batter. Cover for at least 30 minutes or until the batter rises.
4. Pour ½ cup batter onto a medium-hot nonstick skillet or a griddle heated to 450°F, swirling the batter to coat the bottom of the pan. Cook for about 1½ minutes, or until bubbles appear. Do not turn. Place the cooked injera on a clean towel or tablecloth to let cool. Repeat until batter is finished.

Brazilian Cuisine

Brazil is beef country, heaven for the carnivores. There is no place to hide gluten in a steak that comes straight from Brazil's ranches or from the pampas of its neighbor Argentina, except maybe in a sauce or marinade, so ask.

Acarajé are black-eyed pea fritters, which should be made from pure black-eyed pea flour. Ceviche (or cebiche or serviche) is popular all over South and Central America. Whether it is shrimp, scallops, lobster, octopus, bass, or black conch, it is always raw fish that has been marinated or "cooked" in fresh lime or the juice of Seville oranges, peppers, tomatoes, chilies, onion, and other ingredients for at least six hours. The fish loses its translucence and fishy taste in the juice and needs no further cooking. Really.

Quibe is winter squash soup or, sometimes, West Indian pumpkin, but it does not require thickening except for vegetable purée. A true Bahian shrimp stew does not contain flour. Bacalhau is dried, salted codfish and is very popular in Brazil. A good Brazilian restaurant will prepare bacalhau many ways: in chili and almond sauce or Bahia style with coconut milk and tomato, or with cabbage à la mineina, or with eggs.

Roupa velha means "old clothes" in Portuguese. It is also the name for a stew of shredded or leftover flank steak. Before you order it, ask the chef if it has been thickened with flour. Feijoada completa is the national dish of Brazil. The recipe can include everything from dried salt pork, salted beef, pig's ears, tail, and feet; tongue; pork sausage; kielbasa; Brazilian sausage (linguica); and turtle beans. A major discussion is in order before you attempt to order this. There are too many variables here.

Brazilian chocolate mousse is usually made with cashews, and coconut blancmange is typically thickened cornstarch. Remember, this is America, land of shortcuts. Ask the chef. Cha is tea, and guarana is Brazil's favorite soft drink. A not-so-soft drink is the caipirinha, Brazil's national and extremely potent cocktail.

Portuguese cheese rolls are served in many Brazilian restaurants. If they are authentic, they are made with manioc flour and are gluten-free. Shortcut: Buy a package of Chēbē mix and make your own.

CAIPIRINHA COCKTAIL

Caipirinha (pronounced *kye-purr-REEN-yah*) means "country bumpkin," and I suppose a country cousin might give up the farm after a few of these. Coffee's got nothing on this sweet and potent cocktail for being the national fuel. I was given this recipe after an advertising shoot in São Paolo, where I also drank gallons of their seriously high-octane coffee. You'll need a bottle of cachaça, intensely sweet Brazilian rum not easy to find but worth looking for as it makes all the difference in the final result. You'll need a muddler, an essential bar tool with one skinny flat end for mixing and a large, rounded one for mashing. If you don't have one, the flat end of a wooden spoon will do. The secret to this drink is stirring often to keep the sugar evenly mixed.

MAKES 1 COCKTAIL

1. Place lime wedges and sugar in old-fashioned glasses. Muddle well.
2. Fill the glass with ice cubes and pour in the cachaça.
3. Stir well.
4. Say *saúde* ("cheers" in Portuguese).

1 lime, quartered
2 teaspoons fine sugar
2 ounces cachaça

Caribbean Cuisine

The flavors of Africa, Spain, France, and other European colonists predominate and mix with the island abundance of fresh fish and fruit, resulting in a few special dishes worth noting.

Ginger beer is not real beer. This West African import is made with fresh ginger, honey, and lemon. No malt. Sorrel tea is also a wonderful ginger-based refreshment from Jamaica. And there's always Jamaican rum.

Fried plantain is a Caribbean staple. Just make sure it's not breaded and find out what else is fried in the pan or deep fryer. For years I would not order an unfortunately named dish called fungee or fungi, which is also called coo coo or cou cou, depending on whether you are in Trinidad, Antigua, or Barbados. It is not a fungus. It's the Caribbean version of polenta and it's wonderful. Jug jug is the Barbadian version, with chicken and peas, and is gluten-free, and may contain millet.

The conquistadores didn't give the Caribbean much, but they did leave behind a dish called cristiaos y moros, or Christians and Moors, which refers to the white rice and black beans that give it its stunning appearance.

There is always good fish on a Caribbean menu. The highly spiced jerk style of cooking refers to the distinctive Caribbean paste of scallion, chili, and allspice that is rubbed into the flesh before slow cooking over coals. It is wonderful as long as you determine the ingredients in the marinade. "Stew" = "roux," including those made in the Caribbean.

Chinese Cuisine

In order to enjoy good Chinese cooking, you need to buy a wok and learn how or get on speaking terms with the chef. Since many Chinese chefs do not speak English well, or at all, and Mandarin isn't exactly a second language in most American neighborhoods, this may take a little doing. One way to break the language barrier is using the Chinese dining card on page 322.

There is a world of difference between authentic Chinese cuisine and the average sodium-loaded takeout. Still, Chinese cuisine uses an enormous amount of soy sauce and other sauces that contain it.

Mei-fun or chow fun rice noodles are great stir-fried with shrimp and pork curry or with vegetables, but they can't be ordered unless you know exactly what's in the sauce. Nor should you order guon fun, a rice roll with vegetables and meat. You must make sure that the chef has adapted it for you with wheat-free soy sauce, which is why mastering the wok is a good gluten-free move.

As a rule, Chinese dishes are thickened with cornstarch. But many condiments and pickled items are imported from China. Unless you can read a Chinese label, it's virtually impossible to know what's in them. But before you give up on China, look for chrysanthemum soup, a light chicken soup afloat in chrysanthemum petals, or one of the egg drop, egg curd, or ginger broth varieties, which should be free of soy sauce. Forget the Szechuan favorite, hot and sour soup. It's always made with soy sauce, unless you have done your homework and have found a chef willing to make it for you with gluten-free tamari.

As a rule, brown sauces contain soy sauce whereas white sauces, typically thickened with cornstarch, do not.

Peking duck, lacquered to a deep mahogany with honey, is gorgeous when prepared properly. It's made with barley molasses as well. Make sure you know the difference.

Forgo the accompanying plum sauce unless you know what's in it. Pass up the hoisin sauce entirely unless gluten-free varieties are used.

Tea-smoked duck should not be prepared with anything but spiced salt, lemon or orange, rice, brown sugar, and black tea leaves.

Remember what I said about the sauce. Any sauce.

Dim sum is Chinese for "dough." Stay away from these savory dumplings.

If you can handle cracking open your fortune cookie before passing it to someone else, it should say, "Have the dragon eye pudding." This Shanghai classic is usually made with rice flour. The dragon's eyes are really longan berries or guìyuán, also used as a tonic herb.

A TRIO OF AUTHENTIC STIR-FRY SAUCES

There is nothing easier and more flavorful than a Chinese stir-fry. Master a few sauces and forget the takeout with its dubious ingredients. Look for Chinese five-spice powder, star anise, sriracha, and Szechuan peppercorns in Asian markets and international sections of gourmet markets. Use to stir-fry vegetables, beef, pork, chicken, bean thread, or rice noodles. These originally came from *The Frog-Commissary Cookbook* by Steven Poses, Anne Clark, and Becky Roller, with my adaptations over the years. With my thanks and longing for those amazing restaurants.

EACH SAUCE SERVES 2

Orange Ginger Sauce

1½ teaspoons sesame oil
½ teaspoon fresh ginger, minced
½ teaspoon garlic, minced
½ cup gluten-free chicken broth
1 tablespoon low-sodium gluten-free soy
  sauce

1 tablespoon (packed) dark brown
  sugar
⅛ teaspoon Tabasco
½ teaspoon salt
¼ teaspoon freshly ground black
  pepper

1½ teaspoons freshly squeezed orange
  juice
1½ teaspoons cornstarch
1 tablespoon rice wine or dry sherry

1. In a small saucepan, heat the sesame oil over medium heat. Add the ginger and garlic and stir-fry for 15 to 30 seconds, to bring out their fragrance.
2. Add the broth, soy sauce, brown sugar, Tabasco, salt, pepper, and orange juice. Bring to a boil, stirring.
3. Dissolve the cornstarch in the rice wine and whisk into the sauce. Heat until sauce thickens and reaches a full boil. Simmer for 30 seconds.
4. Remove from the heat and reserve for stir-fry.

Garlic Sesame Sauce

½ teaspoon freshly ground black
  pepper
2 tablespoons low-sodium gluten-free
  soy sauce

3 tablespoons gluten-free chicken broth
1 tablespoon sugar
2¼ teaspoons freshly squeezed lemon
  juice

⅓ cup sesame oil
2¼ teaspoons garlic, minced
1 teaspoon cornstarch mixed with 1½
  teaspoons water

1. In a small bowl, combine the pepper, soy sauce, broth, sugar, and lemon juice.
2. In a small saucepan, heat the sesame oil over medium heat. Add the garlic and sauté about 1 minute, until softened but not browned.
3. Add soy sauce mixture, raise heat, and bring to a boil. Whisk in the cornstarch mixture and let boil for 20 seconds.
4. Remove from the heat and reserve for stir-fry.

Szechuan Sauce*

1½ teaspoons sesame oil
½ teaspoon fresh ginger, minced
½ teaspoon garlic, minced
½ cup gluten-free chicken broth
2 whole anise stars
1½ teaspoons red wine vinegar
1 tablespoon low-sodium gluten-free soy
  sauce

½ teaspoon salt
1 teaspoon gluten-free hoisin sauce
⅛ teaspoon sriracha or Tabasco, or
  more to taste
⅛ teaspoon crushed red pepper flakes
¼ teaspoon freshly ground black
  pepper
⅛ teaspoon Chinese five-spice powder

¼ teaspoon Szechuan peppercorns,
  finely chopped
2 teaspoons cornstarch dissolved in 1
  tablespoon water

*Hot and spicy

1. In a small saucepan, heat the sesame oil over medium heat. Add the ginger and garlic and sauté about 1 minute, until softened but not browned.
2. In a small bowl, combine the broth, anise stars, vinegar, soy sauce, salt, hoisin sauce, sriracha, red pepper flakes, black pepper five-spice powder, and peppercorns. Add them to the saucepan, cover, and simmer for 10 minutes.
3. Remove the star anise. Whisk in the cornstarch mixture and let boil for 1 to 2 minutes. Taste and add more sriracha if desired.
4. Remove from the heat and reserve for stir-fry.

German Cuisine

German food is wonderful, hearty, stick-to-the-ribs good. But for those of us on a gluten-free diet, it can be the *wurst*. There's bierwurst, bratwurst, blutwurst, bockwurst, knackwurst, leberwurst, mettwurst, weisswurst, zungenwurst, and just plain wurst—approximately fifteen hundred kinds of wursts, or sausages, all containing who knows what.

Then there's bier: a different beer for every man, woman, and stein in Germany. If the bier and wurst don't get you, the spaetzle and schnitzel (wiener and holsteiner among them) will.

There are dozens of brotes or breads, including pumpernickel, and there is sauerbraten, pfeffernusse, pfannkuchen, pastete, nudeln, nockerl, knödel, kuchen, kasekuchen, lebkuchen, baumkuchen, elisenlebkuchen, and gulasch. If you're gluten-free, this is German for "you can't order it."

Not everything is verboten—you can have cabbage or potatoes, for example, as long as they're not swimming in cream sauce or encrusted with noodles. Bottom line: All the really good German dishes are loaded with flour or bread crumbs or beer or something else that will make you feel queasy right down to your lederhosen.

Have strawberries *mit schlag* or whipped cream. Or maybe some Black Forest ham, a nice ripe Limburger, and a glass of the cherry brandy called kirschwasser.

Greek Cuisine

Forget the kasseri cheese appetizer called saganaki opa. It's delicious. It's dramatic. It's flamed at the table. And it's full of bread crumbs.

Greek dips have become so Americanized, we forget we didn't invent them. Hummus is a garlicky purée of chickpeas. Tahini is puréed sesame seeds with olive oil. Tzatziki is whipped yogurt with cucumbers, lemon juice, and garlic. Taramasalata mixes Greek caviar with olive oil and lemon juice. Baba ghanoush, or baba ghanouj, is a dip of roasted eggplant with garlic, oil, lemon, and tahini. These are traditionally served with pita triangles but are just as delicious with chilled cucumber slices.

The Greeks are known for their briny Greek olives and feta, the salty and reasonably low-fat national cheese. Dolma are grape leaves stuffed with rice, and they are usually gluten-free. Ask first.

Stay away from avgolemono, which is a thick Hellenic lemon and egg soup with rice and chicken both. It is usually thickened with egg yolks only, but maybe not. Avgolemono is also served as a sauce for other Greek dishes, including the more substantial entrée of grape leaves stuffed with beef and lamb and rice, so it is important to establish its ingredients before ordering. Pastitsio and moussaka are the Greek variations of lasagna. Both are held together with béchamel sauce, which is thickened with flour, and pastitsio usually contains pasta called orzo.

Never confuse orzo, which is pasta, with ouzo, a very strong drink.

While spanakopita or spinach pie should be an obvious no-no, some Greek restaurants make a variation that is a bubbly casserole of rice, spinach, and feta cheese minus the filo or phyllo dough. As with every cuisine, all thick sauces are suspect and must be explained before you order any Greek stew or braised dish. *Plaki* means anything on a platter or planked and usually refers to baked or grilled fish. Grilled fish à la Greque usually involves no more than olive oil, garlic, and lemon and is as heart healthy as it is gluten-free. Gyro is marinated, spiced meat, sliced very thinly. Not to be trusted.

Skordelia is another name for garlic mashed potatoes.

The typical Greek dessert is the glutenous baklava and syrupy filo pastries or the baked custard called galaktobouriko. Some almond paste cookies are made with almond paste only, but don't assume they all are. If you find them, get the recipe or the address and phone number of the bakery and send it to me. Traditional raisin rice pudding may or may not be gluten-free, but homemade yogurt, served with honey and walnuts, is a safe and perfect ending to a Greek meal.

Nobody does lamb like the Greeks: the meat is braised for hours until it is succulent and literally falls off the bone. Who needs dessert anyway?

Indian Cuisine

To experience the subtlety of India's culinary principles—fiery hot quenched by soothing and cool, complex spice balanced by sweet—and the perfection of its rice is to appreciate why for centuries Europeans risked life and limb to travel to this magical country. Cardamom, coriander, cumin, ginger, turmeric, cayenne, and cinnamon are the grace notes of Indian cuisine, and, as often as not, the cuisine of this predominantly Hindu culture features vegetarian and dairy-free, as well as gluten-free dishes.

Indian dishes are served all at once, so one can decide how much of each temperature is appropriate. Desserts are deliberately mild and fragrant after a meal of stunning contrasts. In traditional Indian kitchens, curry is based on something called ghee, which is clarified butter, melted and skimmed of its foam several times. Ghee is the foundation for all of the variations, none of which should contain flour. I say *should*, and I will say it until it is fixed in your mind: always ask.

Curries range from mild to incendiary. Never ask for very hot unless you know what that particular chef's definition of this is. You can always ask for something a little hotter next time. If you are sweating from the top of your head to the soles of your feet, it's already too late.

Vindaloo-style of cooking tends to be the spiciest, while *tandoori* refers to the clay oven or tandoor used to prepare milder dishes, such as chicken marinated in lemon, yogurt, garlic, and ginger. Basmati, a lovely short-grain rice, is often the rice of choice and it is sweeter and more fragrant than the standard grain. It should be cooked Indian-style—depending on the quantity, left to soak for twenty minutes or so, boiled for a short time, then set aside so the grains can separate.

Raitas are the yogurt sauces that cool and balance hot dishes. They are usually made with cucumbers and watercress but can be made of bananas, or bananas and coconut, or eggplant and potatoes. They are always soothing and put out the fire nicely.

Biryani is an eggplant and saffron rice casserole based on ghee and can be made with lamb, chicken, or goat. Dal is a thick purée of moong or yellow split peas. Urhad dal is made with lentils, a staple food in India and one of the highest concentrations of protein you can get. Khagina is an Indian omelet; akuri, scrambled eggs; aki, a poaching liquid.

Always ask what chutney contains before trying it. Some exotic versions of this condiment contain pickled fruits and vegetables that have spent time in vinegar, which is safe for all but those who still avoid it. Watch out for uppama. It contains farina.

Pakoras are spicy vegetable fritters, usually held together with lentil, chickpea, or gram flour, all gluten-free. The key word is *usually*. Never order a pakora without first making sure it's safe. Ditto for *dosa*, a rolled lentil flour pancake filled with potatoes and spices. Puri, chapati, naan, kulcha, roti, and paratha are all breads made of excluded flours. The crispy fried spiced wafers called papadam, however, are not. They are traditionally made from lentil flour. At the risk of beating you over the head, ask.

Indian desserts may seem odd to the American palate. Experiment with rasmalai, a sweetened cottage cheese dumpling served with thickened milk, or gulab jamun, cardamom-and-saffron spiced balls of milk curd in sugar syrup served hot. There's always Darjeeling tea or the spicy minted variety called masala, but you really can't call yourself adventurous until you've tasted masala lassi, a traditional spiked buttermilk drink, or mango lassi, a wonderful yogurt drink with mango. I warn you. It's addictive.

GARLIC NAAN

If you think you can never enjoy this savory Indian flat bread, think again. Gluten-free baking wizards Kelli and Peter Bronski have transformed it into something truly special. It's delicious for mopping up all the extra sauce from their Chicken Tikka Masala (page 212) and wonderful warmed and on its own with a bit of chutney or dal. You'll need a pizza stone and the Bronskis' Artisan Gluten-Free Flour Blend (recipe follows).

½ cup warm water (about 115°F)
1 tablespoon plus 2 teaspoons honey
1⅛ teaspoons (½ packet) active dry yeast
1 tablespoon plus 1½ teaspoons milk
1 large egg
1½ cups plus 2 tablespoons Artisan Gluten-Free Flour Blend
1 teaspoon xanthan gum
4 cloves garlic, minced
1 teaspoon salt
2 tablespoons (¼ stick) salted butter, melted
Olive oil

MAKES 4 PIECES

1. Preheat the oven to 400°F with a pizza stone inside. (It's important for the pizza stone to fully preheat.)
2. Combine the warm water, honey, and yeast in a medium bowl and let stand until the mixture foams, about 5 minutes. The foam means your yeast is alive and ready to go.
3. Mix the milk, egg, flour, xanthan gum, half of the garlic, and the salt into the yeast mixture to form a soft dough. The dough will be sticky to the touch.
4. In a small bowl, mix together the melted butter and remaining minced garlic and set aside.

5. Pour 1 to 2 tablespoons olive oil on a cookie sheet and spread with your hand to coat both the cookie sheet and your hand. This will make handling the dough easier. Take one-quarter of the dough, form it into a ball, and flatten it on the baking sheet into a round about 6 to 7 inches in diameter. Repeat with the remaining dough to make 4 pieces of naan. Brush the tops with half of the prepared garlic butter.

6. Let the dough rise on the cookie sheet in a warm location for 20 minutes.

7. Place the cookie sheet on top of the pizza stone in the oven and bake for 4 minutes, then slide the naan directly onto the pizza stone and bake for 1 more minute. Flip the naan, brush the tops with the remaining garlic butter, and bake for an additional 4 minutes, until slightly golden. Serve warm.

Note: For plain naan, simply omit the garlic.

Artisan Gluten-Free Flour Blend

MAKES ABOUT 3 CUPS

Combine the brown rice flour, sorghum flour, cornstarch, potato starch, potato flour, and xanthan gum and store in an airtight container in the refrigerator.

1 ¼ cups brown rice flour
¾ cup sorghum flour
⅔ cup cornstarch
¼ cup potato starch
1 tablespoon plus 1 teaspoon potato flour
1 teaspoon xanthan gum

SWEET AND SPICY CHUTNEY

Chutney and other condiments add sweetness and spice and are essential for their cooling properties. They accompany grilled meats, chicken, fish, and traditional Indian casseroles. This recipe comes courtesy of food writer Sara Pluta and *Living Without* magazine. Look for tamarind concentrate in Indian grocery stores or in the specialty foods section of a large market.

MAKES 1 ½ CUPS

1. In the bowl of a blender, combine the raisins, tamarind concentrate, water, ginger, cayenne, salt, and lemon juice and process until smooth.

2. In a medium saucepan, add the mixture and bring to a boil over high heat. Reduce the heat to medium low and simmer, covered, for 10 minutes.

3. Chill and serve as an accompaniment.

1 cup raisins, currants, prunes, or other dried fruit such as apricots, pears, or pineapple
1 tablespoon tamarind concentrate
6 to 8 tablespoons water
¼ teaspoon ground ginger
¼ teaspoon cayenne pepper
¼ teaspoon salt
1 tablespoon freshly squeezed lemon juice

CUCUMBER RAITA

2 cups plain yogurt (soy or goat's milk yogurt may be substituted)
½ teaspoon ground cumin
Pinch of cayenne pepper or freshly ground black pepper
½ teaspoon salt
2 tablespoons onion, minced
2 cucumbers, seeded and diced
3 tablespoons mint leaves, minced

This cool combination of yogurt, mint, and cucumbers is a staple on the Indian table. Serve alongside meat or vegetable dishes to tame the heat of spicy food. Many thanks to Sara Pluta and *Living Without* magazine.

MAKES 2½ CUPS

In a bowl, mix together the yogurt, cumin, cayenne, salt, onion, cucumbers, and mint. Chill until ready to use.

Italian Cuisine

If you can't see past the pizza, the pasta, and the red sauce, you are missing the joys of traditional Italian cooking. Risotto is a ritual in Northern Italian kitchens, and it is the carbohydrate of choice in Turin, Milan, and Venice, from the Alps all the way down to the Adriatic, where the best short-grained arborio and carnaroli rice are found in the Po River valley. When it is prepared properly, it is rich, creamy, cheesy, savory, satisfying, and everything you miss about pasta. There is nothing better than risotto with wild mushrooms or spring vegetables and Insalata Caprese, a salad in the style of Capri composed of tomatoes, fresh mozzarella, salt, pepper, and basil drizzled with good olive oil.

Polenta or cornmeal mush can be served soft and mixed with cheese or any number of savory sauces. It can be cooked and sliced, then grilled and served as an accompaniment to roasted meats and other dishes. Eating doesn't get better than osso buco, or braised veal shanks, on a bed of soft polenta, as long as the shanks have not been floured first or the brown sauce thickened with flour. Grilled tonno is tuna marinated in olive oil, rosemary, basil, and garlic and served with broccoli rabe and rice.

The perfect gluten-free antipasto plate includes Italian tuna in olive oil, salami, provolone, mozzarella, artichoke hearts, calamari, mushrooms (make sure they are not stuffed with bread crumbs), and hearts of palm, olives, and anchovies. Note: There are many good gluten-free Italian salamis, most notably Genoa, but if you are extremely sensitive and do not know what's in it, don't eat it.

Vitello Tonnato or cold sliced veal with tuna sauce is a masterpiece of poached veal, capers, and anchovies and is likely the most celebrated contribution to the Italian cold table. Milanese almost always means breaded.

La Fiorentina is a grilled T-bone steak, Florentine style, which calls for black peppercorns crushed in a mortar and pestle, garlic, and extra-virgin olive oil. The dark, rich meat sauce of Bologna is not gluten-free unless the cook did not dust the meat in flour before braising. Shrimp or scallops scampi ought to involve olive oil, butter, garlic, and a hot broiler, nothing more, but ask just in case bread crumbs have been added.

Vegetables are a thing of beauty in Italy, cooked simply in olive oil and garlic, which makes them naturally gluten-free, vegan, and delicious. Finocchio or fennel is a much milder version of anise. It is commonly eaten raw in salads but is braised, sautéed, gratinéed, and fried in Italian kitchens.

For dessert, there is croccante, crunchy Italian pralines served with espresso or crushed over gelato. Monte bianco is just that, a mountain of chocolate and chestnuts snowcapped with whipped cream. Zabaglione is an airy concoction made with Marsala wine, egg yolks, and sugar beaten into a froth. Granita is a frozen Italian slush of sugar and very strong espresso, topped with whipped cream or milk. Gelato, the rich ice cream once found only in Italy, has appeared in small cups on every American street corner. The same rules apply to any ice cream: avoid mix-ins and get a clean scoop.

PANNA COTTA

Who cares about cannoli when you can have Davio's owner and star chef Steve DiFillippo's sublime Panna Cotta, Italy's traditional caramel custard? This rich concoction of cream, vanilla, orange peel, and amber caramel is a celebration unto itself. You will need eight to twelve ½-cup aluminum tins, a small pastry brush, and a bowl of ice large enough to accommodate a small saucepan, and maybe some Donizetti playing in the background. Serve it as a sweet conclusion to Chef DiFillippo's Gluten-Free Gnocchi with Wild Mushroom, Garlic, and White Truffle Oil (page 172), and you've got something truly unforgettable.

SERVES 8 TO 12

Amber Caramel

1. In a small saucepan, combine the sugar and water and cook over low heat (do not stir).
2. Use a pastry brush to keep the sugar from sticking to the sides of the saucepan.
3. Watching carefully, cook until sugar dissolves (it's tempting, but do not stir), about 10 minutes or until it turns a light amber color.

1 cup sugar
¼ cup water, plus extra for wetting the pastry brush

4. Remove from the heat and place the bottom of the saucepan in an ice bath to stop cooking.
5. Pour a thin layer of amber caramel into 8×12½-inch aluminum tins, just covering the bottoms.
6. Chill the tins while you prepare the panna cotta mixture.

Panna Cotta

3⅓ cups heavy cream
¾ cup sugar
2 strips orange zest
1 vanilla bean, scraped
1½ teaspoons powdered gelatin
1 cup milk

1. In a small saucepan, bring the heavy cream, sugar, zest, and vanilla bean to a boil.
2. Remove from the heat and stir in the gelatin to dissolve. Add the milk.
3. Let the mixture steep until cool. Strain through a fine-mesh strainer and pour into the chilled ½-cup molds prepared with amber caramel.
4. Refrigerate overnight.
5. Invert the tins onto a plate and pierce the bottoms of the molds to release the contents.
6. Garnish with fresh fruit, if desired.

Japanese Cuisine

If you love sushi or sashimi, you're in luck as long as you remember to bring your own wheat-free soy or tamari sauce or make sure it's provided at the restaurant. Sushi is raw fish with rice. Sashimi is raw fish without rice. I like to order sashimi and a small bowl of brown rice when I eat Japanese. Take a little bit of the rice with a bite of the fish. It's not so filling that way, and brown rice offers more fiber than white. It's always good to bone up on the menu before you jump in. You never know what you might end up with otherwise. If you love raw fish, download these free apps: Guide to Sushi or Sushipedia from Apple. Or Japanese Sushi Guide & Quiz or SuShi for Android devices. Or take this basic course . . .

Akagai: Red clam
Amaebi: Sweet shrimp
Anago: Sea eel
Aoyagi: Skimmer clam
Ebi: Shrimp
Hamachi: Yellowtail
Hirame: Fluke
Hokkigai: Surf clam

Ika: Squid
Ikura: Salmon roe
Katsuo: Bonito
Maguro: Tuna
Mirygai: Giant clam
Saba: Mackerel
Sawakani: Baby octopus
Shake: Salmon

Tako: Octopus
Tamago: Egg omelet
Tobiko: Flying fish egg
Unagi: Clear water eel
Uni: Sea urchin

There are also lobster rolls, California rolls, avocado rolls, Alaska rolls, tuna rolls, crab sticks, and salmon rolls. These are rice, fish, and vegetable combinations that are often sauced. Ask first.

Tofu or soybean curd, a source high in protein, features prominently in Japanese cuisine and can be seasoned, fried, sautéed, or sauced. Always ask how the tofu is prepared because there is a strong probability that it has been soaked or stir-fried in soy sauce. Ditto if you are sensitive to soy. Mozuku is seaweed served with sweet vinegar, which invariably is rice vinegar and should be safe to order if soy sauce has not been added.

Avoid anything that is described as tempura unless you can be sure how the batter is made. Some Japanese chefs use rice flour for their fried dishes to give them a lighter taste, so it is entirely possible that your favorite is one of them. Find out before you cross this dish off your list.

Beware of soba. These buckwheat noodles can be pure buckwheat, which is gluten-free, or a mixture of buckwheat and wheat flour. Never order udon, a wheat noodle. Many Japanese soups or recipes use rice sticks or rice noodles. Ask that they be used in your soup. Miso soup is soybean broth with tofu and wakame. Sumashi is clear chicken broth. Make sure the chicken broth used is gluten-free, check for soy sauce, and always ask which type of miso is being used.

Gyoza is a fried meat dumpling that contains flour and soy sauce. Edamame are steamed soybeans with no soy sauce added. Anything teriyaki is glazed. Yakatori is glazed and skewered. Sukiyaki is a method of preparing vegetables, chicken, beef, or seafood in a soup-like stew à la bouillabaisse. All are full of soy sauce unless you are told otherwise.

There is surprisingly little gluten on a Japanese dessert menu, except fried ice cream tempura style. Green tea ice cream is refreshing and often homemade, with no fillers or stabilizers. Fried bananas with honey are quite good. Yokan or sweet bean jelly is an acquired taste.

MISO SOUP

This is the Japanese equivalent of chicken soup—warm, healing, comforting, and, very often, breakfast. This is the recipe we love at home, adapted from *Cooking the Whole Foods Way* by Christina Pirello, star of *Christina: America's Healthy Cooking Teacher*.

SERVES 4

4 cups dashi (recipe below)
1 3-inch piece of dried
  wakame, soaked and diced
3 green onions or scallions,
  chopped (white and green
  parts), plus extra for garnish
1½ blocks firm Silken tofu,
  cut into 1-inch cubes
1½ teaspoons white rice miso

1. In a small bowl of warm water, reconstitute the dried wakame, about 1 or 2 minutes. It will triple in volume and become bright green.
2. In a medium saucepan, bring the dashi to a simmer over medium heat.
3. Add the wakame and simmer for 1 minute.
4. Add the onions and tofu and simmer 1 to 2 minutes more.
5. Remove a small amount of broth, add the miso, and stir until dissolved.
6. Stir the miso mixture into soup and simmer for 3 to 4 minutes more.
7. Garnish with green onion.

Note: Once miso is added, do not allow soup to boil. Boiling destroys probiotic enzymes and alters the taste.

Dashi

Spring water is fine, but for a real Japanese restaurant broth or dashi, this is worth doing. Kombu is a type of Japanese sea vegetable. Find it and bonito flakes in the international section of a good market or one that specializes in Japanese food products.

MAKES ABOUT 2 QUARTS

2 4-inch pieces kombu
2½ quarts water
2 cups bonito flakes

1. In a 4-quart saucepan, place the kombu. Cover with water, and soak for 30 minutes.
2. Set the pan over medium heat until small bubbles appear around the sides of the pan, about 10 minutes. Remove the kombu from the pan and discard. Raise the heat to high and bring to a boil, about 6 minutes. Reduce the heat to low and add the bonito flakes.
3. Simmer gently, stirring frequently, for 10 minutes.
4. Using a fine-mesh strainer lined with cheesecloth, strain the dashi. Discard the bonito flakes.
5. Stored in an airtight container, dashi will keep in the refrigerator for 1 week or in the freezer for 1 month.

Mexican Cuisine

Enchiladas, tortillas, carne asada, salsa, guacamole, masa harina, huevos rancheros, nachos, tostadas, and good old rice and beans. This is Mexico, land of corn, queso fresca, and mole sauce, a gluten-free paradise. Warning: If you are sensitive to chilis, chili powder, and peppers, don't even think of going Mexican. They are in everything.

Real Mexican cuisine—not the burrito factories dotting the American landscape—uses masa harina, a cornmeal soaked in lime, tomatillos (small green tomatoes), and corn husks, which are traditionally used to serve tamales, guava paste, and hominy, a cereal made from corn. Corn tortillas, soft and homemade, bear no resemblance to the tasteless versions found in fast-food restaurants and on supermarket shelves. Authentic salsas bear little resemblance to those watery concoctions found in the grocery stores.

Corn tortillas are yellow and smaller than flour tortillas. Quesadillas are usually made with large, white flour tortillas but can easily be made with its smaller and gluten-free cousin. Learn to spot them from across the room. It's harder than you think when they are hiding under a sauce. Almost any dish that is made with a flour tortilla can be made with a corn tortilla. Be careful, though, that the rest of the ingredients contain no gluten. Always ask if the chili contains any flour, because some Mexican chefs start their chili from a roux.

A typical Mexican menu might include gazpacho, a spicy chilled soup made of puréed tomatoes, peppers, cucumbers, and spices. Ask the waiter to leave off the croutons that sometimes accompany this dish. If you've forgotten and are served soup with croutons, don't pick them out. Ask for a fresh bowl.

Chile rellenos can be made with bread crumbs or not. Make sure you know which is which. Salsa verde, salsa rojo, and salsa casera do not contain flour. Guacamole sauce or dip is made from avocados. Mole is a spicy sauce that includes cocoa. Frijoles or beans are a mainstay of Mexican cuisine. Frijoles refritos or refried beans are typically not made with any thickening, but they are fried in lard. Beware if you are a vegetarian.

As with all unfamiliar cuisines, avoid any stews or dishes that appear to be enrobed in a thick sauce. They may contain flour. Cornstarch is often used as a thickener in Mexican recipes. Always ask before you rule something out. Chorizo, the spiced Spanish sausage used frequently in Mexican cooking, usually contains tequila, wine vinegar, and hot chilis, among other spices. Never eat a chorizo whose ingredients cannot be accounted for.

The traditional Mexican dessert custard is a caramel pudding called flan, which should be safe if made from scratch. Ask before you order it.

Middle Eastern Cuisine

Warning: Bulgur wheat is a big deal in the Middle East.

Kibbie nayee, the national dish of Lebanon, tabbouleh, and falafel are all made with bulgur wheat. Emjudra is a dish of lentils and rice cooked in onion broth. Ej-jee is a Lebanese omelet flavored with mint and onions. Hummus with tahini is the Israeli and Egyptian version of mashed chickpeas and crushed sesame seeds, and while baba ganoush is spelled differently in Greek, it's still puréed eggplant with sesame dressing. Greek olives are called zatoon in the Middle East.

Laban is said to be an authentic yogurt made from a thousand-year-old culture. I didn't think it tasted a day over five hundred years myself. Cucumbers abound in Middle Eastern restaurants. Use them instead of pita for the dips. *Maza* or *mezze* is the Armenian, Turkish, and Greek answer to antipasto. Mixed dishes are always good because you can discuss their contents when you order and ask that any unsafe dishes be left out and extras of the gluten-free dishes added.

Everybody shares in the Middle East. Not you.

Marinades are usually yogurt, garlic, and lemon in this part of the world, but do check first before you order the kabobs.

Oranges are wonderful for dessert. Or halvah or halawah, Lebanese sugar and sesame paste candy. Kawhwee is a dark Turkish coffee usually served by the thimbleful, for good reason.

Russian Cuisine

With my apologies to Russian friends, this is the land of bitter winters, little sun, and stick-to-the-ribs food that contains enough gluten to make all of Eastern Europe queasy. Siberia is the dumpling and noodle capital of the world with pelmeni, verniki, haluski, and manti. With breads and savories such as kulebiaka, khachapuri, pirozhki, and pirogs, Russian stroganoffs, Ukrainian crepes or blini, and all the thick cabbage and beet dishes of the Baltics, you may ask yourself: *What's left?*

Plentski.

Georgian rice and lamb pilaf are fragrant and filling and are made with nuts and candied orange peel. One pilaf in particular, from Azerbaijan, can be made with an egg, potato, pumpkin, or bread crust. Make sure you know which one is being used.

Borscht or kologniy is a winner. Say *nyet* to tabbouleh. This bulgur wheat is often prepared as a pilaf. Always make sure your pilaf is made only with rice. Have a Russian omelet with sour cream and caviar. Or stuffed prunes. Lamb stew with chestnuts and pomegranates is a traditional Azerbaijani dish that should not contain wheat flour as a thickener, but as you know by now, you must ask.

Every country has its version of polenta, and Moldavian cornmeal mush is really very good. Kasha and wild mushroom casserole is a hearty dish as long as you can be sure the buckwheat groats aren't mixed with unsafe grains.

Rice-stuffed grape leaves are Russian, as are stuffed apples, quinces, peppers, and pumpkins. Lamb is often used for stuffing as well. These dishes should not contain bread crumbs or any flour thickeners, but double-check. Mashkitchiri is literally mashed mung beans, vegetables, and rice. Kabobs are always marinated, which makes them off-limits unless you know what's in the marinade. For dessert, have some halvah with a glass of tea.

Then there's Russian vodka. *Nasdrovia.*

TRADITIONAL RUSSIAN BORSCHT

This is the borscht my brother-in-law, the late Jerzy Kosinski, served to the family when we came to lunch. He claimed the recipe was his grandmother's and that it had survived the war sewn into the lid of the suitcase she carried when she fled Ukraine and, after that, Poland. Then again, it could have been from *Joy of Cooking* or from The Russian Tea Room down the block from his apartment. He was a master storyteller, after all.

Beef stock is more traditional, but I make mine vegetarian. Try to find Russian white cabbage rather than green. It makes for a better texture. Boiling the vegetables first is traditional and also results in a lovely consistency. When puréed and swirled with sour cream, this garnet soup is a showstopper. You can leave it chunky or, if you prefer, purée only half.

MAKES ABOUT 5 CUPS

1. In a large, heavy pan, place the carrots, onions, and beets, and add enough water to cover. Bring to a boil over high heat, then reduce the heat to medium-low, cover, and simmer gently for about 20 minutes, until vegetables are tender.
2. Add the butter, stock, cabbage, and vinegar and simmer for 15 minutes more.
3. With an immersion blender, purée the soup. Transfer the soup to a container and let it chill in the refrigerator. If you prefer to eat the soup warm, place the puréed soup in warm bowls.
4. Garnish with a generous dollop of sour cream, chopped cucumber, and dill.

½ cup carrots, peeled and finely chopped
1 cup onions, peeled and finely chopped
2 cups red beets, peeled and finely chopped
¼ cup (½ stick) unsalted butter
2 cups gluten-free vegetable, chicken, or beef stock
1 cup white cabbage, finely shredded
1 tablespoon red wine vinegar
Salt and freshly ground black pepper to taste
Sour cream, for garnish
½ cup fresh dill, for garnish
1 cucumber, peeled and chopped, for garnish

Scandinavian Cuisine

It's cold in this part of the world, and there is quite a bit of fish, especially codfish. To make the harvest last all year in these chilly climes, there is quite a lot of pickled and salted food. This means vinegar, so if you are avoiding it, you may want to pass on the smorgasbord, the traditional Scandinavian buffet table.

Moving beyond the briny offerings, you will find Danish hot buttermilk soup, apple soup, kirsebaersuppe or cherry soup, and summer vegetable soup thickened with nothing but cornstarch.

Swedish meatballs almost always contain bread crumbs. You won't know until you ask. If you have to ask about beer soup, you need a refresher course in the basics. Gravlax is Swedish marinated salmon, and it's generally worth the high price. You will find reindeer, whale, and venison on menus in Scandinavian countries, and you may find these meats in Scandinavian American restaurants. If you do and can handle it—I draw the line at Rudolph—don't get so caught up in your ability to try new things that you forget to ask how they are prepared.

Danish ham is a real treat. Watch for mustard and bread crumbs in the coating and Madeira sauce in the glaze. Madeira is based on a brown stock that can be based on a roux. As everywhere in the world, watch out for sauces.

The land of the midnight sun is home to a large number of gluten-free Scandinavians, which makes for abundant gluten-free options. Norwegian prune pudding is traditionally thickened with cornstarch. Swedish rice porridge, a traditional Christmas dessert, should be gluten-free. Ditto for prune custard. Akvavit is the traditional firewater of Scandinavia. And Ikea sells a mean gluten-free almond torte.

Spanish Cuisine

While Spain has had an enormous influence on the cuisines of Mexico and Latin America, Spanish food takes its cues from the great cities of Barcelona, Valencia, Malaga, and Granada and from North Africa just beyond Gibraltar. All over Spain, bars and bistros called *tascas* serve the tapas, or small appetizer dishes that are the national snack. Here it is the custom to drink sherry, share gossip, and order from extensive menus of foods served in very small portions. In recent years, tapas and small-plate fever has taken hold all across the United States.

Proceed carefully. It's easy to be overwhelmed by small portions and the speed with which they arrive at the table. In the casual, often-rollicking spirit of these places, some gluten may slip by. Bypass the obvious and maybe not so obvious offenders. Empadillas are turnovers. Emparedos are small sandwiches. Croquettes are called croqetas and are just as crusty and fried.

Stick with simple dishes containing foods you can readily see and don't share. Good choices include Spanish antipasto and garlic shrimp, or gambas al ajillo. Almejas al diablo are clams in tomato sauce. Mussels marinated in red wine, capers, and pimiento are called mejillones a la vinagreta. Angulas a la bilbaina are eels or smelts in garlic sauce. Chorizos are always difficult to divine, but try, they are worth it. In Spain tortillas are not tortillas at all, but flat Spanish omelets served in wedges.

Fillings are another story. Ask. If English is a problem in your local Spanish market or *tasca*, *pregunta* is Spanish for "question." Say, "Yo tengo preguntas." I have questions. Then show them your Spanish dining card (page 331).

There is always paella, the rich dish that is the centerpiece of Spanish cuisine. Paella a la Valenciana is with chicken and seafood; paella marinera is seafood only; paella huertana de murcia with vegetables only; paella de codornices y setas features quail and mushrooms; and fideua de mariscos, a paella of noodles and shellfish, is best avoided. Zarzuela de marisco is a spicy and spectacular shellfish stew served over rice.

Marzipan, almond sugar candy, came to Spain by way of the Moors and is on many Spanish menus. In fact, so many Spanish candies are made with almonds, sugar, coconut, and eggs and no wheat or gluten that it is advisable to find a good Spanish American market and stock up. The Spanish love their baked apples, bananas with honey and pine nuts, and pears in dark Spanish wine, prunes, and apricots. All good.

Thai Cuisine

The contrasts are sharp in this part of the world, and the cuisine is gluten-free-friendly. Four-alarm curries, fiery chili pastes, searing peanut sauces, coconut milk, and lemon grass are the grace notes of this interesting food. Spring rolls are often made with rice wrappers, which can be used for enfolding shrimp and green onions held together with fish sauce and lemon grass. Bean thread or rice sticks are used in place of wheat noodles, with tofu instead of chicken or beef. Pineapple and tapioca make fried rice distinctly Thai.

As a mild prelude to the heat of any number of Thai curries, the coconut-based soup tom ka gai can lull the uninitiated into a false sense of security.

Pad Thai is a classic dish made with rice noodles (ban-pho), egg, bean curd, bean sprouts, and green onion topped with ground peanuts (see Vegetarian Pad Thai, page 222). There are many variations on the rice noodle, as well as rice pancakes and spicy fritters of corn and potato.

The difficulty of dining safely on Thai cuisine is in the sauces. Clear fish sauce contains no wheat, but hoisin sauce does. Soy, tamari, and thick fish and peanut sauces are often used and can be a problem.

If you love this food as I do, my best advice is to master a few gluten-free adaptations or sit down with your local Thai chef and figure out together what you can eat and what you can't. The Thai Gluten Intolerance Dining Card (page 332) will come in handy here. Most Thai dishes are individually stir-fried, so it's not as if your diet is affecting the entire night's business. Naturally, you must be a good-enough customer to make it worthwhile for the restaurant to clean the stir-fry pan and start over for you, and you should be considerate of peak times. You will not be sorry you took the trouble. Fresh, homemade Thai rice noodles alone are worth the effort.

THAI GRAPEFRUIT SALAD WITH TOASTED COCONUT AND FRESH MINT

While Pad Thai may be the national dish, sometimes such a concentration of carbohydrates can be too heavy. This dazzling salad called yum some-oh, from author and expert on Thai cuisine Nancie McDermott, combines traditional ingredients like fish sauce, green chilies, and dried shrimp (which can be found in specialty stores like Import Food Thai Supermarket, www.importfood.com) with the sweet surprise of toasted coconut, mint, and grapefruit. Serve it as a spectacular first course or as a small meal. Thais make it with pomelo, grapefruit's dryer, sweeter, and thick-skinned cousin, but the juicier grapefruit will do nicely. Reprinted here with permission from *Quick and Easy Thai* by Nancie McDermott.

SERVES 4

1. In a small, dry skillet, toast the shredded coconut over medium-high heat for 3 to 4 minutes, tossing often, until most of it turns a rich, soft brown. Turn out into a saucer to cool.

2. In a medium bowl, combine the lime juice, fish sauce, and sugar and stir well to dissolve the sugar and form a smooth sauce. Add the pomelo, toasted coconut, dried shrimp or peanuts (if using), shallots, chilies, and mint and toss gently to combine well.

3. Arrange the salad on lettuce leaves on a serving platter or 4 individual plates. Serve at room temperature.

3 tablespoons shredded coconut

2 tablespoons lime juice, freshly squeezed

2 tablespoons gluten-free fish sauce, such as Thai Kitchen

1 tablespoon sugar

1 cup pomelo or grapefruit, peeled, sectioned, and cut into bite-size chunks

2 tablespoons dried shrimp, coarsely chopped, or 2 tablespoons salted peanuts, coarsely chopped (optional)

1 tablespoon shallots, coarsely chopped

1 teaspoon fresh hot green chilies, finely chopped or dried red pepper flakes

½ cup fresh mint, coarsely chopped

Leaves of Boston or Bibb lettuce for accompaniment

A Word About Shopping

Going gluten-free is a license to explore this great melting pot of ours. With online access and ethnic markets and specialty stores popping up all over the country, you don't have to be in a big city to shop the globe.

THE ASIAN MARKET

Explore your town or city and chances are you will find, nestled at the center of the Asian community, a supermarket that feels distinctly foreign. Among the pickled eels, dried sea urchin, and star anise, you can find rice crackers, rice sticks called haw fun, broken rice, sweet brown rice, cellophane noodles, mi fun or rice vermicelli, and the flat rice noodle of Shanghai called ho fun. You will find rice wrappers thin as onionskin at a third or two-thirds the price seen elsewhere.

A good Asian market may yield a Malaysian cake called tan kim hock, made with coconut flower water, coconut milk, sugar, and glutinous rice. Asian markets stock dried shiitake mushrooms for miso soup and sheets of nori, the crisp seaweed used to wrap sushi. Once you get the hang of making nori rolls, you can duplicate almost any dish in a Japanese restaurant at prices that put stores like Whole Foods to shame. You may also find dulse, another Japanese sea vegetable, which crisps up nicely with a little sesame oil and, with toasted gluten-free bread and mayonnaise, serves as a salty substitute for artery-clogging bacon in my vegan DLTs.

Be warned: Not all foreign products bear English ingredient labels. If you can't read it, don't buy it. Avoid imitation crabsticks and shrimp. They are full of wheat fillers, which is what allows them to be molded into such real-looking shapes.

Against the lovely cacophony of dozens of Vietnamese, Korean, Chinese, Japanese, and Malaysian dialects, you will discover something new every time, and soon your pantry will be stocked with crystallized ginger, protein-rich edamame, wasabi mustards, and exotic teas that cost a mint in specialty stores. Who knows, you may even be emboldened to buy exotic kinds of fresh fish and live poultry the way Asian families do, much closer to the real thing than their packaged and sanitized American cousins.

The housewares aisle is a real bonus, too. Teapots, sushi plates, and shoyu cups and bowls in traditional blue or celadon cost a fraction of what they would elsewhere, not to mention silk slippers, jade bracelets, and embroidered evening bags all at bargain prices.

THE MEXICAN MARKET

Here you will find fresh corn tortillas, ancho chilies, peppers hot enough to make your hair curl, masa harina soaked in lime, and salsa fresca that bears little resemblance to the bland stuff found on supermarket shelves. Tomatillos, jalapeños, serranos, poblanos, and squash blossoms abound.

Look for chipotle purée, or chipotle in adobo seasoning (a blend of garlic, oregano, black pepper, and turmeric); the salty, crumbly Cotija cheese called for in Traci Des Jardin's exquisite Grilled Corn and Squash Salad with Chipotle Crema, Lime Vinaigrette, and Cotija Cheese (page 162), or the Chihuahua cheese for Rick Bayless's Quesadillas Asadas (page 165).

THE ITALIAN MARKET

In Philadelphia's Italian Market neighborhood, scene of Rocky movies and Mummers' warehouses, there are several blocks of Old World cheese shops, fishmongers, butchers, bakers, restaurants, and fruit and vegetable vendors joined by Mexican and Asian markets, as well as Taffets, a gluten-free bakery.

If you can do dairy, cheese is the lure here, ripe Taleggio and aged Reggiannos and Parmesans and homemade pestos for your gluten-free fresh ravioli and linguine and Mediterranean Bean Soup (recipe on page 46). Pick up ready-made gluten-free cannoli shells at Taffets Bakery in the heart of the action. Italian markets yield gluten-free pastas imported from Italy; amaretto cookies, some made from pure almond paste; cured Parma ham; and the most flavorful olive oils and balsamic vinegars in the world. There is short-grain arborio rice for risotto and finely ground corn for polenta, and in some shops you may even get the family recipe to go with them.

Many cities have their versions of my beloved Italian market, most notably Chicago, San Francisco, Boston, and New York, and if you are not near such a neighborhood, ask your local Italian chef and chances are he or she has a few names and addresses for you. Remember, too, good cookbooks usually list their sources for traditional ingredients.

When you get home, crank up the Rossini and stir up a risotto with the abandon of a born Venetian. Whip up some chile rellenos, huevos rancheros, or the perfect winter posole—a silken Mexican stew studded with bits of pork. Forget crackers and nibble on dolma, the grape leaves stuffed with rice the Greeks can't eat just one of. Dream of traveling the world.

COOKBOOKS

These are not the cookbooks du jour. They are classics that teach technique, provide an understanding of essential ingredients, and explain how various cuisines are made, making it easier to render your favorites gluten-free and start you on a well-rounded international library:

The Breath of the Wok by Grace Young and Alan Richardson (Simon and Schuster)

Essentials of Classic Italian Cooking by Marcella Hazan (Knopf)

The Gluten-Free Asian Kitchen by Laura B. Russell (Celestial Arts)

Indian Cooking by Madhur Jaffrey (Barron's)

Mastering the Art of French Cooking by Julia Child, Louisette Bertholle, and Simone Beck (Knopf)

Rick Bayless's Mexican Kitchen by Rick Bayless (Scribner)

Risotto by Pamela Sheldon Johns, from the Williams-Sonoma Series (Simon and Schuster)

The Soul of a New Cuisine: *A Discovery of the Foods and Flavors of Africa* by Marcus Samuelsson (John Wiley and Sons)

Vegetarian Cooking for Everyone, 10th anniversary edition, by Deborah Madison (Ten Speed Press)

Learn more

SHOPPING WEB SITES

Greek, African, Chinese, English, Korean, Italian, Mexican, and Indian specialty foods. www.Amazon.com/International-British-Asian-Foods /b?ie=UTF8&node=376936011

Indian specialty foods like moong dal, chutneys, and spices.
    www.grocerybabu.com
Middle Eastern and Indian chutneys, herbs, and spices.
    www.kalustyans.com
Specialty foods by international region or by country.
    www.internationalfoodshop.com

14

Sprechen Sie Gluten?

You are invited to take advantage of the chambermaid.
—SIGN IN JAPANESE HOTEL ROOM

◆ **Gluten-Intolerance Dining Cards for Travel**

English
Arabic
Chinese
Croatian
Czech
Danish
Dutch
French
German
Greek
Hebrew
Hindi
Italian
Japanese
Korean
Polish
Portuguese
Russian
Spanish
Swahili
Swedish
Thai
Vietnamese

Ladies requested not to have children in the bar. Please leave your values at the front desk.

We've all had a good laugh at signs like these in foreign hotels attempting to translate for their English-speaking guests. Something crucial is lost in translation and the meaning changes, often hilariously so. Funny, yes. But the last thing you want to get lost is a serious request for a gluten-free meal.

If you travel often for business or pleasure, becoming familiar with the many foreign menu terms in Chapter 13 will go a long way in choosing what and where to eat while abroad. Still, the waiter may not speak your language, and that is especially true if you are traveling to far-flung places away from world capitals. If you're like me, your language skills may be too wobbly to get your needs across.

You can always stay home, but how boring is that?

The world is much friendlier to the gluten-free diet than when I penned the first gluten intolerance card, which said in terrible French, *If I have any farine, I'll have a disease in my chair.* I had no idea I was launching a cottage industry or that I would end up putting much better versions in *Against the Grain.* I just knew I wanted to go to Paris, gluten-free or not, and I did not trust my French to get myself anything more than a room and a bar of soap.

Living fully and well should not be dictated by diet or syntax.

The dining cards you will find here are a far cry from my quaint early attempts. They are professionally translated from English into twenty-two languages—Arabic, Chinese, Croatian, Czech, Danish, Dutch, French, German, Greek, Hebrew, Hindi, Italian, Japanese, Korean, Polish, Portuguese, Russian, Spanish, Swahili, Swedish, Thai, and Vietnamese.

Be aware, these cards are as good as the fluency of your waiter in his or her own language. They will not help in remote places where many people cannot read or write. Nor will they prevent lewd practical jokes, as one Westchester tour group discovered at the hands of some frisky Greek island fisherman. That is entirely out of my hands or those of the translator.

Remember these cards are not just for traveling and will also go a long way toward understanding at the ethnic restaurant where the owners are still a bit shaky in English. At home or abroad, most people want to help and appreciate it when you try to communicate in their language, even if it's only on paper.

English Gluten-Intolerance Dining Card

I do not speak your language.

I have a condition called celiac disease/gluten intolerance.

If I eat any food made with gluten, wheat, rye, barley, triticale, malt, oat flour, and any derivatives, fillers, or sauces made with these grains, especially those dishes made with pasta, or coated or dusted with flour or bread crumbs or containing soy sauce or beer, I will become ill.

I am able to eat corn and rice and rice noodles.

If necessary, please check with the chef to make sure my food does not contain any of these ingredients and help me order a meal I can safely enjoy.

Thank you very much.

Arabic Gluten-Intolerance Dining Card

أنا لا أتحدث لغتك.

أنا مصابة بمرض سلياك/حساسية الغلونين.

إذا تناولت أي طعام يحتوي على الغلوتين أو القمح أو الجاودار أو الشعير أو التريتيكال أو منقوع الشعير أو دقيق الشوفان وأي من مشتقاته أو المحاشي أو الصوص المصنوع من هذه الحبوب، وخصوصًا تلك الأطباق المصنوعة من المعكرونة أو الأكلات المغلفة أو المنثور عليها الدقيق أو فتات الخبز (البقسماط) أو التّي تحتوي على صوص الصويا أو الجعة؛ فسوف أُصاب بنوبة حساسية.

يمكنني تناول الذرة والأرز ونودلز الأرز.

إذا لزم الأمر، الرجاء مراجعة المكونات مع رئيس الطهاة للتأكد من عدم احتواء الطعام الخاص بي على أي من هذه المكونات ومساعدتي على طلب وجبة لذيذة لا تسبب لي أي متاعب.

مع خالص الشكر

Chinese Gluten-Intolerance Dining Card

麸质不耐症用餐卡中文版：
新版英语翻译卡片：

我不会说中文。
我有一种叫麸质不耐症（谷物过敏）的疾病，不能吃任何用麦麸、小麦、黑麦、大麦、黑小麦、麦芽或燕麦粉制成的食物。我也不能吃任何用这些谷物原料制成的副产品、馅料或酱汁，尤其是那些以意大利面作为原料的、包裹有面粉或面包屑的、或是含有酱油或啤酒的菜肴。否则我会感到十分不舒服。
我可以吃玉米、大米和米粉（或米线）。
如果可以的话，请您与厨师确认我的食物中不含上面这些我不能吃的成分，帮助我挑选能让我安心享用的菜肴。非常感谢！

Croatian Gluten-Intolerance Dining Card

Ne govorim vaš jezik.
Patim od celijakije/nepodnošenje glutena.
Ako pojedem hranu koja sadrži gluten, pšenicu, raž, ječam, pšenoraž, slad, zobeno brašno i sve proizvode od toga, punila ili umake koji sadrže te žitarice, posebice jela od tjestenine, ili obložena ili posuta brašnom ili krušnim mrvicama ili ako sadrže umak od soje ili pivo, ja ću se razboljeti.
Mogu jesti kukuruz i rižu i tjesteninu od riže.
Ako je potrebno, provjerite s kuharom kako biste bili sigurni da moja hrana ne sadrži bilo koji od ovih sastojaka i pomognite mi naručiti jelo koje ja mogu sigurno jesti.
Puno hvala.

Czech Gluten-Intolerance Dining Card

Nemluvím česky.
Trpím onemocněním zvaným celiakie/nesnášenlivostí lepku.

Pokud budu konzumovat jídlo připravené z lepku, pšenice, žita,
ječmene, tritikale, sladu, ovesné mouky a derivátů těchto látek,
náplní nebo omáček z těchto obilnin, zejména pokrmy připravené z
těstovin nebo obalené či zasypané moukou nebo strouhankou, či
pokrmy obsahující sojovou omáčku nebo pivo, onemocním.
Můžu jíst kukuřici, rýži a rýžové nudle.
Pokud je to nutné, zeptejte se kuchaře, abychom měli jistotu, že moje
jídlo neobsahuje žádnou z výše uvedených látek, a pomozte mi
objednat jídlo, které můžu bezpečně jíst.

Děkuji mnohokrát.

Danish Gluten-Intolerance Dining Card

Jeg taler ikke dit sprog.

Jeg lider af en sygdom der hedder cøliaki/glutenintolerans.

Jeg bliver syg, hvis jeg spiser mad der indeholder gluten, hvede, rug,
byg, rughvede, malt, havre og alle afledte produkter, fyldstoffer eller
saucer fremstillet med disse kornsorter. Dette gælder især retter med
pasta, eller retter som er belagt eller drysset med mel eller rasp eller
indeholder sojasauce eller øl.

Jeg må gerne spise majs og ris og risnudler.

Du bedes om nødvendigt spørge kokken for at være sikker på, at mit
måltid ikke indeholder nogen af disse ingredienser, samt hjælpe mig
med at bestille et måltid, jeg trygt kan spise.

Mange tak.

Dutch Gluten-Intolerance Dining Card

Ik spreek of versta uw taal niet.

Ik heb 'Coeliakie', dat ook wel glutenintolerantie wordt genoemd.

Ik word ernstig ziek als ik maaltijden gebruik waarin gluten, tarwe, rogge, gerst, triticale, mout of havermeel zit. Deze ingrediënten zitten vaak ook in vullingen en sauzen, in pasta en in andere gerechten die zijn bestrooid met bloem of paneermeel of bereid met sojasaus of bier.

Ik kan echter wel maïs, rijst en noedels op basis van rijst eten.

Kunt u tegen de kok zeggen dat mijn bestelling geen van de hierboven vermelde ingrediënten mag bevatten, zodat ik ongerust van mijn maaltijd kan genieten?.

Hartelijk dank!

French Gluten-Intolerance Dining Card

Je ne parle pas votre langue.

Je souffre de la maladie coeliaque ou une intolérance au gluten.

Si je mange une nourriture contenant du gluten, blé, seigle, orge, triticale, malte, farine d'avoine et tous dérivatifs, additifs ou sauces faits avec ces grains, surtout les plats de pâtes ou les plats faits avec de la farine ou une chapelure, ou contenant du soja ou de la bière, je tomberai malade.

Je peux manger du maïs, du riz, et des nouilles de riz.

Si nécessaire, je vous prie de vérifier avec le chef cuisinier que ma nourriture ne contienne aucun de ces ingrédients, et de m'aider à commander un repas que je peux savourer en toute sécurité.

Merci beaucoup.

German Gluten-Intolerance Dining Card

Ich spreche kein Deutsch.

Ich leide an der Erkrankung Zöliakie (eine Gluten-Unverträglichkeit).

Wenn ich Speisen mit Gluten, Weizen, Roggen, Gerste, Triticale, Malz, Hafermehl und aus diesen Getreidesorten hergestellte Produkte, Füllmittel oder Soßen esse, insbesondere Speisen mit Teigwaren, Mehlstaub oder Paniermehl oder Speisen mit Sojasoße oder Bier, werde ich krank.

Ich vertrage Mais, Reis, und Reisnudeln.

Ich bitte Sie, nötigenfalls den Küchenchef zu fragen, um sicherzustellen, dass mein Essen keine der genannten Zutaten enthält, und um mir bei der Auswahl einer Mahlzeit zu helfen, die ich bedenkenlos genießen kann.

Vielen Dank.

Greek Gluten-Intolerance Dining Card

Δεν μιλάω τη γλώσσα σας.

Πάσχω από μια ασθένεια που ονομάζεται κοιλιοκάκη / δυσανεξία στη γλουτένη.

Εάν καταναλώσω οποιαδήποτε τροφή που περιέχει γλουτένη, σιτάρι, σίκαλη, τριτικάλ, βύνη, αλεύρι βρώμης και οποιοδήποτε παράγωγο αυτών, συμπληρώματα ή σάλτσες με αυτά τα συστατικά, ειδικά στα πιάτα με ζυμαρικά, με επικάλυψη ή πασπαλισμένα με αλεύρι ή με ψίχουλα από ψωμί, ή με σάλτσα σόγιας ή μπύρας, θα ασθενήσω.

Μπορώ να φάω καλαμπόκι και χυλοπίτες ρυζιού.

Εάν χρειαστεί, σας παρακαλώ να ελέγξετε μαζί με το σεφ, ώστε το φαγητό μου να μην περιέχει αυτά τα συστατικά και να με βοηθήσετε να παραγγείλω ένα γεύμα που θα μπορώ να απολαύσω με ασφάλεια.

Σας ευχαριστώ πολύ!

Hebrew Gluten-Intolerance Dining Card

אני לא מדברת עברית.

יש לי צליאק, או אלרגיה לגלוטן.

אני לא יכולה לאכול מזון המכיל גלוטן, חיטה, שיפון ,גריסי פנינה, שעורה, שיבולתשועל(קוואקר), לתת, או כל מילוי או רוטב המכיל אותם. מנות המכילות פסטה, או שנזרה עליהם קמח או פרורי לחם, או המכילות רוטב סויה או בירה יגרמו לי התקפת צליאק.

אני יכולה לאכול איטריות אורז ותירס המבושלת בנפרד משאר הדגנים.

אם את/ה לא בטוח בקשר לכול הרכיבים אנא התייעץ/התייעצי עם הטבח ועזרו לי לבחור מנה שאוכל לאכול בבטחה ושלא תגרום לי לחלות.

תודה רבה על ההתחשבות.

Hindi Gluten-Intolerance Dining Card

मैं आपकी भाषा नहीं बोलता/बोलती हूँ।
मैं उदरीय रोग/लस (ग्लूटेन) असहनशीलता नामक अवस्था से पीड़ित हूँ।
मैं लस(ग्लूटेन), गेहूँ, राई, जौ, ट्रिटिकेल (गेहूँ-जौ का संकर दाना), माल्ट, जई का आटा और इन अनाज के दानों से बने कोई पदार्थ, पूरक या सॉस, विशेष रूप से पास्ता मिलाकर बनाए गए व्यंजन, या आटे या ब्रेडक्रंब से लेपित या छिड़काव वाले या सोया सॉस या बियर वाले व्यंजन खाने पर बीमार हो जाता/जाती हूँ।

मैं मक्का और चावल तथा चावल के नूडल खा सकता/सकती हूँ।
यदि आवश्यक हो, तो कृपया शेफ़ से पूछताछ करके यह सुनिश्चित कर लें कि मेरे खाने में इन में से कोई सामग्री शामिल न हो और ऐसे भोजन का आर्डर देने में मेरी मदद करें, जिसका मैं सुरक्षित रूप से आनंद ले सकूँ।

आपका बहुत-बहुत धन्यवाद।

Italian Gluten-Intolerance Dining Card

Non parlo la sua lingua.

Ho una condizione chiamata intolleranza al glutine (celiachia).

Se mangio un qualsiasi alimento a base di glutine, grano, segale, orzo, triticale, malto, farina di avena e tutti i loro derivati o ripieni e salse a base di questi cereali e in particolare piatti a base di pasta, o rivestiti o spolverati con farina o pangrattato o contenenti salsa di soia o birra, mi ammalerò gravemente.

Posso però mangiare mais, riso, e pasta di riso.

Se necessario, può controllare con il cuoco per accertarsi che il mio cibo non contenga nessuno di questi ingredienti? Mi può anche aiutare a ordinare un pasto che possa godere in tutta sicurezza?

Grazie mille!

Japanese Gluten-Intolerance Dining Card

私はあなたの言語を話せません。

私は、セリアック病／グルテン不耐症と呼ばれる病気です。

グルテン、小麦、ライ麦、大麦、ライ小麦、麦芽、オート麦粉の入った食べ物、およびこれらの穀物を使った加工物、詰め物、ソース、特にパスタを使った料理、小麦粉やパン粉をまぶした料理、しょうゆやビールの入った料理を食べると病状が出ます。

とうもろこし、お米、お米でできた麺は食べられます。

必要ならば、私の食べる料理に上記の食材が使われてないことをシェフに確認し、安全に食べられる料理を注文できるよう協力してください。

どうぞよろしくお願いいたします。

Korean Gluten-Intolerance Dining Card

저는 한국 말을 못합니다.

저는 만성 소화장애증/글루텐 편협라는 질환이 있습니다.

전는 필러 또는 쏘스를 만들때 다음과 같은 곡식이
들어가있으면 병에 걸립니다. 글루텐, 밀, 호밀, 보리, 호밀, 밀,
맥아, 귀리 가루, 파스타로 만든 또는 코팅 되있는 음식이거나
밀가루가 뿌려진 또는 빵 부스러기 가루 또는 간장 또는 맥주.

전는 옥수수, 쌀, 쌀 국수는 먹을수 있습니다.

필요한 경우, 제가 안진하게 음식을 즐길수 있도록 주방장과
확인하셔서 재료에 이런것들이 않들어 가있는 음식으로
주문할수 있게 도와주시면 감사하겠 습니다.

정말 감사합니다.

Polish Gluten-Intolerance Dining Card

Nie mówię w Twoim języku.
Choruję na chorobę zwaną celiakią/nietolerancją glutenu.
Jeżeli zjem posiłek zawierający gluten, pszenicę, żyto, jęczmień,
pszenżyto, słód, mąkę owsianą lub ich pochodne, nadzienia lub sosy
sporządzone z tymi ziarnami, a zwłaszcza dania z makaronem,
posypane lub poprószone mąką czy bułką tartą lub dania zawierające
sos sojowy bądź piwo, wystąpią u mnie objawy choroby.
Mogę jeść kukurydzę, ryż i makaron ryżowy.
W razie konieczności proszę skonsultować się z szefem kuchni, by
upewnić się, że mój posiłek nie zawiera któregoś z tych składników.
Dzięki temu będę mógł/mogła zamówić bezpieczne dla mnie danie.
Bardzo dziękuję.

Portuguese Gluten-Intolerance Dining Card

Eu não falo a sua língua.

Eu sofro de uma condição chamada doença celíaca/intolerância
ao glúten.

Se eu comer alguma comida feita com glúten, trigo, centeio, cevada,
triticale, malte, farinha de aveia ou quaisquer derivados, recheios ou
molhos feitos com estes cereais, especialmente os pratos feitos com
massa ou cobertos ou polvilhados com farinha ou pão ralado ou que
contenham molho de soja ou cerveja, eu ficarei doente.

Eu posso comer milho e arroz e massa de arroz.

Caso necessário, por favor verifique com o chefe para ter a certeza de
que a minha comida não contém nenhum destes ingredientes e
ajude-me a pedir uma refeição que eu possa apreciar em segurança.

Muito obrigado.

Russian Gluten-Intolerance Dining Card

Я не говорю на вашем языке.

У меня заболевание, которое называется глютеновой болезнью
или непереносимостью глютена.

Я буду плохо себя чувствовать, если съем что-либо,
содержащее глютен, пшеничную, ржаную или овсяную муку,
ячмень, тритикале, солод и блюда из них, а также начинки и
соусы с
этими злаками, особенно блюда с макаронами, обвалянные в
муке или хлебных крошках или обсыпанные ими, содержащие
соевый соус или пиво.

Я могу кушать кукурузу, рис, рисовую лапшу.

Если нужно, пожалуйста, посоветуйтесь с шеф-поваром и
убедитесь, что предложенное мне меню не содержит этих
ингредиентов, и помогите мне заказать блюда, которыми я
смогу насладиться без опасений.

Большое спасибо.

Spanish Gluten-Intolerance Dining Card

Yo no hablo su idioma.

Tengo una enfermedad llamada enfermedad celíaca o intolerancia al gluten.

Si llego a comer cualquier alimento con gluten, trigo, centeno, cebada, triticale, malta de cebada, harina de avena y sus derivados, rellenos
o salsas hechas con estos granos, especialmente los platos con pasta, o que estén revestidos o espolvoreados con harina o pan rallado o con salsa de soja o de cerveza, me enfermaré.

Puedo comer maíz, arroz y fideos de arroz.

Si es necesario, consulte con el cocinero para asegurarse de que mi comida no contenga ninguno de estos ingredientes y me ayude a ordenar una comida que pueda disfrutar con seguridad.

Muchas gracias.

Swahili Gluten-Intolerance Dining Card

Mimi sizungumzi lugha yako.

Nina hali inaitwa celiac, ni ugonjwa wa kutovumilia gluten.

Nikila chakula chochote kilicho na gluten, kwa mfano ngano, shayiri, triticale, kimea, unga wa oat au michuzi iliyotengenezwa na nafaka hizi, pia vyakula kama pasta na vinginevyo vilivyopakwa unga wa nafaka hizi au mchuzi wa soya au bia, vitanidhuru na kuathiri afya yangu.

Ninaweza kula mahindi na wali na tambi za unga wa mchele.

Kama ni muhimu, tafadhali mjulishe mpishi ahakikishe chakula changu hakina mchanganyiko wa vitu hivi na nisaidie kuagiza mlo nitakaoufurahia na kula kwa usalama.

Asante sana.

Swedish Gluten-Intolerance Dining Card

Jag pratar inte svenska.

Jag lider av glutenallergi/celiaki.

Om jag äter mat med gluten, vete, råg, korn, triticale (en råg-vete-hybrid), malt, havremjöl, eller derivat, fyllnader eller såser tillagade med dessa spannmål, speciellt rätter med pasta eller doppade i eller täckta med mjöl eller brödsmulor, eller som innehåller sojasås eller öl, blir jag sjuk.

Jag kan äta majs, ris eller risnudlar.

Om du inte är säker, vänligen kontrollera med kocken att min mat inte innehåller spår av någon av dessa ingredienser och hjälp mig beställa mat jag kan äta med säkerhet.

Tack så mycket!

Thai Gluten-Intolerance Dining Card

ฉบับปรับปรุงใหม่ การ์ดแปลภาษาอังกฤษเป็นภาษาไทย

ฉันพูดภาษาของคุณไม่ได้
ฉันเป็นโรคแพ้กลูเตน (โปรตีนจากแป้งข้าวสาลี)
ฉันจะเกิดอาการป่วยถ้าฉันรับประทานอาหารที่ทำมาจากกลูเตน ข้าว
สาลี ข้าวไรย์ ข้าวบาร์ลี ข้าวทริทิเคลี มอลท์แป้งข้าวโอ๊ตรวมทั้งส่วน
ผสมอะไรก็ตามที่ทำมาจากธัญพืชเหล่านี้ (โดยเฉพาะอาหารเช่นเส้น
พาสต้า อาหารที่ชุปหรือโรยด้วยแป้งสาลีหรือเกล็ดขนมปัง หรืออาหาร
ที่ใช้ซอสถั่วเหลืองหรือเบียร์)
ฉันสามารถกินข้าวโพด ข้าว และเส้นก๋วยเตี๋ยวที่ทำมาจากข้าวได้
ถ้าไม่แน่ใจ กรุณาเช็คกับพ่อครัวว่าอาหารที่ฉันสั่งไปไม่มีเครื่องปรุงที่
มีกลูเตน ฉันจะได้สามารถทานอาหารจานนั้นได้อย่างปลอดภัย
ขอบคุณมาก

Vietnamese Gluten-Intolerance Dining Card

Tôi không nói ngôn ngư của bạn.

Tôi có một tình trạng gọi là bệnh / gluten celiac không khoan dung.

Nếu tôi ăn bất kỳ thực phẩm được thực hiện với gluten, lúa mì, lúa mạch đen, lúa

mạch, triticale, mạch nha, bột yến mạch và các dẫn xuất, chất độn hoặc nước sốt

làm từ các loại ngũ cốc, đặc biệt là những món ăn được chế với mì ống, hoặc tráng

hoặc rắc bột hoặc vụn bánh mì hoặc chứa nước tương hoặc bia, tôi sẽ bị bệnh.

Tôi có thể ăn ngô và lúa mì và gạo.

Nếu cần thiết, hãy kiểm tra với các đầu bếp để đảm bảo thực phẩm của tôi không

chứa bất kỳ của những thành phần này và giúp tôi đặt một bữa ăn tôi có thể thưởng

thức một cách an toàn.

Cám ơn rất nhiều.

15

Get Outta Here

Only those who will risk going too far
  can possibly find out how far one can go.
  —T. S. ELIOT

I know. You wish you could leave your diet in another time zone. It won't wait patiently at home while you take a little vacation, but there is absolutely no reason to let gluten ground you. Armed with the travel cards in Chapter 14, ample notice, some preparation, and a willingness to try new foods, and except for maybe some obvious danger zones, there's no place in the world that's off-limits to you. Some days will be glorious proof that eating and traveling well is the best revenge. You'll find that the world is more than your oyster; it's the whole gluten-free universe.

That said . . .

Somewhere, sometime, no matter how carefully you've planned, especially in exotic locations, you may find yourself miles away from a safe meal and struggling to make that chocolate bar or emergency bag of nuts and raisins last all day.

Look at it this way: travel is food for the soul. If you do find yourself in that rare situation, suck in your newly flat stomach and realize you may never get another chance to drink in the beauty of an Alpine lake, breathe the saffron-scented air of a bazaar, or see Kilimanjaro at sunrise. In the presence of such wonders, who can swallow anyway?

Flight Risk

First it was a fee for the first checked bag. Soon there was a fee for the second. Now there's a fee for *any* checked bag. Feeling a little chilly in the cabin, grab me that blanket, will you? Eight bucks please and, by the way, here's the bill for the jet fuel.

Rumor has it some airlines are eyeing that pint-sized, rolling carry-on of yours as the newest revenue source. Their rationale: shorter boarding times and fewer delays. What will they think of next, coin-operated toilets? Planning a trip requires making lots of decisions, but choosing between a purse and your underwear shouldn't be one of them.

The word is *monetize*. We are not passengers. We are human profit centers. Bad enough, but now you're gluten-free and you need your snacks.

Why pay extra for a bag stuffed with food you've already paid extra for? Not to mention worrying about whether or not it will end up in Chicago when you are on your way to Tucson. This is why I am a big fan of sending your suitcase to yourself care of the hotel, full of everything you need, including gluten-free items you may not be able to get where you're going. UPS or FedEx costs a bit more than you'll pay in baggage fees, but your bag is guaranteed to get there; it will not be rummaged through, dented, or otherwise manhandled; and you will not run the risk of theft.

Will your airline guarantee that?

On travel day, sail through the airport with a small bag of essentials (always keep your devices and meds with you), fruit, some nuts and raisins, and a gluten-free muffin or a Kind bar, and—once you're through Security—a couple of bottles of water. This not only comes in handy in the air, but it's a lifesaver for long delays on the runway. If you're traveling with children, remember to pack nonsugary, calming snacks. Flying is stressful enough (you did pack some books and games, didn't you?); you really don't want the kids wired up and melting down on a long flight.

Don't forget extra sanitizing hand wipes for sticky fingers; they will go a long way in keeping everyone clean and germ-free.

The Hungry Skies

As you know, airlines have pretty much dispensed with food on all domestic flights lasting four hours or more. Very little is free except juice, water, and a mini bag of pretzels or honey nuts. Everything else, even the most pallid fruit plate, comes at a price. In other words, you're on your own up in the air.

One bright spot is Delta Airlines, who has partnered with Udi's, the popular gluten-free baking company, to supply muffins, bagels, cookies, and/or whole-grain dinner rolls when a passenger requests a gluten-free meal with twenty-four hours' notice. Delta is also adding more gluten-free options in snacks that can be purchased in-flight. JetBlue, too, offers gluten-free complimentary snacks and its Shape Up box, which is available for purchase, includes a gluten-free cookie and crackers.

Things are a bit better on international flights to Europe, Asia, and South America with gluten-free meals available in all cabins with an average of 18-, 24-, 48-, and, in some cases, 72- or even 96-hour notice. Swiss International Air Lines is touting itself as "allergy-friendly" with lactose- and gluten-free food and drinks, zero peanuts, featherless pillows, and unscented soaps in the lavatories. Marketing ploy or big win for our side? Time will tell. On cross-country flights and flights to Hawaii, many airlines will do special meals in first and business class only, leaving the rest of us to fend for ourselves. There is a lot of small print about itineraries changing and food possibly not being available.

What's a gluten-free traveler to do?

+ Book your flight on the airline with the best special meal well in advance.
+ Alert the flight and gate attendants of your special request the minute you check in.
+ Understand you may get the wrong meal.
+ Be aware there's no way to know what you're going to get until it's served to you.
+ Be prepared for a gluten-free meal to be just the opposite.
+ Scrutinize your meal before you eat it.
+ Pack snacks in the event you get stuck with pie in the sky.

Eco Adventures and Exotic Destinations

If you are heading for Africa or the Brazilian rain forest or some other spot off the beaten path where even your dining cards are no help, it's worth the additional fee to pack a bag of gluten-free food. Be sure to ask your airline carrier about security regulations that may apply. To expedite customs on the other end, pack your food in their original packages. To be on the safe side, tuck in a letter from your doctor stating your medical need for these items. And pray.

Domestic Arrangements

If your destination is a major city, either in the United States or abroad, and you've remembered to book a room, rental apartment, cottage, villa, or even a houseboat with a small fridge, by all means send yourself an emergency package care of the hotel or tour manager or concierge. But don't overlook shops, bakeries, restaurants, and food stores in your destination city. It's so much more fun to shop with the locals for regional gluten-free items or those you can't get in the States.

Have a Flight Plan

Before you book your next trip, do your homework and learn each airline's rules for maximizing the odds of getting a safe and special meal. Most airlines will book a meal only after you've confirmed your flight. Always, always bring something safe to eat just in case.

Aer Lingus. www.aerlingus.com   Aerolineas. www.aerolineas.com
Aeroflot. www.aeroflot.com   Air Canada. www.aircanada.com

Ground Stop

There may be no lunch aloft, but gluten-free food in the terminal is giving new meaning to destination dining. Fresh Meadow Bakery & Café offers gluten-free options in Minneapolis–St. Paul, Atlanta, Milwaukee, and Salt Lake City. There's Udi's Café in Denver International, Café Patachou in Indianapolis, Petunia's Pie & Pastries in Portland, and GoPicnic boxes at news kiosks to take on board, not to mention chain restaurants like P.F. Chang's. For a sweet treat—Pinkberry and Red Mango.

Air France. www.airfrance.com

Air India. www.airindia.com

Air Jamaica. www.airjamaica.com

Air New Zealand.
  www.airnewzealand.com

Air Tahiti. www.airtahiti.com

Air Transat. www.airtransat.com

Alaska Airlines. www.alaskaair.com

Alitalia. www.alitalia.com

American Airlines. www.aa.com

Austrian Airlines. www.austrian.com

British Airways.
  www.britishairways.com

Cathay Pacific. www.cathaypacific.com

China Airlines. www.china-airlines.com

Delta. www.delta.com

Dragon Air. www.dragonair.com

El Al Israel Airlines. www.elal.com

Emirates. www.emirates.com

Fiji Airways. www.fijiairways.com

Finnair. www.finnair.com/us

Gulf Air. www.gulfair.com

Iberia Airlines. www.iberia.com

Japan Airlines. www.japanair.com

KLM. www.klm.com

Korean Air. www.koreanair.com

Lan Chile Airlines. www.lan.com

Lufthansa. www.lufthansa-usa.com

Luxair. www.luxair.com

Olympic Airlines. www.olympicair.com

Qantas. www.qantas.com

SAS. www.flysas.com

SATA. www.sata.pt

Singapore Airlines.
  www.singaporeairlines.com

South African Airways. www.flysaa.com

Swiss International Air Lines.
  www.swiss.com

Thai Airways. www.thaiairways.com

Turkish Airlines. www.turkishairlines.com

United Airlines. www.united.com

US Airways. www.usairways.com

Virgin America. www.virginamerica.com

Virgin Atlantic. www.virgin-atlantic.com

Security Issues

Whatever you do, don't wrap a loaf of gluten-free bread in tinfoil and stick it in your suitcase. By the time bomb-sniffing dogs stop drooling on it and the security people rush in, scaring you and everyone else, not to mention wasting everybody's time, you will have missed your flight. If it gets through unnoticed, you may well wonder who or what else is getting through. Either way, it's not good. We live in dangerous times. Gluten is not the worst thing to befall an American abroad.

+ The first stop in any travel itinerary should be the State Department—www.state.gov—for latest warnings and travel advisories for Americans around the world.
+ Check in with the Department of Homeland Security, www.dhs.gov.
+ Rules change constantly. For the latest in what is and what isn't allowed on a plane, go to the Transportation Security Administration Web site, www.tsa.gov.

- ✦ You've already got a sensitive gut and a reactive immune system. It's crucial to get proper vaccinations, get updates about current health alerts on outbreaks in various countries, and pack the appropriate antibiotics just in case—www.cdc.gov/travel/.
- ✦ If you are visiting family for the holiday, carry presents and wrapping paper separately. If the presents are wrapped ahead of time, airport screeners will open them.
- ✦ Keep your devices open and ready for scrutiny.
- ✦ Forget the Swiss Army knife that comes in so handy for fruit and cheese.
- ✦ You don't have to be gluten-free to know you should wear shoes that slip off easily for security checks and to avoid lots of jewelry and other metals. And that means underwire bras, too.
- ✦ In foreign countries, do try to fit in. If women wear skirts, wear one yourself. If men wear a coat and tie to dinner, you do the same. Never wear shorts or skimpy clothing to religious shrines, etc. This is no longer a courtesy. It is a safety precaution.
- ✦ Try not to be demanding when asking for special meals abroad. Many cultures find this offensive, especially the French. Say you are sorry to be a bother, and be grateful for the extra attention. They will fall into your arms.
- ✦ Remember that you are a gluten-free ambassador.

A Tale of Three Cities

PARIS

Paris is no longer the place that took pity on yours truly with my suitcase full of rice cakes, enough phrases to buy the fabulous pair of riding boots I prize today, and the ridiculous French dining card described in Chapter 14. It is no longer the city that taught my husband one of his most valuable lessons—*Never ogle a tart in front of your gluten-challenged wife*. Nor is it the one that was shocked to learn that I could not enjoy the buttery pleasure of a croissant or crusty baguette and consoled me with gorgeous wines and cheeses the likes of which I haven't tasted since.

What I remember most was tables being joined, lovely French voices rising and falling on soft spring air, a couple stopping to dance to music drifting down from an open window, glasses of wine all around, and the little card that made it all happen. It's in tatters now at the bottom of a chest full of mementos, a cherished reminder that a good life is something you invent as you go and that strangers are just friends you haven't met yet.

A new and enlightened Paris awaited me this time. It was one of those gorgeous dreary days where everything is washed in a shade of blue-gray that exists nowhere else in the world. As I made my way to Helmut New-cake, a tiny gluten-free café and patisserie on rue Bichat, I wasn't sure what I was expecting. Certainly not rows and rows of classic French gateaux and pastry—flaky, sublime, and unforgettable. Certainly not a gluten-free éclair that stunned me with its rich authenticity. The geniuses behind this extraordinary café-cum-patisserie, which has become the object of many a gluten-free pilgrimage, are Marie Tagliaferro, a pastry chef with celiac disease, and her husband, François. They have graciously given us the recipe for their transcendent Dark Chocolate Fondant with Ginger and Raspberry Coeur (page 188). I dream of what I'll order on the next trip.

Helmut Newcake
36, rue Bichat, Paris (75010)
www.helmutnewcake.com

In France, and especially in Paris, chefs like advance notice when they are doing something special for you. Remember, too, a little French goes a long way. You may be far from fluent, but making the effort is what counts. Here is the merest soupçon of pleasures awaiting you on the *sans gluten* tour:

Thank You My Deer
(lunch/baked goods)
112, rue Saint-Maur
www.thankyoumydeer.com

Noglu (100% gluten-free
restaurant)
16, passage des Panoramas
www.noglu.fr

Fée Nature (lunch with gluten-free and dairy-free options)
69, rue d'Argout
www.feenature.com

Soya (vegetarian restaurant with
vegan and gluten-free options)
20, rue de la Pierre-Levée

Le Potager du Marais (vegetarian
restaurant with gluten-free and
dairy-free options)
22, rue Rambuteau
www.lepotagerdumarais.fr

Macaroons or *macarons* are the national pastime. They are always gluten-free, but these have been decreed some of the best in Paris.

Ladurée
www.laduree.com

Pain de Sucre
14, rue de Rambuteau
www.patisseriepaindesucre.com

Gluten-free provisions in Paris:

L'Autre Boulange
Biocoop
Naturalia
La Vie Claire

Note: Be aware in some French markets, unwrapped gluten-free bread is shelved next to wheat bread and often made in the same kitchen.

In Burgundy:

Aux Biscuits d'Antoine (gluten-free bakery)
5, Petite Rue
Etivey, Burgundy
www.biscuits-antoine.com

In Cognac:

Le Chêne Vert Bed-and-Breakfast (gluten-free and vegetarian meals prepared on request)
34, rue des Abatis, Chez Primo,
Burie
www.lechenevert.eu.com

Learn More

Gluten-Free Community: L'Association Française Des Intolérants
    Au Gluten, www.afdiag.fr
The Gluten-Free Guide to France by Maria Ann Roglieri,
    www.gfguidefrance.com
Best Blog: *Gluten-Free Paris*—professional chef, baker, author of
    The Sweet Life in Paris (Broadway Books), former pastry chef at
    Chez Panisse, and expatriate David Lebovitz writes dispatches
    from Paris that are a joy to read, whether you are gluten-free or
    not. www.davidlebovitz.com

LONDON

The good news: Gluten sensitivity, or coeliac, as it is known in England, is as common an occurrence as the crowds hoping for a peek at Prince George. The not-so-good news: Where London was once doable on a reasonable budget, it has become one of the most expensive cities in the world for tourists.

Rather than pony up huge sums for a hotel room you won't be spending much time appreciating, you might consider renting a flat for a week or two and put the money into theater and museums, shopping, great restaurants, and that once-in-a-lifetime, could-anything-be-more-British, tea at Claridge's.

Despite the London cab's aura of romance and furled umbrellas, the Tube is the cheapest, most efficient, and most civilized way to get around this magnificent city. If you rent a car and drive down to the West Country or up north on narrow country lanes, know that behind many of those hedges are stone walls, and here and there remnants of Hadrian's ancient wall, which does not give when a lorry driver or one of the locals barrels toward you from the right.

The cider dispensed in rural pubs is not only alcoholic; it's lethal.

Where once requests for gluten-free options were met with a solid loaf of bread, a few crackers, and the occasional scone, there is a new appreciation for special diets, as the idea of healthy and conscious eating spreads around the globe. Even better, there is a focus on fresh, organic, farm-to-country cuisine and, always, the best Indian and Asian fusion in the world.

For stocking up the hotel mini fridge, weekly flat, or bedsit, as the English call a studio with a shared bath, Harrods, Selfridges, and Marks & Spencer have impressive but pricey gluten-free sections in their food halls, and Harrods offers gluten-free afternoon tea. Large food markets, most notably Sainsbury's, Tesco Stores, Ltd., and the flagship Whole Foods Market in the Barkers Building, Kensington High Street, as well as most supermarkets, have dedicated gluten-free and allergy-friendly sections marked FREE FROM.

With that worry aside, and after you've been thoroughly spooked by the ravens at The Tower, you're free to explore Queen Elizabeth Olympic Park, Southwark, and Lime Wharf, and take in the view from The Shard, Western Europe's tallest building. Get a hot ticket at The Shed, the National Theatre's experimental new annex, a pittance compared to most London theaters. Don't get me started on museums and art galleries.

All this activity will make you very hungry. Here are a few good tables.

Inn the Park
A beautiful restaurant in
St. James Park
Serves many gluten-free options
www.innthepark.com

Dishoom
Modern Indian, very cool vibe,
two London locations
Gluten-free menu
www.dishoom.com

Hakkasan
Stunning modern Chinese cuisine
Gluten-free menu, Michelin star,
very expensive
www.hakkasan.com

Claridges, Mayfair
Gluten-free version of the
quintessential English high tea
www.claridges.co.uk
Book at least three months ahead:
dining@claridges.co.uk

La Famiglia
Chelsea, London
Gluten-free Italian
www.lafamiglia.co.uk

The Truscott Arms
Maida Vale, North London
Gluten-free options, including
bottled beer
www.thetruscottarms.com

Manna
Primrose Hill, London
Vegetarian, vegan, gluten-free
www.mannav.com

Fast, casual, budget-friendlier, many London locations:

Pho
Vietnamese, mostly gluten-free
menu
www.phocafe.co.uk

Leon
Gluten-free, soy and other
allergens attended to
www.leonrestaurants.co.uk

Honest Burger
Good clean beef, gluten-free buns,
four London locations
www.honestburger.co.uk

Wahaca Southbank Experiment
Mexican with an extensive
gluten-free menu and view of the
Thames
Several London locations
www.wahaca.co.uk

Otto Pizza
Notting Hill
www.ottopizza.co.uk

Stingray Café
Thin crust gluten-free pizza
and pasta
www.stingraycafe.co.uk

Learn More

Accommodations: www.glutenfreehotelsguide.com
Apartment, country house, and cottage rentals. www.homeaway.com
Bed-and-breakfasts. www.airbnb.com/s/London
Best blog: Jane Cooban is originally from Leeds and lives the life of
    an urban millennial. Great information/fun/hip/a little cheeky.
    www.glutenfreefortea.wordpress.com
Gluten-free community: Coeliac UK. www.coeliac.co.uk
Glutenfree Roads—restaurants, shops, accommodations in UK and
    abroad. www.glutenfreeroads.com

ROME

How can Rome, city of pasta, be paradise for the gluten-free?

All Italians are tested for celiac disease as children. Those who test positive receive a monthly stipend from the government for gluten-free food, plus extra vacation time to shop for and prepare it. So says Maria Ann Roglieri, author of *The Gluten-Free Guide to Italy*, the must-have resource for tasting the pleasures of Rome as well as Venice, Milan, Florence, Sicily, Umbria, and the Italian coast. The Italian Celiac Association and makers of gluten-free products have done a marvelous job educating Italians, and they, in turn, will know how to make sure your meals are safe, gluten-free, and unforgettable.

Two little words: *senza glutine*. Say them and you will have hotels, restaurants, cafes, bakeries, and gelato shops eating out of your hand. When in Rome, you must have an evening stroll while eating gelato, which is always gluten-free, except for mix-ins. Below, an inkling of the many gluten-free pleasures of *cucina romana*:

Gelateria Fatamorgana
Via di Lago de Lesina, 911, and
four other locations
www.gelateriafatamorgana.it

Come Il Latte
Via Silvio Spaventa, 24–26
www.comeillatte.it

Gelateria del Teatro
Via di San Simone, 70, just off
Via dei Coronari
On a dead-end cobblestone
alleyway behind a staircase, this
gelateria is hard to find but worth it.

Il Viaggio
Classic Roman cuisine
Identical menus; one regular, one
senza glutine
www.ristoranteilviaggio.it

Ristorante Nini
In the Fenix Hotel, vegetarian
and gluten-free menus
www.fenixhotel.it

Sans de Blé
Cappuccino and gluten-free
pastries
www.sansdeble.it

Renovatio
Roman cuisine and thin crust
pizza, in the Piazza Risorgimento
www.ristoranterenovatio.it

La Scaletta
Calabrese and Roman dishes,
gluten-free menu
www.lascalettaroma.it

La Piazzetta di Roma
Gluten-free spaghetti carbonara
is a specialty
Piazza dei Visconti, 8

Mama! Eat
Pasta, panini, pizza, fritte,
and beer all *senza glutine*
www.mamaeat.com

Insomnia
Red and white pizzas, foccaccia,
crostini, bruschette, fritte
www.insomnia.roma.it

Learn More

For more restaurants *senza glutine*, www.celiachiaitalia.com/locali-senza-
glutine.html and www.ristosito.com/RistorantiSenzaGlutine.asp
Best blog: Elizabeth Minchilli, food writer, epicure, author of *Private
Tuscany, Italian Rustic*, and *Restoring a Home in Italy*, and lover of
all things Italian offers workshops and culinary tours of her favorite
city and has designed the essential culinary smartphone apps—Eat
Rome, Eat Florence, Eat Venice. www.elizabethminchilliinrome.com
The Gluten-Free Guide to Italy by Maria Ann Roglieri. www.gfguideitaly.com

Gluten-Free Community: Associazione Italiana Celiachia.
www.celiachia.it

International Gluten-Free Community

Why not touch base with the insiders in each country before you leave or, at the very least, the minute you arrive? Some sites can be read in English, some not. Click on the British flag or Tourist. This, combined with your dining cards and a thorough researching of the resources listed throughout this chapter, ought to do the trick.

Argentina—Asistencia al Celiaco de la Argentina, Buenos Aires.
www.acela.org.ar
Australia—Coeliac Australia. www.coeliac.org.au
Canada—Canadian Celiac Association. www.celiac.ca
Croatia—Hrvatsko Društvo za Celijakiju. www.celijakiju.hr
Czech Republic—Czech Celiac Society. www.celiak.cz
Denmark—Danish Coeliac Society. www.coeliaki.dk
Finland—Finnish Coeliac Society. www.keliakialiitto.fi
Germany—German Coeliac Society. www.dzg-online.de
India—Celiac Society for Delhi. www.celiacsocietyindia.com
Ireland—Coeliac Society of Ireland. www.coeliac.ie
Israel—The Israeli Celiac Association. www.celiac.org.il/en.htm
Netherlands—Nederlandse Coeliakie Vereniging. www.glutenvrij.nl
New Zealand—Coeliac New Zealand. www.coeliac.co.nz
Norway—Norsk Cøliakiforening. www.ncf.no
Quebec—Fondation Québecoise de la Maladie Coeliaque. www.fqmc.org
Russia—Saint Petersburg Celiac Society. www.celiac.spb.nu.
South Africa—Allergy Society of South Africa. www.allergysa.org
Spain—Federación de Asociaciones de Celíacos de España.
www.celiacos.org
Sweden—Svenska Celiakiforbündet. www.celiaki.se
Switzerland—Association Suisse Romande de la Coeliakie.
www.coeliakie.ch
Turkey—Living with Celiac Association. www.colyak.org.tr
Uruguay—Associación Celiaca del Uruguay. www.acelu.org

Gluten-Free Goes to Sea

Did you know that the word *posh* comes from the era of steamship travel? To avoid the blazing sun, well-heeled passengers crossing the Atlantic from Liverpool to New York paid dearly for cabins on the port side of the ship going out, on the starboard side going home—portside out; starboard home. Posh.

In the twenty-first century, cruising is a destination unto itself, with many ships, floating cities really, that can and sometimes do eclipse even the most exotic ports of call. Many of these behemoths have a bigger electrical grid than some countries. Some ships are small and offer an intimate experience in the company of like-minded travelers. Some cruises lead to land adventures, others provide leisurely shopping and touring, and still others offer ways to work off the buffet and get you shipshape. Some navigate or barge up and down the world's most majestic rivers, gorges, and glaciers. And one or two duplicate the experience of the great sailing ships.

Know this. Whether you are traveling first-class or on a deck lower down, no amount of money or connections will get you something to eat beyond what's on board when you set sail, especially on small ships with gourmet meals. Always provide plenty of notice of dietary needs when booking. It's always a good idea to remind the kitchen of your next day's meals the night before to avoid any snafu or miscommunication due to a change of shifts in the kitchen. And remember to stash lots of gluten-free goodies in your stateroom.

Pack the Dramamine and wash your hands frequently. Carry along an antibiotic, especially on the big ships, one that will do the job in case there's an outbreak of the Norwalk virus. Cruise ships are love boats for microbes, not great for the gluten-free gut.

Many cruise lines, whether large or small, have gluten-free menus and plenty of options. Companies like Gluten-Free on the Sea (www.gluten freeonthesea.com) and Gluten Free Cruises (GlutenFreeCruises.com) offer dedicated gluten-free cruises in groups or individually.

At this writing, Royal Caribbean International has launched a nutritional program across its fleet for guests with dietary restrictions, and Disney's family-friendly ships (along with its theme parks) are the gold standard for gluten-free traveling. Explore the following cruise companies and set out to sea.

Whatever Floats Your Boat

Pack the Dutch dining card and see Amsterdam from a canal houseboat. Shop for galley essentials in Dutch markets like Albert Heijn Grocery or at the gluten-free food-shops inside Amsterdam's central train station. Not fluent? Food packages are printed with pictures, clearly stating that the food is gluten or dairy-free. Book a table at Lieve Restaurant (www .restaurantlieve.nl), certified gluten-free by Holland's Celiac Association and friendly to nut-free and dairy-free travelers as well. Houseboat rentals: www.houseboathotel.nl

American Queen Steamboat Company. www.americanqueensteam
boatcompany.com

Atlantis All-Gay Cruises. www.atlantisevents.com

Bora Bora Cruises. www.islandsinthesun.com

Carnival Cruise Lines. www.carnival.com

Cunard Line. www.cunard.com

Crystal Cruises. www.crystalcruise.com

Disney Cruise Line. www.disneycruise.com

Holland America Line. www.hollandamerica.com

Norwegian Cruise Line. www.ncl.com

Olivia Lesbian Cruises and Resorts. www.olivia.com

Princess Cruises. www.princess.com

Royal Caribbean Cruises. www.royalcaribbean.com

Seabourn Cruise Line. www.seabourn.com

Silversea Cruises. www.silversea.com

Star Clippers tall sailing ships. www.starclippers.com

Swan Hellenic small-ship luxury cruising. www.swanhellenic.com

Windstar Cruises. www.windstarcruises.com

The All-American Road Trip

Oh, the joys of the open road.

There's nothing like driving through the Painted Desert or the Grand Tetons. Stopping for a big-city weekend along the way. Or getting lost in Brooklyn looking for that gluten-free kosher bakery you've heard about and finding a gluten-free pizza parlor instead. And gas prices aside, it's still the most economical way to travel.

It's always great to plan the itinerary around good gluten-free eating; there's plenty of it in America as well as things to do and see. If you don't want to be stuck with fast food, pack a cooler and refresh it with ice when you stop for the night. Or load up on shelf-stable gluten-free meals and snacks from Go Picnic, available at Target, Wegmans, and other stores.

Always remember to change drivers every two hundred miles and to pack an emergency kit. Don't forget to bring medical supplies and, if possible, book accommodations that include a kitchen, refrigerator, and/or microwave. After that you're on your own, free to roam the countryside, find a gluten-free restaurant or bakery, and picnic by a stream, knowing you've got a trunk full of gluten-free road food or reservations at a hot table and a radio that plays all your favorite traveling music. So what if the map flies out the window and the wind tangles your hair—the kids make you stop at an alligator farm. There is much to be said for the road less traveled.

If you're not the adventurous type, make sure you download the right apps for gluten-free-friendly roadside restaurants along the way. www.gopicnic.com

Big-City Eats

ATLANTA

Yeah! Burger—Gluten-free hot dog and hamburger buns, dedicated fryer for onion rings, French and sweet potato fries. www.yeahburger.com

Arepa Mia—Downtown and Sweet Auburn Curb Market. Lis Hernandez's tribute to traditional Venezuelan arepas, cornmeal patties split in half and stuffed with mouthwatering ingredients. Empanadas, grilled corncakes called cachapas, and Venezuelan-style eggs, everything gluten-free. Catering, too. Muy bueno! www.arepamiaatlanta.com

Wisteria—Fried chicken, collards, mac and cheese, Southern traditional with a gluten-free twist. www.wisteria-atlanta.com

BERKELEY

Chez Panisse—Alice Waters's culinary argument for exquisite farm-to-table simplicity. www.chezpanisse.com

BOSTON

Glutenus Minimus—Glorious baked goods, many of which are nut-free and dairy-free. Many vegan options. www.glutenusminimus.com

Violette Gluten-Free Bakery—Boasts a totally gluten-free facility and organic and locally sourced ingredients. www.violettegf.com

Joe's American Bar and Grill—Hip city casual with gluten-free bread, pizza, and pasta. www.joesamerican.com

Davio's—Gourmet gluten-free dining for special dinners with outposts in several cities. www.davios.com

BROOKFIELD, WISCONSIN

A Gluten Free Frenzy—Café, bakery, and gluten-free grocery store. www.aglutenfreefrenzy.com

CHICAGO

Frontera Grill—Haute Mexican and Chef Rick Bayless at his best. www.fronteragrill.com

Hub 51—Eclectic, modern fare, gluten-free menus and allergy friendly. www.hub51chicago.com

Feast—Gluten-free brunch. www.feastrestaurant.com

Da Luciano—Old-style Chicago Italian and the most extensive gluten-free menu and shop in the city. www.dalucianos.com

DALLAS

Tu Lu's Gluten-Free Bakery—Gluten-free cupcakes, cookies, muffins, panini, and more. www.tu-lusbakery.com

Fireside Pies—Artisanal gluten-free hearth oven pizza. It's been said this is the best in Dallas. www.firesidepies.com

Local Oven—Baguettes, pita, and rolls. www.localoven.com

Nick and Sam's Grill—Great gluten-free lunch and brunch menu. www.nsgrill.com

Asian Mint—Asian fusion with an emphasis on Thai. Gluten-free items marked on menu. www.asianmint.com

Unrefined Bakery—Great breads and baked goods. www.unrefinedbakery.com

DES MOINES, IOWA

Fong's Pizza—Asian fusion meets Italian via Polynesia. Kung Pao chicken, gluten-free and/or dairy-free pizza. www.fongspizza.com

The Club Car Restaurant and Lounge—CSA-approved gluten-free pizza, steaks, pastas, and seafood. www.clubcardining.com

Caché Bake Shoppe—Gluten-free baked sweets in a nondedicated bakery knowledgeable about safe procedures. www.cachebakeshoppe.com

LINCOLN, NEBRASKA

Venue Restaurant and Lounge—Classic menu clearly marked with gluten-free, vegetarian, low-sugar, and vegan, nut-free, and dairy-free options. www.yourvenue.net

Dish—Continental cuisine with a gluten-free option in each category. Dairy-free dishes as well. www.dishdowntown.com

Eazy Eatz—Dedicated gluten-free bakery and café near the University of Nebraska offering breads, as well as sweet treats. Diabetic-friendly whole-grain sandwiches. www.eazyeatzbakerydeli.com

Take Me Out to the Ball Park

Buy me some peanuts and Cracker Jack. And while you're at it, buy me a beer and hard cider and a hot dog and pizza and a steak and some ice cream. From Fenway Park to Dodger Stadium, the gluten-free options are *Outta Here!* You won't care if you ever come back.

LOS ANGELES

The Addiction Bistro—Everything on the menu is available in a gluten-free version. www.theaddictionbistro.com

E.V.O. Kitchen—Huge gluten-free menu, including pizza and five kinds of beer. www.evokitchen.com

Lucifers Pizza—Some say it's the best gluten-free pizza in L.A. www.luciferspizza.com

True Food Kitchen, Santa Monica—Imagine finding a menu designed for an anti-inflammatory diet with extensive gluten-free options like turkey lasagna and flourless chocolate cake drizzled with caramel. Only in L.A.? Dallas, Denver, Phoenix, Scottsdale, Newport Beach, and San Diego, too. www.truefoodkitchen.com

Veggie Grill—Every location has a menu to suit any allergy or intolerance. www.veggiegrill.com

MIAMI/FORT LAUDERDALE

Chart House, Fort Lauderdale and Miami—Fresh fish, gluten-free menu. www.chart-house.com

Fresh First, Fort Lauderdale—South Florida's first 100 percent gluten-, corn-, and peanut-free restaurant and juicery. Panini eggs Benedict, portobello burgers on house-made gluten-free bread, cookies, quinoa cupcakes, superfood smoothies. Organic, vegetarian, and vegan never tasted so good. Breakfast and lunch only. www.freshfirst.com

Rosa Mexicano, Miami—Mexican with separate gluten-free menu. www.rosamexicano.com

NEW YORK CITY

BabyCakes NYC—Erin McKenna launched her gluten-free, mostly vegan cupcake empire from this Lower East Side location. Shops in L.A. and Disney World. www.babycakesnyc.com

Del Posto—Joe and Lidia Bastianich and Mario Batali's Chelsea bastion of sublime Italian and artisanal chef-made gluten-free pasta. Two identical menus: one gluten-free, one not. Pricey and worth it for a special occasion. www.delposto.com

Nizza—This French and Italian restaurant in the theater district is one of the stars in the Gluten-Free Restaurant Awareness Program, and for good reason. www.nizzanyc.com

Pip's Place—Pastries, cakes, cupcakes and more. www.pipsplacenyc.com

Risotteria—This tiny Greenwich Village restaurant is where it all started:

gluten-free pizza, risotto, and the most amazing breadsticks on earth. No reservations, tables fill up fast. www.risotteria.com

Sacred Chow—Animal-free café with many gluten-free offerings. www.sacredchow.com

OMAHA, NEBRASKA

7M Grill—Winner of Omaha's Diner's Choice award, fusion menu with many gluten-free options. www.7mgrill.com

PHILADELPHIA

Barbuzzo—Date-worthy Mediterranean, gluten-free options galore. www.barbuzzo.com

Crêperie Beau Monde—My go-to place for a great meal. Mainly crepes, but glorious gluten-free options abound, including crepe fillings enfolded in omelets. Ask for the "Jax Special" here. www.creperie-beaumonde.com

Davio's—Have them make Gluten-Free Gnocchi with Wild Mushrooms, Garlic, and White Truffle Oil (page 172). www.davios.com

Giorgio on Pine—Authentic Italian trattoria. Gluten-free menu; BYOB. www.giorgioonpine.com

Lolita—This newly reopened, Mexican street food-inspired former BYOB has a slick new interior, liquor license, and pretty much a totally gluten-free menu. Lunch, dinner, and late-night menu until midnight. www.lolitaphilly.com

Pure Fare—Totally gluten-free; organic temple of clean, organic food serves breakfast, lunch, and a mean millet muffin. www.purefare.com

Taffets Bakery and Store—This Italian market and gluten-free bakery specializes in amazing bagels, focaccia, biscotti, baguettes, and teff and quinoa breads. Sweets, too. www.taffets.com

Talula's Garden—Exquisite artisanal farm-to-table, many gluten-free options, gluten-savvy staff. www.talulasgarden.com

SAN FRANCISCO

Daily Grill—Classic American food, kid-friendly, GFRAP-certified. www.dailygrill.com

E&O Asian Kitchen—Hip city Asian. www.eosanfrancisco.com

Mariposa Baking Company, Ferry Building—Uncommon gluten-free bakery. www.mariposabaking.com

Pica Pica Arepa Kitchen—Everything in this casual South American restaurant is gluten-free. www.picapicakitchen.com

The Slanted Door, Ferry Building—A fusion of Vietnamese, Thai, and American. www.slanteddoor.com

SEATTLE

Andaluca—Mediterranean cuisine; tapas and steaks; extensive gluten-free menu. www.andaluca.com

Blue Moon Burgers—Gluten-free buns, onion rings, secret gluten-free coating on the fries, dedicated gluten-free fryer. www.bluemoonburgers.com

Cafe Flora—Fresh gluten-free vegetarian. www.cafeflora.com

Flying Apron Bakery—Gluten-free vegan bread, cakes, sweets. www.flyingapron.com

VANCOUVER, BRITISH COLUMBIA

Panne Rizo—this award-winning bakery and café is a must for gluten-free visitors. Soups, sandwiches, pizzas, panini, cakes, breads, muffins, cookies, and pies made from scratch in a dedicated gluten-free kitchen. If Canada is not in the cards, they ship 2-day FedEx to the United States every Wednesday from Bellingham, Washington. www.pannerizo.com

WASHINGTON, DC

Founding Farmers, DC—Breakfast, brunch, desserts, ice cream. American sustainable farm-to-table. Gluten-free options. www.wearefoundingfarmers.com

The Happy Tart—Tarts, cakes, cupcakes, meringues, baguettes, pastries. Classic patisserie, totally gluten-free. www.happytartbakery.com

Hello Cupcake—They do one thing very well. A different flavor gluten-free cupcake every day. www.hellocupcakeonline.com

P.F. Chang's Bistro—The famous gluten-free lettuce wraps and many other gluten-free choices easy on the wallet. www.pfchangs.com

Oyamel Cocina Mexicana—Chef José Andrés's gloriously corn-based cuisine with an allergy-friendly menu. www.oyamel.com

Zaytinya—Another Andrés restaurant—Turkish, Greek, Lebanese; *mezze* or small plates with a gluten-free menu. www.zaytinya.com

Gourmet Meals on Wheels

Food trucks were once called roach motels and worse. They dispensed grinders, subs, heroes, or hoagies, depending on what part of the country you're from, not to mention *dirty waters*, those New York street hot dogs boiled in the same water for years. We steered clear. Now they are artisanal, organic, vegan, gluten-free, no overhead, chef-driven temples of cutting-edge food at sidewalk prices. It was tempting to list the gluten-free-friendliest, but virtually nomadic, they disappear faster than you can say "Gluten-free meatballs." Look for them on a city sidewalk near you, especially near parks, hospitals, and universities. Or go to FoodTruckDirectory.com.

A Cooks' Tour: Gluten-Free-Friendly Resorts, Ranches, and Bed-and-Breakfasts (with Recipes)

There's a reason why they call it the hospitality industry. Hoteliers, inn-keepers, and the hosts of bed-and-breakfasts who open their homes to you are just that: hospitable. Most will go the extra mile to see that you are well and safely fed, and hope you will return again and again.

Speaking of the extra mile, while staying at Garrick House, a rose-covered hotel high on the cliffs of St. Ives along England's North Sea, I fancied a lobster for dinner. Alas, there were none in the kitchen that night. The next afternoon, as I lay snoozing in a lawn chair, exhausted from hiking a windswept section of the coastal path, my husband nudged me awake and pointed to a large orange crustacean on the grass next to me. Our host had radioed his mates out on a fishing boat, ordered the creature, and drove down to meet them at the pier. And here was a lobster big enough for two dinners and lunch the next day. And what a lunch it was—chilled lobster dressed with a bit of mayonnaise and herbs from the garden. His smile, my delight, and the deluge of requests from other guests, made for a happy situation for everybody.

There may not be a lobster on the lawn, but with a little luck, you will discover freshly baked bread, pastries, and peach and blueberry muffins, indeed entire menus reconfigured just for you.

Harbor no reservations about traveling. Ask and you shall receive. Here are a few ideas to get you started, some with recipes from their generous chefs/owners.

BLACKBERRY FARM, WALLAND, TENNESSEE

In 1939, Mrs. Florida Lasier of Chicago snagged her silk stockings on a wild blackberry bramble while exploring the idyllic Smoky Mountain foothills, and the name Blackberry Farm was born. Once a family farm, this five-star, swoon-worthy, 4200-acre resort run by the Beall family and presided over by executive chef and James Beard Award–winner Joseph Lenn, is luxury at its most satisfying and unobtrusive. The cellars are legendary, the service seamless, and no detail is overlooked. Vegetarian, vegan, and gluten-free menus are available by advance request. Cameron Beall, or Teensy, made her mark on gluten-free baking when she was homeschooled and apprenticed herself in the kitchen to learn how to bake with southern grains. The result is a line of Blackberry Farm gluten-free mixes.

The mountains are too cold to cultivate sugarcane, so the mountain folk press and simmer sorghum for their version of molasses. These waffles are made with corn, buckwheat, rice flour, and oat flour, so much lighter than those made with wheat. If this is breakfast, sign me up.

BLACKBERRY FARM'S TRULY SOUTHERN WAFFLES WITH SORGHUM AND MOONSHINE CHERRIES

MAKES ABOUT 12 WAFFLES

1. Preheat the waffle iron.
2. In a large bowl, whisk together the oat flour, brown rice flour, corn flour, buckwheat flour, baking powder, baking soda, and salt. Set aside.
3. In a medium bowl, place the egg yolks. Add the buttermilk, butter, and sorghum and whisk to combine.
4. Place the egg whites in the center of the dry mixture. Pour in the egg yolk mixture and mix only until combined.
5. Gently fold the egg whites into the batter. Pour a spoonful of batter into the center of the waffle iron and cook until golden brown. (If the first 1 or 2 waffles are softer than you'd like, use less batter and cook a little longer, until nicely browned, for a crisper result.)
6. Place a waffle on a warm plate. Top with a spoonful of Moonshine Cherries and drizzle with sorghum. Serve warm.

1 cup gluten-free oat flour
⅓ cup brown rice flour
⅓ cup corn flour
⅓ cup buckwheat flour
2 teaspoons baking powder
½ teaspoon baking soda
1 teaspoon kosher salt
2 large eggs, separated, at room temperature
2½ cups buttermilk, at room temperature
10 tablespoons unsalted butter, melted and cooled
¼ cup sorghum, maple syrup, or honey, plus sorghum or maple syrup, for serving
Moonshine Cherries (see recipe below), for serving

Moonshine Cherries

If you are out of moonshine (un-aged corn whiskey), the regular kind will do. The large portion of fruit to liquor in this recipe is to the benefit of both, creating pleasantly boozy cherries and tempering the moonshine's sharp bite.

MAKES ABOUT 4 CUPS CHERRIES

1. Clean and thoroughly dry a 1-quart mason jar with a tight-fitting lid.
2. Place the cherries in the jar and pour in the moonshine. Close the jar and let stand in a cool, dark place (such as a liquor cabinet) for at least 24 hours or up to 1 month.

1 pound cherries, stemmed and pitted
About 1⅔ cups moonshine

CANYON RANCH, TUCSON, ARIZONA—LENOX, MASSACHUSETTS—MIAMI, FLORIDA

This world-class spa has much to recommend it, including mountain hiking, tennis, cycling, meditation, yoga, Pilates, and just about every beauty and spa service imaginable. Gluten-free guests will discover a knowledgeable resident nutritionist and a personal dietary needs hotline. Buckwheat bread, pizza, flat bread, and chocolate chip cookies are served in all locations, as well as many gluten-free meal choices. For serious music lovers, the Lenox Canyon Ranch in the Berkshires is a horn's toot away from Tanglewood's summer music festival. Look for gluten-free specials and getaway packages. www.canyonranch.com

THE HOME RANCH, CLARK, COLORADO

Tucked among the aspens and spruce along the Elk River just outside Steamboat Springs lies the ultimate dude ranch, a real live version of a disappeared way of life, complete with squinty-eyed wranglers. Legend has it that Butch Cassidy and the Sundance Kid spent nine winters in this little town. A down-home vibe manages to strike a balance with all-out luxury, and Chef Clyde Nelson has mastered the art of catering to the gluten-free diet, along with any other allergy or preference you care to bring along. Horses, hayrides, trail rides, hiking, or just reading on the porch. Massage after fly-fishing? Not a problem here. Closed October–early December. www.homeranch.com

MAINE STAY INN, KENNEBUNKPORT, MAINE

This magnificent Italianate house on the National Register of Historic Places was built circa 1860 for sea captain Melville Walker and has been home to senators and railroad barons. At the center of Kennebunkport's historical district, near beaches, whale watching, and hiking trails, this gluten-free-friendly retreat is the perfect romantic getaway or family vacation. With a week's notice, the innkeepers will prepare unforgettable gluten-free breakfasts and teas, ensure that the kitchen is free of any cross-contamination, and stock gluten-free snacks, breads, and foods to take to local restaurants. www.mainestay.com

THE INN AT ORMSBY HILL, MANCHESTER, VERMONT

This is where Ethan Allen hid during the Revolutionary War. No wonder. Who would want to fight the British and leave a charming bed-and-breakfast like this? Gluten-free and other special diets are happily accommodated to make sure everyone is cheerful and fortified for snowboarding, skiing, golf, or the Orvis Fly-Fishing School nearby. www.ormsbyhill.com

SWIFT HOUSE INN, MIDDLEBURY, VERMONT

Built in 1815 by Samuel Swift, this historic inn had been a private residence until 1982, when it was transformed into the four-star inn and restaurant that it is today. Near Middlebury College, world-class ski areas like Mad River, Sugarbush, and Killington, and the famous writers' colony, Bread Loaf, and with a kitchen that caters to restrictions like gluten and other common allergens, this is the perfect base for literary, college, and ski weekends. www.swifthouseinn.com

HILTON HEAD HEALTH, HILTON HEAD, SOUTH CAROLINA

This spa and 800-acre resort in gated Shipyard Plantation is serious about wellness, weight loss, exercise, and, even more important, about understanding the emotions that drive unhealthy habits. This is where guests renegotiate their relationships with food and learn that just because it's gluten-dairy-casein-nut-egg-or-sugar-free doesn't mean it's good for you. For those with celiac disease, gluten intolerance, or gluten sensitivity, there is a special meal plan with many fiber-rich and high-protein choices baked on the premises. Special care is taken to eliminate cross-contamination in the kitchen. Cooking classes, lectures, state-of-the-art fitness, world-class tennis center, twenty-seven-hole golf course, nature preserve, gorgeous barrier beaches, lagoons, and yes, alligators. Every sort of special need met. Lives get changed here. www.hhhealth.com

---

HILTON HEAD HEALTH GLUTEN-FREE BLUEBERRY PANCAKES

These wonderful and very light spa pancakes from Chef Jen Welker are gluten-free, nut-free, and soy-free. Each ¼ cup of batter contains a surprisingly satisfying 60 calories, 1.5 grams fat, 11 grams carbohydrate, 1 gram fiber, 1 gram protein, and only 75 mg sodium. The recipe can be halved, if you like.

½ cup gluten-free oats
½ cup water
3 tablespoons (packed) light
  brown sugar
2 tablespoons canola oil
1 cup rice flour
1½ teaspoons baking powder
¼ teaspoon baking soda
¼ teaspoon salt
¼ teaspoon ground cinnamon
¼ teaspoon ground nutmeg
¼ teaspoon ground cloves
½ cup skim milk
¼ cup yogurt, plain, fat-free
1 large egg, beaten
Cooking spray, for the pan
1½ pints fresh blueberries

MAKES 24 PANCAKES

1. In a microwave-safe bowl, combine the oats and water. Microwave on high until the oats are creamy, about 2 minutes.
2. To the oats, add the brown sugar and canola oil. Set aside.
3. In a separate bowl, combine the rice flour, baking powder, baking soda, salt, cinnamon, nutmeg, and cloves. Whisk to blend. Add the milk, yogurt, oats, and egg and mix until just moistened.

4. Spray a nonstick frying pan with cooking spray and place over medium heat.
5. Spoon ¼ cup pancake batter and top with 1½ tablespoons blueberries.
6. Cook until bubbles have surfaced and the edges are lightly browned. Flip and cook the other side, 2 to 3 minutes more.
7. Repeat with remaining batter. Top each pancake with extra blueberries.

TREETOPS SUITE, MALDEN, MASSACHUSETTS

This very private and spacious furnished duplex apartment in a fabulous architect-designed residence is, literally, in the treetops. Fifteen minutes away from Boston, and with its own entrance, an exercise room, bath with skylight, two bedrooms, and a porch overlooking a lush garden, it can easily accommodate two couples or a family and is perfect for long stays and hibernations. While not licensed to serve food, you will find a dedicated kitchen stocked with all the best gluten-free items, including gluten-free bagels, breads, and cereal, fresh fruit from a local natural foods store, and a gift of popovers from the owner's kitchen. Candace Julyan and her architect husband, David Hancock, have seen to everything. www.treetopsboston.com

R. R. THOMPSON HOUSE BED-AND-BREAKFAST, CARLTON, OREGON

To stay at this historic house-cum–romantic Willamette Valley bed-and-breakfast in the heart of Oregon's spectacular wine country is to be surrounded by breathtaking natural beauty amid world-class wineries and tasting rooms. Innkeepers Roselyn and Mike have personal experience with the gluten-free diet and with notice are happy to accommodate (even go well beyond expectations) any dietary restriction. www.rrthompsonhouse.com

RANCHO MAGDALENA, MAGDALENA, NEW MEXICO

In a quiet corner of New Mexico, this 1,000-acre ranch is home to horses, longhorn cattle, goats, dogs, and one high-strung rooster. Offering hunting, hiking, flying lessons, and riding, this is the ultimate sportsperson's experience. The innkeepers treat guests like family and, with a little notice, will produce gluten-free miracles while you visit local artists in their studios. www.ranchomagdalena.com

INN ON RANDOLPH, NAPA, CALIFORNIA

This is not your grandmother's bed-and-breakfast. With its spa room, tasting room, private gardens, whirlpool, heated floors, romantic fireplaces, and couples massage, this stunning, newly renovated inn is soft-spoken luxury at its best. Its gluten-free kitchen is a destination unto itself. Host Karen Lynch, gluten-free herself, has thought of everything, including gluten-free crackers for the day's wine tasting, breakfasts worthy of the inn's rave reviews, and reservations for Pica Pica and C Casa, two totally gluten-free restaurants a short walk away. The Inn offers gourmet gluten-free cooking and baking classes and retreats with Jeffrey Larsen, food stylist and gluten-free baking master. This place is wedding and honeymoon material. Nobody leaves without the granola and guests can't seem to get enough of it, Karen has graciously shared her recipe with us. www.innonrandolph.com

---

INN ON RANDOLPH GLUTEN-FREE GRANOLA

MAKES APPROXIMATELY 5 CUPS

1. In a large bowl, mix the oats, cereal, almonds, hazelnuts, pecans, pumpkin seeds, flaxseeds, cranberries, apricots, cherries, coconut, and orange zest, reserving 1 teaspoon of the orange zest for the liquid mixture. Set aside.

2. Preheat oven to 350°F.

3. In a large saucepan, stir the molasses, maple syrup, canola oil, brown sugar, vanilla, cinnamon, nutmeg, orange juice, and the remaining orange zest until well blended.

4. Place the saucepan over medium heat. Bring the mixture to a slow and even boil, stirring constantly.

5. Continuing to stir, pour the syrup ingredients over the dry ingredients and mix well.

6. Turn the mixture onto a rimmed baking sheet. Bake for about 45 minutes, turning every 10 minutes or until it is light brown in color and smells fragrant. The granola should be moist and somewhat chewy.

7. Let cool and store in an airtight container. Do not refrigerate. Will keep for 7–10 days.

Dry Ingredients:

3½ cups gluten-free oats
1½ cups gluten-free cereal
½ cup almonds, chopped
½ cup hazelnuts, chopped
½ cup pecans, chopped
¼ cup pumpkin seeds
¼ cup sunflower seeds
⅛ cup flaxseeds
½ cup dried cranberries
½ cup dried apricots, chopped
½ cup cherries, chopped
¾ cup shredded coconut
Zest of 2 oranges, approximately 1 teaspoon reserved for mixing with the wet ingredients

Syrup Ingredients:

⅓ cup gluten free molasses
⅓ cup maple syrup
¼ cup canola or other flavorless oil
½ cup (packed) light brown sugar
1 teaspoon vanilla extract
2 teaspoons ground cinnamon
1 teaspoon ground nutmeg
¼ teaspoon freshly squeezed orange juice
1 teaspoon orange zest, reserved from Dry Ingredients

LOCUST GROVE RANCH BED-AND-BREAKFAST, MOUNT VERNON, OHIO

This lovely, gluten-free-friendly ranch in the heart of Amish country will not only see to it that you eat safely and well, it will board your horse for the night. www.locustgroveranch.com

THE ARTIST'S INN AND GALLERY, TERRE HILL, PENNSYLVANIA

Nestled among Amish farms in Lancaster County, Pennsylvania, this is the place to hear the clip-clop of a bygone way of life. Whether you go for the antiques in nearby Adamstown, admire the local handmade quilts, or browse the innkeeper's lovely drawings, you will find this romantic inn charming, intimate, and completely accommodating of your gluten-free needs. www.artistinn.com

IRON MOUNTAIN INN, BUTLER, TENNESSEE

Deep in the Smoky Mountains and tucked away in a remote corner of northeast Tennessee, this is the perfect casual gluten-free getaway. The inn is rustic and the surrounding countryside serene. There are hiking trails of varying difficulties, including the challenging Damascus, Virginia, to Hampton, Tennessee, leg of the Appalachian Trail nearby. Other sports include golf and fly-fishing, swimming in Watauga Lake, or just rocking on the porch and drinking in the sweeping views. Let them know you're gluten-free and they'll do the rest. www.ironmountaininn.com

TWO BARS SEVEN RANCH, TIE SIDING, WYOMING

This 7,000-acre ranch near Laramie knows how to take care of guests with gluten intolerance and dairy allergies and can accommodate soy-free, sugar-free, and corn-free diets. Near a small town called Tie Siding, there is horseback riding, fishing, hiking, and dining in the great outdoors. (307) 742-6072, www.twobarssevenranch.com

CHICKEN PARADISE, SAN ANTONIO, TEXAS

Yes, there are chickens at Chicken Paradise. Fancy, award-winning chickens. You'll remember more than the Alamo on Anne and Joe Barfield's twenties-era Texas ranch with its spectacular and very private single guest suite, farm-to-table cuisine, and the biggest little ole pool in the county. The host, a long-standing celiac and gluten-free whiz, caters not only to the gluten-free diet but to vegan, vegetarian, low-fat, low-carb, casein-free, diabetic, and dairy-free restrictions as well. And she will steer you to all the gluten-free-friendly restaurants in the area. Deep in the heart of Texas's most historic sights and near San Antonio's River Walk, this is down-home hospitality meets big-city excitement. Expect to be served farm-fresh eggs, herbs and vegetables from the garden, and Joe's Chicken Paradise French Toast Bananas Foster (recipe follows). Chicken Paradise is listed in the Gluten Intolerance Groups Restaurant Awareness Program. www.chickenparadise.com

JOE'S CHICKEN PARADISE FRENCH TOAST BANANAS FOSTER

SERVES 4

1. Heat an oiled griddle to 325°F over medium low.
2. In a medium-size bowl, whisk together the eggs, cinnamon, vanilla, salt, and honey until well mixed. Add the coconut milk.
3. In a large bowl, soak the bread in the egg mixture, turning occasionally and pricking the bread with a fork, allowing the bread to absorb as much liquid as possible. Spoon any remaining egg mixture onto the bread and flip again.
4. Grill the bread slices on each side, being careful not to scorch it. Spoon any remaining egg mixture onto the bread and flip again. Reserve in a warm oven.
5. In a cast-iron skillet, melt the butter over low heat. Add the brown sugar. Allow the brown sugar to partially dissolve in the butter, and then add the maple syrup.
6. Using a flat whisk, whisk the butter mixture and add the cinnamon. Cook over medium-low heat for 3 minutes, until well blended.
7. Add the bananas. When they begin to brown, add the pecans. Remove the skillet from the heat and carefully add the rum. With a stick flame, using the utmost care, ignite the rum and wait for the flames to die down.
8. Place the warm French toast on plates and top with the syrup.

Butter or dairy-free Earth Balance for greasing the griddle
5 large eggs
½ teaspoon ground cinnamon
1 teaspoon vanilla extract
Pinch of salt
2 to 3 tablespoons honey, maple, or agave syrup
½ can coconut milk or 1 cup regular milk
4 thick slices gluten-free bread

Syrup:
3 tablespoons unsalted butter
¼ cup (packed) light brown sugar
¼ cup maple syrup
¼ teaspoon ground cinnamon
2 bananas, cut in half lengthwise, then halved again
2 tablespoons pecans, toasted lightly
2 tablespoons dark rum

CALA LUNA RESORT, TAMARINDO, COSTA RICA

This exotic paradise will bend over backward to accommodate a gluten-free diet. All you have to do is contact the chef and work together to create a menu and you will have an idyllic yoga retreat, or the first or second honeymoon of a lifetime. www.calaluna.com

RANCHO LA PUERTA, TECATE, MEXICO

This has been my go-to place to reinvigorate, relax, and recover from life's challenges. I've seen it go from nuts and sprouts to all-out luxury, but it has always stayed true to the vision of its founders—natural whole foods, tranquility, and plenty of exercise. The food here is mainly vegetarian, natural, and unprocessed and comes from the spa's legendary organic gardens. The kitchen caters to allergies, with gluten-free, soy-free, and dairy-free options at breakfast, lunch, and dinner. There are cooking classes and demonstrations, too, along with a dizzying array of spa services and exercise classes. With a simple request, a gluten-free backpack will be ready to accompany you on the unforgettable, all-day hike up Mount Kuchumaa, one of Mexico's holiest places. If you're lucky, you may catch a glimpse of wild horses. www.rancholapuerta.com

ROASTED CHILI POLENTA WITH SHIITAKE TOMATILLO SAUCE

1 onion, diced
1 rib celery, diced
1 red bell pepper, diced
½ teaspoon olive oil, plus more to coat the ovenproof casserole
3 cloves garlic, minced
1 teaspoon ground cumin
¼ teaspoon red pepper flakes
2 cups fresh corn kernels
¼ cup polenta
2 cups carrots, shredded
2 tablespoons fresh oregano, chopped
1 cup gluten-free nonfat yogurt
10 ounces (2½ cups) Parmesan cheese, grated
10 ounces (2½ cups) Monterey Jack cheese, grated
Pinch of freshly ground black pepper
Low-sodium gluten-free soy sauce to taste
6 large egg whites, lightly beaten
2 cups gluten-free vegetable stock
Anaheim or Ortego chilies, washed, roasted, peeled, and seeded

One reason I returned to the ranch year after year was Bill Wavrin, author of the award-winning *Rancho La Puerta Spa Cookbook*. He packed my backpack with gluten-free hiking essentials, made sure I had my quinoa porridge every morning, and served this authentic Mexican polenta, which, for all its silkiness and heat, manages to be low-fat. The secret is fresh Anaheim or Ortego chilies and roasting the peppers over an open flame to give them their smoky flavor.

SERVES 8 TO 10

1. Preheat the oven to 375°F.
2. In a sauté pan over medium heat, sauté the onion, celery, and bell pepper in the olive oil until the onion is golden, about 6–8 minutes. Add the garlic, cumin, and red pepper flakes and cook an additional 2 to 3 minutes.
2. Place mixture in a large mixing bowl, add l cup corn, the polenta, carrots, oregano, yogurt, the cheeses, black pepper, soy sauce to taste and egg whites and set aside.
3. In the bowl of a blender, place the stock or water and the 1 cup of the remaining corn and purée until smooth. Add to the onion mixture. Blend well. Adjust the seasoning to taste with soy sauce.
4. Coat an ovenproof casserole with olive oil. Layer the chilies on the bottom of the pan and pour the mixture carefully into the casserole, smoothing with a spoon to even out the top.

5. Cover with foil and bake for about 1 hour and 15 minutes, until cheese is bubbly and vegetables are cooked through. Allow casserole to rest 15 minutes before serving. Top each serving with Shiitake Tomatillo Sauce.

Shiitake Tomatillo Sauce

1. In a saucepan over medium heat, sauté the onion and leek in olive oil until the onions are very brown, about 8–10 minutes, taking care not to burn. Add the mushrooms, one-half of the garlic, and the oregano and sauté 5 minutes more, or until the mushrooms are soft. Set aside in a mixing bowl.

2. In a separate saucepan, combine the tomatillos, stock, and remaining garlic. Simmer over medium heat for 15 minutes. Strain the tomatillos from the stock, reserving the stock.

3. Place the tomatillos in the bowl of a blender. Add the bell peppers and a little stock and blend to purée (take special care when blending because the tomatillos are hot). Mix with the onion-mushroom mixture. Adjust the seasoning.

4. In a saucepan, add the sauce and bring to a simmer over medium heat for 1 to 2 minutes. Serve hot over the roasted chili polenta.

¼ teaspoon olive oil
1 onion, julienned
1 leek, white section only, julienned
2 shiitake mushrooms, stems removed, julienned
4 cloves garlic, minced
2 tablespoons fresh oregano, stemmed and chopped
2 tomatillos, husked (if not available, substitute green tomatoes)
2 cups gluten-free vegetable or chicken broth, plus more to blend the tomatillos
2 red bell peppers, stemmed, seeded, and roasted
Salt and freshly ground black pepper to taste

TURTLE ISLAND RESORT, FIJI

Candlelit dinners on the beach, sailing, snorkeling, dancing the night away, and yes, turtles. This eco-friendly resort will serve you just about anything with a little notice, including gluten-free meals. This South Pacific paradise is the place for an unforgettable honeymoon. www.turtlefiji.com

CEDAR HOUSE BED-AND-BREAKFAST, GISBORNE, NEW ZEALAND

Once the starchy St. Winifred's private school for girls, this gabled Edwardian mansion was originally built in 1909. Steps away from spectacular Pacific beaches, wilderness trekking, and exploring Maori culture, with a little notice (who just pops down to New Zealand?) they'll be glad to serve you a fortifying gluten-free breakfast before you set off on a tour of this magical and rugged countryside. FYI, Gisborne is the first city in the world to see the sun each day. www.cedarhouse.co.nz

BRIDGE VIEW FARMHOUSE BED-AND-BREAKFAST,
KILBRITTAIN PARISH, WEST CORK, IRELAND

There are many reasons to visit Bridge View Farmhouse with its breath-taking views of Courtmacsherry Bay on the Atlantic coast of Ireland. The beaches are spectacular, the fly-fishing excellent, not to mention hiking trails, castles, golf, and gardens, and, of course, the bridge. But it may just be innkeeper Marion Moloney's amazing gluten-free scones and break-fast pancakes that make this lovely farmhouse the emerald in the Emerald Isle. www.bridgeviewfarmhouse.com

BEACHES: SANDALS RESORTS

This popular family and couples resort company tells us that with a bit of advance notice, they will accommodate many special diets, including gluten-free, at all their properties, so you can get on with golf, snorkeling, family excursions, and romantic walks on the beach. www.sandals.com

The Grand-to-Somewhat-Grand Tour

Sometimes we just want to let someone else worry about dinner reservations, hotel accommodations, language barriers, kitchen contamination, and all the obstacles that can occur away from home.

If you like organized vacations, the following companies are pros at marshaling kitchen staff, inspecting cooking conditions, ordering entrées, and sending them back if necessary. You may even get to sing *A hundred bottles of gluten-free beer on the wall* as you tour Tuscany, Paris, and the wine country.

As with any travel tour, ask about cancellation policies, taxes, insurance, and other fees, travel partners and connections, accommodations, and, depending on where you are going, security precautions.

Bob and Ruth's Gluten-Free Dining and Travel Club.
www.bobandruths.com

Gluten-Free Globetrotter—Blog about gluten-free travel planning/
upcoming tours. www.glutenfreeglobetrotter.com

Lotus Tours. www.lotustours.com

Untours European Vacation Packages—Everything but the tour bus
and those corny dinners with locals. Packages include apartments,
cottages, villas, and savvy go-to hosts in each location who will
arrange anything, including gluten-free shopping and restaurants.
www.untours.com

Culinary Getaways

Talk about a cook's tour.

Cooking is a big deal nowadays, especially among chefs who want to get in on the gluten-free restaurant revolution. The rest of us simply need some skills. What better way to tune up the repertoire and celebrate a healthy new life than mastering the joys of the gluten-free kitchen. Think of it as a vacation with edible homework.

The Culinary Institute of America
Hyde Park, New York; Napa, California; New York City
Noncredit classes in gluten-free, vegan, and vegetarian cooking and baking taught by professional chefs.
www.ciachef.edu

Le Cordon Bleu
Sixteen American cities and, of course, Paris
Special courses in gluten-free cooking
www.chefs.edu

Leith's School of Food and Wine, London
Gluten-free baking classes
www.leiths.com

The Chopping Block, Chicago
www.thechoppingblock.net

Cook, Philadelphia
Cooking and baking classes with visiting chefs specializing in gluten-free cuisine
www.audreyclaire.com

Bob's Red Mill Cooking School, Milwaukie, Oregon
Gluten-free baking classes with Carol Fenster
www.bobsredmill.com/cooking-classes

Leslie Cerier Cooking Classes, Amherst, Massachusetts
Gluten-free with the organic gourmet. Leslie teams up with Melinda Dennis, RD, nutrition coordinator for Boston's Celiac Center at Beth Israel Deaconess for wellness weekends of great food and nutrition at fabulous places like Canyon Ranch in Lenox, Massachusetts, and Omega in Rhinebeck, New York.
www.lesliecerier.com
www.deletethewheat.com

The Cooking School at Jungle Jim's, Cincinnati, Ohio
Courses in gluten-free and special diets
www.junglejims.com/cookingschool

Gluten Free School
Online cooking courses
www.glutenfreeschool.com

Learn More

It would take a lifetime of traveling to visit all the wonderful places here, but no matter how exhaustive these listings are, every day more and restaurants, hotels, resorts, cruises, bakeries, tours, and so on, are seeing the value in offering gluten-free choices to their customers.

COOKBOOKS

The Foothills Cuisine of Blackberry Farm: Recipes and Wisdom from Our Artisans, Chefs, and Smoky Mountain Ancestors, by Sam Beall and Marah Stets (Clarkson Potter)

To get the latest dispatches from parts unknown:

www.glutenfreeroads.com—Find restaurants, shops, and accommodations close to home and everywhere in the world.

www.glutenfreetravelsite.com—Peruse restaurant menus and find bakeries, stores, hotels, resorts, and cruises. App for iPhone and Android smartphones.

www.spafinder.com—This site offers worldwide wellness, spa, fitness vacations, and luxury accommodations.

www.allergyeats.com—This app includes a peer-reviewed database of US restaurants.

www.gluten.net—Search for restaurants certified by the stringent standards of the Gluten Intolerance Group's Gluten-Free Restaurant Awareness Program.

www.canieathere.com—Restaurant finder and recipes.

www.allergictraveler.net—Because it isn't always gluten that can ground us.

www.mymagicjourneys.com—Disney's guide to family-friendly vacations.

Part IV

Can We Talk?

Emotional, Social,
and Family Issues

16

Your Cheating Heart

You always hurt the one you love.
—THE MILLS BROTHERS

- ◆ Recognizing the Triggers
- ◆ Beating Denial at Its Own Game
- ◆ Saving Yourself from Yourself
- ◆ Weighty Issues
- ◆ Gluten Accidents and Other Tough Situations
- ◆ Avoiding Unwelcome Questions
- ◆ Drinks with the Gang
- ◆ Communion
- ◆ Going to College
- ◆ The Disability Decision
- ◆ Dating
- ◆ The Holiday Family Dinner
- ◆ Enablers, Worry Warts, and Other Oddballs
- ◆ Let's Play Emotional Football
- ◆ When Worry Turns to Control
- ◆ Saboteurs

Some of us, myself included, suffer mightily when we eat gluten.

When we cheat, we consign ourselves to long stays in the bathroom, extreme fatigue, hives, vomiting, stomach pain, esophageal distress, a pervasive feeling of malaise. And we are the lucky ones.

The unlucky ones have no reaction at all. With no way to measure the harm, injury may be silent and cumulative. We have no idea until the damage is done.

So why would anyone in his or her right mind want to cheat?

It's not because we're dumb, or dense, or more self-destructive than the next person. We are sad. We are in shock. We want our old lives back. We feel isolated and sorry for ourselves. We're not good with change. Our social lives revolve around food. We resent the lack of spontaneity the diet imposes. We want to be normal, whatever that is. Breaking up with bread is hard to do.

It's hard to accept that this diet is for life, no free passes, no exceptions.

What about those of you who have tested negative for celiac disease and fall somewhere on the sensitivity spectrum? Gluten doesn't make you sick, but you do feel better not eating it. This was your choice. What's the harm in eating a slice of pizza today and going back to being gluten-free tomorrow? You're not really sick, right? The reason is simple. If you feel better not eating gluten, there's a good reason for it. If you are negative for celiac disease today, you may not be tomorrow.

A small percentage of you suffer from something called refractory celiac disease. You just don't get better, no matter how careful you are, and you get so sick at the slightest whiff of gluten, the idea of deliberately eating gluten is anathema. My heart goes out to you.

Cheating is never a good idea, no matter what your reason for avoiding gluten. Food, however, is not a practical issue. It is the most primal instinct we have. It warms us in places that need warming, emotional places, old places, places that have nothing to do with what's on our plates. When we feel the loss of foods we associate with childhood—which represent comfort, family, spontaneity, fun, and socializing—we lose our equilibrium. We push back.

Crazy as it may seem, we stash cookies in kitchen drawers, order a cheeseburger, roll and all. Those who worry about us are confounded and wonder why there are crumbs on the front seat of our car, chocolate chips in our purse. We shave the sides of a lemon pound cake, telling ourselves that the thinner the slice, the safer the serving.

Denial is a powerful river that must run its course. Until such time, here are some strategies for defusing the urge to self-sabotage.

Recognize the Triggers

- Flying through time zones. Rules get suspended in the air and on vacation.
- Passing a bakery and getting a whiff of buttery sweetness
- Going to the mall (especially when hungry)
- Watching a child eat an ice cream cone
- Cold or flu coming on. You want the chicken noodle soup your mother gave you when you were sick.
- Family gatherings, especially Thanksgiving
- The holidays in general
- Dating and its kissing cousin, Falling in Love
- Breakups and other relationship problems
- Conflict of any kind
- Loneliness
- Sadness
- Change—even the good kind
- Natural and man-made disasters. *The world is ending anyway. Why would I worry about gluten?*
- Dieting
- Quitting smoking
- Drinking
- Weddings and other big parties
- Peer pressure
- Overwork
- Not enough exercise
- Too much sugar
- Not enough sleep
- Stress at home
- Stress at work
- Stress, stress, stress

How to Beat Denial at Its Own Game

Review the above list of triggers, make note of those that ring true for you, and add some of your own. As the Boy Scouts like to say, "Be prepared."

+ If passing a bakery (pizza parlor, soft-pretzel vendor, burger joint) triggers the urge to cheat, change your route.
+ Never allow yourself to get truly hungry. Hunger will trump common sense every time and make fast work of willpower.
+ Eat frequent, small meals. Fullness is your friend.
+ Get a good night's sleep. Fatigue is *not* your friend.
+ Get plenty of exercise. You want those endorphins kicking in.
+ Make sure you are getting the kind of protein that stays with you for several hours.
+ Avoid sugary foods and fruits that raise insulin levels and leave you ravenous an hour later.
+ If you drink, avoid alcohol for the time being.
+ Always have a healthy snack on hand for sudden urges.
+ Reward yourself when you've successfully resisted.
+ Get rid of every no-no in the house. Donate to a food bank.
+ Stock your workplace and office fridge with shelf-stable snacks, peanut butter, and microwavable lunches from home.
+ Busy yourself with sports, hobbies, and community work. Volunteer at a women's shelter. There's nothing like real need to help you with your own.
+ Take up needlepoint, knitting, squash, or juggling.
+ Meditate for a few minutes each morning.
+ Become a picky eater. Assess food choices, not just for their gluten-freeness but for the freshness of their ingredients, lack of processing, chemicals, fillers, calorie-fiber-protein-fat content. Choose only the most fortifying.
+ Make a list of foods you would never stoop to eat.
+ Consider GMOs, trans fats, diet sodas, high-fructose corn syrup, partially hydrogenated oils, excessive sodium, empty white flour (gluten-free flour can be just as empty as your old stuff)—any food you can't find in nature. This will disqualify many temptations.
+ If you can afford it, hire a gluten-free chef or catering service until you're over the hump.

✦ If you can't, look for like-minded souls for meal sharing.
✦ Review Chapter 3, "Necessary Losses," and make friends with your feelings.

Place the Blame Where It Belongs

Don't you love it when someone says, "You made me forget my appointment"? Well, actually, it was *your* appointment and *you* forgot it. We teach our children to be responsible for their mistakes and not to blame others. Why can't we do the same?

It's so much easier to say the chef put that Gruyère crouton in your onion soup, when, in fact, you *knew* it was there and ate it anyway. Or to blame the waiter who didn't tell you there were bread crumbs on the chili rellenos. You know perfectly well you saw them and made a choice.

Just to be clear—I am *not* talking about cross-contamination or getting inadvertent gluten. But even here it's better to use the first person rather than to blame: *I'll be more careful next time, I'll not go to that restaurant again, I'll try to explain my diet a bit better.*

Owning the consequences is half the battle.

Save Yourself from Yourself

LEARN TO COOK

I'm not talking about a fancy course at Cordon Bleu. I'm saying get some skills. The more you know about food, the less reliant you will be on the boxed, bagged, packaged, or otherwise processed varieties. The more comfortable you are in the kitchen, the more likely you are to eat fresh, healthy, and naturally gluten-free foods. Review Chapter 6, "Essential Skills."

ELIMINATE AVENUES OF SELF-DECEPTION

Tell someone you trust about your diet.

Even if you lie to yourself, you won't be able to lie to them. Know that you may get mad at those who try to intervene. Apologize ahead of time. Ask that they stick to their guns even if you get snarky and that you will love them for it. If you are in a big social group, tell someone at your table that you're gluten-free. How could you possibly cheat after that?

DO SOMETHING FOR SOMEONE ELSE

There is nothing like an act of kindness and generosity to forget about our own challenges. Volunteer to deliver Meals On Wheels to the ill or housebound. Contact gluten-free food companies on behalf of a food bank, church, or a community organization for donations of healthy and nutritionally dense gluten-free food for those who can't afford it.

LEARN THE DIFFERENCE BETWEEN PHYSICAL AND EMOTIONAL HUNGER

There's an old saying in diet circles: *It's not what you're eating; it's what's eating you.*

Emotional hunger creeps up on you while you are watching television, in the middle of an argument, during a moment of sadness and loss. It takes advantage of you when you have too much work and too little time; when you have the flu, a broken foot, tennis elbow, a dented fender; or whenever you feel most sorry for yourself. It arrives with your new car agreement, the mortgage application, the promotion, the pink slip, and the divorce papers. It explodes in a sudden desire to eat everything in sight because it doesn't come from the belly but from wherever we keep our pain.

The following chart may help you sort out some of the land mines that drive us to cheat, and to, literally, eat our emotions. When a truck hits you, get the license plate and a good description of the driver.

Emotional Issue → Expressed as →	Physical Hunger
My life is empty	I can't stop eating
I can't have anything	I'll have this cookie
I'm so angry I could kill somebody	I need to crunch pretzels
There is no one to comfort me	I must have macaroni and cheese
I want to hurt you	Let me hurt myself instead
You don't care about me	I'll eat this cake; *then* you'll worry
You're always trying to control me	I'll show *you*
I'm sick and alone	Grilled cheese and tomato soup
Nobody loves me	So what if I eat a bagel?
Why me?	Why not?

Keep a Food Journal

I know. You're way too busy. But the results may surprise you. Patterns will emerge. A particular time of day may reveal itself to be more fraught with temptation than another. Issues that seem to have nothing to do with food may suddenly come into focus. Certain foods are associated with good behavior while others ratchet up the urge to cheat. A big protein day, for example, may leave you satisfied and virtuous, while an afternoon of sweet snacks may make you ache for gluten. You may discover that eating with certain friends or family members causes some discomfort.

Buy a notebook and keep track for two or three weeks. I know it sounds corny, but use the Daily Cheat Sheet on the next page. If Dr. Sanjay Gupta can keep a food journal—he did it, not for reasons of gluten, but to get into the best shape he could at a milestone birthday—so can you. Be specific. If you ate standing up, say so. How you feel is as important as what you eat on any given day.

Let's Review

Not only does a food journal prevent you from underestimating or even forgetting that which you don't want to remember; with careful observation you may be able to match the food craving with the emotional cue that prompts it. It's different for everyone, but the list below may strike a familiar chord. Make sure you have the gluten-free equivalents on hand for those cravings that ring true.

Pretzels, chips, bread sticks = Anger
Pasta, noodles = Sadness
Cocktail mix, trail mix = Denial
Ice cream, anything frozen = Pain
Muffins, toast, cereal = Romantic love
Gravy, stuffing, sandwiches = Mother love
Anything with butter fat = Unrequited love
Bite-size cookies, nuts, M&M's, or other miniature foods = Anxiety

Weighty Issues

There are two kinds of gluten-free people: those who lose weight on the diet and those who gain it.

DAILY CHEAT SHEET   Date _____

	Foods Eaten	Time Eaten	Where Eaten	With Whom	In Response to Physical Hunger? (Rate level from 1 to 10)	In Response to Emotional Hunger? (Rate level from 1 to 10)	Symptoms
Breakfast							
Midmorning Snack							
Lunch							
Afternoon Snack							
Dinner							
Miscellaneous Food Consumed (List of all picking, nibbling, noshing, vendor food. Remember, eating over the sink, cleaning plates, and finishing the kids' sandwiches count!)							

_____ I did not cheat at all today.   _____ I cheated a little today.   _____ Gluten disaster.

_____ I resolve to forgive myself the weaknesses of today and to start again tomorrow, committed to my health, determined to end my self-destructive behavior, and to be as resourceful in finding gluten-free foods I will enjoy as I am in finding the foods I sneak.

_____ Not perfect, but better than before. I will try harder tomorrow.

_____ Congratulations! Keep up the great gluten-free work.

Comments:

Why is that? The ones who lose weight usually see gluten-free eating as a change from a not-so-healthy diet to a healthy one. Along with the banishment of gluten, there is renewed focus on low-fat, whole-grain, protein-fiber-vitamin-rich meals with fewer sweets and the occasional gluten-free treat.

Those who gain weight most likely miss the empty breads and sweets and starches no longer allowed and have substituted equally empty gluten-free breads and sweets and starches. The emphasis is on making dishes over rather than revamping everything. Many, but not all, gluten-free products are good for us. Some contain compensatory amounts of sugar, fat, and even higher calories than the original food. No wonder the pounds pile on.

To further complicate the weight issue, gluten itself may cause some to gain, causing the double whammy of going gluten-free while trying to shed the excess poundage.

Those with severe gluten intolerance are often malnourished when they start living gluten-free. Their bodies haven't been absorbing properly for a long time. After such a diagnosis, the emphasis is on rebuilding health, strength, and muscle, which means resuming a normal body weight, which in turn means eating pretty much anything you want for a while. But now every calorie and fat gram is getting in.

How do you know how much you can eat before you begin to put on weight? You have no idea. Some people are able to find a healthy balance on the scale and others just keep gaining. Why? If you see the gluten-free diet as an opportunity to eat healthier, more nutrient-dense foods, chances are you'll slim down. If you see it as substituting one packaged product for another, chances are you won't.

Dieting is never easy. Doing it while learning to be gluten-free and susceptible to cheating is a double whammy.

+ Forget the fast fix. Take your time. You're learning to eat for the rest of your life.
+ Eat simply for a while: whole grains, vegetables, fruits, small amounts of meat and cheese.
+ Avoid liquid diets and shakes. They are full of chemicals and can lead to serious metabolic imbalances. The minute you resume solid food, the weight comes back.
+ Be suspicious of diet programs that require you to buy food at franchised centers. Most do not offer gluten-free options and these companies rely on recidivism. When you are ready to go it alone, you'll have no clue as to what to eat except prepackaged food.

✦ Join Weight Watchers. This is a pretty good gluten-free option. You eat real food and stay within a point range to reach your goal. (Points may have to be adjusted upward for some gluten-free foods.) While it's true that packaged products are pitched at weekly meetings, the plan is not dependent on them. There's nothing like a weekly public weighing to keep you honest.

✦ Book an appointment with a registered dietician to help you design a healthy and balanced diet you can happily live on.

✦ Eat close to nature, and those foods that are naturally gluten-free. Eat a Mediterranean diet.

✦ Avoid the quick fix and go for something you can enjoy and live on.

✦ Have a good checkup for vitamins and minerals, and supplement if necessary.

The Difference Between Pain and Suffering

Pain, even the most extreme physical and emotional pain, waxes and wanes. It changes from moment to moment. It feels dense and unmovable, but it isn't.

Consider the cliché *Roll with the punches.* We use this common expression but don't often think about what it means. When we stiffen up and try to keep from getting hurt, it hurts more. When we keep our feelings at arm's length, our arms are stiff; we are not flexible.

This is what suffering is. It is the brick wall that keeps our feelings from their natural course. Shinzen Young, an American Buddhist monk, Vipassana meditation teacher, and mathematician, puts it this way:

Pain x Resistance = Suffering

As a culture, we have dedicated ourselves to the notion that psychic pain is preventable. An entire pharmaceutical industry has sprung up around the misguided belief that we can deflect, defer, postpone, or even wipe out difficult sensations altogether. Loss, loneliness, a sense of isolation, sadness, or grief—any number of uncomfortable emotions can arise with a serious change in the way we have to eat. Instead of sitting with the uncomfortable feelings that lead to craving, we push hard against them.

No wonder we suffer.

The next time you experience the urge to cheat, resist the impulse to push it away.

Let your feelings happen instead.

Breathe.

Offer no resistance.

I'm guessing that when you fully experience the emotion, no matter how painful, it will dissipate on its own and take with it the craving.

Forgive Yourself and Move On

If you do have a lapse, accept that you are human and fallible and cut yourself a break. Give yourself a hug, acknowledge how hard this gluten-free thing really is, and start over. Success is getting up one more time than you fall down.

Fear of Frying, Gluten Accidents, and Other Tough Situations

Murphy's law is immutable. If anything can go wrong, it will.

Life, love, business, family tradition, sibling rivalry, spiritual belief, and organized eating buffet us. We fall prey to irrational fears. Life's milestones, such as going to college, falling in love, and getting married, are especially difficult. It's all about equilibrium, perspective, emotional honesty, knowing where the pitfalls are, and, always, moving forward with a healthy sense of humor.

GUSTAPHOBIA

This is the fear of eating in other people's homes and/or restaurants. Those who were severely sick before going gluten-free are particularly prone to this problem. In its advanced stages, the sufferer becomes reclusive and unable to engage in the most innocent breakfast, lunch, or dinner without sneaking into friends' pantries to read labels. Paranoia becomes a way of life.

It's human nature to get a little nervous about gluten in the early stages of the diet, especially if you have celiac disease, but when it becomes a way of life, it can be disabling, not to mention socially isolating.

The Cure for Gustaphobia

- ✦ Watch a pro eat. Include another gluten-tolerant in the party plans and bask in their confidence.
- ✦ Ask pals for their recipes. Study the labels on the products they use. Watch as they prepare your food.

- Be honest. Tell people you're picking at your dinner because you're just getting the hang of eating again.
- Learn how to cook gluten-free yourself. There's nothing like developing skills to allay anxiety.
- Go out with a gluten-free friend and learn how ordering a good and safe meal is done.
- Study the menu together and learn where the pitfalls and pleasures are. If your buddy is on friendly terms with the chef, ask for an introduction. A tutorial never tasted so good.
- Shopping with a partner helps a lot, too. Along the way, discuss the fears that crop up—How can you trust the label? What if the product has been cross-contaminated? Is the staff lying to me?
- If you don't know anyone, ask the manager of your local organic market for a gluten-free tour.
- Get on the gluten-free grapevine (see Chapter 23, "Community") and ask to be introduced to an experienced gluten-free shopping buddy in your area. Shadow this person for a while.
- Conversely, there is such a thing as too much community. Take a vacation from the blogosphere and chat sites. For every person who posts a reasonable answer to your question, there are ten vitriolic and otherwise dumb responses. The Web can be confusing and, often, mean-spirited.
- If you're still afraid to leave the house, wondering if the breeze can spread hot dog bun particulate matter from your neighbor's barbecue, it may be time to talk to a professional. Seriously. No shame in it.
- Pay it forward. When your own training wheels come off, offer to partner with a newbie.

We're all afraid of something. Truth is a two-way street. After cooking heart-healthy salmon steaks for your best friend, she may tell you she's terrified of fish bones.

Avoiding Unwelcome Questions

Sooner or later, someone will ask you why you're not eating. There is nothing wrong with saying you're gluten-free, given so many people are these days. But sometimes we don't want to be spokespeople for the entire gluten-free community or subject our plumbing issues to the spotlight. We'd rather not defend the diet to naysayers or discuss personal health issues with gossipy industry colleagues or coworkers. And we especially don't want some kind-hearted person flagging down a waiter or scurrying into the kitchen to try to help. Social networking aside, sometimes we just want some privacy.

True story.

When I was first diagnosed with celiac disease, I attended an advertising award ceremony during which clever little microphone-shaped ravioli were served. The person next to me asked why I wasn't eating mine. I said, "I guess you didn't see the *60 Minutes* story on ravioli. It's a miracle we're all still alive."

You'll never see these people again. Have some fun with it.

Some Unconventional Answers to the Age-Old Question: Why Aren't You Eating?

+ I have a bet with my husband-sister-best friend-boss that I can lose the most weight in one week, which ends tomorrow.
+ This isn't a chicken; it's a Hazardous Materials site.
+ My hypothalamus is on the fritz.
+ Have you seen the kitchen?
+ Say you're politically opposed to mass feeding; then go to the restroom when the fight breaks out.
+ "How could anyone swallow after that speech?" is always nice. Just make sure the speaker's spouse is not sitting at your table.

GLUTEN ACCIDENTS

Sounds like a toxic spill, doesn't it? It is in a way. But is getting *glutenized* as serious as some say?

Doctors disagree. Most say if it's an isolated incident, you may not feel so hot, but a dose of accidental gluten won't cause lasting damage. If you are exquisitely sensitive, however, getting an inadvertent crouton or crumb may cause an immediate and nasty reaction such as cramping, dizziness, vomiting, or a painful mouth ulcer.

You are the lucky ones, in my opinion—lucky because you *know* when you've gotten gluten. You can trace what you've eaten and track down the problem, thereby preventing another accidental glutening.

An accident is just that—something temporary, a teachable moment.

The first time it happened to me, common sense told me I needed to move the stuff out of my gastrointestinal tract as quickly as possible. My solution was to drink gallons of water and take a ton of fiber, which is exactly what my doctor would have said to do if I'd asked him. He also

Oops

Before I had the hang of the diet and knew better, I decided it would be healthy for me to add brewer's yeast to my morning tonic. At first I felt fine. Then I noticed, to put it as gracefully as possible, that bathroom visits were increasing while the rest of me was decreasing at a fairly steady rate. It wasn't long before I realized that my morning drink was the culprit. I tell you this not to be indelicate but to illustrate how easy it is to miss the obvious. There is no shame in not knowing.

would have said to do nothing and wait for nature to take its course. Still, I like to think I got better sooner because I took action. As it happens, I am not alone in my need to be proactive.

Here's what other gluten-free citizens have posted as their go-to solutions:

Unsanctioned Home Remedies for a Gluten Accident

+ Psyllium husks or some other fiber will do the trick.
+ Some say charcoal "sucks the gluten right out of the intestines."
+ Pepto-Bismol
+ L-glutamine
+ Papaya
+ Pineapple
+ Digestive enzymes/probiotics
+ Bananas
+ Avoidance of rich foods (light foods to rest the stomach)
+ Avoidance of light foods (logic here is heavy moves gluten out of the system faster)
+ Wine for cramping
+ Tons of water
+ Extra B$_{12}$
+ Acidophilus
+ Ginger
+ Soothing teas like chamomile or mint
+ Extra calcium, magnesium, and zinc

Note: Never make the situation worse, that is, if you have diarrhea, don't take laxatives.

Best Practice

Have your doctor do periodic screenings. If you *are* getting gluten, whether unwittingly or not, it will show up on the test. If it doesn't show up, you can rest easy knowing that while a rare accident may cause a reaction, it won't cause irreparable harm.

Before you rush out and buy supplements, teas, fruit, and wine, you should know that there is absolutely no proof that any of these remedies work better than doing nothing and waiting for the gluten to leave your system naturally. Understand that this isn't just about getting symptoms for a brief period of time; it's about being afraid they won't go away. The urge to self-treat is often about regaining control. That's not necessarily a bad thing.

Drinks with the Gang

I have been a nonsmoker for so long, I can't remember when I quit. Despite the fact that smoking was considered sophisticated, even attractive, I knew I ought to cut it out. After a few days of going cold turkey, and before the smoking ban in public places, I accepted an invitation from a friend who owned a very popular bar.

I was never one for hard liquor, but I do enjoy a glass of wine. Knowing how obnoxious an ex-smoker can be, I sipped a nice cabernet and tried not to mention the fog around me. By the second glass, I was attempting to swallow the smoke rings floating by, and by the third, I was mooching cigarettes from everybody around me. I quickly learned that alcohol weakens resolve and is not a friend to someone trying to kick a lifelong habit. I did not have another sip of wine until I was well over cigarettes. I avoided it again when I had to give up gluten.

Bars and restaurants may forbid smoking, but there's no rule about the bowls of pretzel nuggets, nuts, pigs in blankets, nachos, and those little pizza things set out for happy hour. Of course, you can go out with the gang and belly up to the bar. Just do some planning first.

Best Drinking Strategies Bar None

+ Don't drink until you've got your diet under control. Order iced tea, soda, or fizzy water.
+ If you do have something alcoholic, forget mixed drinks. You really don't want to have to climb over the bar to read a label.
+ Friends don't let friends eat gluten. If you find yourself with a little buzz, designate a pal to pull you away from the pretzels.
+ Even better, put it in writing—this person has your permission to prevent you from eating gluten.
+ Carry a snack-size bag of something nice and salty for when the munchies hit. Ask the bartender for a clean bowl. Put it in front of you. Nosh away.
+ If you're really hungry, order something safe from the appetizer menu and have it served to you at the bar.
+ Wrap it up quickly. Talk to everyone you can, especially the one who organized the evening, then do a fast fade.
+ If clients are present who will report back to your boss, make sure they see you, *then* skedaddle.

✦ Follow the above strategy for company events. Talk to everyone at cocktails, especially VIPs and clients. Disappear as soon as everyone goes in to dinner.

✦ Volunteer to make the arrangements for the next get-together. Pick a place that has gluten-free pizza and safe snacks.

Communion

One of my earliest gluten accidents took place in a Catholic church.

While attending Mass at the National Shrine of St. John Neumann in Philadelphia with my husband and parents, both of whom were ill and needed a bit of saintly intercession, I went up to the rail, received the wafer in my hand, lowered my head, and walked away. Right or wrong, my plan was to give it to one of my parents who sat to my right.

A voice boomed at my back. "Consume the host!"

I froze in my tracks and popped the wafer straight into my mouth. Sheepish, I told my shocked family, "I thought it was God."

Weren't we in the spiritual presence of a saint who was credited for more than one miracle? I figured anything could happen. But you know from reading the previous section on gluten accidents what I did when I got home.

Being gluten-free and taking the Eucharist is relatively easy in many Protestant churches. Anglican, United Methodist, Baptist, Christian Reform, Lutheran, Presbyterian, Episcopal, and other denominations will accommodate the special diets of its parishioners. Ask and you shall receive.

However, for many Catholics, especially for those with celiac disease, participating in the central mystery of the Mass can be a troubling issue. You may find yourself in conflict with Church authority as you find your way. What matters most is your faith, how you feel about your participation in the ritual, and your personal relationship with your priest.

How to Safely Receive Communion

✦ Sit down with your priest or minister and decide together what to do.
✦ If you are comfortable taking wine and skipping the bread, do so.
✦ Always ask if you can take the first sip to avoid crumbs in the chalice.
✦ If you would prefer a more traditional host, ask if you can supply a gluten-free wafer for consecration.

✦ If there are enough gluten-free members of your church community and the ritual includes the breaking of leavened bread, ask that it be made by a local gluten-free baker and prepared for Communion.

✦ If your congregation is large, post a note on the church bulletin board and you may find yourself with more company than you imagine.

✦ Order gluten-free hosts and ask the priest to keep them for you in the appropriate receptacle.

✦ If you and your doctor agree that you may eat the low-gluten host sanctioned by the Roman Catholic Church and allowed by canon law, ask that these be ordered for you.

✦ Find a Catholic priest who will bend the rules and consecrate the gluten-free host quietly and out of public view. Ask that he put it in a pyx, a small container usually used for transporting a consecrated host to the ill and housebound, and give it to you at Mass.

✦ Decide what's best for you. If you choose not to partake, don't let anybody make you feel guilty. Heaven knows this is a matter between you and the Boss.

Learn More

Benedictine Sisters of Perpetual Adoration—Catholic Church–sanctioned altar breads. www.benedictinesisters.org

Celebrate Communion—Gluten-free communion wafers in crushproof containers. www.celebratecommunion.com

Communion wafers for Protestant denominations. www.cph.org/p-4137 -gluten-free-communion-wafers-1-12-pack-of-50.aspy

Gluten-Free Hosts—zero-gluten hosts and gluten-free hosts for Catholics under 20 parts per million. www.glutenfreehosts.com

F. C. Ziegler Company—Shop online for sanctioned receptacles and other religious articles. www.zieglers.com

Going to College

Finding, then getting into, the right college is stressful enough. Add being on your own for the first time, making new friends, and the fact that gluten-free accommodations aren't very high on the list of reasons for choosing a school, and the transition can be difficult.

In college we are totally responsible for our meals. It's easy to sleep through breakfast and fall prey to late-night junk food, binge eating, and constant grazing on high-calorie, high-fat foods. No wonder most students pile on the dreaded *freshman fifteen*. It can also be challenging to eat gluten-free in college dining halls.

Things are getting better. One reason is the explosion of awareness of the gluten-free diet and the fact that many young people are not only gluten-free but have multiple food allergies. Another is a 2012 settlement between the Department of Justice and a Massachusetts university over a student's right to receive safe, gluten-free options in the dining hall, giving teeth to the Americans with Disabilities Act with regard to medically necessary diets. This could be a wake-up call for all colleges and universities. Down the road, it could put restaurants on notice as well.

Still Visiting Schools?

+ Visit each school's residential and/or dining hall Web page to see how special diets are dealt with.
+ Get in touch with the head of student dining services and ask about gluten-free options. Request a sit-down when you visit the school.
+ Have lunch in the dining halls when you're on campus and grade them.
+ Search sites for student-written reviews of the schools you are considering. You may find that the kitchen has been certified by one of the national gluten-free organizations.
+ Check out student groups and ask about eating gluten-free on campus.
+ Address the issue of dining hall fees and negotiating them downward if your needs cannot be accommodated to your satisfaction.
+ Ask if you will be allowed to bring your own mini fridge and microwave or if you will be required to rent one from the school. Check on rules for toasters and hot plates and see if accommodations can be made.
+ Check in with a local support group for gluten-free shopping and cheap eats near the campus.
+ As soon as you decide and have been assigned a roommate, get in touch and take a reading on his or her attitude toward sharing with a gluten-free student. It could be a match made in heaven. If not, ask for a reassignment before it's too late.

Already on Campus?

+ Keep a stash of nonperishable gluten-free staples you don't have to cook, such as cereal energy bars, crackers, peanut butter, and snacks, the more the merrier. A student's metabolism burns hot.
+ If you have a small refrigerator in your room, stock the freezer with ready-to-eat meals, as many as you can cram in.
+ Don't forget food trucks. Many of the best gluten-free trucks around are found on campuses around the country. Buy extra and freeze.
+ You can never have enough bananas or any other fresh fruit. Buy reusable plastic produce protector bags and keep the brown spots at bay.
+ Keep a gluten-free beer or two on hand for BYOB parties. Yes, I know you have to be twenty-one. No exceptions unless you want an unpleasant visit from your RA.
+ Ditto for wine or other gluten-free spirits. This will keep you from accidentally drinking frat-house punch laced with who knows what and waking up in the rosebushes.

The Disability Decision

If you have celiac disease and a letter from your doctor proving it, you can register with the Students with Disabilities Office. Under Section 504 of the Americans with Disabilities Act, you are entitled to special-needs accommodations, priority housing, and a medically mandated diet. This is a very personal decision, one that should be made with a thorough understanding that while this designation gets you immediate and legally mandated support, it can also stigmatize.

Learn More

The Everything Gluten-Free College Cookbook (Adams Media) by Carrie S. Forbes, blogger, and creator of *Gingerlemongirl.blogspot.com.*

FARE (Food Allergy Research & Education) College Food Allergy Program—Searchable database for school contacts and managing food allergies on campus. www.foodallergy.org/resources/college-students

Gluten Free Travel Site—For student reviews of colleges and universities. www.glutenfreetravelsite.com

Udi's—Top ten college campuses for gluten-free students from the people who make gluten-free bread and rolls. www.udisglutenfree.com

STUDENT COMMUNITY

While student blogs tend to disappear or change after four years, books like mine stay around for a lot longer. The following will take you through school, graduate school, and out into the world of work, roommates, and dating. Depending on when you open these pages, there may be a whole new gluten-free community. You're in college. You know your way around a search engine.

AntiWheat Girl. www.antiwheatgirl.com
CC Gluten Freed. www.ccglutenfreed.com
Celiac Chicks. www.celiacchicks.com
Celiac Sisters. www.celiacsisters.net
Young, Wild and Gfree. www.youngwildandgfree.wordpress.com

Dating

Dating and falling in love. Both are fraught with food.

Lots of candlelight and cheese and wine and general nibbling around the edges of what may be a serious relationship. Hard to pay attention to what you're eating while canoodling. How does a well-adjusted, gluten-free person go about experiencing love and all its derangements?

For starters, never lie about being gluten-free, even on the first date. But don't make it the central topic of conversation, either. Who wants to hear about diet restrictions when you could be flirting? You are gluten-free. Lots of people are. No big deal.

Actually, you can learn a lot about a person by observing how he or she responds to your ordering safely from a menu. Do you detect a bit of derision or condescension? Is there outright making fun? Does your request for a clean grill inspire a rant about diet neuroses? If there is no respect or consideration for another's dietary needs, imagine how this person might respond to a real emergency. You can go back to the drawing board and save yourself the pain of a breakup.

My husband's mother was more than a little strange. When I look back, I see that my clever boy added a little something about her with each successive date. By the time she and I met, there was nothing she could do that would shock me—and she did plenty—or change how I felt about her son.

Being gluten-free is like that. A little information goes a long way until the relationship develops. By the time you've gotten to the embarrassing bits, if there are any, you've built up a solid foundation of trust.

Pointers for Gluten-Free Singles

✦ Avoid food altogether on a first date. Meet for coffee or at a museum. Attend a gallery opening. Go cycling or running, or just sit in the park.
✦ Cliché as it may be, time stands still when two like-minded people meet. Make sure you've got a gluten-free protein bar or snack and another to offer your date.

- ✦ If you end up meeting at a restaurant, arrive full. This way you can order a salad and give your full concentration to getting to know your date.

- ✦ Or make the reservations yourself and pick a place that's easy for you.

- ✦ Tell the truth eventually. How would you feel if you found out months later that he or she was a little phobic in tight places, an orphan, afraid of the dark, or liked to eat foods in alphabetical order?

- ✦ As painful as it may be, understand that someone who is disrespectful about your diet probably isn't going to respect other areas of your life.

- ✦ Our differences are what make us unique, special, lovable, ourselves. Repeat that ten times before your next date.

- ✦ If you are looking for love online, don't put your diet in your profile, unless you are very good at breezy copy. You don't want to come off as ill. Save it for the face-to-face.

- ✦ As things progress, make dinner or cook with your date. Make something shockingly good that he or she will not believe is gluten-free.

Setting the Date

There are many gifted bakers and chefs, some on these very pages, who'd be happy to pipe rosettes onto a gluten-free extravaganza and create some seriously good food for the engagement party. And yes, the wedding reception can and should be gluten-free. Don't alter a standard menu; find a caterer who'll do a gluten-free party no one will ever forget. If you can't get a glorious meal on your own wedding day, when can you?

The Holiday Family Dinner

Drum roll, please.

The list of uninvited guests is long. There is sibling rivalry, passive-aggressive behavior, oedipal struggle, withholding of love, dispensing of love, mother love, father love, competition, overfeeding, avoidance issues, you-love-him-best issues, love-me-love-my-stuffing, your sister's pregnant and you're not even married yet, and the ever popular, *If you're special then I must not be,* and its close relative, *If you're damaged, maybe I am, too.* None of these things are on the table where you can see them. All anybody can see is brisket, turkey, stuffing, lasagna, plum pudding, matzo balls, and gluten as far as the eye can see.

I hear the horror stories. A sister promises to make a gluten-free stuffing, then denies she ever offered to make it. One woman is asked to bring

Love at First Site

The era of segmentation is upon us. There are dating sites for farmers, Christians who want to mingle, mid-lifers who are starting over. Now there's GlutenfreeSingles, a place to bond and possibly fall in love with a celiac, gluten-sensitive, or dairy-free other. While I mostly like the idea, it could be deadly dull living with someone who has your identical plumbing, not to mention the Darwinian implications. Wouldn't two gluten-intolerants having a baby pretty much guarantee an autoimmune slam dunk? Food for thought. www.glutenfreesingles.com

her own food to her brother's house. Another is asked to arrive after everyone has eaten. Some families simply stonewall the problem, serving the meal with no alternatives, as if nothing has changed. Others make such a big, eye-rolling deal of it, who could eat?

We would drop friends who behaved half as badly. The plain truth is blood gets away with more than water does.

First let's take a good, hard look at ourselves.

+ How would you rate your response and willingness to attend to the needs, whether dietary or not, of other family members?
+ Are you willing to change your routine for others?
+ Do you make special dishes for your dairy-free nephew?
+ Do you make sure to buy pasteurized cheeses for your pregnant sister-in-law?
+ Have you ever forgotten Uncle Ray's lactose intolerance or Auntie Kay's aversion to cigarette smoke?
+ Are you as flexible as you want others to be?
+ Have you explained in great detail, and preferably with examples, your diet to the family?
+ Be honest. Have you set them up to fail?
+ Has your family experienced a really good gluten-free meal at your house?
+ Have you offered to pay for the extra expense for gluten-free foods?
+ Do you always phone well ahead of the holidays and offer to make something?
+ Have you shared, not hinted, in an open and non-adversarial way how important it is for you to feel included in your family's holidays?

If you've answered mostly yes and you can honestly say you've been as truthful about your feelings and expectations and you are still made to feel unwelcome, it's time to bring the situation to a head.

+ Turn down the next family invitation and say why.
+ No fair telling them you're busy or you're going elsewhere. Leave no room for interpretation.
+ Ask, simply, what this is really about.

Be prepared for an honest answer.

You may be told it's about the time your brother's best friend wasn't welcomed warmly at your house. Or how you got all the attention as a child. Or that you are accomplished and successful and gorgeous and food is the only way your siblings can feel superior to you. Or how Grandma would turn over in her grave if her family didn't keep eating green bean casserole. Or they don't know what the hell gluten is, much less how to cook without it.

+ Listen respectfully and do not be defensive.
+ Offer to have the holiday meal at your house next year.
+ Include something you'd never eat but another family member loves.
+ Don't tell them what is gluten-free and what is not. Let them love everything first.

Cruelties to people you love come from places so dark and tangled, it would take an army of Dr. Phils to shed some light on them. If the relationship matters, it's incumbent upon you to work on it.

+ Hand out holiday gift subscriptions to *Living Without* magazine or *Gluten-Free Living*.
+ Send a box ahead of your arrival. Pack it with the best-tasting gluten-free treats you can find and share it with everyone.
+ Buy the family troublemaker a copy of this book. I know. This sounds like a shameless plug, but I suggest it because the family of a certain founder of a celiac research foundation was treating her abysmally until they heard me on the radio.
+ Sometimes, the best way to be heard is to stop speaking.
+ Make it plain that you will not be accepting any more invitations until such time as the family takes your diet seriously.
+ Be grateful when people change. Love them for it.

Note: There is no reason to write about all the wonderful, loving families who wouldn't dream of giving sons and daughters and siblings a hard time. Those of you who are made to feel drenched in gluten-free love are more than lucky. Say thank you often and loudly.

Three-Strikes-and-You're-Out Rule

It's normal to find that someone has forgotten your gluten-free diet the first time. After all, it's new to you, too. The second time is iffy. Maybe you don't see them that much. Maybe you didn't explain as well as you should have how important it is to your health. You should give them a pass. They have a lot more on their plates than your needs. If it happens a third time, and each time after that, odds are it's not about food. It's about why they have a hard time giving you special treatment. Sad, but true.

Enablers, Worry Warts, and Other Oddballs

These are the grandparents who can't stand to see their little darling go without. The friends who never could lose that twenty pounds and enable you to eat right along with them. The woman who infantilizes her gluten-free husband to the point of tasting his food before he picks up his fork. The mother who's so afraid you'll get sick, she won't feed you anything. The sister who sees danger everywhere, and no matter how many times you explain, asks, *Doesn't coffee have gluten in it?* The husband afraid to lose the intimacy of the midnight raids on the cookie jar—just the two of you in the middle of the night, talking yourselves into falling in love again. Everyone who ever teased you into having just one bite.

Going gluten-free can send a shudder through those closest to us. Will you still be friends if you can't stop for pizza while you shop? Any change as important and defining as this one shakes the foundation upon which a relationship rests. It's not just life-changing for you, it changes the rules for everyone in your world.

Let's Play Emotional Football

Understand that a child is often the flash point for adult problems. A common area of conflict is between young parents seen as overbearing by disapproving grandparents. But often the real issue is generational, with one side arguing the finer points of child rearing and the other asserting new lives and rules of their own. Otherwise-sane adults turn a child into an emotional football.

+ Defuse this dangerous and confusing situation by having a family conference.
+ Make it clear little Henry is to be gluten-free no matter whose opinions are to the contrary.
+ Be open to hearing how dismissive and dictatorial you may sound to grandparents who managed to raise you without dire consequences.
+ Find common ground.
+ Ask Henry how he feels.
+ Love is the key here. And respect.

When Worry Turns to Control

Overly nurturing people are another breed of problem. You have a gluten accident and they say, "How could I have let this happen to you?" While this kind of concern is seductive, it's also a form of manipulation.

Just as the bully is often insecure, so the nurturer often has control issues. It's important to know the difference between genuine care and something not quite right. I hate to make generalizations, but men on gluten-free diets (except those who choose it voluntarily) often let their wives or mothers or even daughters do it for them. In my experience, women seem to be hardwired to go along with this. I've found myself counting grams of fat for a husband who couldn't care less. If you don't believe me, go to a health spa and see how many women offer the odd male guest one of the measly four shrimps on their plates.

We've all seen the wife out for dinner with her husband telling the waiter what he can and can't eat. The husband sits passively by, until she nixes something he really wants, and then he calls her a nag. This is called buttering both sides of your gluten-free bread. You can't relinquish control and keep it at the same time.

In some circles, this is called codependency. We become furious with the person who is trying to help us, but we keep the situation in motion by not helping ourselves. It's not so hot for the worrywart, either, taking on another person's diet and being resented for it. It's easy to be sucked into being taken care of by a nurturing partner because it taps into the universal need to be loved and attended to. Conversely, sometimes the desire to be admired and appreciated is so large that we step over boundaries and give too much in order to get it.

This is a deeply complex situation that goes far beyond my pay grade. Suffice it to say, it takes two to tango.

Saboteurs

We've seen it all before. One partner quits cigarettes and the other smokes at the computer they share. One goes on the wagon and the other one sweetly asks, "Pour me a drink, will you?" Little bits of chicken turn up in the vegan lentil stew. Flour turns up in the paleo pie. Seitan passes itself off as beef.

A friend of mine whose career depended upon her thinness on camera came home furious and humiliated after her boss took her out to dinner, an interesting choice of venue, to tell her she was getting a little too plump for the anchor chair. She took to her bed and her husband, whose own career wasn't as stellar, coaxed her out of it with a big pot of spaghetti.

What about the one who can't seem to shed those twenty pounds even if her career is on the line? She may tempt you to cheat, not because she is inherently evil, but because your gluten-free diet has made her feel alone in her weakness.

No grandparent, husband, wife, friend, lover, sister, or brother ever deliberately sets out to sabotage, enable, smother, pacify, confuse, undermine, deliberately misunderstand, or turn on you because they want to see you suffer. They do it because they feel threatened, excluded, abandoned.

Old Joke

Husband and wife eating dinner in a fancy restaurant:

Waiter: "Are you enjoying your meal, sir?"

Husband: "I don't know. Ask her."

Bada-Boom

Empathy Always Saves the Day

The answer to all of these situations, my friend, is simple.

Ask yourself, *In what ways has my gluten-free life affected those close to me?* and speak to that. Always speak to that.

Put on a pot of coffee, cut two slices of Jilly and Jessie's Spiced Carrot Cake with Sweet Mascarpone Frosting (page 215) and listen. Really listen.

You'll be fine.

17

Sex and the Celiac

I'll have what she's having.
—NORA EPHRON, *WHEN HARRY MET SALLY*

A gluten-free fable:

Love in the Time of Semolina

Once upon a time, Byron, a handsome young poet with faulty plumbing, fell for Teresa, a robustly beautiful Italian girl with doe eyes, glossy black hair, and skin the color of the Umbrian earth.

Celiac disease had hit Byron hard. He'd lost a lot of weight. Until he met Teresa, he rarely ate out, preferring to cook his own food or defrost one of the meals his mother prepared and delivered to him every Sunday. His focus, up to that point, had been on regaining his strength and learning how to live gluten-free, scrupulously avoiding even the slightest whiff of anything that could keep him sick.

In Teresa's big Southern Italian family, pasta wasn't merely a food; it was part of their DNA. Pasta with olive oil, anchovy, and garlic; Livornese with olives and capers; puttanesca with fresh tomatoes and hot peppers; Bolognese with ground pork, veal, and beef—all were made with nothing but the finest semolina flour. When told Byron could not partake of their boisterous Sunday meals, Teresa's family shook their heads sadly.

But Teresa's Nonna knew. "*Celiachia,*" she said, remembering how many children were affected by this odd complaint when she was a girl in Naples.

Teresa wanted nothing more than to make her beloved well and strong again. She turned her kitchen into a gluten-free zone, hand-stirring risotto and polenta and cooking big pots of gluten-free lasagna and brown rice pasta. She even made gnocchi from scratch the way her grandmother had taught her, cutting out the dumplings with a whiskey glass.

Byron knew how lucky he was.

"You are the most wonderful woman in the world," he told her, kissing the tips of her fingers.

To put it as delicately as possible, it wasn't long before the pair got past the hand-holding stage. But whenever things became amorous, Byron's stomach churned and he had to rush to the bathroom with the kind of problem that can really take the bloom off a budding romance. Too embarrassed to reveal his sensitive plumbing to Teresa, Byron made a hasty retreat, leaving her to wonder, as many young girls would in her situation, what she'd done to drive him away.

He couldn't imagine what he was reacting to. He was scrupulous about his diet. He carried his lunch to work and avoided unknown restaurants as he had been warned to do. He ate before going to parties and checked the ingredients of all the vitamins, cold remedies, and prescriptions in his medicine cabinet.

The only time he truly enjoyed eating was with Teresa, who never mixed her food with his, was careful to cook his pasta in a fresh pot of water, and even bought a second toaster oven for her tiny apartment, so her crumbs wouldn't mingle with his. No one else cared for him like that, except, of course, his mother.

Byron's mother did not want to meddle in the personal matters of her grown son, but this was her baby, after all. Privately she wondered if a girl raised on that much pasta exuded it through her pores. She remembered her own courtship with Byron's father, how fascinated they were with every freckle, finger and toe, earlobe and dimple. They wanted to eat each other up, not unlike toddlers who put every object of their desire into their mouths.

She wished her husband were here to talk to Byron, but he'd died young and she always suspected his illness was related to their son's problems.

"Does Teresa brush and floss her teeth before kissing you?" she asked.

"Ma!"

"Well, does she?"

Byron glared, but she would not be dissuaded.

"It could be her lipstick you're sensitive to, or her face cream or body lotion or talcum powder. Whatever it is, you need to talk to her about it. And you need to tell her the truth."

Byron knew his mother was right.

"There's something I have to tell you," he said when he saw Teresa next.

She listened quietly as Byron stumbled through his explanation of what happens to him after they kiss.

"I thought it was me," she said, relief swimming in her beautiful eyes.

"Oh God, no," he said. "I love you."

Out went Teresa's old cosmetics. In came a new supply of gluten-free, hypoallergenic lotions, creams, cosmetics, and pretty lipsticks that did not change Byron's desire to kiss her. With a lifetime supply of plain dental floss, and his-and-hers electric toothbrushes, the young couple found an unlikely and surprisingly sexy source of togetherness. Teresa washed carefully after touching unsafe foods and they often showered together to avoid wasting water and time. There were no more embarrassing incidents.

In the spring, Byron proposed, presenting Teresa with a new poem and a modest diamond solitaire. They started planning a big fat gluten-free wedding and a honeymoon in Teresa's ancestral village where much brushing and flossing and kissing *senza glutine* would go on.

The moral of the story, dear reader, is this: When you are seriously affected by gluten, the concept of being lovesick takes on a whole new meaning.

How to Love Your Gluten-Free Lover

When bees do it, it's cross-pollination. When allergic humans do it, it's cross-contamination. Not a romantic phrase, but nevertheless apt.

We know how much can happen to a food before it hits your plate— French fries cooked in a bath of oil used for onion rings, an errant crouton, a flour-dusted raisin, a knife that's just cut another sandwich, a grill or a cutting board that didn't get wiped down.

What about food that was never on a plate?

A kiss stolen over a plate of pasta and, before you know it, you're ingesting something you hadn't bargained for.

Where does lipstick color go when it fades?

It goes straight into your stomach. Unless, of course, it goes into his. Or hers.

To compound the problem, many of you are sensitive to other substances besides gluten. Peanut and wheat germ oil–based cosmetics, skin creams, aluminum in deodorants, talc made from wheat starch, fragrance and chemical-laden air fresheners, toxic cleaning products, and formaldehyde in carpeting all contribute to problems. For the truly sensitive, just breathing something toxic is enough to cause itchy throats, wheezing, and yes, kissing fingers that have just licked the cake batter out of the mixing bowl can really put a pall on any romantic plans.

We've all heard the stories.

A woman with shellfish allergy goes into anaphylactic shock after kissing her boyfriend. A teenager with a peanut allergy steals a kiss and keels over. Or, as poor Byron well knows, a little fooling around and wham, an hour in the bathroom.

The only way to avoid a nasty and potentially embarrassing situation is to do what our young friend so bravely did. Have a frank conversation with your partner about the following hygiene matters and intimate behavior; then have some good, clean fun.

- ✦ Brush, floss, and rinse your mouth after eating foods your partner is sensitive to; not only will your breath be sweeter, your mouth will be healthier and even more kissable.
- ✦ Make sure all of your shared vitamins and supplements are gluten-free.
- ✦ Never use another's napkin or cutlery or glass.
- ✦ Use hypoallergenic and fragrance-free soap, cosmetics, shampoo, styling aids, and personal products.
- ✦ Wash any body part that has been powdered, creamed, conditioned, shampooed, gelled, made up, dusted, fluffed, or slicked or has touched any gluten-containing substance that can get into the wrong place.

I won't go into all the ways one can unwittingly share food or list how otherwise inedible products can get into your stomach. Besides, if I have to tell you, this chapter isn't for you. I am no prude, but this is *The Gluten-Free Revolution*, not *Fifty Shades of Grey*.

Kahlil Gibran said, *Let there be spaces in your togetherness*. I would add, *Let there be no gluten in your spaces*.

Fertility Problems

Inevitably, all this fooling around leads somewhere. With good planning and a little luck, baby makes three.

Maybe. Maybe not.

Sometimes, no matter how hard you try, no matter that you have taken your temperature, figured out when you're ovulating, or stood on your head to help matters along, good news eludes you.

The experts say infertility is one of the most commonly overlooked problems in those not yet diagnosed with gluten intolerance. In fact, research points to such an increased incidence of infertility, miscarriage, and other problems of pregnancy, anyone experiencing these troubles would be smart to see a gastroenterologist and be tested for celiac disease or gluten intolerance.

In celiac disease, malabsorption can cause a deficiency of the key nutrients crucial for female hormone production, which regulates ovulation. Celiac disease can also increase the odds of endocrine or hormonal disorders, such as thyroid disease, which disrupts ovarian function.

One recent study at Thomas Jefferson University Hospital in Philadelphia found that the rate of miscarriage and infertility in celiac patients is at least four times higher than in the general population. In an interview with *Living Without* magazine, Dr. Anthony J. DiMarino, chief of the Division of Gastroenterology and director of Jefferson's Celiac Center, says this increased susceptibility to fertility issues makes sense because of the nutritional problems in women with undiagnosed celiac disease: "If the placenta is attacked by antibodies, you can see how this could directly affect its ability to sustain a pregnancy." In the same article, Daniel A. Leffler, MD, director of clinical research at the Celiac Center at Beth Israel Deaconess Medical Center in Boston, says that many of the early studies on infertility and celiac disease didn't target women with unexplained fertility but instead lumped all causes of infertility together.

Researchers at the Celiac Disease Center at Columbia University agree. When they screened 188 women with infertility for celiac, there was no higher risk of celiac disease until that group was narrowed down to just those with unexplained infertility. Of that group, as many as 6 percent had celiac disease, nearly six times higher than expected.

A UK study found that late onset of menstruation and early menopause in gluten-intolerant females not following a gluten-free diet may contribute to infertility by shortening the reproductive period in a woman's life. Further, men with celiac disease may have reversible infertility due to impotence, hypogonadism (decreased functional activity of the testes), abnormal sperm motility, or androgen resistance that resolves or improves when gluten is withdrawn.

At Tampere University Hospital and the School of Medicine at the University of Tampere, Finland, researchers found the rate of celiac disease among women reporting infertility was 4.1 percent higher than in the control population, and they were more likely to have shortened reproductive periods and early menopause as well. Researchers further correlate noncompliance with the gluten-free diet and increased risk for spontaneous abortion, low-birth-weight babies, and shorter periods of breast-feeding.

In an article in the *Lancet*, Dr. Peter H. R. Green, director of the Celiac Disease Center at Columbia University, says that undiagnosed celiac disease is indeed associated with delayed periods, cessation of periods (amenorrhea), premature menopause, recurrent miscarriages, increased infant mortality, and fewer children. Dr. Green further states that infertility in men can be associated with celiac disease and that male celiacs tend to have children with a shorter gestation and lower birth weight than those without the disease.

It's safe to say that undocumented celiac disease in either parent can have a negative effect on your ability to get pregnant.

Scratch below the surface of the gluten-free community and you will hear tragic stories of miscarriages, infertility, and even stillbirths. Post a question online, and tales of difficult pregnancies, miscarriages, and fetal defects will inundate you. You'll hear from one woman after another desperately trying to get pregnant and finding out, years too late, that undiagnosed problems with gluten were the culprits.

Most experts agree that more research needs to be done. At this writing, new studies are under way. At Thomas Jefferson University Hospital, Anthony J. DiMarino is overseeing a large study on the reproductive health of women with celiac disease, and preliminary data was presented at the American College of Gastroenterology's annual meeting. Researchers at the Celiac Center at Boston's Beth Israel Deaconess Medical Center are teaming up with a Boston fertility clinic on what will be the largest screening to date in women with unexplained infertility.

A physician survey fielded at Thomas Jefferson University Hospital in Philadelphia points to a large discrepancy between clinical investigation and practice in an effort to more precisely identify and treat individuals with gluten intolerance and infertility screening with the goal of getting the internist, gynecologist, and fertility specialist on the same page.

Is That Your Biological Clock I Hear Ticking?

+ If there is a history of digestive problems, celiac disease, miscarriage, or difficult pregnancy in your family tree, run—do not walk—to your gastroenterologist for testing.
+ If you have tested positive for celiac disease, wait until your symptoms are under control and your blood work (see page 500–501 for appropriate tests) has returned to normal before planning to conceive. This could take six months to a year of strict adherence to the gluten-free diet.
+ Discuss your plans with your gastroenterologist and, if necessary, redo blood tests to make sure you are not getting any gluten.
+ Make sure any problems with anemia, iron, zinc, folate, and other important vitamin and mineral deficiencies have been brought into normal range before you try to conceive.
+ Have his hormone levels taken as well, check for testosterone problems and androgen resistance, and remember, malabsorption can affect sperm production as well.

✦ Follow the gluten-free diet as scrupulously and as nutritiously as you can.

✦ If you drink or smoke, don't.

✦ Easy for me to say: *relax.*

Deborah S. Simmons, PhD, in an article on the American Fertility Association Web site, suggests that those with unexplained infertility, who have sensitivity to gluten and who test negative for celiac disease should consider eating gluten-free anyway and see if bowel function and brain fog, or other manifestations of non-celiac gluten sensitivity, improve.

If this is the course you take, I would strongly suggest retesting for celiac disease and waiting a good long time until improvement is noticeable before attempting to conceive.

What About Non-Celiac Gluten Sensitivity and Infertility?

As we go to press, we don't know enough about gluten sensitivity to safely say how it may affect a pregnancy. The experts agree that research is far behind in this area.

Alice Bast, director of the National Foundation for Celiac Awareness, who has experienced firsthand the tragedy of celiac disease–related birth complications, is optimistic that new research on celiac disease will shed light on what seems to be an epidemic of gluten sensitivity.

To that end, Bana Jabri, MD, director of research at the University of Chicago Celiac Disease Center, is currently focusing all of her efforts on discovering markers that can identify gluten sensitivity before antibodies to gluten are present, which would be a huge breakthrough for those who have suffered the many reproductive complications of silent gluten intolerance. Dr. Jabri's work and that of other researchers in this important field will have enormous implications for the millions of us who are avoiding gluten without any real diagnosis or warning of impending problems.

I Just Feel Better Without Gluten

At the very least, you are sensitive to gluten. Why else would you avoid it? Your body may know something you don't. If you are planning a family, I can't think of a better reason to have what may be an unnecessary medical test.

Danish researchers studied 211 infants and 127 mothers with celiac disease and found that the mean birth weight of children born to mothers on a gluten-containing diet was significantly lower than babies born to mothers without celiac disease. Interestingly, the same study determined that women on the gluten-free diet gave birth to children weighing more than those born to mothers without celiac disease.

In a study that looked at the effect of the gluten-free diet on pregnancy and lactation, investigators learned that women with celiac disease who were not on the gluten-free diet experienced pregnancy loss at a rate of 17.8 percent, compared to 2.4 percent of women with celiac disease who were on the gluten-free diet.

In a letter to the editors of *Gut* emphasizing the need for health care professionals to recognize and treat the manifestations of celiac disease in women of reproductive age, Dr. K. K. Hozyasz, of the National Research Institute of Mother and Child in Warsaw, suggests that "coeliac disease should be considered as a cause of birth defects associated with folic acid deficiency, for example, spina bifida, orofacial clefts, heart defects, in the offspring of women of short stature."

He goes on to say that "a low plasma level of folic acid is a common finding in newly diagnosed patients and there are good theoretical reasons for hypothesizing that coeliac disease could also be a maternal risk factor for birth defects."

The article further states that, although spontaneous abortion has no specific cause, celiac disease may be suspected in the presence of persistent iron deficiency and abnormal weight loss during a first, but more often a second, pregnancy. Women with undiagnosed celiac disease seem to have an 8.9-fold relative risk of multiple spontaneous abortions and low-birth-weight babies compared with treated patients.

An Italian study at the University of Naples concluded that a gluten-free diet resulted in a 9.18-fold reduction in the miscarriage rate and a reduction in the prevalence of low-birth-rate babies from 29.4 percent to zero. Of 112 pregnancies in women with untreated celiac disease, 20 ended in miscarriages compared with 2 of 22 in patients on a gluten-free diet. Similarly, six babies were stillborn in an undiagnosed group compared with none in a group on a gluten-free diet. The researchers put a finer point on the issue: they found sufficient proof to say that after one year on the gluten-free diet the majority of these women enjoy a successful pregnancy.

It's safe to say that the odds of having an uneventful pregnancy are not so good for the undiagnosed celiac. I can't think of a better reason for getting tested before getting pregnant.

But you are on the gluten-free diet already. Isn't that enough?

Afraid not.

The reasons are simple. For one thing, you may not be as careful with your diet, making the assumption you don't *really* have to be. You may have celiac disease and not know it. Or you may be in that gray area of pre-celiac disease, sensitive to gluten but having no antibodies. Worse, you have no idea what nutritional deficits you may be dealing with when you decide to try to conceive. Or you may have none of the above. You are simply avoiding gluten.

The point is, you don't know. Get tested—there is a brand-new life on the line.

There's More to Eating for Two Than Avoiding Gluten

You're pregnant. Congratulations are in order.

What's on the menu besides avoiding gluten? Registered dietician Gloria Scarparo suggests:

+ Rigorously adhering to your gluten-free diet.
+ Eating five small meals instead of three big ones.
+ Aiming for a normal weight gain of twenty to twenty-six pounds.
+ Washing all fruits and vegetables.
+ Avoiding raw or undercooked meat, which can increase the risk of toxoplasmosis.

Anyone who is pregnant and gluten-intolerant should get enough of the following:

+ **Calcium**—A daily dose of 1,200 milligrams of calcium combined with low-fat dairy products and calcium-rich foods like soybeans, sunflower seeds, carrots, cabbage, cauliflower, and citrus fruit.
+ **Iron**—Iron deficiency is relatively common in pregnant women. Take at least 30 milligrams of iron daily. Good sources of iron are spinach, peanuts, and dried fruit. If eaten with foods that are high in vitamin C, such as bell peppers, broccoli, citrus fruit, kiwis, and strawberries, the iron will be absorbed more efficiently.
+ **Folate**—Folate or folic acid is one of the most vital vitamins for the unborn child in the first trimester, is crucial for the embryo during its growth phases, and works to prevent serious birth defects. Those who are planning to get pregnant and are gluten-intolerant should get at

least 400 micrograms daily for at least three to six months before trying to conceive and thereafter during the pregnancy. In its natural state, folic acid is found in hazelnuts, walnuts, almonds, cabbage, beets, asparagus, spinach, gluten-free grains and cereals, citrus fruits, bananas, melons, and kiwis.

+ **Protein**—Choose lean meat, fish, eggs, and poultry or combine beans with whole grains.
+ **Fiber**—To avoid constipation, which is common in pregnancy, eat whole grains like brown rice, quinoa, millet, and buckwheat; add coarsely ground flaxseed to meals; and drink plenty of liquids, at least 68 ounces a day.

Gluten isn't the only troublesome food. The American Pregnancy Association recommends avoiding the following foods during pregnancy:

+ **Raw meat**—This includes sushi, undercooked seafood like seared ahi tuna, or uncooked beef or poultry because it puts the mother-to-be at a higher risk of toxoplasmosis and salmonella.
+ **Deli meat**—Deli products pose their own problems for the gluten-free, but for the pregnant and gluten-free they're a no-no. These products may be contaminated with *Listeria*, a bacterium that can cross the placenta and may infect the baby or cause life-threatening blood poisoning.
+ **Liver**—There is some concern about the amounts of vitamin A in liver. Large amounts of vitamin A have the potential to pose a risk to an unborn baby. The safest approach is to avoid eating liver.
+ **Fish**—Fish containing high levels of mercury should be avoided. These include shark, swordfish, king mackerel, fresh tuna, sea bass, and tilefish. Canned tuna is considered safe, but no more than six ounces of albacore tuna a week should be eaten. Mercury consumed during pregnancy has been linked to developmental delays and brain damage. Avoid fish exposed to industrial pollutants from contaminated lakes and rivers that may be exposed to high levels of polychlorinated biphenyls (PCBs). These fish include bluefish, striped bass, salmon, pike, trout, and walleye. Contact the local health department or Environmental Protection Agency to find out which fish are safe to eat in your area.
+ **Raw shellfish**—The majority of seafood-borne illness is caused by undercooked shellfish, which includes oysters, clams, and mussels. Cooking helps prevent some types of infections, but it does not prevent

the algae-related infections associated with red tides. Raw shellfish pose a concern for everybody and should be avoided altogether.

✦ **Raw eggs**—Raw eggs or foods containing raw eggs should be avoided during pregnancy because of the potential exposure to salmonella. Caesar dressings, mayonnaise, homemade ice cream or custards, hollandaise sauces, and unpasteurized eggnog should be avoided.

✦ **Soft cheeses**—Unpasteurized and raw cheeses may contain bacteria called *Listeria*. Soft cheeses to avoid are Brie, Camembert, Roquefort, feta, Gorgonzola, and Mexican-style queso blanco and queso fresco. Soft nonimported cheeses made with pasteurized milk are safe to eat as long as they do not contain gluten.

✦ **Unpasteurized milk**—This may also contain *Listeria*, which crosses the placenta and may lead to infections or blood poisoning.

✦ **Pâté**—Another possible source for the bacteria *Listeria*.

✦ **Caffeine**—Although most studies show that caffeine intake in moderation is okay, it seems counterintuitive to give an unborn baby a stimulant. Some say caffeine may be related to miscarriages. Avoid caffeine during the first trimester to reduce the likelihood and afterward limit caffeine to fewer than 300 milligrams per day. Caffeine is a diuretic, which can result in water and calcium loss, so make sure you are drinking plenty of water, juice, or milk if you do consume caffeinated beverages.

✦ **Alcohol**—There is *no* amount of alcohol known to be safe during pregnancy and during breast-feeding. Prenatal exposure to alcohol can interfere with the healthy development of the baby and, depending on the amount, timing, and pattern of use, alcohol consumption during pregnancy can lead to fetal alcohol syndrome.

✦ **Unwashed vegetables**—While vegetables are safe to eat, it's essential to scrub them thoroughly in order to avoid exposure to toxoplasmosis, which may contaminate the soil in which they are grown.

✦ **Herbal remedies**—Certain herbal remedies, such as goldenseal and mugwort, may be associated with uterine contractions and should be avoided. Take nothing without checking with your doctor first.

✦ **Cigarettes**—Don't even breathe near one.

A *New York Times* article by Alex Kuczynski aptly called "The Nine Months of Living Anxiously" cites the growing list of edible and environmental worries that add to the paranoia of a mommy-to-be. Among the purported no-nos:

Why Such a Big Mama?

Fascinating facts from the American Pregnancy Association:

Baby = 7 pounds   Maternal breast tissue = 2 pounds
Placenta = 1 to 2 pounds   Maternal blood flow = 2 pounds
Amniotic fluid = 2 pounds   Fluids in maternal tissue = 4 pounds
Uterine enlargement = 2 pounds   Maternal fat stores = 7 pounds

That's a whopping 28 pounds, not counting pickles and gluten-free ice cream.

Thongs   Pedicures
Tanning salons   Kitty litter boxes
Underwire bras   Aspirin
Botox   Paint
Chocolate mousse   Chemical hair dyes
Manicures   Hot tubs

Not to mention phthalates, found in many industrial and seemingly benign cosmetic products such as nail polish, perfume, hand and body lotions, creams, and hair products.

The FDA puts farm-raised salmon on the list of banned foods because it contains higher levels of PCBs and dioxins than what is considered safe by the Environmental Protection Agency. Safe levels of PCBs and dioxins? Now there's an oxymoron.

One study, reported in the *American Journal of Clinical Nutrition*, found foods high on the glycemic index—white bread, highly processed grains, potatoes, and the like—may increase a woman's chances of having a baby with spina bifida or some other neural tube defect, and the strongest link was seen among obese participants. Women in the group who ate the most high-glycemic foods had four times the risk of delivering a baby with spina bifida. There are many high-glycemic and highly processed gluten-free foods. Avoid them.

Then there's the issue of safe water. To be brutally honest, government water standards are a whole lot lower than yours. Filtered or bottled water is always a good idea. For gluten-free mothers-to-be, it's a must.

To Breast-Feed or Not

There are breast pumps and embarrassing leaks back at the office and the problem of what to do when baby is hungry in public (tuck yourself in a corner somewhere and wrap a shawl around both of you). Some friends won't invite you out (dump them!) and some husbands feel just plain left out of all that bonding. You can't leave the little tyke with anybody for very long because you're dinner for the next year or so.

Still, the good reasons far outweigh the inconveniences, not the least of which, according to ProMom.org, is that a breast-feeding mom will lose the baby fat much more quickly than a formula girl. Besides, there is nothing like looking at your chubby, healthy baby and knowing you did that all by yourself.

An interesting study done by a group of Polish researchers looks at the best times to introduce gluten to infants as well as the protective effect of breast-feeding. Results suggest that gluten introduction during the time of breast-feeding makes for a lower risk for celiac disease than among infants introduced to gluten when on formula. While it was unclear whether or not breast-feeding provides permanent protection from celiac disease or delays the onset, the researchers felt it was reasonable to avoid giving infants gluten before four to seven months of age and to be breast-feeding at the time of introduction.

Many experts disagree about the protective effect of breast milk, and there is more work to be done regarding the short window in which to expose infants to gluten. The role of breast milk and intestinal bacteria in an infant's developing immune system will be the focus of much more research in years to come.

The American Academy of Pediatrics says that the average length of time for breast-feeding is twelve months or longer, depending on the mutual desire of the parties. This is another good reason to be at least a year out from a celiac disease diagnosis. Undiagnosed celiac disease often cuts short a woman's period of lactation. The longer you are on the gluten-free diet, the more likely you will have enough milk for the whole time.

From ProMom, ten good reasons to consider breast-feeding:

1. Breast milk is the perfect food. It can never be tampered with. There are no nutrients missing, nor are there ingredients that will be proven to give rats a headache in years to come. Its safety can never be questioned, nor can it ever be recalled.

2. According to the Academy of Nutrition and Dietetics, breast-feeding encourages bonding and stimulates the release of the hormone oxytocin, which is responsible for stimulating milk ejection and for maternal behavior.

3. Breast-feeding helps decrease insulin requirements in diabetic mothers.

4. Breast milk is always the right temperature: no bottles to heat up, no accidental burns.

5. Breast-feeding makes for less smelly diaper changes. In side-by-side tests of breast-fed versus formula-fed babies, the natural baby won by a nose.

6. Breast-feeding satisfies baby's emotional need to be held, cuddled, and cradled. Some hospitals have programs where volunteers hold sick babies whose families cannot come every day.

7. Not breast-feeding may increase a mother's risk of breast cancer.

8. Breast milk lowers the risk of the baby developing asthma.

9. Breast-fed babies get fewer cavities.

10. Breast milk, because of its protective antibodies, is believed to confer immunity to some diseases and aids in the development of a healthy immune system. Breast-feeding may delay or reduce the risk of developing celiac disease.

In case you're wondering, breast milk is 100 percent gluten-free.

You've said hello to your feet again. And to the creature you can't stop marveling at, whose tiny toes and fingers and perfect mother-of-pearl nails are a miracle in miniature.

You want to raise a happy, healthy, well-adjusted, generous little person who will thrive and be all that he or she can be, even if there are issues with gluten. You are full of dreams and up to the challenge parenthood imposes. You are brimming with hope, a healthy dose of nerves, and more questions than you even know to ask.

What if My Baby Is a Celiac?

Ritu Verma, MD, section chief of Gastroenterology, associate professor of Clinical Pediatrics, and director of the Celiac Center of Children's Hospital of Philadelphia, has guided hundreds of children and their families through testing, diagnosis, and adjustment to the gluten-free diet. She has raised three children, two with celiac disease, one of whom has grown up to be the wildly popular blogger AntiWheat Girl. Herewith, she offers a short course in . . .

RECOGNIZING, DIAGNOSING, AND MANAGING
CELIAC DISEASE IN CHILDREN

To put it simply, celiac disease is an autoimmune condition that runs in families and occurs when certain genetically susceptible individuals eat gluten, which triggers a mechanism that, in turn, causes the body to attack normal healthy tissue, primarily the gastrointestinal tract.

Diagnosis starts with being aware of the potential for celiac disease and therefore thinking about the symptoms, especially if a parent, grandparent, or sibling suffers from CD or non-celiac gluten sensitivity. We think of the classic presentation as a skinny child losing weight with a distended belly, a loss of fat stores, and muscle-wasting from constant diarrhea and vomiting.

Not hard to spot.

However, celiac disease can affect virtually any organ system in the body and is currently seen more often in children who don't have those classic symptoms. Celiac disease should be considered in a child with short stature, dental enamel defects, thyroid problems, chronic headaches, elevated liver enzymes, anemia, leg pains, joint pains, alopecia, early osteoporosis or osteopenia, or dermatitis herpetiformis, the skin's reaction to gluten. There may even be chronic constipation and excessive weight gain.

The central nervous system may also be affected, with depression, seizures, anxiety, irritability, behavioral problems, and attention deficit and sensory integration disorders. If one or more of these atypical and often puzzling symptoms cannot be explained by another disease or condition, one should think about testing for celiac disease.

All children with type 1 diabetes should be screened. Almost 10 percent to 20 percent of type 1 diabetic children also have celiac disease. So, too, children with Down's syndrome, Turner's syndrome, and Williams syndrome also have a higher genetic predisposition. Hypothyroidism and many other autoimmune rheumatologic conditions should make a parent suspicious of celiac disease, as well.

Because celiac disease is a genetic condition, and there is a much higher predisposition among first-degree (mother, father, brother, sister, son, daughter) and second-degree relatives (grandmother, grandfather, aunt, uncle, niece, nephew cousin, grandchild), and regardless of the presence or absence of particular symptoms, these close family members must be screened.

What does screening involve?

A simple blood test, taken by your doctor, should include the total immunoglobulin A (IgA) level, tissue transglutaminase (TTg) antibody, endomysial antibody (EMA), and, more currently, deamidated gliadin (DGP). If the IgA level is abnormally low, then other antibodies must be measured. These are all elevated in children or adults with active celiac disease. In the presence of low IgA or IgA deficiency, IgG versions should be obtained.

It is important that the child be eating adequate gluten—approximately two slices of bread a day or a tablespoon of regular flour mixed into the child's food—for at least a month prior to testing in order to ensure the accuracy of the results.

In families with a high incidence of gluten intolerance, or history of GI cancers or autoimmune diseases, genetic testing may be helpful, especially of those who are already gluten-free. Two HLA genes, DQ2 and DQ8, are responsible for the majority of celiac disease. One or both genes need to be present in the majority of cases for celiac disease to develop.

However, 30 percent to 40 percent of the general population have one or both genes and never develop the disease. Genetic testing is not routine, and certainly not necessary for everyone, but it can be helpful in the presence of a diagnostic dilemma—false-positive screening and a borderline biopsy—or in a family with several symptomatic members. It is an individual decision and clearly a conversation one should have with one's physician.

In the presence of positive blood antibodies, the only way to confirm a diagnosis of celiac disease is to perform a small bowel biopsy, still the irrefutable gold standard. This involves an upper endoscopic outpatient procedure, which requires the child to fast overnight.

During the procedure, several biopsies from the small intestine need to be taken to assess the level of damage from gluten. In order to make a diagnosis of celiac disease, the biopsies must demonstrate an increase in intraepithelial lymphocytes and varying degrees of villous atrophy. Once a physician sees this combination along with positive blood work, a definitive diagnosis can be made.

Why subject a child to an invasive procedure so early?

Why not just put the child on a gluten-free diet?

For one thing, blood work can be falsely positive in the presence of food allergy, infections, and other autoimmune conditions. Removing rye and barley isn't necessary for children in the case of wheat allergy. Blood work can be falsely negative, too, so biopsy is helpful. The child may have non-celiac gluten sensitivity, which may cause symptoms but does not pose the same risks as celiac disease, at least as far as we know right now. As I write this, much research is being done in that area, and these assumptions may not stand in the future. The jury is still out.

Children with untreated celiac disease have a much higher incidence of serious problems. The longer one eats gluten, the higher the risk of certain GI cancers, including a rare enteropathy-associated T-cell lymphoma.

There can be nutritional complications like night blindness, neuropathy, bleeding problems, and anemia. Delayed diagnosis increases the possibility of developing other autoimmune diseases in adulthood, for example, Sjögren's syndrome, thyroid disease, or rheumatoid arthritis, and also poses a higher risk of morbidity and mortality.

A child diagnosed with celiac disease after the age of ten years faces a 25 percent higher risk of developing these complications later in life. The risk only increases with age. Put simply, children have nothing to fear when celiac disease is detected and confirmed early.

In the face of this, I ask parents who do not want to submit their children to an invasive procedure if they are absolutely sure in their mind their child has celiac disease. If they are convinced with just a positive blood test, then they can start the gluten-free diet under the guidance of a dietician. A biopsy is the only way to know for sure.

Perhaps the most compelling reason to do the biopsy is future compliance. When children become teenagers subject to the peer pressure of eating with their friends, they will ask, as my own daughter did, "Do I really have celiac disease?" She was asymptomatic. Her CD was picked up in screening. Was I reacting to her brother's diagnosis and his classic and severe symptoms? All those years later, I wondered. I was able to look up her chart and review her biopsy, and answer her question with total confidence. Yes, you do.

If there is any doubt, and especially in the absence of symptoms, the gluten-free diet may be abandoned with devastating results. Dots may not be connected as other conditions develop.

Many parents ask when a child should be screened. My answer is always the earlier, the better.

In a family where a parent or sibling has celiac disease or is suspected of having it, a child who displays symptoms can and should be tested as early as possible. If a child with a first-degree relationship to celiac disease displays no symptoms, screening should be considered between two and three years of age, so long as the child is eating gluten-containing foods.

Family members need to be tested for celiac disease. There are no hard-and-fast guidelines for retesting, but I recommend that children be tested yearly until puberty. If a child demonstrates no outward symptoms, I would repeat the testing every three years.

As we are seeing more and more cases of adult-onset celiac disease, I would even go so far as to say that anyone who was a child in a family affected by celiac disease or gluten intolerance and continues to eat gluten should ask that a celiac panel be done as part of his or her annual checkup at the same time his or her cholesterol is checked.

I see many parents devastated by this diagnosis. They are justifiably fearful. Their babies are in need of so much protection, too small to be so sick. I encourage families to see how fortunate they are to have a child with a condition that requires no medicine or surgical intervention, only a gluten-free diet, which, if followed to the letter, is guaranteed to reverse damage to the intestine and decrease the odds of any further complications.

I am happy to tell them that, with early diagnosis, good nutrition, and strict adherence to the diet, their children will be as normal as any other child. And these days, they will have plenty of company and a far easier time keeping their kids from unsafe foods in a society so fluent in what it means to be gluten-free.

My only caveat is vigilance.

Gluten irritates and damages the immune system, so any trace of it, or small amount of cross-contamination, can cause the problems to come right back.

As a physician, I cannot overemphasize the importance of education and follow-up until the training wheels come off. That really does make all the difference between feeling isolated and confident. At Children's Hospital Center for Celiac Disease, we have dieticians, social workers, psychologists, and support groups where children can meet other children who are dealing with the gluten-free diet and share experiences.

As a mother myself, of two children with celiac disease, now grown and perfectly healthy, I know how important education and community can be.

Yes, it may seem daunting at first. But if you have determined, unequivocally and in a way that's right for your family, that your child is or is not a celiac, you can stand down knowing the future holds no hidden threats or surprises.

I would venture you are ahead of the game already. You or someone in the family is gluten-free, otherwise you would not be reading this excellent book, wondering and asking questions, doing your homework.

I will never forget the Sunday Jax Lowell came to a meeting at Children's Hospital of Philadelphia for no reason other than to volunteer her time and give back to the gluten-free community. Listening to her talk to the families and read to the children that day, my own among them, rapt and thrilled to meet an adult who knew how they felt and who understood them perfectly, I saw there is another kind of healing.

The real cure for celiac disease isn't just a healed intestine and compliance with the gluten-free diet; it's growing up knowing we are special.

Let me assure you that you are in the capable hands of a gifted and generous writer, one who has not only researched her subject thoroughly, but who has lived it, too, without ever having lost her optimism or her sense of humor, or forgotten what it is to be a child.

—Ritu Verma, MD

Learn More

American Congress of Obstetricians and Gynecologists. www.acog.org

Academy of Nutrition and Dietetics. www.eatright.org

An Epidemic of Absence: A New Way of Understanding Allergies and Autoimmune Diseases by Moises Velasques-Manoff (Scribner)

The American Fertility Association. www.theafa.org

American Pregnancy Association. www.americanpregnancy.org

American Society for Reproductive Medicine. www.asrm.org

Centers for Disease Control and Prevention Reproductive Health publications. www.cdc.gov

Children's Hospital of Philadelphia Center for Celiac Disease. www.chop.edu/service/center-for-celiac-disease/

International Council on Infertility Information Dissemination, Inc. www.inciid.org

La Leche League. www.lalecheleague.org

Maternal and Child Health Bureau. www.mchb.hrsa.gov

National Institutes of Health. www.nih.gov

Nursing Mothers Counsel. www.nursingmothers.org

101 Reasons to Breast-feed Your Child. www.notmilk.com

Promotion of Mother's Milk, Inc. www.naturalchildbirth.org

RESOLVE: The National Fertility Association. www.resolve.org

Sher Institutes for Reproductive Medicine. www.haveababy.com

USDA—Food and Nutrition Information Center National Agricultural Library. www.fnic.nal.usda.gov

Vegetarian Resource Group. www.vrg.org

And Baby Makes Three

18

Monday's child is gluten-free,
Tuesday's child gets hives from tea,
Wednesday's child can't bear cat hair,
Thursday's child must gasp for air,
Friday's child will wheeze and sneeze,
Saturday's child is eggless, please.
But the child born on the Sabbath day,
Fair and wise, loves to say,
"I'm glad I'm specially made this way."
—Variation on a Nursery Rhyme

One parent tells me she has put her autistic son on a gluten-free, casein-free diet and his concentration and behavioral symptoms seem to have improved. Another says her son's depression and violent outbursts have all but stopped in the absence of gluten. Still more are raising their children gluten-free and casein-free because of attention deficit disorder, attention deficit/hyperactivity disorder, and sensory integration disorders.

Every day I hear of a family that has removed gluten and soy and, to the best of their ability, GMOs from their kids' diets and have been rewarded with calmer, more focused, and emotionally and neurologically stable children. This doesn't take into account those families whose children have documented celiac disease, non-celiac gluten intolerance, and various degrees of gluten sensitivity.

Something is afoot.

The groundswell of interest in raising kids gluten-free may speak to the frustration parents feel about the quality of the food their children are getting or the pace of the research regarding these serious problems. It may be a backlash to neurologic and psychological labels and pharmaceutical solutions with long-term implications. Or it may be that gluten intolerance and sensitivity cause different problems in children, ones that are easily mistaken for developmental and behavioral issues. Could it be the babies, with their small bodies and big problems, are telling us genetically altered wheat and corn and soy are toxic to a developing digestive system? Perhaps brain fog, inability to concentrate, depression, and mood swings common to gluten-sensitive adults are more dramatic in children and therefore more likely to be called a disorder rather than a symptom.

So many parents can't be wrong.

But science does not concern itself with anecdotal evidence. Research is strictly controlled and evidence-based. That is as it should be.

Childhood is a window that closes quickly. Until hypotheses become settled science, many families are seeing the irrefutable fact that their children do better without gluten. I have no doubt that these pioneering families will teach us lessons and advance what we know about the mind-body connection in children.

In the meantime, I would caution everyone to test for celiac disease and gluten intolerance and other food sensitivities as early as possible and before starting their kids on the gluten-free diet. Given new studies on the brain-gut connection, I would urge you to keep your pediatrician, neurologist, allergist, and gastroenterologist all on the same page. We are a large, diverse, and curious family with much to learn from the littlest among us.

Baby's First Foods

Here are a handful of gluten-free foods that will go down easily, and won't cause trouble while gluten issues are being sorted out.

A TWICE-BAKED TEETHING BISCUIT

When my mother wasn't looking, my grandmother rubbed whiskey on my sore gums to ease the pain of a tooth cutting through. This teething biscuit, developed by Joe Garrera, master baker and consultant to more than one gluten-free bakery, is the perfect solution for baby's justifiable bad mood. The secret is letting the biscuit cool and dry thoroughly before baking it a second time. For uniform shape, pipe the dough through a No. 8 pastry bag with no tip.

MAKES 3 DOZEN BISCUITS

1. Preheat oven to 375°F. Line 2 baking sheets with parchment paper.
2. In the bowl of a stand mixer, combine the eggs, vanilla, and vegetable oil on low speed. Add the sugar gradually and mix until the sugar is no longer grainy.
3. In a separate bowl, combine baking mix and baking powder. Add to the egg mixture and beat on low speed until a thick but pipeable batter develops.
4. Pipe through a No. 8 pastry bag with a 1-inch hole (do not use the tip) about 3 inches apart onto the prepared baking sheets.
5. Bake 14 to 16 minutes, or until golden.
6. Cool for 15 to 20 minutes and slice into desired widths.
7. Reduce the oven temperature to 275°F and bake the biscuits another 15 to 20 minutes.
8. Cool completely.
9. Store in the refrigerator in a sealed container, or freeze.

12 large eggs
1 tablespoon vanilla extract
1¾ cups vegetable oil
2 cups sugar
5 cups all-purpose gluten-free baking mix
5 teaspoons baking powder

CORNMEAL PORRIDGE FOR BABY AND ME

Eloise always said, *You have to eat oatmeal, or you'll dry up. Everybody knows that.* This classic children's gluten-free porridge is even better. Dried chopped apricots are optional, depending on the age of the child. This came from the much missed *Gourmet Magazine*.

SERVES 2

2 tablespoons golden raisins
½ cup yellow cornmeal
½ cup cold water plus
  1½ cups boiling water
¼ teaspoon salt
½ cup whole milk or almond,
  rice, or soy milk, plus
  additional to pour into the
  cereal
1 tablespoon unsalted butter,
  halved
8 dried apricots, cut into small
  pieces
Light brown sugar or maple
  syrup

1. In a small bowl, cover the raisins with cold water and let them soak for 10 minutes.
2. In a medium saucepan, whisk together the cornmeal, cold water, and salt until the mixture is smooth.
3. Add the boiling water and the milk in a slow stream, whisking all the time.
4. Cook the mixture over a pan of simmering water, stirring often, for 10 to 15 minutes, or until the liquid is absorbed and the porridge is thickened.
5. Divide the porridge between 2 bowls and top it with the butter, the apricots, and the raisins that have been drained of their water.
6. Serve the porridge with brown sugar and milk.

RICE PUDDING

Mild enough for a child's budding palate, this silky smooth nursery pudding comes from Emmy Award–winning host of *Christina: America's Healthy Cooking Teacher*, Christina Pirello. Nuts are optional, age- and allergy-dependent. A general rule: the smaller the child, the smoother the pudding. From *Christina Cooks*, with thanks to Christina.

4 cups gluten-free vanilla soy
  milk
1 cup almond milk
1 cup arborio rice
⅔ cup maple syrup
1 teaspoon vanilla extract
Generous pinch of sea salt
½ cup currants
¼ teaspoon ground cinnamon,
  plus an extra pinch
½ teaspoon ground
  cardamom
½ teaspoon ground nutmeg
⅛ teaspoon ground allspice
½ cup slivered almonds,
  toasted (optional)
3 tablespoons gluten-free
  granulated sweetener

MAKES 6 TO 8 SERVINGS

1. In a heavy saucepan, combine the soy milk, almond milk, rice, maple syrup, vanilla, and salt. Cook, stirring constantly, until the mixture boils.
2. Stir in the currants, ¼ teaspoon cinnamon, the cardamom, nutmeg, and allspice.
3. Reduce the heat to low and cook, covered, stirring often, until the rice is creamy and the pudding thickens, about 1 hour.

4. Optional step: In a hot skillet over medium heat, place the almonds, a pinch of cinnamon, and the sweetener and pan toast, watching carefully, until the almonds are coated, about 1 to 2 minutes. Transfer to a small bowl to cool and set aside.

5. Spoon the pudding into bowls or dessert cups and sprinkle with the almonds if using.

Into the Mouths of Babes

Ask any mom. Not everything that gets into a toddler's mouth is supposed to be there. To be a child is to be tactile, messy, creative, silly, experimental, and free. Parenting a gluten-free child means knowing everything on sticky, curious fingers and toes eventually ends up on faces and in little mouths and ears. Art supplies like crayons and markers, play dough, and glue need to be safe, nontoxic, gluten-free, *and* fun.

With thanks to Connie Sarros, author of *Wheat-Free, Gluten-Free Cookbook for Kids and Busy Adults* (Contemporary Books), you can make it child's play.

PLAYDATE PLAY DOUGH

Made with lick-your-fingers ingredients, this yummy hand-mixed play dough is good enough to eat and safe for gluten-sensitive tummies. Remember to wash your hands thoroughly before squishing it up.

MAKES 1 QUART

1. In a medium bowl, put the peanut butter, corn syrup, honey, confectioners' sugar, and dry milk.

2. With clean hands, mix the ingredients thoroughly. Do not refrigerate.

3. Keep this yummy play dough in an airtight container for up to 3 days.

1 cup gluten-free peanut butter
¾ cup light corn syrup
¼ cup honey
1¼ cups confectioners' sugar
1¼ cups nonfat dry milk or dry milk substitute

Refrigerator Art Alert

Make sure the art supplies you buy your child are free of common allergens, as well as gluten. All Crayola markers, finger paints, and crayons are gluten-free. Crayola Dough is *not*. Elmer's products are also a safe choice. Go to the company Web site frequently for any changes or alerts. www.crayola.com

BUBBLES

What child doesn't love blowing bubbles? Connie Sarros suggests blowing these with a slotted spoon if you don't have an empty spool.

2 cups warm water
2 tablespoons nontoxic, environmentally friendly dish detergent
1 tablespoon sugar
1 empty thread spool or slotted spoon

MAKES 1 PINT

1. In a bowl, stir together the water, dish detergent, and sugar.
2. Dip one end of the spool into the soapy mixture.
3. Blow bubbles through the spool from the dry end.

BATHTUB PAINT

No more tears at bath time. This toddler-friendly recipe comes courtesy of Elaine Monarch, founder of California's Celiac Disease Foundation. Have a handy sponge or rag for quick cleanups, and by all means involve your bathing beauty. Did Matisse's mother make this for him?

½ cup allergy-free liquid hand soap
1 teaspoon cornstarch
Assorted food coloring
Cloth or sponge for cleanup

MAKES ABOUT 4 ICE TRAY CUBES

1. In a container, mix the soap and cornstarch.
2. Pour into ice cube trays.
3. Let your child put drops of food coloring in each cube and experiment mixing the colors.
4. Play to your heart's content. Use the rag or sponge to clean the walls afterward.

GLUTEN-FREE PAPIER-MÂCHÉ

2 parts gluten-free glue
1 part water

1. Combine the glue and water.
2. Dip paper into the mixture and wipe off any excess.

Language Matters

My friend Louise has been afraid of bananas all her life. As a child, she couldn't digest them properly and got a terrible rash. Instead of telling little Lou bananas weren't inherently bad but just something that didn't agree with her, Louise's parents warned that even one whiff of a banana could kill her. When the dancing Chiquita Banana shimmied across the TV screen, they sang their own jingle: *A banana will kill you in the most horrible way.*

They didn't mean their daughter harm. They just couldn't tell her how afraid they were and made her afraid instead.

Today Louise gives the smoothie counter a wide birth. She considers the idea of a Caribbean vacation with all those plantains and banana trees tantamount to a trip to Dante's inner circle. Her first husband took her to a fancy New Orleans restaurant specializing in Bananas Foster. Let's just say her second never made that mistake.

Louise is an example, albeit extreme, of how presenting a dietary restriction to your child as something to be fearful of can have a lasting affect on the adult he or she becomes

Children are like tofu. They tend to absorb whatever flavor they are exposed to. And they have very big ears. If you are fearful, they will get that and be afraid. If you blame others, they will follow suit. Take responsibility and they will learn to do the same. In other words, your child is an emotional sponge and will feel about his diet what he hears and senses about it from you.

- Respect the offending food and its place in the lives of others without demonizing it.
- Explain that there really are no bad foods, only tummies that have trouble digesting them. Just as there are no bad animals and flowers and trees, only skin and eyes and noses and respiratory systems that are sensitive to them.
- Food isn't the allergy, the allergy is.
- Reinforce the idea that our individual characteristics are what make us special. Like blue eyes, brown skin, freckles, the proclivity to play the piano or tell stories, so too our difficulties with certain foods are as unique as a snowflake.
- Make gluten-free meals a positive experience. A child who grows up seeing his sensitivity to gluten or dairy or peanuts as something foisted upon him by a hostile world is more likely to grow up feeling victimized.
- Children taught to see themselves through the prism of that which makes them special are more likely to grow up honoring this part of themselves.

Perspective is important. One accident does not death by gluten make. This is your fear, not your child's. There's a fine line between teaching a healthy respect for the repercussions and creating a person who's afraid to eat.

Much as you want to, you can't guarantee your child safe passage in a dangerous world. No one can do that. But you can raise a person who's not afraid of it. Take a good look at a child who picks the brightest crayons and boldly colors outside the lines. You'll see a parent willing to do the same.

Why Does Ritchie Get Itchy?

Empathy—the ability to get out of oneself to intuit and attend to the needs of others—is one of the most important life skills a compassionate human being can have. As author Ian McEwan puts it, "Imagining what it is like to be someone else other than oneself is at the core of our humanity."

For a child struggling to fit in, empathy can be the difference between feeling isolated by a special diet and being part of a group of kids who are challenged in different ways. Big or little, it helps to know that others struggle, too.

I venture that if we tossed our troubles into a big pile and exchanged them for someone else's, we'd get to see what our friends and neighbors carry and probably take back our own. This is hard to understand at an age where conformity equals social acceptance.

Explain that Ritchie gets itchy when he's near a peanut and may have to use his EpiPen or that Lizzie gets dizzy from dog dander and can't have a puppy. While Janey may be able to eat pizza and grilled cheese sandwiches, she can't play outside when the pollen count is high.

Some Empathy-Building Activities

+ Make an imaginary pet for the friend who is allergic to cat or dog dander.
+ Invent a passive indoor sport for your child's asthmatic or environmentally sensitive friends to play when the air is unhealthy.
+ Devise an allergy buddy system.
+ Dip dairy-free ice cream on gluten-free cones. Make nut-free gluten-free brownies for your child to take to school.

- Volunteer to make nut-free, dairy-free, and gluten-free pizza for everyone.
- Make sure "no child is left behind." Network with parents of soy-free, casein-free, and chemical-free kids.
- Start an allergy club and create a membership directory with Polaroid pictures.
- Host a special allergy "show and tell."

Teaching a child to see their friends' frailties and watching out for them can go a long way in countering the natural self-absorption that comes with any health issue or lifelong diet. What better antidote to isolation than celebrating everyone's differences?

When you encourage empathy, you are teaching generosity and good manners, the most valuable lessons any parent can impart to a child.

Labels Have a Way of Sticking

As a child in England, my friend James was horribly allergic to cow's milk and wheat. His belly was distended and he was pale and listless. He was a celiac, of course, but no one knew it yet. The only things that didn't make him sick were rice and bananas. Period.

When James was barely a year old, the family attended a church picnic, where everyone in the village brought a covered dish. Children and adults played lawn games and ate their fill. Fearful that little Jimmy would get the wrong food from a well-meaning neighbor, his father fashioned a sign, complete with pictures of little monkeys and bunches of bananas, and hung it around the baby's neck.

To James's everlasting embarrassment, the yellowed photograph of him wearing this sign survives in the family album. A thin child in a diaper and a dopey sun hat sits on a plaid blanket on a patch of grass, solemnly staring into the camera. A sign around his neck bears the words PLEASE DON'T FEED ME, I'VE GOT MY OWN BANANAS.

While it may be tempting, no child, no matter how small, should be turned into a living Post-it note.

- By all means, send your darling off to school with a follow-up note reminding the teacher of his or her special needs, but only after you've made an appointment and explained the problem in person and offered to participate in the solution.

- A private signal between your child and the teacher can save a child a world of embarrassment.
- Ditto for the bathroom monitor.
- Ask the teacher to avoid giving your child undue attention in front of the class.
- Explain to the teacher in adult terms. "You know how it feels when you're trying to lose a few pounds and the waiter shouts, 'Who gets the diet plate?' That's how my child feels."
- Ask that no announcements be made regarding his or her diet.
- Make special place mats for the whole family, not just the gluten-free child.
- Resist the temptation to rush into every lunch, dinner, sleepover, school trip, picnic, party, and snack situation like a gluten-sniffing dog. All you are doing is making things worse.
- You wouldn't say, *Don't give Henry a glass of wine, he's an alcoholic.* The idea is to protect your child, not to humiliate him.

Little People—Big Feelings

Just as adults new to the gluten-free diet may experience a sense of sadness and loss and may be depressed, angry, moody, or just plain ornery, so do children.

Your toddler doesn't have the verbal skills or insight to be able to articulate this, so the feelings take many forms—tantrums, anger, loss of appetite, moodiness, decline in school performance, feigned illnesses, picking fights, tears, and refusing to eat or to play with other children. The reaction may even manifest itself as a cold, fevers, headache, lethargy, and the thing you fear most, eating gluten.

There is a period of mourning for children, too. In our haste to see them get well, we forget that all they want is for things to be the way they were before. If a child is to take responsibility for his diet, he has to know that it's okay to honor the sadness, anger, and loss of control that come with it.

Some Thoughts on Easing the Transition

- Create a safe place for your child to talk about these feelings with no judgment about how they are being expressed.

+ Do not respond with fear or your child will quickly get the message that only feelings that don't scare Mommy and Daddy are okay.
+ Try not to look at the behavior, but attempt to see what's behind it.
+ Remember that difficult children are usually those who are having a difficult time.
+ Repeat after me: *Bad* rhymes with *sad*.
+ Create a chain of understanding and support for your child and include family members, teachers, child care professionals, and physicians.

In the age of kiddy antidepressants and one-size-fits-all behavioral diagnoses, you may be afraid, and justifiably so, of having your child labeled *difficult* and unnecessarily stigmatized. It's easy to want to say nothing and hope for the best when your child is acting out.

The danger in waiting is that the behavior becomes the issue, not the reasons motivating it. Sometimes the best way to protect a child from assumptions is to simply explain to the professionals that it's taking a while for him or her to be okay with a new diet—as it would with anyone, large or small.

A child's tantrum is like watching a summer storm. First comes the boom of thunder, then the crack of lightning, and finally the rain, cleansing and necessary.

Playdates and Other Danger Zones

Hard as it is to believe, there are parents who will not invite your child to a party because making something special is too much work. Worse, there are parents who will break a playdate when they get wind of special requirements. Alas, an increasingly stressful and work-intensive world has made this kind of insensitive behavior more commonplace than we'd like to believe.

Most parents couldn't be more solicitous and will go to great effort to make sure your child feels welcome, but some can be cruel to children whose special needs make their lives difficult.

I would not advise confrontation as a means of getting these parents to include your child in activities or to take his or her requirements seriously. That will make things worse and leave your child feeling friendless and ostracized.

Grace and Good Manners Carry the Day

✦ When your child is invited somewhere, send a friendly e-mail thanking the parent for the invitation and take the opportunity to explain your child's diet. Do this in a way that doesn't make the other mother afraid to host him.

✦ Offer to make something and be available for questions when the menu is being planned.

✦ Volunteer to supply pizza crusts, cupcakes, or other snacks for the party.

✦ Offer to supply foods that can be kept in his or her freezer.

✦ And don't forget nonedibles as described above.

✦ Never ask another a parent to do something that you are not willing to do for his or her child.

✦ Conversely, when your youngster has a new friend over, always ask about his special needs and requirements beforehand.

✦ Share your child's gluten-free foods when the date's at your house. Serve gluten-free pizza, cupcakes, cookies, and snacks. It may cost a bit more, but it's worth it.

✦ Word of mouth travels fast.

Home Plate

Some foods make you fat.
Some foods make you thin.
Some foods taste so good,
They make you want to grin.

Kids love to help in the kitchen.

Not every child is a chef-in-the-making, but by all means teach your child to cook. The more participation, the more fun, and the more fun, the better your chances are of teaching your little one what's safe and delicious to eat, as well as what isn't.

Food writer Mark Bittman agrees. In his column for the *New York Times*, he concedes cooking isn't for everyone, but that children are more likely to develop healthier eating habits if their parents cook. He further opines that "one of the few benefits of food television has been to increase kids' interest in food and even in cooking," and he frequently meets seven- and ten-year-olds who actually spend time in the kitchen.

It must be true. Just the other day, the proud parents of the eight-year-old upstairs told me he'd made them a pretty decent shepherd's pie.

Bittman sings the praises of a new magazine aimed at kids called *Chop-Chop: The Fun Cooking Magazine for Families,* named 2013 Publication of the Year by the James Beard Foundation. I would add that while magazines like *ChopChop*, Alice Waters's classic children's cookbook, *Fanny at Chez Panisse*, and Mollie Katzen's vegetarian cookbook, *Pretend Soup*, will offer some recipes that contain gluten, you are better off adapting them and giving your children a thorough grounding in healthy, farm-to-table foods. For the little ones, there is nothing like *Eloise Breaks Some Eggs*, based on Kay Thompson's Eloise and Hilary Knight's wonderful drawings.

Janet Rinehart, president of the Houston CSA (see Chapter 23, "Community"), offers the following advice:

+ Make sure the recipe you choose is appropriate for the age level of your child.
+ Read the recipe all the way through and make sure you have all the ingredients and equipment on hand, then lay it all out on the counter.
+ Calculate how much time the job will take, including cooling time. Ask yourself if it will be finished for supper.
+ Wash your hands.
+ If you stop in the middle to pet the dog, wash your hands again.
+ Ditto if you are touching raw meat, chicken, eggs, and the like. Remember, you are teaching kitchen hygiene, too.
+ Have towels at the ready—one for wiping up spills, the other for hand washing.
+ Make sure everything is child height. Step stools come in handy here.
+ If the recipe calls for an herb, teach your child to learn its smell. Ditto for cheese. Decide if you like mild, medium, or sharp.
+ Be patient. Perfection isn't the point here.
+ Explain as you go.
+ Don't dominate; be part of the team.
+ Don't yell, even if the potholder catches fire and the dog runs off with a chicken leg.
+ Laugh, clean up the mess, and laugh some more.
+ Remember that the only way to learn is by making mistakes.

NO MORE TUMMY ACHES CUPCAKES WITH RASPBERRY FROSTING

Izzie O'Brien, cupcake lover and heroine of my illustrated children's book, *No More Cupcakes & Tummy Aches*, is sure she'll never grow up if she can't have birthday cake. And if she never grows up, she'll never be tall enough to be a ballerina. What better way to teach that gluten-free is nothing to be sad about than to make cupcakes together.

Created by Chef Lee Tobin, founder of Whole Foods Gluten Free Bakehouse, these girly pink cupcakes are proof that happy endings aren't only found in storybooks. Egg yolks are the secret of their golden yellow color, and raspberry purée gives the icing its pretty pink hue. For those tummies that are lactose-intolerant as well, Chef Tobin offers a dairy-free variation.

MAKES ABOUT A DOZEN CUPCAKES

For the cupcakes:

Nonstick spray or cupcake papers for the muffin tin
1½ cups rice flour
1 cup potato starch
½ cup tapioca starch
1 tablespoon plus 1 teaspoon baking powder
1½ teaspoons xanthan gum
½ teaspoon salt
6 large egg yolks
1 cup milk (or dairy-free soy, rice, or almond milk)
2¼ teaspoons vanilla extract
¾ cup (1½ sticks) unsalted butter, at room temperature (or dairy-free Spectrum shortening)
1½ cups sugar

1. Preheat the oven to 350°F. Spray a 12-cup muffin tin with non-stick spray or line with cupcake papers.
2. In a large bowl, combine the rice flour, potato starch, tapioca starch, baking powder, xanthan gum, and salt. Set aside.
3. In a separate bowl, combine the egg yolks, milk, and vanilla.
4. In the bowl of a stand mixer or in a bowl using a hand mixer, cream the butter with the sugar on medium speed until light and fluffy, 2 to 3 minutes. Add, alternately, the wet and dry ingredients, scraping down the sides of the bowl with a spatula and mixing well to thoroughly combine the ingredients.
5. Fill the cupcake tins two-thirds full and bake for about 25 minutes, or until golden brown and springy to the touch.
6. When cool, remove the cupcakes from the tin and frost.

Raspberry Purée

1 12-ounce bag of frozen raspberries

1. Thaw the contents in a microwave oven.
2. When the berries are completely softened, strain through a fine-mesh sieve to remove the seeds. Extra purée can be frozen for future use.

Raspberry Frosting

1. In the bowl of a stand mixer, combine the confectioners' sugar and the butter on low speed.
2. Scrape down the sides of the bowl with a spatula and add the milk.

3. Continue mixing, adding raspberry purée to taste. (More milk and/or purée can be added for the frosting consistency you prefer.)
4. Frost the cooled cupcakes.
5. Have a party.

They Always Loved You Best: Sibling Rivalry

As a boy, my father was as healthy as a horse. His brother George was allergic to everything. George got the cream. Dad got the milk. George got the nutrient-rich broth. Dad got the pallid remains of the chicken that made it. George was shipped off to an aunt's seaside cottage for his summer vacation, while Dad got to go to tar beach up on the roof.

Daddy grew up to be an athlete who wouldn't think twice about going back into the game with a broken bone. Uncle George grew up afraid to open an umbrella.

Can anyone tell me why these two brothers hated each other?

Sibling rivalry. As Anna Quindlen so eloquently put it, "They are, therefore I am not." When one child is the focus of so much special attention, it's easy for the others to feel slighted. Here are a few ideas for keeping siblings from brooding:

+ Set up a kitchen cabinet or a separate shelf just for the gluten-free sibling. Stock it with everything he needs and likes and put it within easy reach.
+ Set up something equally special for the non-gluten-free sibling.
+ Encourage sharing and don't make gluten-free goodies so sacrosanct that they become an argument one child always wins.
+ Allow your gluten-free child to opt out of family events that are too difficult. A sibling's ice cream and cake birthday can be torture for a child who has to eat something different from the others. Never cancel the event itself. And never make the non-gluten-free child feel guilty for enjoying it. Ask yourself how sad it would be to grow up never having a birthday cake because your sibling couldn't eat it.
+ Find ways to give the others equal attention. If you send one to gluten-free summer camp, arrange an equally wonderful experience for the other.

There is nothing better for a mom or a dad than seeing brother taking care of sister or sister tucking little brother under her wing, reading

1 16-ounce box confectioners' sugar

½ cup (1 stick) unsalted butter, at room temperature (or Spectrum palm oil shortening)

2 tablespoons milk (or use dairy-free soy, almond, or rice milk)

2 to 4 tablespoons Raspberry Purée (recipe above)

labels for him, explaining why he can't eat what others are enjoying. Watching them become friends as they grow, each one separate and unique, not resenting, but respecting and loving each other's differences as much as their similarities—this is what makes empathic parenting worth all the fuss.

Which brings me back to my father and his brother. No mystery why my smart and otherwise generous dad would buy a beach house to which he never invited his brother, or why, for his entire life, he refused to be in the same room with a chicken.

Gluten and Behavior

More and more parents are putting their children on gluten-free diets because of behavioral problems. There are many reasons for hyperactivity, mood swings, depression, and angry outbursts in children, some of them serious enough to warrant medical and psychiatric attention. But just as more and more adults are having a problem with gluten, you've got to wonder if the ever-increasing number of children labeled with mood disorders and in counseling may also be reacting to the toxic effect of gluten in their diets.

In a paper entitled "Celiac Disease Presenting as Autism," published in the *Journal of Child Neurology*, researchers discussed the case of a five-year-old boy with digestive problems and diagnosed with severe autism. When put on the gluten-free diet, the child's digestive problems resolved quickly, along with the symptoms and signs of autism. The study concluded, "All children with neurodevelopmental problems should be assessed for nutritional deficiency and malabsorption syndromes such as celiac disease."

The *Journal of Pediatric Gastroenterology and Nutrition* presented a study supporting a well-known fact that the gut is hardwired to the brain. This one measured the incidence of leaky gut (intestinal lining that has become hyperpermeable, resulting in larger food molecules, yeast, and other toxins the body doesn't normally allow through to get into the blood circulation, leading to inflammation) in children with autism as well as their first-degree relatives and compared them to a normal, unaffected population. Researchers found a much higher percentage of leaky gut, 36.7 percent, in the first group as compared to 4.8 percent in the control subjects, and a high percentage of autistic children presenting with GI problems such as constipation and diarrhea. The study concluded, "Results support the leaky gut hypothesis and indicate that measuring intestinal permeability could help identify a subgroup of patients with autism who could benefit from the gluten-free diet."

Neurologic problems such as anger and depression are well documented in adult gluten intolerance. So why not look for it in children who aren't responding to counseling, medications, or other mood disorder interventions? Kelly Dorfman, author of *Cure Your Child with Food*, says that three or more positive responses to the following questions may suggest gluten intolerance as the reason for your child's behavior problems.

+ Does your child crave or strongly prefer gluten-based foods, such as bread, pasta, cereal, and pizza?
+ Have psychological and/or behavioral strategies to control your child's outbursts been mostly unsuccessful?
+ Do any of your child's immediate family members have gluten sensitivity or celiac disease?
+ Does your child currently have or has he or she in the past had chronic digestive symptoms, such as excessive gas, diarrhea, or stomach pain?
+ Is your child on the small side, despite eating plenty of food?

Neurologist David Perlmutter, in his excellent book *Grain Brain*, cites a virtual epidemic of neurologic disorders not seen in previous generations and tells of treating many young patients diagnosed with neurologic problems like ADHD, developmental delay, learning difficulties, tic disorders, even autism and Tourette's syndrome with a gluten-free diet. He reports improvements in test scores, emotional stability, and concentration. In the case of one toddler, the results were so dramatic that the school nurse who had called the parents to ask if they would consider putting the child on medication and had been refused, called back to thank them for changing their minds and doing so.

There does seem to be a troubling uptick in pediatric neurological problems. Many parents worry that their children are being given medications that may affect their long-term health. Any concerned parent would want to take matters into his or her own hands.

But I would add one strong caveat here. In your eagerness to see the depression lift and the behavior resolve, you don't want to overlook celiac disease and the serious ramifications for your child's future of letting it go undiagnosed.

Test before you toss the gluten. And test again periodically.

Bullying

If you're like me, you may think first grade is all adding, subtracting, show-and-tell, and painting rainbows on craft paper. Here's a shocking statistic:

According to a study published in the *Annals of Allergy, Asthma, and Immunology*, the first ever to look at food bullying, about 35 percent of children over age five with food allergies have been bullied, teased, or harassed. Worse, one-third of parents have no idea what their child is enduring. In grades six through ten, that number goes up to a full 50 percent.

I thought bullying didn't happen until high school, when girls and boys get mean and tribal until their hormones straighten out.

Study coauthor Scott H. Sicherer, MD, professor of pediatrics and researcher at the Jaffe Food Institute at New York's Mount Sinai Hospital, says most of the bullying was verbal, but kids reported having gluten and other allergens thrown and waved at them, and intentionally mixed with their food. Often teachers unwittingly enable bullying by singling out a child as the reason why the class can't have birthday cake or pizza.

Ritu Verma, MD, director of the Center for Celiac Disease at Children's Hospital of Philadelphia (See "Recognizing, Diagnosing, and Managing Celiac Disease in Children," page 410), is no stranger to the subject. As mother of two children growing up with celiac disease, she remembers that when her son Pranav Chugh was in sixth grade, kids pushed a doughnut into his face and teased him so mercilessly about the gluten-free bread in his lunch box that he stopped eating.

Signs of Bullying

+ Your child may appear sad, withdrawn, or anxious.
+ There may be sudden angry outbursts or crying.
+ He or she may experience frequent nightmares and have difficulty sleeping.
+ He or she may avoid social situations.
+ Your child exhibits a sudden lack of interest in school.
+ There is a drop in your child's grades.
+ Your child feigns illness to avoid going to school.
+ Your child has stomachaches and other symptoms of going off the gluten-free diet to try to fit in.

If you suspect bullying, the best thing you can do is to encourage your child to talk by taking a calm and comforting, nonthreatening tone. Outrage or invasive questioning only worsens the situation. The child may worry that you will embarrass him or her further at school, ensuring worse treatment at the hands of the bullies. Reassure your child gently that he or she can tell you anything and that you are here to help. Dr. Verma recommends asking direct questions, such as: Is someone bothering you about your food?

Preventative Measures

+ Discuss your child's gluten-free diet with the school administrator, nurse, dietician, teachers, and cafeteria workers in person and follow up with something in writing.
+ Ask about the school's food allergies policies, emergency action plan, and its bullying prevention plan and how it's being implemented.
+ Prepare an emergency action plan and file it with the school.
+ Give the teacher a book about gluten-free living on your child's grade level to share with the class.
+ Include a letter from your child's pediatrician explaining the medical necessity of the gluten-free diet.
+ Ask the school to send out a letter on official letterhead to inform parents that a food-allergic student is in their child's class.
+ Volunteer to be a room parent or to plan holiday parties.
+ Consider filing an ADA 504 Plan, which requires the school to accommodate your child's diet and is legally enforceable. Under the Americans with Disabilities Act, food allergies are considered an invisible disability because they affect crucial life functions such as eating, breathing, and digestion.

If Your Child Is Bullied

+ Discuss the bullying episode with the school principal, guidance counselor, psychologist, and teacher.
+ Document the incident or incidents—names, dates, and details.
+ Keep a journal of every time you have talked to school administrators about bullying—again, names, dates, and details of the conversation.

✦ Make sure to keep accurate notes on the school's compliance with the procedures spelled out in your 504 plan.

✦ If appropriate action is not taken, write to the school board superintendent and the school board attorney and include all documentation.

Safe@School: 504 Plans

The Americans with Disabilities Act ensures special diet accommodations for students with celiac disease under the National Lunch Program. 504 plans, named for Section 504 of the Rehabilitation Act of 1973, a civil rights law guaranteeing equal opportunity for Americans with disabilities, applies to all institutions receiving federal financial assistance, such as public schools.

504 plans typically accommodate gluten-free cafeteria lunches, but also cover food-related activities such as school parties, field trips, licking of envelopes and stickers, and the handling of gluten-containing materials in art class.

A good plan addresses proper hand washing, cross-contamination issues, staff education, menu review, positive role modeling, peer support, and, just in case, recognizing the signs of a reaction and treating it promptly.

To file a 504 plan, you will need to provide documentation of your child's medical issues. Bear in mind, documentation rules vary from state to state and from one school district to another. To get the process started, a parent or guardian must contact the child's school and request a 504 evaluation. A meeting is then scheduled during which the principal, a counselor, the school nurse, and the teacher determine whether or not the child is eligible. If the child qualifies, the team will draft a plan and subject it to annual review and revision.

Some parents fear the "special needs" label and worry that a 504 plan may unnecessarily stigmatize their children. These are justifiable concerns. On the other hand, experts say, a 504 plan assures continuity should there be a new teacher, new principal, new superintendent, or a move to another school or town. Without it, changes can render verbal agreements invalid. A 504 plan is always in place and any new staff must learn to accommodate the student.

It's a lot to consider.

If you *do* choose a 504 plan, know that the more comprehensive the plan, the safer the child, and the happier the parent. Do some homework.

Learn More

American Celiac Disease Alliance—School Resources Page.
www.americanceliac.org
National Foundation for Celiac Awareness—504 Road Map—Navigating
the School System page. www.celiaccentral.org

Grandma's House

No more stiff Sunday dinners at Grandma's house. These days, grandparents are familiar with childproof locks and the latest toys and games. They have more energy than most parents. They take the kids on cruises, vacations, to the mall, to the beach, and home from school. They arrange playdates at their homes and, in fact, sometimes have to be gently told the parents would like a little time with their child.

These are the grandparents who will do whatever it takes to provide a safe, gluten-free environment. They need guidance from their children on exactly how to do that.

But sometimes grandparents are not so perfect.

GRANDMA IN DENIAL

A distraught mother asked me what she should do about the mother-in-law who deliberately fed her celiac grandchild gluten every chance she got.

"She doesn't believe me," she said. "She thinks I'm a hypochondriac and doesn't want her granddaughter growing up without foods other children eat."

It didn't make sense. Why would a grandparent deliberately set out to hurt a child she claimed to love? Careful listening unearthed some clues. The grandmother claimed her son had no such problems as a child and often referred to her daughter-in-law's allergies. Was it possible that in denying the baby's condition, she was denying the possibility that she may have had a role in it?

I suggested mother and daughter sit down and write Grandma a letter.

Why not tell her that being allergic to gluten isn't any different from Grandpa not being able to have salt, or having asthma or arthritic knees. Be loving and kind.

"It's okay if you gave me celiac disease," the child wrote with her mother's help. "You gave me freckles, too, and your red hair. If it weren't for you I wouldn't have my mommy and daddy and grandpa, too."

A few days later, the mother received a surprise visit from her mother-in-law.

"I'm so sorry," she sobbed. "I was so ashamed that maybe it was something on my side that made her sick. I blamed you instead of helping her."

Sometimes all it takes is love and being told it's okay.

AARON

Take Aaron.

He is the gluten-dairy-sugar-and-junk-food-free vegetarian child of macro-vegan-hyper-allergic-organic-composting parents, that rare and serene toddler who is partial to greens and tofu. He has never had refined sugar.

Enter Aaron's grandparents, steak-mashed-potatoes-bacon-and-eggs people who think raising a vegetarian baby is dangerous. They offer him ice cream, candy, and chocolate milk every chance they get.

"They eat like animals," Aaron's mother tells me.

"They're killing themselves," growls Aaron's dad.

I asked them if they ever served Aaron's grandparents meat. They are horrified.

"I don't drink," I say, "but does that make it all right not to offer a glass of wine to my guests?"

They got the point.

"Maybe if you showed respect for their food choices, they might do the same for you. Besides, would it kill you to cook a free-range chicken or fry an organic egg?"

Aaron's grandparents didn't want to see him sick. They felt judged and made to feel unhealthy, outdated, politically incorrect, irrelevant, and old-fashioned. Conversely, Aaron's parents had no idea they were being rude, self-righteous, rigid, and downright obnoxious. It was their way or the highway. Everybody was playing emotional football with Aaron.

Now Grandma and Grandpa look forward to chicken at their children's house, the hormone-free, free-range organic variety. For their part, they are becoming quite adept at making gluten-free tofu sandwiches for family picnics. The last time I looked, they were keeping a sharp eye on anyone who might inadvertently give little Aaron white sugar.

Scratch below the surface of these stories and you will find guilt, fear of failing, suspicion, and resentment of different ways of parenting—a big dose of the if-it-was-good-enough-for-us syndrome. With the rare sociopathic exception, everybody wants to make gluten-free grandkids safe and happy.

✦ Gather your clan around you and explain the seriousness of the problem.
✦ Offer comments from your child's doctor and pass out copies of articles on pediatric celiac disease, gluten intolerance, and sensitivity.
✦ Teach grandparents the basics of what gluten-free means and where gluten may hide in the supermarket.
✦ Give grandparents a crash course in kitchen hygiene and how to avoid cross-contamination.
✦ Take grandparents shopping for a supply of safe, gluten-free foods for your child's visit. Show them the gluten-free aisle and freezer case to familiarize them with gluten-free labeling and certified products.
✦ Offer to stock a shelf of your child's favorite treats when visiting.
✦ Be willing to teach your child's grandparents everything you know.
✦ If Grandma likes to bake, show her how easy it is to use gluten-free flour blends in her favorite recipes.
✦ Make sure grandparents have safe art supplies on hand, too.
✦ Grandchildren should never feel strain between their parents and grandparents.
✦ If there is some disagreement, disagree and settle it privately.
✦ Under no circumstances should grandparents suggest that a little gluten couldn't hurt.
✦ Drop hints *and* brochures. Disneyland does a great job with gluten-free options.

Boo! Safe Trick-or-Treating

Halloween is a big deal these days.

Put yourself in Spider-Man's tights. You're standing there in your mask and cape, looking like the real deal. The door opens.

You shout, "Trick or treat!"

You hold out your bag and in go all sorts of goodies, only to be confiscated when you get home. You end up with a lousy apple or a lollipop. Is this any way to treat a superhero?

Between gluten, dairy, peanuts, lactose, casein, and cross-contamination fears, Halloween candy is pretty much off-limits for kids with gluten sensitivity and food allergies, mainly because you don't know where it's coming from and many miniature candies have no labels. The whole idea is just plain spooky.

That's no consolation for a butterfly princess and her pals. How do you make sure your child gets a pirate's share of the booty? FoodAllergy .org posts the following tips for safe trick-or-treating:

+ Stock up on gluten-free treats or inexpensive trinkets to trade for any unsafe candies your child may receive. Sorting through the candy together and trading for safe treats and toys helps your child identify dangerous and gluten-free treats.
+ Set a no-eating-while-trick-or-treating rule, so you can check all booty.
+ Toss everything without a label.
+ Bear in mind that mini, fun-size, or bite-size candy may not contain the same ingredients as the full-size version.
+ Before the big night, make up a big batch of your child's favorite gluten-free treats in a sealed bag and pass them around to the neighbors to give to your child. Remember to describe your little pirate or princess so they know which kid to give it to.
+ Better still, make up a name tag in the spirit of the costume. Say pirates and fairies did this to avoid confusion.
+ Remember that the emphasis is on fun, not so much on candy.
+ Start a new tradition by having an uncle or a family friend arrive in costume and transform all unsafe treats into gluten-free ones. Choose someone who's good at sleight of hand, is a bit theatrical, and doesn't mind wearing something silly.
+ Or leave the inedible candies for the Good Witch to collect and leave behind small gifts for the donors.
+ Forget trick-or-treating and have a party, featuring safe and delicious treats instead.
+ If your child is out after dark, don't forget reflective tape (in keeping with her costume, of course).
+ Skin-test any makeup for a reaction before applying.
+ No sharp objects. But you knew that.

Party Themes That Guarantee Attendance

It's competitive out there in toddler land.

One well-known chef asked what kind of party her kids wanted and they said a cocktail party. They and their friends dressed like grown-ups and, even better, acted like them—big lessons here about how we sound to our children. The children sipped juice "cocktails" from martini glasses while grown-ups dressed as waiters tended bar and served the children canapés from trays. Eloise couldn't have done it better.

Why not a Hollywood premiere party?

+ Roll a red carpet down the front walk and let all the kids dress up as their favorite star, movie character, super hero, or animated character.
+ Rent a small klieg light to sweep your front door.
+ Let each parent wear a chauffeur's cap and drive each guest to your house.
+ Interview each child as he or she arrives and film the event for posterity.
+ Keep the fun going inside with prizes for best costume, best imitation, best performance—you get the idea.
+ Go to a trophy shop and buy some cheap Oscar look-a-likes for the prizes.

Why not transform your own house into a haunted tour?

+ Change all the lightbulbs to eerie red or purple.
+ Hang a "body" from the shower nozzle.
+ Put a monster in a closet.
+ Make a tape of something being dragged, a bureau door slamming, a squeaky screen door, spooky voices, and play it as background.
+ Serve "eyeball" soup, wolf's bane, witches' brew. Be advised that dry ice will make a punch bowl smoke.
+ Go to a magic shop and get fake blood, cobwebs, fright wigs, and a disembodied hand to put in the dishwasher or in the bathroom sink.
+ Obviously, this party is not for toddlers prone to nightmares. Bigger kids will love it, though—the gorier, the better.

Whatever the theme, a party puts you in control, start to finish, and no gluten-free gremlin will be the wiser.

FACE PAINT

Halloween goblins, rock stars, superheroes, princesses, and witches—face painting lets pint-size imaginations run wild. Let the kids paint each other or hire a professional to paint them for memorable parties and photo ops. Connie Sarros suggests using an all-purpose gluten-free flour mix for this one.

ENOUGH TO PAINT 1 OR 2 LITTLE FACES

2 teaspoons solid vegetable shortening
5 teaspoons cornstarch
1 teaspoon all-purpose gluten-free flour mix
3 to 4 drops of glycerin (available at pharmacies)
Food coloring

1. Put the shortening, cornstarch, and flour mix on a large dinner plate. Stir with a small spoon to form a smooth paste.
2. Add 3 to 4 drops of glycerin for a creamy texture.
3. The mixture will be an eerie white. Apply as is.
4. If you wish to color your paint, divide the mixture into several small piles on your dish. Stir 2 drops of food coloring into each pile.

Camp Separation Anxiety

For many of us, going to camp and returning year after year is an important part of childhood. We cherish memories of soggy bunks, poison ivy, one-legged races, s'mores, and crushes on counselors. Much as we pretended we missed our parents, we dreaded the day they packed up our moccasins and swimming trophies and drove us home.

Packing a child off to camp is hard enough. Sending one who is gluten-free can be downright terrifying. But thanks to the many gluten-free groups and associations that organize such things, it is now entirely possible to feel just as guilty sending your gluten-free darling off to a few weeks of marshmallows on a stick as any other parent.

While the gluten-free diet is a life-changer for kids, so is finding a new gang of gluten-free friends who know the ropes. Some gluten-free camps run for only a few days, others much longer. Some are exclusively gluten-free. Others include non-gluten-free kids. Age ranges vary. No matter, they fill up quickly.

Celiac Disease Foundation. Offers camperships to gluten-free camps all over the country. www.celiac.org

CALIFORNIA
Camp Celiac, Livermore. www.celiaccamp.com

GEORGIA

Camp Weekaneatit, Warm Springs. www.glutenfreecamp.org

INDIANA

Camp Gluten Freedom, Indianapolis. www.glutenfreelivingnow.org

MICHIGAN

Camp Westminster/Free to Be Camp, Roscommon.
    www.campwestminster.com/summer-camp/food-allergies
Celiac Support Association Gluten Free Camp at Manitou-Lin in
    Middleville. www.csaceliacs.info/camps.jsp
Habonim Dror Camp Tavor, Three Rivers. www.camptavor.org

MINNESOTA

Gluten Detectives Camp, Bloomington. www.celiaccenterofminnesota.org
Gluten-Free Fun Camp, Annandale. www.twincitiesrock.org/camp

NEW YORK

Camp Eagle Hill, Elizaville. www.campeaglehill.com

NORTH CAROLINA

Gluten Intolerance Group Kids Camp East, Camp Kanata, Wake Forest.
    www.gluten.net/programs/social-programs/gig-kids/kids-camp

PENNSYLVANIA

Emma Kaufmann Camp, Pittsburgh. www.emmakaufmanncamp.com
International Sports Training Camp, Stroudsburg.
    www.international-sports.com
NJY Camps, Milford. www.njycamps.org

RHODE ISLAND

CSA Camp Aldersgate, North Scituate. www.csaceliacs.info/camps.jsp

TEXAS

The Great Gluten Escape Camp, Gilmer. www.campgilmont.org/gge

UTAH

FCYD Camp, West Jordan. www.fcydcamputada.org

WASHINGTON

Gluten Intolerance Group Kids Camp West, Camp Sealth, Vashon Island. www.gluten.net/programs/social-programs/gig-kids/kids-camp

WEST VIRGINIA

Emma Kaufmann Camp, Morgantown. www.emmakaufmanncamp.com

Food for Thought: The Myth of Perfection

Maybe you drank a cup of coffee or enjoyed a glass of wine during pregnancy. You forgot to play Chopin piano concertos or read Shakespeare's sonnets to her in utero, dooming your darling to zero artistic ability. And there was that time you let a phone call interrupt his dissertation on *Captain Underpants*, cutting short a career on the stage.

We are smart, rational people, and yet we think that if we find the perfect gluten-free cookie or brownie and the store stops carrying it, our child will never have another as good. If we can't find the perfect flour blend for the artisanal, allergen-free birthday cake we want to bake, our toddler's party will be a disaster and our children will have no friends and their parents will doubt our skills. We remember that time we fell short and forgot to supply the gluten-free cupcake when all the other kids got one—and see it as the pivotal preschool moment from which every disappointment can be traced.

We tell ourselves a story about the kind of parent we should be. Then we try to live up to it. We chase down an ideal that doesn't exist.

This is the myth of perfection.

As much as we want it to, life doesn't give out gluten-free cookies every day. Nor should everyone get a trophy at kick ball. Or get a standing ovation at show-and-tell. Entitlement is not the lesson we want to impart. Hard as you work to make it otherwise, some days being gluten-free means your child may miss out on something.

Not getting what they want all the time is how our children learn equanimity and gratitude. Accepting the occasional disappointment is how they are not crushed by it.

"Losing Is Good for You," an article in the *New York Times* by Carol Dweck, a psychology professor at Stanford University, bears this out. Kids, she says, respond positively to praise; but after hearing they are talented, smart, and so on, they collapse at the first experience of difficulty. Demoralized by their failure, they say they'd rather cheat than risk failing again.

But they are so little, and their needs are so large. You want to kiss away their tears. You want to believe it is within your power to make everything right all of the time. And if you fail just once, it negates all of the times you didn't. Perfection allows no room for balance. And balance is not a zero-sum game.

Some days we coast along in the zone. Others are a struggle from the second we open our eyes. Why, we ask, when we've learned all the rules of parenting a child with a dietary restriction, shouldn't every day be like the one before?

Parenting well and with intention is not a sprint; it's a long-distance race. The goal is not to allow oneself to be driven by an unrealistic need to be perfect but to remain, cliché that it is, connected to what matters most— friends, family, being part of a circle unbroken by special requirements.

When we have balance, we know our successes can't be canceled by the inevitable setbacks, only made stronger by them. When we let go of our all-or-nothing approach, we discover what we haven't been looking for. Instead of clinging to the idea that there is one cereal our child *must* have, a lunch box treat that will make him feel part of the class, one way only to throw a pizza party, we discover our ability to improvise. We find something so good, we can't believe it was our second choice.

Of course, you are going to protect your child from gluten in any form. You are going to work hard to keep day care workers, teachers, dieticians, and other parents informed and on your child's side. A good parent keeps her child from danger, no matter the cost. One crumb or a stray peanut may as well be a bullet. We are human shields.

But we can't keep them from disappointment, nor should we try.

It may sound corny, but difficulty is what creates character, stiffens the spine. It's what allows them to grow into flexible, inventive, and realistic adults, and it is often the motivation for real achievement. It's what sweetens the triumph when it comes. How can we keep our children from that?

Here's the catch. If we want our kids to be well-adjusted adults who see disappointment as opportunity, we have to see it that way ourselves.

Most agree that a happy childhood is not one or two experiences we can point to. It accumulates. We look back and see we were given permission to fail as well as to succeed. We were loved unconditionally, but not to the exclusion of others. We were attended to, listened to, and taken seriously. And for a brief time, we floated in a cocoon of total safety. I don't know anyone whose happy childhood involved perfect parents.

It's Okay

- ✦ To make eggs for dinner when you're too tired to cook anything else.
- ✦ To stay in your pajamas until lunchtime.
- ✦ To cancel a playdate because you're too tired to get her there.
- ✦ To blow off homework until after a walk in the park.
- ✦ To buy something for the bake sale and pretend you made it.
- ✦ To let him stay up late because you got home from work late and wanted to play.
- ✦ To fib about the time to get her to go to sleep early.
- ✦ To create a diversion while you talk on the phone, check your e-mail, answer a text.
- ✦ To make up a fast ending to a bedtime story because you want to go to bed, too.

When I was a child, my mother and I walked in freshly fallen snow the moment it stopped falling, no matter what time that was, even two in the morning. She'd wake me up, bundle me into my snowsuit, and take me into a world that was ours alone.

This is one of the most vivid memories I have of her—muffled sound, crystalline white, softly swirling flakes, just the two of us wrapped in a warm baffle of sweaters, gleeful in our abridgement of the rules.

How delicious it was to know my father was sleeping soundly, unaware of our adventure.

Nobody else's mother did that.

I asked her once who taught her how to play.

"You," she said.

I think this is what happens when we don't try so hard to be what we think the perfect parent should be. And just be.

Learn More

Department of Health and Human Services. www.stopbullying.gov
Allergic Child. www.home.allergicchild.com
American Academy of Allergy, Asthma, and Immunology. www.aaaai.org

American Academy of Pediatrics—Physician Referrals. www.aap.org

FAAN—Food Allergy Action Plans. www.foodallergy.org

Family Food Allergy Action Plans. www.allergykids.com

Feingold Association of the United States—Information regarding the
    role of foods and synthetic additives in behavior, learning, and
    health problems. www.feingold.org

FARE Food Allergy Research and Education. www.foodallergy.org

Food Allergy Initiative. www.faiusa.org

SUPPORT, PARENTS' NETWORKING, KIDS' GROUPS

Allergy Moms. www.allergymoms.com

Anaphylaxis and Food Allergy Association of Minnesota.
    www.minnesotafoodallergy.org

Autism Speaks. www.autismspeaks.org

Autism Spectrum Disorder Foundation. www.myasdf.org

Celiac Disease Foundation. www.celiac.org

Celiac Disease Foundation Kids Korner and Teens and Young Adults
    For information (818) 716-1513 or use contact format www.celiac.org

Celiac Support Association. www.csaceliacs.info

Celiac Support Association Cel-Kids Network.
    www.csaceliacs.info/children.jsp

Gluten Intolerance Group. www.gluten.net

Kids with Food Allergies. www.kidswithfoodallergies.org

MOCHA (Mothers of Children Having Allergies). www.mochallergies.org

National Foundation for Celiac Awareness Kids Central.
    www.celiaccentral.org/kids/home

NC FACES. www.ncfaces.org

Parents of Allergic Kids. blog.pakcharlotte.org

Raising Our Celiac Kids. www.celiac.com

Teens Living with Celiac Foundation. www.teenslivingwithceliac.org

GLUTEN-FREE ART SUPPLIES

Crayola. www.crayola.com

Elmer's Glues. www.elmers.com

COMMUNITY/BLOGS

The Edible Schoolyard Project—Alice Waters's food foundation for
    children funds school programs, organic community gardening,
    lessons on sustainability. www.edibleschoolyard.org

Food Farm Health—Perspective from a mom, aspiring farmer, and real-food advocate. www.shanonhilton.blogspot.com

Gluten Freek by Gluten-Free Mama. www.glutenfreeguy.com

Gluten-Free Vegan Mom. www.glutenfreeveganmom.com

Kids with Food Allergies Community. www.kidswithfoodallergies.org

Kim's Welcoming Kitchen. www.welcomingkitchen.com

Raising Jack with Celiac. www.raisingjackwithceliac.blogspot.com

BOOKS

Cure Your Child with Food: The Hidden Connection Between Nutrition and Childhood Ailments by Kelly Dorfman (Workman)

Eloise Breaks Some Eggs, based on Kay Thompson's Eloise and Hilary Knight's drawings (Ready-to-Read)

Fanny at Chez Panisse by Alice Waters (William Morrow Cookbooks)

The Kitchen Classroom: 32 Visual GFCF Recipes to Boost Developmental Skills by Gabrielle Kaplan-Mayer (Woodbine House)

No More Cupcakes & Tummy Aches by Jax Peters Lowell, illustrated by Jane Kirkwood, foreword by Alessio Fasano, MD

Pretend Soup and Other Real Recipes: A Cookbook for Preschoolers and Up by Mollie Katzen and Ann L. Henderson (Tricycle Press)

Wheat-Free, Gluten-Free Cookbook for Kids and Busy Adults, 2nd ed., by Connie Sarros (McGraw-Hill)

The Unhealthy Truth: How Our Food Is Making Us Sick and What We Can Do About It by Robyn O'Brien (Broadway Books), for kids who need help with sensory integration, motor, language, communication, and attention skills

MAGAZINES

Autism Parenting Magazine. www.autismparenting.com

Autism Speaks—magazines and newsletters. www.autismspeaks.org

ChopChop magazine—Cooking with kids. www.chopchopmag.org

Gluten-Free Living. www.glutenfreeliving.com

Kids Magazine for Autistic Children. www.autismlovetoknow.com

Living Without magazine. www.livingwithout.com

Simply Gluten-Free. www.simplygluten-free.com

Part V

Medical Matters

19

The Seven-Year Itch and Other Associated Conditions

*The foot bone's connected to the leg bone,
the leg bone's connected to the knee bone . . .*
—JAMES WELDON JOHNSON, "DEM BONES"

- ◆ A Cautionary Tale
- ◆ Dermatitis Herpetiformis
- ◆ Asthma
- ◆ Osteoporosis
- ◆ Osteomalacia
- ◆ Addison's Disease
- ◆ Systemic Lupus Erythematosus (SLE)
- ◆ Sjögren's Syndrome
- ◆ Rheumatoid Arthritis
- ◆ Diabetes Mellitus
- ◆ Thyroid Disease
- ◆ Lymphoma
- ◆ A Short List of Celiac Disease Symptoms
- ◆ Associations, Information, and Support

Every day gluten-free bulletin boards and chat sites buzz with questions.

I'm tired all the time.

I have a rash across my nose and cheeks.

Has anyone else experienced a gluten reaction like this?

My bones ache. Could there be gluten in my calcium supplements?

One person complains of weight gain and is sure she's getting microscopic bits of gluten in her breakfast smoothie. Another believes gluten is responsible for her swollen joints, as well as for the debilitating fatigue holding her hostage. Bellies bloat, bones ache, eyes sting, energy levels lag, joints hurt, skin erupts and blisters, glands swell, mouths ulcerate, hearts pound, and brains fog over. While it's true that gluten causes a long list of problems, it isn't always the culprit.

The simple fact is that celiac disease is an autoimmune condition and, as such, predisposes us to other autoimmune conditions, diseases, and syndromes, many quite difficult to diagnose, even by the experts.

To make matters more complicated, those of you who avoid gluten without benefit of formal testing may also be dealing with an associated condition you do not yet know you have. It's not uncommon to hear of diabetes or lupus or dermatitis or even infertility preceding by several years a diagnosis of a problem with gluten. It's important to know the symptoms and signs of these associated conditions, some of which develop over months and sometimes years, often insidious and silent.

It's crucial to know what kind of specialist to seek and what kinds of tests to expect. It can be tricky getting to the right person in the age of managed—or should I say *mis*managed—care, but if you arm yourself with knowledge about whom you need to see and why, if you are able to present your symptoms in the context of how they relate to gluten intolerance, and if you insist on it, you've got a better shot at a referral.

As with all conditions, the earlier you get a diagnosis and begin treatment, the better.

Still, gluten can be protean in the mayhem it can cause. It can defy the most educated patient. Even the best doctors may have trouble connecting the dots.

A Cautionary Tale

In the late nineties I found myself in the middle of JFK Boulevard, a green light ticking off the seconds to red. I should have been sprinting, channeling the aggressive New York pedestrian gene that has never failed me, even after all these years in Philadelphia. But my legs felt heavy, alien. There was pain in my upper back at the sharp edge of each breath.

I asked my doctor why a gym-going tennis player in great shape suddenly felt like she was walking through molasses.

"On a scale of one to ten, what is your stress level?" he asked.

"A hundred and thirty-seven," I said.

I was working too hard, doing too much. I'd just completed two manuscripts due the same day to different publishers, all the while being a good and dutiful daughter to ailing parents. My husband had had a heart attack that year. I was sure I was suffering from exhaustion, the mysterious illness of Hollywood starlets. Maybe all I needed was to buy a pair of Ray-Bans and go into seclusion. I wondered if I had rickets like the child laborers in Upton Sinclair's books.

The word *autoimmune* rose in the stagnant air of the examining room. Celiac disease lurked in the background like a suspect the police were not finished questioning. Its associates—the pancreas, thyroid, liver, and kidneys—were fingerprinted, microscopic bits of my lungs explored. Knees, elbows, wrists, hips, and other moving parts were palpated and measured for inflammation. My blood was screened for parasites and antinuclear antibodies, telltale signs of a besieged immune system attacking itself. At one point, my carotid arteries came under scrutiny; beriberi considered, lupus discussed, and, inevitably, the dreaded amyotrophic lateral sclerosis (ALS) that killed my father.

Soon, the walk from the front door to the curb left me winded. I had become a world-class napper.

I found myself in the electromyography lab, where *velocity* is the operative word in the world of the nervous system. How fast were messages being sent along nerve sheaths, axons, and neurons? A breakdown along the telephone poles that tell muscles to move and twitch could account for drooping eyelids and eyebrows, blurry vision, feet that slap on the sidewalk, spoons clattering into the sink, and legs that give out on JFK Boulevard.

I was tested for ALS and myasthenia gravis, which involves electric shocks and the sticking of thin and very sharp needles into my legs and hands and the delicate flesh of my upper arms, during which I composed a letter to the surgeon general demanding that American medical practice conform to the rules of the Geneva Convention.

To my everlasting relief, I did not have my father's disease. But neither did I have a diagnosis.

In a dream, the ghost of my grandmother stood on the porch of our old family cottage, her thin white hair, poker straight, the hated walker parked on the summer rug like a taxicab with the meter running.

"It's time you showed up," she said.

I wanted to ask her what it was like to be dead, and if she still missed us, but she led me down the hallway to my parents' bedroom, egging me on with a knuckle in my back. A small raised area, no bigger than a fist, pulsed under the bedspread.

She drew back the cover.

A human heart, more like a piece of liver than a valentine, wet and shining with dark blood, its circumference a maze of arteries and vessels feeding the chambers, valves opening and closing with a sticky *bump-squish*, beat like a pneumatic pump where my father once curled into my mother like a contented snail.

She gave me a crooked look.

Do I have to tell you everything?

The room filled with fragrance, heavy and sweet; underneath it; the fishy smell of a beached sea creature. It seemed to sense my presence and propelled itself across the spread toward my hand.

Just as it reached me, the bubble of the dream popped.

"I think it's my heart," I told my husband the next morning.

"How can you be sure?"

"I dreamt of Nana and she showed me."

This is a man who takes the subconscious as seriously as a diagnosis from Sloan Kettering.

"We'd better find a good cardiologist," he said.

Things happened fast after this.

EKG, normal, echocardiogram, not so much. An angiogram was scheduled in which a catheter with a little camera snaked up to my heart from the femoral artery. It was looking for occlusions, clots, structural anomalies, blockages, abnormal blood flow, problems within the heart muscle itself.

My arteries were whistle clean, but there was muscle damage, evidence of previous myocardial infarction, MI in the medical lingo. I can't imagine when I had a heart attack and didn't know it, but there was that time in Washington Square when I felt squeezing in my back and the pain went straight to my jaw. Why didn't I go to the emergency room? I'm a woman. I sat on a bench and drank a bottle of water.

The doctor's tone was somber as he delivered the news. *Cardiomyopathy of unknown origin.*

I was put on a calcium channel blocker, which slows down the heart's workload and is just fine if you don't mind sleeping all day and not being able to compose a coherent English sentence. I can tolerate pretty much anything except not being able to write. After three months, I discontinued the medicine. The doctor did not argue, but I could tell he thought I was crazy.

I became one of those people you have to tiptoe around, avoid upsetting. For the first time I thought about dying.

A year later, another catheterization revealed an even weaker heart, as did a biopsy during which Janis Joplin's "Take Another Little Piece of My Heart" blared. The following spring, a third catheterization showed even more damage.

"So, what's the deal? Do I keep getting worse and, at some point in the not-too-distant future, drop dead?"

"I wouldn't put it that way," my cardiologist said, "but you're young and a good candidate. If I were you, I'd think about getting on the waiting list for a new heart."

He couldn't point to a cause, an infection, a virus, a congenital condition, a fluky valve, an occluded artery, electrical storms, something, anything. He scoffed at the idea that this was in some way related to *food allergy*, as he characterized it.

I'm not a person who gives up.

The first thing you notice when you fly into Rochester, Minnesota, are the private jets from Jordan, Dubai, Saudi Arabia, and the Arab Emirates lined up on the tarmac. For all the acrimony and mistrust, Middle Easterners sure know where to go in an emergency. I'm told the Mayo Clinic draws the richest, most powerful, and most desperate patients in the world. Thanks to Dr. Joseph Murray, a world-renowned expert on celiac disease, who had agreed to conduct my investigation, I was one of them.

As the hotel shuttle approached the clinics with its new load of pilgrims, I was struck by neat lawns, wide porches—the scrubbed normalcy of the place. There is an understated, almost prim, sense of money here, and I wonder if this is because sensible Norwegian people settled the area or because it's unseemly to advertise gains gotten from sickness. No Kiwanis Club sign, WELCOME SICK-O's. No bar and grill called the Final Opinion.

We passed Gift of Life Transplant House, a gracious Georgian colonial with long windows and serene gardens. I imagined sitting in its sunny day room scouring the papers for news of a train wreck, or a twelve-car pileup, hoping the young Minneapolis mother struck down by a bus was A-negative. I pondered the etiquette of thanking the grieving family for their loved one's heart and considered the difference between living and just being alive.

Dr. Murray ordered all the usual and not-so-usual tests and in short order ruled out active celiac disease and other GI problems.

Lung experts found my respiratory muscles weak and were not convinced it wasn't ALS. They ordered another round of electric shocks and needles, this time between exquisitely tender ribs. Just when I was sure I had the family curse, the word *asthma* was breathed into the air. I was given my own oxygen/blood gas machine in a sleek silver case that made me feel like Faye Dunaway in *The Thomas Crown Affair*.

Rheumatologists plunged my hands into ice gloves and stuck them in a humid little terrarium, which measured the ability of capillaries to expand and contract during extremes of temperature. My red, white, and blue fingertips told them I had Raynaud's, a constriction of these tiny vessels. After that, another doctor got another bright idea and I began to fully grasp the meaning of being thoroughly investigated.

When she heard I was going to the Mayo Clinic, my friend Cordelia took off the small dented gold cross she is never without and fastened it around my neck. She did not offer details but inferred that this little bit of gold had powerful magic.

By week four, I've got asthma and Raynaud's, but only theories about my heart. They suspect I have Prinzmetal's angina, which causes the artery that feeds the heart to constrict, cut off the supply of oxygen-rich blood, and trigger myocardial damage. Enough of these little heart attacks and the heart muscle eventually weakens and dies.

My angiogram would be done by a German cardiologist, one of the world's experts on this problem. At a certain point, ergometrine or ergonovine would be injected into my heart. This would or would not cause a spasm and prove or disprove the theory.

I remember lying on a table in a cold room wearing nothing but a thin gown and Cordelia's cross taped to my chest. The doctor entered the room and, with a brusque explanation, opened the femoral artery. In seconds, the wire was in and snaking up to my heart, snapping photos along the way. It wasn't so bad and I relaxed a little.

Suddenly, I couldn't swallow.

I don't mean that funny feeling at the back of your throat. *I really couldn't swallow.* There was a searing pain in my chest; a squeezing that literally took my breath away. I gulped for air. Panic ran though my arms, legs, neck. The nurses urged me to hang on, told me I'd be okay. They worked fast and none too gently. The doctor barked orders, and he, too, was rough.

I wanted to say, *You're hurting me*, but I couldn't talk. Mixed with the pain was terror; I still couldn't breathe. There was a moment, clichéd as it sounds, that I saw a body attached to monitors, swaddled in blankets, and surrounded by people, a cross taped to its chest, and thought *No, that can't be me.*

I woke up in St. Mary's Hospital. My mouth was cottony and I had the beginnings of a hematoma that would eventually go from hip to hip and interfere with walking. I wanted to go home.

The famous cardiologist walked in and perched on the edge of my bed.

"You must have an angel on your shoulder," he said. "If I'd given you ergonovine, I don't think I would have gotten you back.

"Seconds before the injection, you had a massive spontaneous spasm, which took one hundred milligrams of nitroglycerine injected directly into your heart to stop. In other words, you had a heart attack. If you'd had that ergonovine, I doubt very much I would have gotten you back."

"After all that, you don't know what's wrong with me?"

"I don't need ergonovine to tell me you have Prinzmetal's angina," he said. "You showed me yourself."

Not much is known about this condition that causes the involuntary contractions of the arteries of the heart. Extremes of temperature can trigger it, as can fear, emotion, a heavy meal, a broken heart, too much work. I am convinced it is related to celiac disease, but medical science is not interested in patient opinions, not even from someone who is good at teasing narrative threads.

I was given nitroglycerin patches, Cardizem, a calcium channel blocker that wouldn't interfere with creativity, baby aspirin, some L-arginine to keep the vessels warm, and a prescription for cardiopulmonary rehab. I was told to go to the ER every time I got the squeezing in the back that is my heart's odd way of telling me it's in trouble.

At home I took morning walks, meditated, wore my heart monitor, and learned exactly how long I could get away with wearing my nitro patch before the headache kicked in.

I returned Cordelia's cross and, with it, another story for its legend.

I swore off sugar, fat, and processed food and started back up the steep cliff that is reconditioning.

That was almost ten years ago.

I no longer wear nitroglycerin patches, no longer get breathless crossing streets, no longer use my asthma inhaler. I am able to hike long distances, lift weights, write books, play tennis. I have torn up my frequent visitor card for the ER.

How did that happen?

Maybe I wasn't so far off thinking I had rickets. The nervous system requires calcium for smooth functioning. Vitamin D is necessary for calcium absorption. As a celiac, I do not properly absorb these vital nutrients. After a bout of achy hip pain, I booked an appointment with an endocrinologist who discovered I had dangerously low levels of vitamin D. Perhaps all of those stressful months indoors and at the computer depleted whatever little reserves I had left. With no vitamin D to help calcium get into my body, my body's computer malfunctioned.

Doctors insist there is no known cause of Prinzmetal's angina.

I think it was malabsorption caused by celiac disease informed by a perfect storm of external stress. I know because I take a large, prescription dose of vitamin D weekly (along with magnesium and calcium) and haven't had a spasm since. Nor have I had an asthma attack or red, white, and blue fingers. I think coronary artery spasm, asthma, and possibly Raynaud's were due, in my case, to compromised absorption of those minerals and vitamins that ensure the smooth running of my involuntary nervous system.

WHY HAVE I TOLD YOU MY STORY?

Reason #1: Never give up, even if your doctor does. No matter what.

Reason #2: If there is a more compelling argument for getting tested for celiac disease before going gluten-free, I don't know what it is.

Many of you say you feel horrible when you eat gluten, so why not skip the ordeal of having to eat a lot of it for the tests and just follow the gluten-free diet? It sounds good on the surface, but as Dr. Peter Green, director of the Columbia Celiac Center in New York, says, "It should be shouted from the rooftops that early diagnosis is protective."

Knowing we have an autoimmune response to gluten and therefore increased chances of developing an associated autoimmune condition can help us avert an even greater health disaster. It's that simple.

Getting tested is essential.

Not everyone is as stubborn as I am, as assertive with professionals, or as good at plowing through complicated information. I am not a doctor, nor am I an expert on any of these conditions. I am not suggesting you will develop any of the problems described in this chapter or experience anything like what happened to me. My purpose here is to provide a quick profile of each of the conditions related to celiac disease and possibly other forms of gluten intolerance.

It's important to know who to see, what tests to expect, and how and where to turn for more information and support. In the increasingly narrow world of health care choices, specialized medicine, and overworked and overscheduled doctors, it's dogged, pit-bull-on-your-pant-leg tenacity that gets the job done. Patient knowledge has never been more crucial to seeing the whole picture and getting a good diagnosis.

Here, from my faithful *Merck* and other professional sources, and with guidance from the medical experts who reviewed the following sections, I've done a bit of the homework for you.

Let's start with the "Seven-Year Itch."

Dermatitis Herpetiformis

DH, as it is commonly called, is an intensely itchy, blistering, burning skin rash that is, literally, one of the skin's reactions to gluten. It has driven more than one celiac to distraction. When a person with celiac disease consumes gluten, says the National Institutes of Health, the mucosal immune system in the intestine responds by producing a type of antibody called immunoglobulin A (IgA). This enters the bloodstream and deposits in the skin, triggering further inflammation that results in the blistering rash of DH. According to Dr. John Zone, professor of dermatology at the University of Utah, virtually all DH patients have celiac disease or gluten intolerance.

DH usually starts off gradually. Tiny red bumps appear across the elbows, knees, back, buttocks, and scalp with tiny blisters on the surface of the lesions. There is burning. And itching. Incessant scratching often causes the blisters to open and crust over, obscuring the original outbreak and creating new injury.

Dermatitis herpetiformis is often mistaken for eczema, psoriasis, and various other forms of dermatitis, which is why it's important to find a dermatologist who is familiar with the condition and its relationship to celiac disease. Help the dermatologist connect the dots—or the bumps, in this case. Provide a context for suspicion by informing the doctor that there is, or may be, celiac disease or gluten intolerance lurking in the background.

After examining the lesions, the dermatologist most likely will ask permission to take a small specimen for biopsy, usually from an area near the outbreak but not directly on it. After freezing the area, the tissue will be sent to a lab to be examined for antibodies within the skin, specifically IgA granules, which are diagnostic of DH.

It is critical for the lab your doctor uses to be familiar with DH. Specimen kits are available to patients and their doctors from the University of Utah's Immunodermatology Laboratory, which specializes in DH.

Often strict adherence to the gluten-free diet is enough to keep DH under control. In some cases, a drug like dapsone or sulfapyridine is given to relieve the itch. It's important to know that these medications come with potentially serious side effects—including liver damage, kidney stones, and lowering of white and red blood cell counts with long-term use. If you are given one of these drugs, expect to be asked to have a CBC (complete blood count) and liver functioning tests done from time to time in order to monitor organ functioning. If you are not asked to have this blood work done, it would be wise to request it.

If dapsone and sulfapyradine are used correctly and monitored by a physician who is on the lookout for side effects, and used in concert with the gluten-free diet, they can produce complete improvement of the skin symptoms in greater than 90 percent of patients; however, they will effect no improvements on the surface of the intestine skin.

Many DH patients avoid drugs altogether and use over-the-counter and home remedies to soothe the itch. One person I know wears gloves to bed in order to minimize the damage from scratching. Others take long baths followed by a thick slather of a rich skin cream such as Cetaphil, Eucerin, Neutrogena, or Bag Balm. Some swear by bath oils in lukewarm water, or use Aveeno oatmeal soaks, Epsom salts, and gentle salt scrubs, and many use mild body washes instead of soap. A few people report that drinking plenty of water, taking omega-3 fatty acids, and taking flaxseed oil all help. Still others are convinced that humidifiers and various anti-itch gels, including old-fashioned calamine lotion, do the trick.

The point is: What works for one person may not work for another.

If you're reading this, you already know you can't tolerate gluten, but I would advise sharing this with any relatives who might be at risk for celiac disease and who complain of intense itching and ugly, blistered skin. DH, I am told, often appears in the absence of gastrointestinal symptoms.

Leading Specialist in Dermatitis Herpetiformis:

John J. Zone, MD
Chair, Department of Dermatology
University of Utah Health Care
50 North Medical Drive
Salt Lake City, UT 84132
(801) 581-2955

For other doctors specializing in dermatitis herpetiformis, contact:

American Academy of Dermatology
P.O. Box 4014
Schaumberg, IL 60168
(886) 503-7546
International: (847) 240-1280
www.aad.org

For specimen kits and skin testing information:

Immunodermatology Laboratory
University of Utah/Health Sciences Center
4A330 School of Medicine
30 North 1900 East
Salt Lake City, UT 84132
(866) 266-5699
E-mail: immunoderm@hsc.utah.edu
www.healthcare.utah.edu/dermatology

Asthma

Once upon a time, doctors thought there was little connection between asthma and celiac disease. But according to a 2011 Swedish study published in the *Journal of Allergy and Clinical Immunology*, people with gluten intolerance are 60 percent more likely to develop asthma than those not affected by gluten. The study showed that for every 100,000 people with celiac disease, 147 will have asthma that would not have occurred in the absence of the digestive disorder. Conversely, those with asthma are more likely to develop celiac disease. In an article written by Jefferson Adams for Celiac.com, Dr. Jonas Ludvigsson, lead researcher in the study, says, "The association between these two diseases is unclear, but the role of Vitamin D should be stressed. If a person with CD also has low levels of D, this could affect the immune system, which could increase the risk of asthma." Another possibility Ludvigsson told Celiac.com, "is that asthma and celiac disease share some immunological features. If you have it, you are at increased risk of both diseases."

Talk about an *Aha!* moment. Fifteen years after my own brush with asthma, I feel vindicated by science. Most likely the culprit *was* vitamin D. Not only did my airways narrow; the tiny capillaries in my fingers and my coronary arteries did, too.

If you've ever had an asthma attack, you're not likely to forget it.

According to the Mayo Clinic, asthma is a condition in which your airways constrict and swell and produce extra mucus. This can make breathing difficult and trigger coughing, wheezing, and shortness of breath. For some, asthma is a minor nuisance. For others, it can be a life-threatening event.

Some signs of an impending attack are increasing difficulty getting a breath, chest tightness, and pain, and a wheezing or whistling sound caused by narrowing airways and often made worse by colds, congestion, and upper respiratory infections. Please note: some people do not wheeze or are not aware of wheezing and mistake asthma symptoms for cardiac problems.

Asthma can be induced by exercise, especially when the air is cold and dry. Workplace irritants, such as chemical fumes, paint, gases, dust, and, most commonly, air-conditioning and heating vents and poorly circulated air, can cause occupational asthma. Allergy-induced asthma is triggered by particular allergens, such as pet dander, tree pollen, grass, roses, cockroaches, cigarette smoke, fragrances, and sulfites in wine and other products. A severe asthma attack that does not respond to or is not eased by using a rescue inhaler warrants a trip to the emergency room.

If you think you are suffering from asthma, a specialist in pulmonary medicine is the person to see. A complete medical history will be taken, including questions about your home, such as rugs versus wood floors, heating and venting systems, mold and moisture issues, seasonal issues, and food and other allergies, both chemical and natural. This is definitely the time to bring up celiac disease and gluten sensitivity. And that moldy summer cottage you open up and air out every year in May.

Expect to take the following lung function tests:

Spirometry—Involves breathing into a tube that measures how much air you can exhale after a deep breath and how fast you can get it out. This test is usually administered before and after a puff of a bronchodilator. If your numbers improve by more than 15 percent after the inhaled medicine, you can pretty much assume you have asthma.

Peak flow—Similar to the spirometry, this is done to measure how hard and how fast you can exhale and to establish what your best numbers are. Low readings will tell your doctor your lungs are not operating at their peak performance. You may be given a take-home version of this test so that you can chart your numbers daily. With a little luck, faithful and proper use of this device, and calling your doctor at the first sign of a cold or upper respiratory infection, you may never have to take corticosteroids.

Other tests include:

Methacholine challenge—Methacholine is a known asthma trigger that, when inhaled, will cause a mild narrowing of your airways. The test is pretty straightforward, but it does trigger an attack that is easily reversed, so it should be done only if you are stable at the outset.

Nitric oxide test—If your airways are inflamed, nitric oxide levels in your breath will be higher than normal.

Imaging tests—You may be asked to submit to a chest X-ray or a CT (computerized tomography) scan of your lungs and sinus cavities to see if there are any structural abnormalities, masses, or infections causing breathing problems.

Sputum eosinophils—This test involves spitting into a cup and looking for white blood cells called eosinophils in the saliva and mucous after staining it with rose-colored dye.

Provocative testing—Your doctor will measure your lung function during exercise and/or after taking several gulps of cold air.

MEDICATIONS

Asthma medications fall into two categories, (1) long-term control medications, such as inhaled corticosteroids, that are generally taken daily and (2) short-term rescue inhalers that can open the airways and abort an impending attack.

Corticosteroids always come with some risk, especially for the bones, but these metered inhaled drugs have fewer side effects than oral corticosteroids.

Still, make sure you are getting regular bone density or DEXA (dual-energy X-ray absorptiometry) scans while taking this medication.

Long-acting beta agonists like Serevent open the airways and are meant to be taken in concert with inhaled corticosteroids. If taken alone, some research shows these medications may increase the risk of a severe attack. Never take them for an acute asthma attack.

Short-acting beta agonists are meant for quick relief and can rapidly ease symptoms. Ventolin and Atrovent are examples of these rescue inhalers, which should be carried at all times for emergencies.

For severe asthma, oral and intravenous corticosteroids are indicated, but because they can cause severe side effects, they are taken for a short time and then tapered off.

There are many nonmedical things you can do to improve your odds of not having an asthma attack. Always use your air conditioner, and if you live in a damp climate, think about getting a dehumidifier. Root out and destroy mold, especially in showers, sinks, tubs, and basements. Wear a mask when cleaning, raking, and gardening, and get rid of leaves and firewood. Don't go near anyone who smokes and carry a portable fan when circumstances do not allow you to flee. Rethink down pillows and replace them with hypoallergenic versions. Encase mattresses and box springs in dust-proof covers. Wear a big muffler and pull it up over your mouth and nose when it's cold. Regular exercise can strengthen your lungs, as can eating plenty of omega-3 fatty acids found in fish, flaxseed, and salmon. Take breathing lessons; Buteyko, Papworth, and yoga breathing techniques may reduce the amount of medication you need. Acupuncture can help.

Before you and your doctor decide what treatment is best for you, get tested for celiac disease and have your vitamin D levels taken.

Osteoporosis

As we age, osteoporosis is a problem many of us will face, especially those diagnosed with celiac disease and gluten intolerance as adults. According to *The Merck Manual*, osteoporosis is a generalized progressive diminution in bone tissue mass, causing skeletal weakness, even though the ratio of mineral or organic elements is unchanged in the remaining normal bone. This is really a fancy way of saying osteoporosis is a thinning of the bones that can result in pain, a loss of height, and fractures of the hip, spine, and other bones.

There is drug-induced osteoporosis, typically caused by corticosteroid use, smoking, barbiturates, and blood thinners. There is endocrine osteoporosis, which occurs in hyperthyroidism, hypogonadism, diabetes mellitus, and other glandular conditions. And there is a kind of osteoporosis those with celiac disease or gluten intolerance should take a special interest in, which falls into the category of miscellaneous osteoporosis and can be induced by anything from prolonged periods of weightlessness, such as found in space travel (or sitting on our fannies in front of a computer every day for hours on end), to kidney and liver failure and malabsorption syndrome.

Malabsorption is what happens when the intestine is injured by gluten. Nutrients can't get through. We may be taking our calcium and vitamin D (and faithfully doing our weight-bearing exercise), but we may not be absorbing enough of each to keep our bones healthy, or we may be coming from too far behind to catch up. The longer celiac disease and gluten intolerance go without diagnosis, the higher the risk of developing osteoporosis. In fact, very often celiac disease is discovered only after we seek treatment for our aching bones. If ever there was a case for getting blood tests for family members who may be at risk for celiac disease, it's this insidious and potentially disabling condition.

Osteoporosis may be silent for many years, often doing nothing more than causing a low-level ache. By the time pain sets in or fractures occur, the condition is usually advanced.

There are two ways to seek a diagnosis of and treatment for osteoporosis. One is through a rheumatologist and the other is through an endocrinologist. As part of your workup, either specialist should rule out osteomalacia, a softening of the bones usually caused by a vitamin D deficiency, and other metabolic diseases of the bone.

You may be issued a jug with a stinky chemical in the bottom and asked to use it to collect your urine for twenty-four hours. It's inconvenient (you must keep this on ice or in the refrigerator between uses), but it is the way to find out if you have any other problems with calcium.

The Merck Manual further states that standard X-rays are not sensitive enough to reveal osteoporosis until 30 percent of bone has been lost. The DEXA scan is a brief, painless test that measures the density of the spine and hip and is the gold standard for detecting osteoporosis or osteopenia, a condition that occurs before full-blown osteoporosis sets in.

Anyone with long-standing problems with gluten should insist on a DEXA scan. Depending on the results and your age, a follow-up every year to measure improvements is wise. An expert in the interpretation of these test results tells me that it's important to have this test on the same machine each time. Different scanners may interpret or measure results differently, making it difficult to compare results from year to year.

Calcium, magnesium, and vitamin D supplementation, coupled with a gluten-free diet rich in calcium, may arrest bone loss or even help to reverse it. In other cases, a class of drugs called bisphosphonates (Fosamax, Boniva, Actonel, Reclast) may be prescribed for you. Many of these drugs, while highly effective, come with risks and contraindications. Some experience chest or throat pain and heartburn and many doctors recommend quarterly or semiannual or annual infusions to bypass the esophagus altogether. Rare but serious and long-standing side effects include abnormal heart rhythm or atrial fibrillation; incapacitating bone, joint, and muscle pain; and bone loss in the jaw called osteonecrosis. Even more troubling, a report published in the *Journal of Bone and Mineral Research* studied 310 people who sustained atypical femur breaks and 94 percent had been taking Fosamax for five years or longer.

For pre-osteoporosis or osteopenia, many doctors advise against drug therapy at all and prescribe calcium, magnesium, and vitamin D supplementation, in addition to walking, dancing, jumping, and other weight-bearing exercises, all of which can strengthen bones. To avoid the very real risk of thigh fractures, some doctors recommend taking a drug holiday after two or more years on bisphosphonates.

Miacalcin, a calcitonin-salmon nasal spray, or Evista, an estrogen-based drug that mimics estrogen's beneficial effect on bone density, may be prescribed, but these, too, come with a long list of side effects and contraindications. These are decisions not to be made lightly and must be weighed against the seriousness of your condition, your family history, and your current health, and always with input from your doctor. Once you decide which course is best for you, remember to verify the gluten-free status of your medication.

The National Academy of Sciences recommends the following daily intake of dietary calcium and vitamin D for healthy Americans:

Calcium

0–6 months, 210 mg/day
7–12 months, 270 mg/day
1–3 years, 500 mg/day
4–8 years, 800 mg/day
9–18 years, 1,300 mg/day
19–50 years, 1,000 mg/day
51 years plus, 1,200 mg/day until menopause
51 years plus, 1,500 mg/day after menopause

Vitamin D

0–50 years, 200 IU/day
51–70 years, 400–600 IU/day
71 years plus, 600–800 IU/day

Note: These figures apply to the general population. Newly diagnosed celiacs often need to take higher doses of calcium, vitamin D, magnesium, and other minerals in order to make up for years of not absorbing these important bone-building elements. Supplementation and/or correction of any deficiency should be undertaken with your doctor's supervision.

A WORD ABOUT VITAMIN D

The National Institutes of Health tell us that vitamin D is vital for proper absorption of calcium and other minerals. The best source for this vitamin, which the body stores in the fat cells against a rainy, dark day, is exposure to direct sunlight (glass interferes with vitamin D absorption, so sitting in front of a sunny window won't help). But don't think you have to fry yourself to a crisp. Approximately twenty minutes of exposure without sunscreen in the morning or afternoon, when ultraviolet rays are the least damaging, should do the trick.

Few food sources besides cod liver oil (ugh), eel (double ugh), salmon, mackerel, sardines, and other oily fish provide vitamin D. Some foods are fortified with vitamin D, but many of these are cereals and cereal bars that are not gluten-free. Most people absorb enough vitamin D during the summer to last through the winter, but long hours indoors at computers and use of sunscreens have cut down on sun exposure. Add to this the absorption difficulties in people with gluten intolerance and it's wise to have vitamin D levels (as well as other vitamin and minerals) measured. There is a dark side to taking too much vitamin D. Excessive amounts can cause nausea, loss of appetite, weight loss, and serious muscle weakness, so it's best to have your doctor prescribe the dose that's right for you and monitor your progress from time to time.

Osteomalacia

Osteomalacia means "soft bones." The Cleveland Clinic describes this condition as a metabolic disease that weakens bones and can cause them to fracture more easily. In osteomalacia, the bone breaks down faster than it can rebuild, leaving the patient with pain in all bones and especially the hip, frequent bone fractures, and muscle weakness.

Anyone with intestinal absorption problems caused by celiac disease and gluten sensitivity is at risk for osteomalacia, and almost always the culprit is vitamin D deficiency. Osteomalacia can also occur in the elderly and at any age among those who don't drink milk and, in particular, those who are lactose-intolerant.

In children, the condition is called rickets and in the early stages of development, soft bones are more likely to bow and fracture than harder, healthy ones. Once upon a time, rickets was rampant in children working all day in gloomy sweatshops. Today, we have only to look as far as the eerie and artificial light of the computer screen and our zealous use of high-SPF (sun protection factor) sunscreens for the source of sunlight deficiency.

Other conditions that may cause osteomalacia are cancer, kidney failure, and acidosis, liver disease, and lack of phosphates in the diet (whole wheat and bran, cottage cheese or cheddar cheese, peanut butter, corn, broccoli, chicken, and turkey contain phosphates). It can also occur as a side effect of antiseizure medication. Tell your doctor if you have had gastric bypass surgery, because this procedure seriously inhibits absorption.

In its early stages, the condition is silent and is seen only on X-ray or MRI (magnetic resonance imaging). As it worsens, dull, aching pain becomes widespread and muscle weakness is apparent. Bone fractures happen with no injury or trauma. There is constant bone pain, especially in the hips, lower spine, pelvis, legs, and ribs. As calcium requires vitamin D to maintain healthy levels, other symptoms, such as numbness around the mouth and arms and legs and spasms of the hands or feet, occur due to low levels of calcium. Muscle weakness can cause decreased muscle tone and strength and result in a waddling gait. In extreme cases, weak limbs must be braced for stability and to prevent falls.

Osteomalacia is diagnosed and treated by a specialist in endocrinology or rheumatology. As always, the more complete the history, the faster and more accurate the diagnosis.

The following tests may be ordered:

72-hour urine collection—In cases of osteomalacia caused by vitamin D deficiency or phosphorus loss, abnormal levels of D, calcium, and phosphorus are often seen in the urine.

Blood work—Vitamin D, creatinine, calcium, and phosphate levels.

Bone X-ray—To detect pseudo fractures.

Bone density—To show bone softening and loss.

ALP (alkaline phosphatase) **isoenzyme** and **PTH** (parathyroid hormone)—
May be done to see if a kidney problem or other disorder is causing osteomalacia.

Bone biopsy—The most accurate test for osteomalacia, in which your doctor will insert a slender needle through your skin into your bone to withdraw a small sample to view under a microscope. While the biopsy is very accurate in detecting osteomalacia, it is invasive and uncomfortable and rarely needed.

Good news. The prognosis for osteomalacia is excellent. Most will require supplements of vitamin D, calcium, and phosphorus and will see improvement within weeks, although those with impaired absorption of the intestines may need larger doses to heal completely within six months.

For information on osteoporosis *and* osteomalacia contact:

National Osteoporosis Foundation
1150 17th Street NW #850
Washington, DC 20036
(800) 231-4222
www.nof.org

Addison's Disease

Rumors abound that John F. Kennedy had a problem with gluten. Given his Irish heritage and the fact that in childhood he suffered from severe gastrointestinal distress, weight, and growth problems, it's a fair guess. As an adult, abdominal pain, migraines, weight loss, and osteoporosis plagued him. Over the course of his lifetime and during his presidency, he underwent evaluations at major medical centers in Boston, New Haven, and New York, as well as at the Mayo Clinic. Among his multiple diagnoses were ulcers, colitis, spastic colitis, irritable bowel syndrome, and food allergies.

Imagine what a gluten-free Camelot would have been like. We'll never know. What we do know is that among his many problems, JFK suffered from Addison's disease, a chronic, insidious, and rare insufficiency of the adrenal glands that can be associated with celiac disease and gluten intolerance.

To paraphrase *The Merck Manual*, Addison's disease is an endocrine disorder caused by atrophy of the adrenal cortex, most likely by an auto-immune process, resulting in an insufficient amount of an important hormone called cortisol. In the absence of cortisol, insufficient carbohydrate is formed from protein. Hypoglycemia (low blood sugar) and diminished liver function results. This leads to serious neuromuscular weakness. Resistance to infection, stress, and trauma is diminished because of reduced adrenal output.

Symptoms of Addison's disease include weakness, fatigue, low blood pressure, and increased pigmentation, which is characterized by tanning of both exposed and unexposed portions of the body, especially on pressure points (bony areas), skin folds, and scars. Black freckles appear over the forehead, face, neck, and shoulders, and often bluish-black discoloration appears on the lips, mouth, rectum, vagina, and other mucous membranes. Addison's can cause a decreased tolerance to cold. Dizziness and fainting attacks can occur, as can weight loss, dehydration, vomiting, and diarrhea. There also may be some abnormalities on the EKG (electrocardiogram).

If Addison's is suspected, a referral to an endocrinologist is crucial. Blood levels of sodium and potassium and BUN (a measurement of kidney function) will be taken. Cortisol levels are measured, and tests for adrenal insufficiency may be ordered. Other tests that may be ordered are WBC (white blood count) and fasting blood glucose. X-rays or CT scans may be used to examine the heart, to look for calcifications in the adrenal glands, and to screen for kidney or lung problems.

Addison's is a serious disease, but with carefully monitored substitution of the missing or insufficient hormones by an endocrinologist, the prognosis is excellent.

For information, support, and referrals, contact:

National Adrenal Disease Foundation
505 Northern Boulevard, Suite 303
Great Neck, NY 11021
(516) 487-4992
www.nadf.us

Systemic Lupus Erythematosus (SLE)

According to the Lupus Foundation, lupus is "a chronic inflammatory disease that can affect various parts of the body, i.e., skin, joints, blood, and kidneys." The body's immune system normally makes antibodies to protect against viruses, bacteria, and other foreign materials. These foreign materials are called antigens. In an autoimmune disorder such as lupus, the immune system loses its ability to tell the difference between foreign substances and its own cells and tissues. The immune system then makes antibodies directed against "self." These antibodies, called auto-antibodies, then react with the "self" antigens to form immune complexes. The immune complexes build up in the tissues and can cause inflammation, injury to tissues, and, in some cases, organ failure.

For most people, lupus is a mild disease affecting only a few organs, but for others it can cause serious and even life-threatening problems such as kidney failure. Lupus can begin abruptly with fever, resembling an acute infection, or it may develop insidiously over months or years with episodes of fever or malaise. The National Institutes of Health tell us the most common symptoms are painful or swollen joints, unexplained fever, skin rashes, and extreme fatigue. The Lupus Foundation adds to the list the classic "butterfly" rash across the cheeks and nose. This rash, resembling the markings of a wolf, *lupus* in Latin, is how the disease got its name. Anemia, kidney involvement, pleurisy (pain in the chest on deep breathing), skin photosensitivity to sun or UV (ultraviolet) light, hair loss, abnormal blood clotting problems, Raynaud's phenomenon (fingers turning white and/or blue in response to cold), low blood counts (white cells, red cells, platelets), seizures, and mouth or nose ulcers are among the many signs pointing to this condition.

When a patient has many symptoms and positive blood test results, the rheumatologist has few problems making a correct diagnosis and initiating treatment. But more often than not, lupus shows itself over time with vague, seemingly unrelated complaints like achy joints, fever, fatigue, or pains. Lupus can be mistaken for other types of arthritis, fibromyalgia, chronic fatigue, rosacea, and that great catchall diagnosis, stress. It takes tenacity on the part of the patient and patience on the part of the doctor when lupus is suspected. Often the picture forms over a period of months or years.

Blood tests for lupus include the LE (lupus erythematosus) cell test. This was the first diagnostic test for lupus, but it is rarely done nowadays because of its lack of sensitivity. The ANA (immunofluorescent antinuclear antibody) test is the best screening test for lupus because virtually all people with lupus have a positive ANA. On the other hand, a positive ANA by itself is not diagnostic, since the test may also be positive in individuals taking certain medications, in other autoimmune diseases (scleroderma, Sjögren's, rheumatoid arthritis, autoimmune thyroid disease, or

Hashimoto's thyroiditis), liver disease, and chronic infectious diseases such as leprosy and malaria. Therefore, more specific blood tests that measure individual antigen antibody reaction are also helpful. The anti-dsDNA antibody test, as well as the anti-Sm, anti-RNP, anti-Ro (SSA), and anti-La (SSA) antibody tests will most likely also need to be done.

Other helpful laboratory tests are ones that measure the complement levels in the blood. Complement is a blood protein that, with antibodies, destroys bacteria. If the total blood complement is low or the specific C3 or C4 complement values are low and the person has a positive ANA, some weight is added to a diagnosis of lupus. Low C3 or C4 in people with positive anti-dsDNA may also point to lupus kidney disease or active disease in other organs.

If a skin rash is present, a biopsy may be performed to assist in the diagnosis. A test may be positive one time and negative the next. The disease may be active one time, quiescent another. While no one test is diagnostic, all results are considered for diagnosis.

Bottom line: Like the wolf, lupus is elusive.

While a cure has not yet been found for lupus, management includes nonsteroidal anti-inflammatory drugs (NSAIDs) and drugs like Tylenol for joint and muscle pain. For serious inflammation, corticosteroids (e.g., prednisone) may be used. If you use steroids, short treatment periods are recommended to avoid serious side effects. Anticoagulants may be required for people with recurrent blood clots. And antimalarials such as hydroxychloroquine (Plaquenil) or chloroquine (Aralen) are prescribed for skin, oral, or nasal ulcers and joint systems. Since these medications can cause serious complications in the eyes, an eye exam is suggested before beginning a course of antimalarials. A yearly or twice-yearly follow-up with the ophthalmologist for repeat testing and examination is a sensible precaution. Anticancer drugs (methotrexate, azathioprine, or cyclophosphamide) are only used in patients with life-threatening manifestations. As always, gluten-free status must be considered along with the potential risks of these medications. For more information, doctor referrals, research, support, local chapters and subscriptions to the magazine *Lupus Now*, contact:

Lupus Foundation of America
2000 L Street NW, Suite 410
Washington, DC 20036
(202) 349-1155
www.lupus.org

Sjögren's Syndrome

Sjögren's syndrome, also known as the sicca syndrome, is defined as a chronic, autoimmune, inflammatory, rheumatic disorder that primarily affects the body's own moisture producing (exocrine) glands. Experts can't say what causes it. It's characterized by dryness of the mouth, eyes, and other mucous membranes, musculoskeletal pain, and fatigue. It shares overlapping features with other autoimmune or connective tissue disorders, including rheumatoid arthritis, lupus, and scleroderma. Sjögren's syndrome is the second most common autoimmune rheumatic disease after rheumatoid arthritis. Ninety percent of Sjögren's patients are women.

Like lupus, Sjögren's can attack almost all of the body's organs since the exocrine glands are found all over the body, producing moisture (tears, saliva, and the like) for normal functioning of the eyes, mouth, digestive and respiratory tracts, skin, and vagina. In Sjögren's, these glands are invaded by lymphocytes and are gradually destroyed. Sjögren's may be primary, which means it occurs in a previously healthy individual, or secondary, which means it can also develop in an individual with a pre-existing connective tissue disease such as rheumatoid arthritis.

Symptoms of this serious, annoying, but rarely fatal condition include a dry, gritty, or burning sensation in the eyes due to decreased tear production, dryness of the mouth (the sensation of cotton in the mouth), and whole-body dryness (the feeling that one is turning into a tumbleweed). Sjögren's may cause difficulty talking, chewing, or swallowing; a sore or cracked tongue; a change or a loss of taste or smell; increased dental decay; joint pain; digestive problems, dry nose, dry lungs, recurring respiratory infections, dry skin, swollen salivary glands, fatigue, and sensitivity of eyes and skin to light. In 10 to 25 percent of cases, experts say, the lymphocytic infiltration may spread to the internal organs and lead to serious complications from inflammation of the lungs, kidneys, or central nervous system.

Lymphoma risk in Sjögren's is up to forty-four times higher than that of the general population. Combined with the lymphoma risk associated with undiagnosed celiac or noncompliance with the gluten-free diet, there is no better incentive to be scrupulous with your gluten-free diet. Other problems associated with Sjögren's are Raynaud's phenomenon (cold-induced color changes of the hands and feet caused by painful constriction of small vessels), corneal damage, accelerated tooth decay, and salivary duct stones. Sjögren's can also cause liver disease, pancreatitis, sensory neuropathy, kidney problems, and alopecia. Dryness of the respiratory tract can lead to chronic lung infections and pneumonia.

Sjögren's syndrome is difficult to diagnose and is best managed by a rheumatologist. As with celiac disease, the average time from onset of symptoms to diagnosis is about six years. A good ophthalmologist and a knowledgeable dentist also play important roles in this condition. The former conducts diagnostic tests and periodically evaluates the eyes for outer surface damage, and the latter attends to the problems caused by a lack of saliva.

The Sjögren's Syndrome Foundation's new patient FAQ lists the following blood tests to expect when you're seeking a diagnosis:

ANA (antinuclear antibody)—As in lupus, the presence of ANA in your blood is not diagnostic but is a marker for the presence of autoimmune reaction.

Anti-SS-A (or Ro) and SS-B (La)—Up to 70 percent of Sjögren's patients are positive for SS-A and up to 40 percent are positive for SS-B. These antibodies may also be found, though less often, in lupus.

RF (rheumatoid factor)—Many Sjögren's patients have a positive RF, just as do people with rheumatoid arthritis. That is why one disorder is sometimes confused with the other.

ESR (erythrocyte sedimentation rate)—This test measures inflammation. An elevated ESR may indicate an inflammatory disorder such as Sjögren's.

Igs (immunoglobulins)—This test measures blood proteins that participate in immune reactions and may be elevated in Sjögren's and related immune system diseases.

An ophthalmologist may be asked to conduct all or some the following:

Schirmer's test—Measures tear production, which is reduced in Sjögren's.

Rose bengal, fluorescein, and/or **lissamine green** corneal staining—Used to find dry spots on the surface of the eye.

Slit-lamp exam—May show a reduced volume of tears or mucous filaments that can sometimes form as a complication of dry eyes.

Other tests that may be ordered:

Sialiometry—Measures the amount of saliva produced during a certain period and reflects salivary gland function.

Sialography—An X-ray of the parotid salivary-duct system performed after injecting contrast into the duct.

Salivary scintigraphy—A nuclear medicine test also used to assess salivary gland function.

Lip biopsy—Confirms lymphocytic infiltration (that is, inflammation) of the minor salivary glands. A fifteen-minute procedure requiring local anesthesia, this is the most specific test for Sjögren's.

Once pinpointed, Sjögren's management often requires comprehensive care. For the mouth, this includes fastidious dental hygiene and frequent cleanings. Frequent small sips of water and sugar-free mints and gum stimulate salivary flow. Artificial tears and saliva (yes, there is such a thing) help ease symptoms of dry mouth and eyes. Household humidifiers, periodic naps, medications that reduce joint pain, avoidance of sugary food and drinks, alcohol in any form (i.e., mouthwashes), rinses, even the wearing of gloves to avoid vessel constriction (especially when shopping in the supermarket freezer case) are all ways to accommodate and reduce symptoms. Frequent slathering with emollient creams helps manage dry skin.

Drugs that decrease salivary secretion, such as decongestants and antihistamines, should be avoided. Ditto for sunbathing because many Sjögren's patients develop skin photosensitivity. Relocation to the desert should be reconsidered.

There are two drugs available to stimulate saliva flow: pilocarpine (Salagen) and cevimeline (Evoxac). Although only FDA-approved for dry mouth, published studies suggest that these drugs may help dryness in other body parts as well.

Antimalarials, such as those used in lupus, have shown promise in treating fatigue, joint pain, muscle pain, and swollen glands. The eyes must be checked periodically for rare but serious side effects. Corticosteroids are reserved for disabling pain, fatigue, or serious internal organ involvement. In the worst cases, stronger immunosuppressants may also be used.

Is there a cure? No.

The Sjögren's Syndrome Foundation puts out a newsletter called *The Moisture Seekers* that is full of tips, conference news, the latest research, and support. *The Sjögren's Book*, edited by Daniel J. Wallace, is a valuable resource. For more information:

Sjögren's Syndrome Foundation
6707 Democracy Blvd., Suite 325
Bethesda, MD 20817
(301) 718-0300
www. sjögrens.org

Frederick B. Vivino, MD, MS, FACR
Director, Penn Sjögren's
      Syndrome Center
Penn Presbyterian Medical Center
3910 Building, Suite 200
51 North 39th Street
Philadelphia, PA 19104
(800) 789-7366

Rheumatoid Arthritis

According to *Mosby's Medical Dictionary*, rheumatoid arthritis, or RA, is a chronic, inflammatory, destructive, and sometimes deforming connective tissue disease that has an autoimmune component. It attacks the synovium (membrane lining the joints) and is characterized by symmetric inflammation of multiple joints leading to severe pain and swelling. The normally delicate synovial membrane is invaded by huge numbers of inflammatory cells. Over time it develops many villous folds (not unlike the intestinal villous atrophy found in gluten intolerance), and becomes more engorged, larger, thicker, and eventually fibrous. This inflamed tissue acts like a tumor and then begins to erode into adjacent structures such as bone, cartilage, and ligaments, destroying everything in its path. The course of the disease is highly variable but is most frequently marked by alternating periods of remission and exacerbation.

An autoimmune disorder associated with celiac disease and gluten sensitivity, RA's cardinal signs are tender, warm, and swollen joints, morning stiffness that may linger for hours, firm nodules under the skin, and systemic symptoms such as fever, fatigue, and weight loss. If you've ever experienced a painful flare of rheumatoid arthritis, you know why it's called "fire in the joints."

In the beginning, diagnosis can be challenging because a rheumatoid-like arthritis can also occur in lupus, Sjögren's syndrome, scleroderma, polymyositis, and mixed connective disease, but it is typically nonerosive and much less destructive. A similar pattern of symmetrical polyarthritis may even be seen in Lyme disease. A proper diagnosis, therefore, requires an appointment with a rheumatologist skilled at assessing the condition and its many manifestations.

Expect a thorough examination of the affected joints, a discussion of your medical history and that of your immediate family, especially allergies, autoimmune conditions, medications, and supplements you are currently taking (don't forget to mention travel to areas where you may have been exposed to deer ticks). This is the time to bring up any problems you may be having with gluten, either documented celiac disease or GI symptoms due to gluten sensitivity. After evaluating the possibilities, the doctor will most likely order a series of blood tests and X-rays to look for signs of more advanced disease, such as erosions and joint space narrowing. Depending on the severity of your symptoms, you may be asked to submit to an aspiration of synovial fluid (small needle inserted into a joint to withdraw fluid). No one test confirms a diagnosis of RA, but rather it is a combination of clinical signs and laboratory tests.

Blood work should include:

CBC—Complete blood count

C-reactive protein—This is a nondiagnostic measure of the presence and level of inflammation.

RF (rheumatoid factor)—These are antiglobulin antibodies commonly found in up to 80 percent of patients with rheumatoid arthritis. The higher the titer, or concentration of an antibody, the higher the odds it's RA, but lower abnormal levels of RF may also point to Sjögren's syndrome, scleroderma, lupus, and other autoimmune conditions.

ESR—In rheumatoid arthritis, the erythrocyte sedimentation rate, another gauge of inflammation and not diagnostic on its own, is elevated in 90 percent of the cases.

Joint ultrasound or **MRI** or **X-ray**—May be ordered in cases where erosions are not seen on X-ray.

Aspiration of synovial fluid—Synovial fluid, abnormal during active joint inflammation, is cloudy and sterile and usually contains a high level of white blood cells. If crystals are seen, polyarticular gout or pseudorheumatoid arthritis or pseudogout may be an alternate diagnostic possibility. I won't lie. This hurts, but only for a second.

Anemia—Normochromic/normocytic anemia (that is, anemia with normal appearing red blood cells) is typical of many chronic inflammatory diseases, including celiac disease and is also found in 80 percent of RA patients.

Additionally, if rheumatoid factor is present, the American College of Rheumatology also recommends testing for:

Anti-CCP (anti-cyclic citrullinated peptide)—Antibodies that, when also present, significantly increase the chances that rheumatoid arthritis is the correct and final diagnosis.

Treatment for RA depends on its severity. As with all inflammatory diseases, the earlier it is caught and treated, the better. Conservative therapy might include a high dose of aspirin or other salicylates taken with meals and snacks. For those patients who do not tolerate aspirin, NSAIDs (nonsteroidal anti-inflammatory drugs) such as ibuprofen and naproxen are often given. This class of drugs can produce stomach upset, gastric ulcers, and gastrointestinal bleeding at high doses. Prescription NSAIDs such as Celebrex may be safer on the stomach but also come with a long list of side effects, some of which may be life-threatening in those with cardiac problems. Never start a course of drugs like this without discussing all of your medical problems with your doctor. Corticosteroids, most notably prednisone, are the strongest and most dramatically effective short-term anti-inflammatory drugs, but they also have serious side effects and should be used for the shortest possible time and only for the worst cases.

Many integrative medical practices offer complementary and alternative treatments. According to the Mayo Clinic Web site, the seeds of evening primrose, borage, and black currant contain a fatty acid that may help lessen rheumatoid arthritis pain and morning stiffness. These plants' oils are not without their side effects, which may include nausea, diarrhea, gas, and liver damage, or they may interfere with prescription medications. Never assume these treatments are benign just because they are "natural." Always check with your doctor first.

Movement therapy is also beneficial for RA. Tai chi, which involves a gentle and graceful series of exercises and stretches combined with deep breathing, is especially effective. One only has to look in the parks near Asian communities to see robust and flexible Chinese elders practicing this ancient healing art. Traditional physical therapy works as well.

The Mayo Clinic further points to studies showing that fish oil supplements and other sources of omega-3 fatty acids may reduce joint pain and stiffness. One must weigh indigestion and a fishy taste in the mouth as the cost of such a regimen. Again, having your doctor on board ensures you are getting the most out of all therapies.

Diet and food allergy as a trigger for RA is no longer a fringe idea. Many physicians now believe that joint inflammation is an autoimmune response triggered by food allergy and sensitivity, and routinely recommend an anti-inflammatory diet to their patients. More and more doctors consider these factors in prescribing treatment for RA and there is much to be said for trying an elimination diet before embarking on a course of prescription drugs. And yes, gluten wreaks all sorts of havoc, whether full-out celiac disease or undocumented sensitivity.

Jean Carper, in her landmark book *Food: Your Miracle Medicine*, lists the inflammation-causing culprits—the worst being corn, wheat, or, more specifically, gluten, followed by bacon and pork, oranges, milk, oats, rye, eggs, cheese, and cane sugar, among the offenders. A better case for a plant-based, gluten-free, organic diet has not been presented. Carper also cites those foods that may soothe the symptoms: fatty fish such as mackerel, salmon, sardines, herring, and tuna, and ginger. For more information, further reading, and to find a doctor near you, contact:

Arthritis Foundation. www.arthritis.org
Arthritis Today. www.arthritistoday.org

Diabetes Mellitus

Mosby's Medical Dictionary defines diabetes mellitus as "a complex disorder of carbohydrate, fat, and protein metabolism that is primarily a result of a deficiency or complete lack of insulin secretion by the beta cells of the pancreas or resistance to insulin."

The *Report of the Expert Committee on the Diagnosis and Classification of Diabetes Mellitus* of the American Diabetes Association describes the various types of diabetes: "Type 1 Diabetes includes patients with diabetes caused by an autoimmune process and who are dependent on insulin to prevent ketosis," which *Mosby's* further defines as "an abnormal accumulation of ketones in the body as a result of excessive breakdown of fats caused by a deficiency or inadequate use of carbohydrates, characterized by ketonuria, a loss of potassium in the urine which can lead to life-threatening ketoacidosis, coma, even death."

According to the National Diabetes Information Clearinghouse (NDIC), type 1 diabetes (formerly called juvenile diabetes or brittle diabetes or insulin-dependent diabetes) is caused when the beta cells of the pancreas no longer make insulin because the body's immune system has attacked and destroyed them. Symptoms include frequent thirst and urination, extreme hunger or fatigue, weight loss, sores that heal slowly, dry itchy skin, loss of feeling or tingling in the feet, and blurry vision. Treatment includes taking insulin shots or using an insulin pump, making wise food choices, exercising regularly, and controlling blood pressure and cholesterol. Given the autoimmune nature of the condition, this form of diabetes is believed to be associated with celiac disease. In fact, Dr. Stefano Guandalini, medical director of the University of Chicago Celiac Disease Center, says every patient diagnosed with type 1 diabetes should be screened for celiac disease, not once, but every two to three years, because the 7 to 8 percent of patients with type 1 diabetes and celiac disease progressively rises to 8 to 10 percent ten years after initial testing.

But that doesn't let us off the hook. Obesity, sedentary lifestyle, and a steady diet of fast and processed foods and humongous portions of fat, sugar, high-fructose corn syrup, and calories are contributing to a virtual epidemic of type 2 diabetes, even among young children. Not just those with celiac disease, but those with varying levels of gluten sensitivity, may be prone to this problem because of the high fat, sugar, and carbohydrate contents of many gluten-free breads, cakes, and cookies.

The NDIC further tells us that type 2 diabetes, formerly called adult-onset or non-insulin-dependent diabetes, is the most common form of diabetes. People can develop type 2 diabetes at any age—even during childhood. This form of diabetes usually begins with insulin resistance, a condition in which fat, muscle, and liver cells do not use insulin properly. At first the pancreas keeps up with the added demand by producing more insulin. In time, however, it loses the ability to secrete enough insulin in response to meals. Obesity and inactivity increase the chances of developing this type of diabetes, as do high levels of cholesterol and high blood pressure.

Gestational diabetes is another form of diabetes that may occur in the third trimester of pregnancy. It may be a sign of latent diabetes or it may disappear with the birth of the child.

All types of diabetes require the care and monitoring of an endocrinologist. Periodic eye exams, cholesterol-lowering medications, and diet, as well as frequent foot examinations and care on the part of an experienced podiatrist can go a long way toward avoiding serious complications.

Proper nutrition makes all the difference. Combining the gluten-free and diabetic diets won't be easy, but it will result in better health. For diabetes information, diet, and management and support:

American Diabetes Association
www.diabetes.org

National Diabetes Information
Clearinghouse
1 Information Way
Bethesda, MD 20892
(800) 860-8747
www.diabetes.niddk.nih.gov
ndic@info.niddk.nih.gov

Thyroid Disease

The thyroid gland, as described by *Mosby's Medical Dictionary*, is "a pea-sized, ductless gland at the front of the neck that is part of the endocrine system and which secretes the hormone thyroxine (T4) and triiodothyronine (T3), an iodine-containing compound, as well as produces the hormone calcitonin." These substances are essential to normal body growth, normal metabolic rate, carbohydrate catabolism (the bodily process of breaking down carbohydrates for energy storage and heat production), skeletal maturation, that is, growth in infancy and childhood, and cardiac rate, force, and output. Thyroid hormones promote central nervous system development and the synthesis of many enzymes essential for muscle tone and vigor. In other words, it's a small but important pea-sized gland.

Hyperthyroidism (*hyper* meaning "too much") or Graves' disease is characterized by *The Merck Manual* as an "overproduction of these hormones resulting in rapid heart rate, moist skin, tremors, bulging eyes, increased sweating, palpitations, fatigue, increased appetite and weight loss, frequent bowel movements, insomnia, and atrial fibrillation or sudden, fast heart rhythm." A qualified endocrinologist will measure the levels of thyroid hormone and treat this condition with drugs that will inhibit and normalize the release of what is overproduced. The right dosage comes from careful monitoring of thyroid hormone and adjusting doses accordingly.

Hypothyroidism (*hypo* meaning "too little") or myxedema is just the opposite. Too little thyroid hormone in circulation can contribute to a dull facial expression; hoarse voice; slow speech; puffiness and swelling around the eyes; cold intolerance; drooping eyelids; sparse, coarse, and dry hair; and coarse, dry, scaly, and thickened skin. Weight gain is another sign of hypothyroidism, as are forgetfulness and other evidence of intellectual impairment (the "brain fog" celiacs often complain of may be related to hypothyroiditis). There are often deposits of carotene on the palms of hands and soles of feet, and macroglossia or enlargement of the tongue. Undiagnosed myxedema can lead to seizures or coma. Hypothyroidism is thought to be an autoimmune disease, related to celiac disease, and often occurs as a prelude to Hashimoto's thyroiditis. Lifelong supplementation with thyroid hormone compensates for the deficiency and, again, is carefully monitored for the correct amount.

Hashimoto's thyroiditis, or autoimmune thyroiditis, is a chronic inflammation of the thyroid gland with lymphocytic infiltration much like the exocrine and salivary gland destruction in Sjögren's. Symptoms often take the form of a painless enlargement of the gland or fullness in the throat. When the doctor examines the gland, it is usually not tender and it is smooth, firm, and more rubbery in consistency than a normal thyroid. Other forms of autoimmune disease are common in people with Hashimoto's, including Addison's disease, diabetes, hypoparathyroidism, and yes, celiac disease. Treatment for Hashimoto's thyroiditis is straightforward, with a lifelong replacement of thyroid hormone and strict adherence to the gluten-free diet. For referrals and information, contact:

American Association of Clinical Endocrinologists
245 Riverside Avenue, Suite 200
Jacksonville, FL 32202
(904) 353-7878
www.aace.com

Lymphoma

Whew. Just writing the word gives one pause.

Okay. Let's face the fear head-on. We've all been told that there is an association between undiagnosed celiac disease and increased risk from lymphoma or adenocarcinoma, in particular T-cell lymphoma of the small intestine.

According to the Lymphoma Research Foundation, there are more than thirty subtypes of lymphoma. These consist of five types of Hodgkin's lymphoma, which arise from abnormal white cells that spread along the lymph nodes, as well as organs outside the lymphatic vessels. Lymphoma also includes twenty-four types of non-Hodgkin's lymphoma, a more common form that starts in the spleen or in lymph tissue found in organs like the stomach or small intestine.

While we are assured by the foundation that most people who have the following complaints will not have lymphoma, anyone (especially with celiac disease or gluten intolerance) with persistent symptoms should be examined to make sure lymphoma is not present. These are chills, painless swelling of the lymph nodes, fever, night sweats, unexplained weight loss, lack of energy, and generalized itching. The development of anemia, low blood albumin, or recurring steatorrhea, a diarrhea caused by malabsorption, in a previously healthy celiac should prompt further investigation in the form of blood work, CT scanning of the abdomen, and, in some cases, a segment of the bowel obtained surgically under anesthesia through a laparoscope in order to examine the excised tissue for proliferation of T cells. The doctor best suited to pursue an investigation of this kind is a gastroenterologist with a specialty in oncology.

An article in the *American Journal of Clinical Nutrition* suggests that in diagnosed celiacs, malignancy may appear as a return of malabsorptive symptoms or a surgical emergency associated with obstruction, perforation, and, sometimes, bleeding. The same article goes on to say that the risk for developing lymphoma diminishes with duration and compliance with the gluten-free diet and that malignancy rarely occurs before forty years of age. Patients diagnosed as children and who are compliant have a lower risk of malignancy.

However, a more recent article in the *American Journal of Medicine*, reporting on a study conducted at New York–Presbyterian Hospital between 1981 and 2000, concludes that "the risk of non-Hodgkin's lymphoma among its study subjects persisted despite a gluten-free diet." Also observed was an increased risk of small intestinal adenocarcinoma, esophageal cancer, and melanoma.

A new Swedish study published in the August 5, 2013, edition of the *Annals of Internal Medicine* shows that unhealed intestines in celiac disease is tied to a higher risk of lymphoma. The study included 7,625 people who were diagnosed with celiac disease and had intestinal biopsies one year later. Of those, 43 percent still had damage to their intestines on the follow-up exam. They were tracked for nine years, and during that span 53 were diagnosed with lymphoma.

So what's a gluten-intolerant to do? If you have never been tested for celiac disease, do it. If you test positive on biopsy and have intestinal damage, follow a diet that promotes healing and follow up with another biopsy. Once you know the extent of the severity of your gluten sensitivity, follow the diet religiously, have frequent checkups, and insist that other first- and second-degree relatives get tested for celiac disease. My own unprofessional opinion is this: be smart, be aware of the symptoms, but don't obsess.

I'll say it again. Get tested. Arm yourself with information. But don't worry unnecessarily. Stress contributes to many illnesses, including cancer. All the more reason to eat healthy, high-quality, preferably organic gluten-free foods; exercise; take your vitamins; keep your fat and sugar and calorie intake low (whether gluten-free or not); maintain a healthy weight; and pat yourself on the back for getting rid of the gluten. For more information, contact:

The Lymphoma Research
Foundation
115 Broadway, Suite 1301
New York, NY 10006
(212) 349-2910
www.lymphoma.org

Help:
LRF@lymphoma.org
LRF Helpline:
(800) 500-9976
Helpline@lymphoma.org

I have focused on conditions in the preceding section, rather than symptoms associated with gluten intolerance and celiac disease, because the latter often resolve once gluten is removed from the diet. These troublesome associates of gluten intolerance can range from the obvious digestive complaints—gas, bloating, diarrhea, constipation, heartburn—to autoimmune reactions such as hives and apthous ulcers to neurologic issues such as fatigue, headache, brain fog, and even foot drop (gluten ataxia), which are often mistaken for separate conditions. It's important to recognize all of the ways gluten can harm you if you are intolerant of it or sensitive to it.

Here is a short list of weird problems/symptoms and other conditions that should raise red flags:

Iron deficiency anemia/pernicious anemia
Alopecia
Anxiety and depression
Aphthous ulcers
Attention deficit disorder/attention deficit/hyperactivity disorder
Chronic fatigue syndrome
Dental enamel defects
Folic acid deficiency
Food allergy other than gluten

Heartburn or GERD (gastroesophageal reflux disease)
Inflammatory bowel disease (IBS)
Impotency
Infertility
Lactose intolerance
Migraines
Peripheral neuropathy
Short stature/delayed puberty

Learn More

American College of
Rheumatology
2200 Lake Boulevard NE
Atlanta, GA 30319
(404) 633-3777
www.rheumatology.org

Medic Alert Foundation
2323 Colorado Avenue
Turlock, CA 95382
(888) 633-4298
www.medicalert.org

CDC/Centers for Disease Control
and Prevention
www.cdc.gov

U.S. National Library of Medicine
www.nlm.nih.gov

American Prinzmetal's Angina
Association
18610 Sea Turtle Lane
Boca Raton/Palm Beach,
FL 33498
(561) 477-3515
www.prinzmetal.us
info@prinzmetal.us

National Institute of Arthritis
and Musculoskeletal and Skin
Diseases
Information Clearinghouse
National Institutes of Health
1 AMS Circle
Bethesda, MD 20892
(301) 495-4484
www.niams.nih.gov
e-mail: NIAMSinfo@mail.nih.gov

Raynaud's Association, Inc.
94 Mercer Avenue
Hartsdale, NY 10530
(800) 280-8055
www.raynauds.org
info@raynauds.org

20

The Doctor Will See You Now

Never go to a doctor whose office plants have died.

—ERMA BOMBECK

Fact of modern life:

The doctor who listened to all of your problems and gave you limitless time has gone the way of the Walkman. His or her replacement is overburdened, buried in paperwork, frustrated, frazzled, and threatening to quit medicine altogether.

Insurance companies run the show. And the show is not a pretty one.

Many physicians have slimmed down their practices and gone to what some call *concierge* or *tiered* care, which means you have to pay them a fee *over* what you pay for insurance premiums to get their undivided attention—the bigger the fee, the more access.

One friend who has been with her internist for over twenty years was asked to pay $5,000 extra a year for the privilege of calling him at his beach house.

Afraid not to, she forked it over.

Other doctors are coming down with a case of the haves and the have-nots, dividing their practices between those who pay more and get special treatment and those who don't and get less. You can't blame them. There are just so many hours in the day. The system is failing them, too.

What are the rest of us supposed to do?

The idea of paying even more than we do now for medical care is not only out of the question, it's outrageous. It isn't feasible to move to France.

With any luck, the Affordable Care Act will emerge out of the storm of political enmity surrounding it, weed out the bad policies, loosen the choke hold insurance has over patients and physicians alike, and provide a safety net for the uninsured. Moving forward, insurance companies cannot put a lifetime cap on the amount of money paid out, leaving those who suffer catastrophic illness with few options aside from bankruptcy.

Those with gluten intolerance and the problems associated with it will no longer have to face being dropped or denied coverage because of a preexisting condition clause. A ridiculous situation, really, because celiac disease requires no medical intervention, only GI checkups and the gluten-free diet.

Reimbursement for nutritional counseling, crucial to those new to the gluten-free diet, is still a work in progress under the Affordable Care Act. While obesity, kidney disease, and diabetes counseling are covered at no cost to the patient under the new plans, the services of a registered dietician for those with gluten and other self-managed dictary issues are not. Many organizations, among them the American Celiac Disease Alliance, are lobbying hard for inclusion. I hope this will be remedied soon, but at this writing, your best shot is to get your gastroenterologist to order a short course of gluten-free counseling and to make it clear that it is medically necessary.

For those of you not sure about which kind of gluten sensitivity you have, it helps to have your family doctor or gastroenterologist write *rule out celiac disease* whenever ordering testing. Food allergy and gluten sensitivity is still a murky area in terms of insurance reimbursement.

For now, you've got your fifteen minutes. And you'd better make it count.

In an informal survey, I asked several doctors at Thomas Jefferson University Hospital in Philadelphia what makes a patient a good patient. Almost to a person, they said someone actively engaged in their treatment, one who participates in their own care, who listens keenly and sees the patient-doctor relationship as a partnership. Passive and compliant patients, and especially those who, for reasons of age and infirmity, do not communicate well, pose the biggest challenges. All stressed the importance of arriving with a complete and up-to-date list of all medications. There was general agreement that a good patient is focused and arrives at the appointment with no more than three questions or issues to discuss.

One doctor emphasized the value of electronic records. A simple click and all blood work, lab tests, and clinical notes are at the physician's fingertips. He said it was the difference between "flying into O'Hare" and "looking out the cockpit window."

But what if a patient sees doctors at different hospitals? And what if, in the spirit of competition, those hospitals do not share records and, in fact, make it pretty darn hard for one doctor to access the findings of another?

Until there is a universal medical records database, and all the privacy issues that attend such a step are addressed, doctors say the burden is on the individual patient and not on the hospital network to gather his or her records and make copies for their doctors. This eliminates duplication and nasty surprises, such as finding out after the fact that your insurance company won't reimburse you for a test you've already had. Keeping good records also decreases the chances of getting the wrong diagnosis.

That's a good reason to hope we're all on the same electronic page in the near future.

False Positives

Regarding the problem of misdiagnoses, Evan Falchuk, vice-chairman of Best Doctors, Inc., cites data that shows 29 percent of US patients had been misdiagnosed and 60 percent require a change in treatment. He points to a greatly fragmented health care system with a growing number of sub-specialties, overconfidence in the accuracy of tests, a rigid reliance on evidence-based medicine, and the fact that most physicians see more than a hundred patients a week.

To lower the odds of getting the wrong diagnosis, he suggests that patients get to know their family medical history and make sure the doctor is aware of it. Getting a second opinion is a must, says Falchuk, and he urges patients not to lead the witness. "Share your symptoms," he says, "but not your diagnosis." If cancer is involved, patients must always have the pathology rechecked.

Complicating the matter of diagnosis for the gluten-free community is the fact that you may be gluten-sensitive today and gluten-intolerant tomorrow. Staying on top of your diagnosis and retesting is crucial.

Some Dos and Don'ts at the Doctor's Office

+ Don't walk in with a chip on your shoulder the size of Cleveland. Yes, you waited for a while. Yes, you are frustrated. You only get one chance to make a first impression.
+ Do pass on compliments from other doctors. Flattery will get you everywhere.
+ Say why you chose this person. "I hear you are really good at solving mysteries and I really want to work with you to figure this out."
+ Do arrive with clear questions and issues you would like to discuss during the visit.
+ Do let your doctor know what you expect from the visit. Start with the number of questions you have brought. The idea is to keep your doctor focused on you, not on the next patient.
+ Don't drift. If asked if you are under any stress, say yes. Skip divorce details.
+ If your appointment is tomorrow, prepare for it today.
+ Make copies of test results and any reports pertinent to the visit.
+ Do list current medications, including vitamins and other supplements, complete with dosages.

The GI Bill of Rights

1. You have the right to have your symptoms taken seriously.
2. If you suspect a sensitivity to gluten-containing foods, you have the right to insist that diagnostic blood work be done, even if the doctor doesn't agree.
3. You have the right to request that a teaching fellow not be allowed to do your procedure.
4. You have the right to a second opinion.
5. You have the right to make a formal complaint if you feel you have been denied treatment that is necessary.

✦ If this is a first visit, list all allergies, conditions, surgeries, family history, anything medically relevant.

✦ If you have a life-threatening allergy to certain medications, ask that it be written in block letters in your chart. For example: NO EPINEPHRINE!!! NO GLUTEN!!!

✦ If you are feeling too overwhelmed or too sick to organize everything, ask your family doctor to phone ahead of your appointment and explain your situation to the specialist.

✦ If you're not assertive or have trouble talking, ask your partner or a close relative to come with you to present your case and take notes.

✦ Do ask one doctor to help you get in to see another doctor.

✦ If you have an issue with asking for special treatment, ask someone to ask for you.

✦ Do tell the truth. It's amazing how many people lie to their doctors about smoking, drinking, bad eating habits, sexual partners, cheating on the gluten-free diet, and the like.

✦ Don't waste precious appointment time discussing the old doctor's missteps.

✦ You will be asked how long you have been feeling bloated, tired, gassy, feverish, or have had diarrhea or constipation. Keeping a symptom log will help you be precise.

✦ Help your doctor connect the dots. For a GI appointment, write down what you ate that may have triggered symptoms. Mention that your mother had stomach trouble all her life; your big sister can't get pregnant; your grandfather died of colon cancer.

✦ If you are seeing a specialist, do ask that a written or electronic report be sent to your family doctor or internist and to you if you have gone outside your doctor's health system.

✦ Many physicians prefer to give patients copies of reports at the end of the appointment. Don't forget to ask for them.

✦ Do not leave without another appointment or clear steps for follow-up.

Your Family Doctor, Your Quarterback

This is the person you will see more than any other medical professional. Take your time finding the right one for you. Book several appointments and don't be shy about saying you are meeting with two or three other people. Ask about their fee structures before you fall in love. If you can afford a concierge relationship, fine. If you can't, you'll be disappointed.

Familiarize yourself with the doctor's area of interest and see if it's a good fit for you. I once had the good fortune of being seen by one of the most brilliant internists in Philadelphia, but his interest was deep vein thrombosis, a condition that has never troubled me. This, combined with a busy schedule as chief medical officer of the hospital, made it clear to both of us he didn't have time for me.

You need someone willing to help you manage your gluten issues, but also to be around when you get the flu. Say so if you don't want to see somebody you don't know when you need immediate care.

If your insurance company insists that you stay within their network, by all means, interview candidates within the network. If you have celiac disease and one of the conditions associated with it, you may have to see a gastroenterologist or a rheumatologist or even an endocrinologist from time to time. Even if you have non-celiac gluten intolerance or some other level of sensitivity, you're going to need some follow-up care. If your plan requires a referral in order for you to see a specialist, make sure the doctor you choose understands that he or she will have to provide them.

Sad as it may be, some doctors are incentivized for rationing care. If you detect the slightest hint of argument, condescension, or minimizing of your gut issues, keep walking.

Your family doctor or internist will be your interlocutor, translator, strategist, detective, cheerleader, and quarterback who can run with the ball. Choose wisely.

Building a Good Relationship

My ophthalmologist is one of those rare doctors who will give a patient three hours if the situation warrants and, as a result, is often behind schedule and overworked. In order to get my computer glasses right, she took apart and readjusted her own computer according to my measurements and tested my eyes on the spot. Once she called me from a wedding to ask if my eye was feeling better after a nasty scratch on the cornea.

"I don't have to go in to dinner if you need me," she said.

The mountains of candy boxes, plants, and flowers in her office attest to the fact that those of us lucky enough to be in her care, know it.

Doctor Checkup

- American Board of Medical Specialties, a not-for-profit, has the lowdown on your doctor's certification. www.abms.org
- Public Citizen, an advocacy group, lists doctors disciplined by state and federal agencies. www .questionabledoctors.org
- Federation of State Medical Boards will tell you if your physician is licensed and board certified, as well as if there have been any legal or disciplinary actions taken against them. www.fsmb.org
- Quality-check the hospital with which your doctor is affiliated at the Joint Commission, regarding accreditation of health care organizations. www.jointcommission.org
- Find ratings and contact information for gastroenterologists. www .healthgrades.com /gastroenterology -directory

The last time I saw her, she was frantic. Her brother, who lives in another state and relies on her for everything, was quite ill. She had several patient emergencies to attend to before driving several hours to be by his side.

"You wouldn't believe how many people just don't care," she told me, "and insist on being seen even though their visits could be postponed."

It's amazing how many patients never see the person inside the white coat.

✦ Empathy is what you are asking for from your physician. Give some yourself.
✦ Acknowledge how hard it must be to be so overworked and have to follow rules created by insurance company bean counters.
✦ Send a thank-you note when something goes well.
✦ Be appreciative.
✦ Be kind.

The Case of the Dour Doctor

A stony demeanor can be a good defense.

Such was the case with my mother's oncologist. A brilliant doctor whose considerable skill was often bested by the cancer he'd made a career of battling, he often had to tell people they didn't have much time.

My mother teased him, told him he ought to take a day off or else he'd get sick and be of no help to anybody. She brought him her homemade raspberry jam. I tried to make him laugh, too, but he never cracked.

He could not cure my mother's illness, but he found a drug that shrank it down to nothing, giving her four more years with us—good, symptom-free years. By the time the medicine stopped working, a heart problem had intervened, and she slipped quietly away.

I wrote to Dr. D., not only to tell him that my mother had died but also to say I knew how few thanks he got in his particular line of work; I expressed my deep gratitude for the years of grace he gave her.

The minute the dour doctor received my letter, he called and we both had a good cry. Moral of the story: Be as human as you want your doctor to be.

How to Fire Your Doctor

Sometimes we have no choice.

When I returned from the Mayo Clinic with the diagnosis that saved my life, not all my doctors were as over the moon as I. The cardiologist who missed the problem said, "If we spent as much as Mayo does on every patient, medicine would be bankrupt."

I gently pointed out that while he must have felt badly about not being able to figure it out himself, he should have been glad somebody did. Out went the internist who ran out of tests and told me it was all in my head. Ditto for the GI doc who downplayed the gluten connection.

I did not slam their doors. I closed them gently and set about finding people who would respect what I had done. I took my time and did the homework. Now I have the smartest and most caring doctors on the planet. I don't have expensive insurance or pay extra to see them. With two exceptions, they are all at Thomas Jefferson University Hospital in Phila-delphia, a great teaching and research institution making its mark in many fields, including gluten intolerance.

I don't mind the medical students and interns that trail after my doc-tors like ducklings. I like them, actually. Patients can teach, too, and I try to impart something to these eager young healers.

Let's review.

+ Never leave a doctor without explaining why.
+ Be respectful and polite.
+ Resist parting shots, like, *My brother Vinnie, the malpractice attorney, says . . .*
+ Better to say, *I don't feel you are interested in my digestive issues* or *I need someone willing to spend more time with me.*
+ Or, *You seem not to like it when I ask you questions or challenge your opinions.*
+ Don't ask for another recommendation. You will get someone like the one you are leaving.
+ Never speak badly, tweet about, or otherwise trash and embarrass the person you have left.

Ladies and Germs

Autoimmune conditions like those associated with gluten intolerance can make one particularly vulnerable to germs. If you're not careful, a long wait in a doctor's reception room can make you sicker than what brought you in. It's a serious issue with antibiotic-resistant microbes proliferating all over the globe.

Look around.

People are sneezing and coughing and spraying germs into the air, which is usually dry and overheated, the perfect medium for spreading bugs. They are clutching tissues and touching everything around them. Others are sleeping and looking quite feverish. And it's not just the patients. A secretary once coughed right into my receipt and then handed it over with the same hand she used to wipe her nose.

How do you avoid getting more than you bargained for?

+ Definitely use one of the masks dispensed at many clinic front desks.
+ Use a hand sanitizer or alcohol wipe before and after any contact with employees.
+ Make it a rule never to read a magazine or newspaper in a waiting room. Consider how many sick people have handled that piece of paper.
+ Bring a book or an iPad to pass the time.
+ Never sit on a chair that has a discarded tissue on the seat.
+ *Never* pick up a tissue and throw it away.
+ Try to find a chair in a corner away from the crowd, preferably one without arms. Or keep your hands in your lap.
+ If that's not possible, check in with the receptionist and tell her you'll wait in the hall.
+ If the office is willing, ask that you be called on your cell, then go downstairs and have a cup of coffee while you wait.
+ Try not to use the bathroom.
+ If you must use the facilities, wash your hands carefully and use the paper towel to wipe the seat, another to turn off the tap and open the door. (Most people think the seat is where the problem lies, but who ever washes the faucet and the doorknob?)
+ If possible, wait until you are called back to where the doctor's offices are and use a toilet not designated for the public. Same procedure in there.

✦ Use your own pen.
✦ If you've used a credit card, wipe it down.

Even Dirtier in the Hospital

I was in the hospital for a weekend last year. Nothing serious, but my doctor wanted to admit me, just to make sure. I was bored out of my skull and needed a walk around the hallway. The second I touched a naked but nicely polished toe to the linoleum, the nurse rushed in with gripper socks.

"*Never* put your feet on the floor! It's the dirtiest place in the hospital."

I found this surprising, given the loud floor mopping that went on under my bed in the middle of the night.

The woman who shared my room and my bathroom had a serious infection. I overheard her doctor discussing it with her family. Shouldn't I have been told? Or did privacy concerns trump my need to know? I could ignore it and hope I didn't catch anything. Or I could make a fuss.

I chose the latter.

Out of my roommate's earshot, I told the resident what I had heard and asked to be moved. He said he had to speak with the attending. I held firm in the blowback that ensued. A few hours later, they moved my roommate. I wasn't the most popular patient for the hours remaining until my discharge, but I did not get a hospital infection either.

According to *U.S. News and World Report*, 1 out of every 20 patients falls victim to an infection they pick up while in the hospital. *Time* magazine reports that hospital infections contribute to the deaths of nearly ninety thousand patients in the United States each year, costing over $10 billion.

Infections from *Clostridium difficile* (also called *C. diff*), caused by prolonged use of antibiotics, can be life-threatening, and strike 4 in every 1,000 patients who spend the day in the hospital. And you've already got a fluky gut. MRSA (methicillin-resistant *Staphylococcus aureus*) and pneumonia take their toll, especially among the elderly and children and those with compromised immune systems.

Most infections arise at surgical or procedure sites. Needle sticks, catheters, and postsurgical breathing tubes become the entry point. Less than meticulous hand washing spreads them from patient to patient. *Time* reports hospital staff follows hand-washing rules less than 40 percent of the time. Nurses are more apt to wash their hands than doctors.

The CDC recommends:

Yogurt for Hospital Infections?

Dannon yogurt contains *Streptococcus thermophilus*, *Lactobacillus bulgaricus*, and *L. acidophilus*, the beneficial bacteria powerful antibiotics strip away. At Holy Redeemer Hospital in Philadelphia, dieticians meet with patients on these powerful antibiotics to ask them to eat yogurt and explain why two cups a day can keep the *C. diff.* away. Cases of *C. diff.* have fallen by two-thirds over previous years. Naturally, there are naysayers. They laughed at Lister, too.

✦ Patients ask hospital staff to clean their hands in front of you.

✦ Ditto for visitors.

✦ If you have an IV line or urinary catheter, ask if you still need it.

✦ Ask about the hospital's safe injection practices, that is, is the syringe changed as well as the needle for each patient? Both should be discarded.

✦ Ask how long you will be taking a particular antibiotic.

✦ Know the signs of infection: redness or fluid coming from the procedure or injection site. Tell the nurse you are worried it may be infected.

✦ If you are too sick to look for these signs, familiarize a family member before you are admitted.

✦ If you have diarrhea, mention it immediately.

Good Hospital Hygiene Requires:

✦ Cleaning skin where catheter is being inserted

✦ Cleaning skin at surgical site

✦ The use of catheters only when necessary

✦ Hand washing before and after every patient

✦ Hair covers, masks, gowns, and gloves when necessary

You want to make sure everyone follows the rules, but you're also the one in the bed. You don't want to be ignored or treated badly because you're a stickler. Use a light touch here, maybe even a little humor, when asking staff to conform to the rules.

I know I'm weird, but do you mind washing your hands?

While you're in the bathroom washing up, would you mind putting a little Ajax in the sink?

If I have to walk around in this getup, you have to wash your hands.

The minute you get home, if you are able, take a hot shower, wash your hair, and launder your clothes in hot water. Do *not* soak in the bathtub. If you remembered to wear an old pair of shoes for the trip home, throw them away. Do *not* save the hospital slipper socks or the gown as a souvenir.

Eating Safely in the Hospital

Gluten-free tonsils have to come out, as do ruptured appendixes. Babies have to be born, gallbladders removed, knees replaced, and everybody's got to eat.

The good news is you won't be there long. What with insurance companies sending even the frail and the elderly home with tubes and shunts, staples, and things best taken care of by trained professionals, one wonders why they just don't do surgery in the parking lot. But for the short and getting shorter time you're there, you may ask, What's for dinner?

More and more hospitals, particularly large medical systems, have jumped on the gluten-free bandwagon. At Beth Israel Deaconess Medical Center in Boston, you can expect to be served in-patient gluten-free meals, and your visitors can expect the same in the cafeteria.

In some New York area hospitals you can expect in-patient gluten-free meals and trays for visitors. Others, such as Philadelphia's Thomas Jefferson University Hospital, offer gluten-free snacks following GI procedures. The University of Chicago Medical Center has gone so far as to seek and qualify for accreditation from the rigorous Gluten Intolerance Group's gluten-free food service program.

As more and more star toques turn up running big hospital kitchens, hospital fare is beating its bad rap and, in some places, is actually good, even for those on restricted diets.

However.

Many hospitals, particularly those in small or rural communities, are still way behind. You may be offered a gluten-free menu and tick all the right boxes, but you may end up with your dinner slathered in thick gravy or unsafe crackers, chicken noodle soup, or ice cream sandwiches. Depending on who's running the kitchen, and if there is a dietician on call when you arrive, you may end up with a high-fat and high-sodium diet or find they've overcompensated with a bland, boring, and unnecessary low-fat, low-sodium one.

If they do have a dietician, by all means ask to see him or her and discuss what you can and cannot eat for the duration. You might take advantage of the patient advocate in your hospital, but bear in mind that it is his or her job to help you negotiate all aspects of the hospital experience in a way that doesn't open the hospital up to legal action.

The best thing to do is not to expect good or even gluten-free food and to enjoy it if it's offered. Add to your overnight bag of personal necessities your list of medications with dose and frequency, smartphone charger, reading material, a nice robe for hallway strolling, and the following emergency food supplies:

✦ Gluten-free energy bars
✦ Crackers and cheese—A cold windowsill should keep the cheese fresh for a day or two.
✦ A few slices of gluten-free bread or a couple of rolls that will hold up on that same windowsill.
✦ Nuts and raisins
✦ All the fresh fruit you can carry.

When the menu arrives, check off things like:

✦ Fresh fruit, as much as they'll give you
✦ Eggs—soft boiled, scrambled, or poached
✦ Applesauce and juice

In addition:

✦ Ask to see the box before you order gluten-free cereal, pudding, or ice cream.
✦ Some hospital kitchens have cream of rice cereal. Ask.
✦ Order a plain baked potato with a little butter, or steamed vegetables— not tasty, but safe.
✦ Cottage cheese is boring but will fit the bill. Ask for a fruit cocktail to dump into it. Or bring your own caraway seeds or chives.
✦ Yogurt, if you know what brand. Mix with fresh fruit from your tray.
✦ Avoid the whole thing and ask if your family can bring you takeout from a reliable restaurant.

Prescription Meds—Theirs or Yours?

I understand why hospitals insist on giving you their medications. After all, they are accountable for the efficacy of their own pharmacy, not yours. And let's be honest, some patients are not exactly taking them as prescribed.

But you know what you're taking is gluten-free and you have no such assurances about the hospital brand. It's bad enough being in the hospital; you don't want to get glutened in the bargain.

Ask your doctor to write an order allowing you to take your own medications. Forget the little weekly dispenser and bring them in their original bottles. Give your medicine to the nurse with dosage instructions so they are dispensed back to you properly.

Having said that, be prepared for the attending to overrule the whole thing and for your meds to be confiscated or sent home with a loved one. All is not lost. If you have to take the generic versions of your medications, ask the staff to look up the ingredients in their pharmacy before giving them to you.

Nurses' stations have a reference for the doctor to check before ordering your medication. (FYI: This is why you bring a current list and doses, so any new medications can be checked against possible drug interactions.)

When my husband had heart surgery several years ago, I went over all of his meds with the thoracic surgeon and the hospital cardiologist before a duplicate list was submitted. It isn't difficult and it could save you a world of trouble.

Doctors pop in and out as needed and often do their rounds before you are fully conscious, leaving the nurses pretty much in control of everything that happens to you. These nightingales are often doing the work of three people. Resist buzzing every thirty seconds unless you really need to. Be appreciative of special treatment. Like everything else, with few exceptions, you will get back what you give.

Gluten Isn't the Only Accident That Can Happen in a Hospital

Many years ago when I was hospitalized for my as-yet-undiagnosed celiac disease, my roommate was an Italian grandmother in a leg cast up to the hip. Like many women of her generation who scrubbed their front stoops, and whose floors you could actually eat off of, she grumbled about our bathroom not being up to her standards.

A few minutes after I arrived, she took a bottle of Windex and a spray can of disinfectant out of her purse and thumped off to clean the bathroom.

"What happened to your leg?" I asked, too weak to offer any help.

"Nothing," she said. "I'm here for my gallbladder and two idiots just put me in a cast."

I was incredulous.

"You let them do that?"

She shrugged.

"Whattaya gonna do?"

Just then two sheepish residents walked into our room. My roommate stuck her head out of the bathroom.

"I was wondering when you two would be back."

Then she let them take off the cast that belonged to another patient. You can't make this stuff up.

In 1999 the Institute of Medicine published *To Err Is Human*, shocking the medical community by reporting that 98,000 people a year died annually as a result of medical error. In September 2013, ProPublica.org reported on a new study in the *Journal of Patient Safety* that puts that figure somewhere between 210,000 to 440,000 patients who go to the hospital and suffer some kind of preventable harm.

Not everybody gets off as easily as my roommate, white with plaster dust but no worse for the error. Many of the people you will meet in the hospital are suffering from coffee nerves, no backup, overwork, and sleep deprivation; they are running on automatic pilot. Here are some ways to minimize your risks:

◆ Assume nothing. In your flimsy gown, you look like everyone else they will see today.
◆ Learn how to distinguish between a student, a first-year resident, a senior resident, an attending physician, consultants, and those lay workers who are often mistaken for medical or nursing personnel.
◆ If you don't see a name tag with job identification, ask. "What's your job here?" is good opener.
◆ Ask the person in your room what they are about to do. And why.
◆ If the person in your room has not looked at your ID bracelet, show it to them.
◆ Ask to see the order for the procedure.
◆ Ask if your doctor has approved.
◆ Don't save your questions for the juniors. Ask your surgeon what she's doing, too.
◆ Put a big fat X on the arm, leg, foot, or boob in need of attention.
◆ Write "left kidney" on your belly.

I had a little neuroma (a tiny, benign nerve tumor that hurts a lot and is usually caused by wearing high heels) removed from between the fourth and pinky toe on my left foot. The surgeon was a jokester and said more than once, "It's your left foot, right?"

He wouldn't stop.

So freaked out was I that I folded the good foot under my body before they knocked me out. Under sedation I muttered about it the whole time.

Remember Murphy's Law. *What can go wrong will go wrong.*

+ If you're scared and in pain or otherwise woozy, make sure there is someone with you who isn't.
+ Anonymous people in the know say never to opt for an elective procedure at the end of the week. Something goes wrong and everybody who can help is either swatting tennis balls or on the golf course.
+ Don't schedule anything in late June and early July, either. That's when the green first-year residents show up at the teaching hospitals. Wait until they find out where the defibrillators are.

Testing, Testing, One, Two, Three

Up to this point, I've suggested, nagged, wheedled, warned, and cajoled you to get tested. And tested again periodically. I've given you good reasons for doing so, even if you've given up gluten for the heck of it.

Let's summarize.

Ten Reasons to Get Tested

1. You've got a first-degree relative with celiac disease.
2. You are planning to start a family.
3. You couldn't get pregnant if you stood on your head, and you tried that, too.
4. You have low iron, unexplained anemia, or liver problems.
5. You are on the gluten-free diet but still have symptoms.
6. You are a young man with osteoporosis.
7. You are losing weight without trying.
8. You are gaining weight without trying.
9. You have an itchy rash that won't go away.
10. You are sluggish and tired all the time.

The keys to getting accurate test results are threefold:

1. You **MUST** be eating gluten for at least a month or two when you are tested.
2. Getting to a gastroenterologist (not an allergist and not your GP) familiar with the newest testing methods.

3. Getting your blood work to a lab that is familiar with gluten antibody testing.

Blood Tests for Celiac Disease and Non-Celiac
Gluten Intolerance

(IgG) antigliadin antibody (AGA)
IgA antigliadin antibody (AGA)
IgG anti-tissue transglutaminase antibody
IgA anti-tissue transglutaminase antibody
Endomysial antibodies (EMA)
Total IgA immunoglobulin
Anti-deamidated gliadin peptide (DGP)

Other Tests to Consider

A new test, the anti-deamidated gliadin peptide (DGP) test, has been developed to replace the anti-gliadin antibody test (AGA), a primary test commonly ordered in the past but that has limited accuracy.

As reported on their Web site, the Celiac Center at Beth Israel Deaconess Medical Center has replaced the traditional AGA test with the IgA anti-tissue transglutaminase (IgA-tTG), whose sensitivity and measures of accuracy are excellent. Even so, they say, there are occasional individuals whose IgA anti-tTG results may be misleading.

For the vast majority of screening and follow-up cases, the Center's lab will continue to use IgA anti-iTG and, in addition, order total IgA levels. If a patient has IgA deficiency, more common among celiac patients than in the general population (that is, more than 1 in 400 individuals), this may cause a falsely negative IgA-tTG.

On occasion, a physician may order a gene test called HLA-DQ2 and HLA-DQ8. If blood work is negative, but there is still enough suspicion, perhaps a familial connection, these may be done. Except in very rare cases, being positive for the gene precludes the need for a diagnostic small bowel biopsy or endoscopy because 98 to 99 percent of those with celiac disease carry the gene.

The Celiac Center at Beth Israel Deaconess Medical Center recommends an IgG deamidated gliadin peptide (IgGDGP) if:

✦ There is known IgA deficiency in the initial evaluation for celiac disease.

+ There is known IgA deficiency with celiac disease to monitor the response to a gluten-free diet.
+ When IgA anti-tTG is normal in patients with villous atrophy or damage in the small intestine.
+ In patients with a moderate to high risk of celiac disease, but a normal IgA anti-tTG, to guide a decision regarding the need for endoscopy and biopsy.
+ In patients with a low risk of celiac disease, a normal anti-tTG, but a positive AGA.

It bears repeating: These tests, like all others, normalize on a gluten-free diet. Only those continuing to eat gluten can expect accurate results.

TEST FOR GLUTEN SENSITIVITY

At present there is no test for non-celiac gluten sensitivity. Doctors make this diagnosis by excluding other possibilities, such as celiac disease or wheat allergy. However, there are interesting possibilities on the horizon.

In a study reported by *Living Without* magazine and presented at Digestive Disease Week, May 2013, researchers at the University of Rome applied a patch containing 1.2 milligrams of gluten inside the upper lips of twenty patients who had tested negative for celiac disease and food allergy. Two hours later, 80 percent experienced swelling, wheals, and/or blistering at the application side. Half of the subjects experienced bloating and 11 percent experienced diarrhea within twenty-four hours of taking the tests. The study concludes that the same gluten-related inflammation seen in the oral mucosa could be occurring in the intestinal mucosa. Obviously, more research is necessary, but this is an interesting finding.

ABOUT THE SMALL BOWEL BIOPSY

The small bowel biopsy is the gold standard for diagnosing celiac disease and assessing damage or atrophy of the intestinal villi, fingerlike projections necessary for the absorption of nutrients. Many are not willing to take this test, especially parents not wanting to put their little ones through it, relying instead on blood work. Still, this procedure is invaluable when tests are difficult to interpret or symptoms have not resolved despite following a gluten-free diet.

The biopsy is a painless outpatient procedure conducted under local anesthesia. A tube is inserted and several tissue samples are taken from different sections of the intestine to look for the characteristic flattening and scarring that take place in response to the insult of gluten. It can confirm celiac disease and is also used, in the presence of continuing symptoms, to assess healing from a previous positive biopsy.

My own biopsy was done many years ago, and I've had two more over the course of twenty years, one to confirm healing and the other to rule out a relapse. I repeat the blood work as part of my annual GI exam in order to ensure that I am not getting any accidental gluten. It makes good sense.

As a biopsy-proven celiac, it's comforting to know that hidden gluten or the rare accident is not turning up on the radar in any meaningful way.

STOOL TESTS

Stool tests, such as those offered by Dr. Kenneth Fine's EnteroLab, look for signs of gluten sensitivity and intolerance in fecal matter. While Dr. Fine has patented this method and touts its ability to pick up gluten antibodies in earlier stages than current blood tests do, no published research supports this claim. These tests are not widely accepted by the medical community and most insurance companies won't cover them. Important to note: This method does not detect celiac disease.

TESTS FOR ASSOCIATED CONDITIONS

Let's say you have tested positive for celiac disease or you are just plain worn out from gluten intolerance and sensitivity. It's wise to spend some time with a registered dietician, wherever you are on the spectrum. Depending on how old you are, it might be years since you absorbed your vitamins and minerals properly. As you know from the previous chapter, you may even be at greater risk for developing certain other disorders.

Talk to your doctor about making some or all of the following tests part of your annual routine.

- CBC (complete blood count)
- Blood tests to monitor the levels of B_{12}, albumin, calcium, vitamin D, magnesium, and zinc
- Thyroid functioning
- Blood sugar
- DEXA (bone density scan)
- Antinuclear antibody (ANA) testing

✦ C-reactive protein (CRP) or erythrocyte sedimentation rate (ESR) to measure the presence and level of inflammation

TESTING FOR GENERAL GOOD HEALTH

If you haven't felt up to par for a while, depending on your age, medical history, and your doctor's inclinations, items on the annual checklist may include:

✦ Lipid panel to measure blood cholesterol, including HDL (good) and LDL (bad) levels
✦ Pap smear
✦ Blood pressure
✦ Mammogram (for women)
✦ PSA (prostate-specific antigen) level and digital prostrate exam (for men)
✦ Colon cancer screening
✦ Flu and pneumonia immunizations
✦ Dental checkups and cleanings
✦ EKG and/or stress echocardiogram of the heart

VOCABULARY TEST

Does your doctor use ten-dollar words when twenty-five-cent ones will do?

Admit it, you pretend you know what the heck he or she is talking about, then you run home and look it up, only to forget exactly how it was used in the sentence. Even worse, there's no headache (cephalgia) like the headache you get trying to make sense of your medical report, or an article in a medical journal where every third word is Greek to you.

Short of lugging around a medical dictionary; enrolling in a crash course on Medspeak, or getting a free Medical Source Dictionary app for your iPhone, iPad, or iPod, here, with the help of my dog-eared *Mosby's Medical Dictionary*, is a handy translation of some of the common conditions behind the fancy terms that come with an expensive medical education.

Achalasia: A spasm in which the muscle cannot relax, usually the lower end of the esophagus
Adenopathy: Swollen glands
Angina pectoris: Chest pain originating in the heart
Bruxism: Involuntary grinding or gnashing of the teeth

Cephalgia: Headache
Dyspepsia: Indigestion
Dysphagia: Difficulty swallowing
Dyspnea: Shortness of breath
Ecchymosis: A bruise
Edema: Swelling caused by water retention

Emesis: Vomit

Eructation: Belching

Erythema: Redness

Excipient: A nonmedicinal ingredient in prescription medicine

Febrile: Having a fever or feverish

Hyperhidrosis: Excessive sweating (the prefix *hyper* means "too much"; *hypo* means "too little")

Hypertension: High blood pressure

Hypotension: Low blood pressure

Intermetatarsal neuritis: Pain and numbness in the toes

Lesion: Wound, sore, or infected patch of skin

Lipid: Fat

Myalgia: Muscle pain

Myocardial infarction: Heart attack

Nephrotoxic: Poisonous to the kidneys

Nocturia: Peeing a lot at night

Oncologist: Doctor who treats cancer

Onychomycosis: Nail fungus

Pallor: Pale skin

Paresthesia: Numbness, tingling, or pins-and-needles sensation

Paronychia: Hangnail

Pathogenesis: The mode of origin or development of a disease

Pityriasis sicca: Dandruff

Postprandial somnolence: Sleepiness after a big meal

Rhinitis: Inflammation of the mucous membranes of the nose

Steatorrhea: Fatty diarrhea common in celiac disease

Stomatitis: Mouth infection

Syncope: Loss of consciousness, fainting, blackout

Pruritus: Itching

Purpura: Purplish skin discoloration caused by bleeding under the skin

Purulent: Infection containing pus

Rhinorrhea: Runny nose

Tetany: Muscle spasms, twitches, and cramps

Tinea pedis: Athlete's foot

Ventilation: Breathing

Vertigo: Dizziness

Villi: Fingerlike projections in the intestine involved in absorbing nutrients

Xerosis: Dry, itchy skin

If only someone would come up with a way to decipher your doctor's handwriting!

Learn More

A-LIST MEDICAL CENTERS FOR GLUTEN INTOLERANCE

Directors of these centers read like a *Who's Who* of the best minds in the field—Alessio Fasano, Joseph Murray, Stefano Guandalini, Anthony J. DiMarino, Ritu Verma, Karoly Horvath, Peter Green, Michelle Pietzak, Cynthia Rudert, Sheila Crow, Ciaran Kelly, and Dan Leffler, among others.

If you live in a rural area or your doctor is unfamiliar with the latest antibody testing, some centers offer lab kits with self-addressed labels, so all you have to do is have your blood drawn and send it to the experts. One center in Chicago provides patients new to the gluten-free diet with starter care packages of gluten-free products.

All offer the latest research, testing services, physician referrals, nutritional counseling, and support for adult and pediatric gluten intolerance.

Baltimore, Maryland

The University of Maryland Medical Center—Research, diagnosis, and patient care. www.umm.edu

Boston, Massachusetts

Celiac Center at Beth Israel Deaconess Medical Center. www.bidmc.org/celiaccenter

Center for Celiac Research and Treatment, MassGeneral Hospital for Children. www.celiaccenter.org

Charlottesville, Virginia

University of Virginia Health System Digestive Health Center. www.healthsystem.virginia.edu/digestivehealth

Chicago, Illinois

The University of Chicago Celiac Disease Center. www.uchospitals.edu/specialities/celiac

Rush University Medical Center Adult Celiac Disease Program. www.rush.edu/celiac

Iowa City, Iowa

University of Iowa Celiac Disease Clinic. www.uihealthcare.org/celiac

La Jolla, California

University of California at San Diego William K. Warren Medical Research Center for Celiac Disease. www.health.ucsd.edu/specialties/gastro/areas-expertise/Pages/celiac-disease-clinic.aspx

Livingston, New Jersey

Kogan Celiac Center of the Barnabas Health Ambulatory Care Center. www.barnabashealth.org/services/celiac

Long Island, New York

Stony Brook Celiac Disease and Gluten Sensitivity Center.
www.stonybrookchildrens.org/specialties-services/clinical-programs
/celiac-gluten

Los Angeles, California

Children's Hospital Los Angeles, Division of Pediatric Gastroenterology.
www.chla.org

New York, New York

Celiac Disease Center at Columbia University.
www.celiacdiseasecenter.columbia.edu

Philadelphia, Pennsylvania

Children's Hospital of Philadelphia Center for Celiac Disease.
www.chop.edu/service/center-for-celiacdisease
Thomas Jefferson University Hospital Celiac Center. www.jefferson
hospital.org/departments-and-services/celiac-center

Pittsburgh, Pennsylvania

Allegheny Health Network Multidisciplinary Center for Management
of Celiac Disease.
www.ahn.org/specialties/celiac-disease

Rochester, Minnesota

Mayo Celiac Clinic (Mayo also has clinics in Scottsdale, Arizona, and
Jacksonville, Florida). www.mayoclinic.org/diseases-conditions
/celiac-disease/basics/definition/con-20030410

San Diego, California

University of California at San Diego Wm. K. Warren Medical Research
Center for Celiac Disease. celiaccenter.ucsd.edu

Wilmington, Delaware

Alfred I. duPont Hospital for Children, Pediatric GI Division.
www.nemours.org/content/derm/nemours/www/filebox
/healthpub/patientreferral/gastro.pdf

LAB

IMMCO Diagnostics—Autoimmune and celiac disease antibody testing. www.immco.com

INFORMATION YOU CAN TRUST

Celiac Disease Foundation Healthcare Practitioner Directory. celiac.org
Find a doctor based on specialty or ailment. www.vitals.com
Hospital Guide—Gluten Intolerance Group. www.gluten.net

The last thing you want to do is go to Wikipedia when you are looking for information on your own health. Online searches should never replace a face-to-face meeting with your doctor, but it can make that meeting more productive. Here are some reliable sources:

Mayo Clinic—This site offers the latest medical news and health articles from the venerable Rochester, Minnesota, institution. Sign up for e-mail on subjects of interest. www.mayoclinic.com

MedlinePlus—This site, operated by the U.S. National Library of Medicine, offers encyclopedic information on all diseases and conditions, including definitions of medical terms and referrals to organizations that deal with specific illnesses. It is also helpful for searching for the top doctors in each field. www.medlineplus.gov

WebMD—This easy-to-navigate site guides you from general information to more specific links to possible causes and treatments. www.webmd.com

Apples are gluten-free.
One a day may keep the you-know-who away.

21

Winning the Drug War

One pill makes you larger,
   and one pill makes you small,
      And the ones that mother gives you,
         don't do anything at all.
            —GRACE SLICK, "WHITE RABBIT"

Those of you new to the gluten-free diet may well say that food is the cure, no medication required.

True. But even the healthiest among us may have to pop a cold pill, take an antibiotic, lose the cholesterol, and build up our bones from time to time. And therein lies the gluten. Or not.

From now on you have to ensure that all of your prescription and over-the-counter medications are free of gluten.

If you've heard that very few medications contain gluten, you heard right.

It's not the actual medicine you have to worry about. It's the excipients—fillers used to bind the drugs and deliver the medication—that may be suspect. To complicate matters, generic forms of medications may source different excipients than the brand name, which means that even if the brand name is determined gluten-free, the generic form must be verified. Each time you receive a generic made by a different manufacturer, a switch made with maddening frequency these days, you must verify again.

If you've ever tried to read the mice type on the list of ingredients, side effects, and reactions with other drugs in the product literature, you know that rooting out gluten in the medicine cabinet can be a blinding exercise.

Drug company research and development departments rival the CIA for secrecy—with intracompany espionage and dirty tricks, not to mention allegations of price fixing, suppressing research about dangerous drug reactions, and all-around socking it to the consumer. With piracy a billion-dollar business, requests for drug company formulas are routinely met with suspicion.

Like all good marketers, pharmaceutical companies are clever at increasing usage of their product. For example, take restless leg syndrome. Is this really a condition or just some weird neurologic side effect caused by medication? Why not double your profits by calling a side effect a condition, then market another medicine to take it away? Just saying.

The most famous example of this strategy is Alka-Seltzer. No need to tell consumers one tablet does the job. Put two in a package, launch the most brilliant advertising campaign in history—*Plop, Plop, Fizz, Fizz, Oh, What a Relief It Is!*—and double your sales overnight.

Let's just say Big Pharma is about as forthcoming as the food industry is about GMOs.

There Oughta Be a Law

Congressman Tim Ryan (D-OH) and Congresswoman Nita Lowey (D-NY) cosponsored the Gluten in Medicine Identification Act of 2012 (H.R. 4972) to "require the labeling of drugs for human use to contain a parenthetical statement identifying the source of any ingredient constituting or derived from grain or starch-containing ingredient."

The bill was endorsed by all of the big gluten-intolerance groups—the American Celiac Disease Alliance, Celiac Disease Foundation, Celiac Support Association (CSA/USA), Gluten Intolerance Group, and the National Foundation for Celiac Awareness. Over six thousand letters were written urging Congress to act. Slam dunk, right?

Wrong.

This important bill, which would ensure the safety of prescription medications and over-the-counter drugs for millions of gluten-intolerant Americans, stalled and eventually was killed by the 112th Congress, voted the most partisan and ineffective in history.

In May 2013, Ryan and Lowey tried again. This time, they introduced an identical bill, H.R. 2003, with a new name, Gluten in Medicine Disclosure Act of 2013. With only nine supporters in the House, this, too, has met with a tepid response.

If not now, when?

Until such time as there is an act of Congress to make gluten-free drug taking easier, you are on your own. Nevertheless, you must persevere, either by using one of the sources for gluten-free medications listed here or by phoning the drug company yourself, a frustrating but necessary evil.

If you do buy one of the available and often reliable gluten-free drug guides, the information is only as good as the day it was verified. If you are able to get a drug company on the phone and you find a willing ear, try to resist ranting about their excessive profit margins or the strength of their lobby. You're trying to find out about gluten. Count to ten before you make the call.

Sometimes a drug maker will list certain ingredients on the label as *unspecified*. To disclose them would be giving away trade secrets. While the manufacturer won't reveal these proprietary ingredients, they should be able to tell you if gluten is involved.

I emphasize the word *should*. The key to getting the information you need lies in your approach. Honey gets a lot more than vinegar.

Rx for Zero Gluten

+ Start by telling all of your doctors and your pharmacist you are gluten-free and what that means in terms of medications. And don't forget the dentist. Do not assume the word *gluten* will ring a bell.

+ Arm yourself with a short description of the problem and explain how it can pertain to both over-the-counter and prescription medicine.

+ Write it on an index card, make copies, and leave one with each of your health care providers, along with your contact information, to keep as a permanent record in your file.

+ It's always a good idea to investigate the gluten-free status of drugs you may be required to take or are considering taking at some future date. This way, should the need arise, you'll know which ones are gluten-free ahead of time.

+ Go through all of your existing medications and verify their safety, either by using one of the guides listed in this chapter or by contacting the manufacturer yourself.

+ This is a good time to clean out the medicine chest and toss the Cipro you've been hoarding since the anthrax scare and those eye drops you've forgotten the reason for.

+ Don't overlook over-the-counter products like baby aspirin, vitamins, and other supplements. Review even the most innocuous-sounding stuff and switch to a gluten-free brand if necessary.

+ Before you fill any new prescriptions, ask the pharmacist to give you the product insert. Even better, ask her to check all of the ingredients for you.

+ When you verify that a brand-name drug is gluten-free, have the doctor specify *brand name necessary* on the prescription. You may have to argue with your insurance company, but it's worth the peace of mind.

+ Periodically check to make sure its gluten-free status remains unchanged.

+ Develop a relationship with the pharmacist filling your prescriptions. He or she can be an important advocate.

+ Do ask your pharmacist to call the manufacturer of a particular medicine and check on its gluten-free status for you if necessary. If you're very nice, he or she may even fight with the insurance company for you, or give you a shortcut to getting it done.

+ If you must take generics, as so many of us must, ask with each refill if the same company is still making it.

+ Always use the same pharmacy. People are much more likely to help if they know you are a good customer.

Contraindication!

If you notice a difference in the color or look of a particular medication you take, call the company or check with your pharmacist right away. The company may have reformulated the drug, which in turn means you have to check for gluten all over again. If you take a generic drug, it may mean a different manufacturer is making your medication.

Compounding the Problem

One way to be sure you're avoiding gluten is to find a good compounding pharmacy that can prepare gluten-free medications for you. Most have gone the way of the buffalo, but they're not entirely impossible to find and most offer mail-order services.

Specially compounded medications and gluten-free vitamins and supplements cost a bit more, but they're well worth it in terms of peace of mind. After the meningitis outbreak at the New England Compounding Center in Framingham, Massachusetts, that killed fifty people, compounding pharmacies are more strictly monitored. Make sure the one you choose is regulated by the FDA.

Many of these specialty companies specialize in sugar-free, yeast-free, dye-free, lactose-free, casein-free, and wheat-free formations as well:

College Pharmacy, Colorado Springs, Colorado.
   www.collegepharmacy.com
Compounded Solutions in Pharmacy, Monroe, Connecticut.
   www.compoundedsolutions.com
Meyer Pharmacy, Waverly, Iowa. www.meyerpharmacy.com
Pine Pharmacy, Niagara Falls, New York. www.pinepharmacy.com
San Diego Compounding Pharmacy, San Diego California.
   www.sandiegocompoundingpharmacy.com
Stokes Pharmacy, Mount Laurel, New Jersey. www.stokesrx.com

FIND MORE

Directory of Compounding Pharmacies.
   www.ecompoundingpharmacy.com
International Academy of Compounding Pharmacists. www.iacprx.org

Warning: Do Not Swallow While Taking This Medication

What exactly is going down with that glass of water?

Just as you study a new medication's information sheet for possible reactions, contraindications, side effects, signs of overdose, and so on, now you must become equally familiar with the names for the starches, fillers, sweeteners, coloring and suspension agents, and other strange-sounding and possibly glutenous ingredients that make prescription and over-the-counter medications palatable.

One way to do that is to buy a current *PDR* (*Physicians' Desk Reference*), a doorstop of a book listing all of the package inserts that are included with prescription medication. Go to the section on inactive ingredients and familiarize yourself with those ingredients that may hold the potential for trouble.

GlutenFreeDrugs.com lists the following inactive or excipient ingredients as gluten-free. Please note that I did not say chemical-free or free of substances you might be reluctant to touch, much less swallow.

Benzyl alcohol is made from benzyl chloride from tar oil, not gluten.

Cellulose (methylcellulose, hydroxymethylcellulose, or microcrystalline cellulose) can be made from plant fiber, woody pulp, or chemical cotton, but not gluten.

Cetyl alcohol is a substance derived from spermaceti, the waxy substance from the head of the sperm whale. Gluten sounds almost palatable by contrast.

Croscarmellose sodium is an internally cross-linked sodium carboxymethylcellulose for use as a disintegrant in pharmaceutical formulations.

Dextrans are sugar molecules.

Dextrates is a mixture of sugars resulting from the hydrolysis of starch.

Dextrins result from the hydrolysis of cornstarch by heat or hydrochloric acid.

Gelatin is gotten from boiling the skin, connective tissue, and bones of animals. Ugh.

Glycerin can be made in the following ways: saponification of fats and oils in the manufacturing of soaps; hydrolysis of fats and oils through pressure and superheated steam; or fermentation of beet sugar molasses in the presence of large amounts of sodium sulfite or from propylene, a petroleum product—none of which involves gluten.

Glycerols are obtained from fats and oils as by-products in the manufacture of soaps and fatty acids.

Glycols are products of ethylene oxide gas.

Iron oxide is just that, rust used as a coloring agent.

Mannitol is a sweetener derived from monosaccharides.

Polysorbates come from a chemically altered sugar called sorbitol.

Povidone or crospovidone is a synthetic polymer.

Silicon dioxide is a dispersing agent made from silicon.

Sodium lauryl sulfate is a derivative of the fatty acids of coconut oil.

Stearates are derived from stearic acid, a fat that occurs as a glyceride in tallow and other animal fats and oils, as well as some vegetables, and is made by hydrogenation of cottonseed and other vegetable oils.

Titanium dioxide is a chemical not derived from any starch source. It's used as a white pigment.

Triacetin is a derivative of glycerin.

Sister Jeanne Crowe, PharmD, RPh, and Nancy Patin Falini, MA, RD, tell us in their *American Journal of Health-System Pharmacy* article, "Gluten in Pharmaceutical Products," that only those medications that come into direct contact with the intestinal tract, that is, tablets, capsules, syrups, oral solutions, and rectal suppositories, must be checked for possible sources of gluten. Medications that are injected, delivered as transdermal skin patches, or inhaled (as long as the medicine is not swallowed) generally do not cause problems.

INGREDIENTS THAT SHOULD AROUSE SUSPICION

Starch

Steven Plogsted, PharmD, of Nationwide Children's Hospital in Columbus, Ohio, warns that starch is the single most suspicious source of gluten in the medicine cabinet. This binding agent can be made from corn, potatoes, wheat, rice, or tapioca, and its origin may not be readily identifiable on the label. Unidentified starch requires further investigation. If a particular drug does not contain starch, Dr. Plogsted says, chances are very good, 99.9 percent, that it will be gluten-free as well.

Pregelatinized Starch

This, too, may be derived from wheat starch, cornstarch, or tapioca starch.

Dextri-Maltose

This is a mixture of dextrin and maltose produced by the enzymatic action of barley malt and corn flour. Any presence of barley malt in the manufacturing process makes this ingredient highly suspicious.

Flour, Gluten, Dusting Powder

The first two should be obvious, but dusting powder from an undisclosed source can be trouble. Verify with the manufacturer before using.

Malt, Malt Syrup

These ingredients are derived from barley and are often used in the making of other inactive ingredients, such as dextrimaltose.

NOT LIKELY TO CONTAIN GLUTEN, BUT ASK ANYWAY

Dextrin

Although wheat starch can be used in the manufacture of dextrin, most dextrins manufactured in the United States are corn-based and gluten-free.

Maltodextrin

Maltodextrin found in medication is almost always derived from cornstarch and therefore gluten-free.

Caramel Color

Almost all caramel color produced in the United States is gluten-free. However, imported products containing caramel color should be checked. It is always a good idea to use *dye-free* medications.

Look for the Silver Lining

Drug companies have to go through an enormous amount of red tape and expense to change a brand-name formulation after FDA approval, so if you do find a gluten-free medication, chances are very good that it will stay that way. That is not to say you can be complacent or drop your guard with generics. Just don't be paranoid.

What About Cross-Contamination?

Don't worry about it.

Drug companies are bound by federal regulation to use one room and one production line to manufacture one product. All equipment is stainless-steel, everything is sterilized, and sophisticated ventilation systems eliminate any chance of airborne contamination. These places are more sterile than the average operating room. If only we could get big food processors to follow the same rule.

In Case of Emergency

If you find yourself hospitalized with a serious infection and have not been able to verify the gluten content of a particular antibiotic, request that you be given the drug intravenously until a safe substitute can be found. Get well. Argue with the insurance company later.

Common-sense Check

If you're having chest pain, *do not* refuse to take nitroglycerin until you're sure a particular brand is gluten-free. If you're having a heart attack, gluten should be the last thing on your mind. Verify the gluten-free status of just-in-case meds as well as those you take regularly. We'll both sleep better knowing you've done this.

With so much attention being paid to gluten, more drug companies are making gluten-free medications. Still, some won't verify the gluten-free status of raw materials from their suppliers. Others say their drugs aren't gluten-free because they don't want you potentially taking a dose of gluten every day. The key word here is *daily*. Anything you take every day, verify.

Note: In the previous edition I listed the status of many popular prescription drugs and over-the-counter medications and formulas, never realizing that the information would be in print so long that many readers would come to it years after those formulas had changed. Determined to provide detailed information, I didn't take into account this is a book that doesn't end up on the remainder table. I apologize to those who came late and were confused or frustrated.

I provide no such list here.

In order to ensure the ongoing veracity of this edition, I will leave you to the information and sources below. This way, you'll know your homework is up-to-date.

Okay.

You've gone through your prescriptions and the over-the-counter stuff in your medicine chest. Here are some of the companies that may be in your collection.

Abbott Laboratories	Genentech	Roche USA
www.abbott.com	www.gene.com	www.rocheusa.com
AstraZeneca	GlaxoSmithKline	Roxane Laboratories
www.astrazeneca-us.com	www.gsk.com	www.roxane.com
Bristol-Myers Squibb	Merck	Sandoz
www.bms.com	www.merck.com	www.us.sandoz.com
Eli Lilly	Pfizer	Wyeth
www.lilly.com	www.pfizer.com	www.pfizer.com

Prescription-Speak

Just as medical terms leave us in the dark, so does the shorthand surrounding the dosage of our prescription meds. Sometimes I just think all of it is Latin for *I'm smarter than you.*

With a little help from the School of Pharmacy and as a public service, I've decoded the arcane instructions, abbreviations, and notations found on prescription pads, medicine bottles, tubes, sprays, and dispensers.

aa: of each

a.c.: before meals

ad: up to

a.d.: right ear

ad lib.: at pleasure, freely

a.m.: morning (we knew that)

amp.: ampoule (glass or plastic tube containing medicine)

aq: water

a.s.: left ear

ASA: aspirin

ATC: around the clock

a.u.: each ear

b.i.d.: twice a day

BM: bowel movement

BP: blood pressure

BSA: body surface area

c.: with

cap: capsule

CHF: congestive heart failure

D5W: dextrose 5% in water

dil.: dilute

disc. or D/C: discontinue

disp.: dispense

div.: divide

d.t.d.: give of such doses

DW: distilled water

elix.: elixir

et: and

ex aq.: in water

fl or fld: fluid

ft.: make; let it be made

g. or Gm. or g: gram

gr. or gr: grain

gtt.: drop

H: hypodermic

h. or hr.: hour

HA: headache

HBP: high blood pressure

HC: hydrocortisone

h.s.: at bedtime

HT: hypertension

ID: intradermal

IM: intramuscular

inj.: injection

IV: intravenous

IVBP: intravenous piggyback

IVP: intravenous push

LCD: coal tar solution

M.: mix

mcg. or mcg: microgram

mEq: milliequivalent

mg. or mg: milligram

ml. or ml: milliliter

mOsm or mOsmol: milliosmol

MS: morphine sulfate

N & V: nausea and vomiting

NF: national formulary

NMT: not more than

noct.: night

non rep. or N.R.: do not repeat

NPO: nothing by mouth

N.S. or NS: normal saline

½ NS: half-strength normal saline

NTG: nitroglycerin

O: pint

o.d.: right eye

oint.: ointment

o.l.: left eye

o.s.: left eye

o2: both eyes

o.u.: each eye

p.c.: after meals

p.m.: afternoon, evening

p.o.: by mouth

p.r.n.: as needed

pulv.: powder
q: every
qd: every day
qh: every hour
qid: four times a day
R: rectal
R.L. or R/L: No. This is not Ralph Lauren, it's Ringer's lactate.
Sig.: write on label
SL: sublingual
SOB: shortness of breath
sol.: solution
s.o.s.: if there is need
ss.: one-half
stat.: immediately
subc or subq or s.c.: subcutaneously (under the skin)
sup.: suppository
susp.: suspension
syr.: syrup
tab.: tablet
tal.: such

tal. dos.: such doses
tbsp: tablespoonful
tid: three times a day
tiw: three times a week
top: topically
TPN: total parenteral nutrition
tr.: tincture
tsp.: teaspoonful
U or u: unit
u.d. or ut dict: as directed
ung.: ointment
URI: upper respiratory infection
USP: United States Pharmacopeia
UTI: urinary tract infection
VS: vital signs
w/: with
WBC: white blood cell count
w/o: without
X: times
y.o.: year old
ZnO: zinc oxide

Take an ASA and call me in the a.m.

While You're in the Drugstore

Remember that over-the-counter drugs, vitamins, minerals, toothpaste, stomach remedies, cough syrups, pain preparations, allergy medications, antidiarrheal products, laxatives, decongestants, cold and flu formulas, digestive enzymes, lip balms, and nasal sprays all have to be investigated for gluten.

These, too, use inactive or excipient ingredients to sweeten, color, suspend, or otherwise make palatable these products. Always, always, always call the company to verify, and if you are buying the generic brand, let's say Rite Aid or Walgreen's versus the brand name, to save some money, and if it isn't labeled gluten-free, make sure you ask the pharmacist or company rep to verify that the cheaper alternative is gluten-free.

Don't wait until you have to run out in the middle of the night in your pajamas for a bottle of decongestant. It's best to educate yourself now, before the emergency.

CVS has a list of gluten-free over-the-counter products available through Customer Relations; go to www.cvs.com.

Reliable Sources for Gluten-Free Vitamins and Other Supplements

Country Life—Certified gluten-free. www.countrylifevitamins.com

Freeda Vitamins. www.freedavitamins.com

Kirkman Labs—Hypoallergenic products tested for gluten. www.kirkmanlabs.com

Nature Made Vitamins—Gluten-free products are labeled as such. www.naturemade.com

Pioneer Nutritional Formulas—Below 10 parts per million of gluten. www.pioneernutritional.com

Solgar Vitamins—Claims most of its products are gluten-free. www.solgar.com

Lactose Alert!

If you are sensitive to gluten, you may be intolerant of lactose, too. Be aware that lactose is a common filler in prescription medications. If you take something containing lactose every day or several times a day, you're looking at a lot of lactose. Do your homework.

Learn More

AdverseEvents—Searchable database of millions of prescription drug side effects sent to the FDA by doctors, nurses, pharmacists, patients, and drug companies. www.adverseevents.com

ConsumerLab.com—An independent laboratory testing vitamins, minerals, supplements, and nutritional products for quality and safety of ingredients. Consider it the *Consumer Reports* for over-the-counter products. www.consumerlab.com

Gluten-Free Drugs—Dr. Steven Plogsted and his pharmacy students at Nationwide Children's Hospital, Columbus, Ohio, maintain this excellent list. www.glutenfreedrugs.com

The Physicians' Desk Reference (Thompson Healthcare)—This reference is available in prescription and over-the-counter editions and is updated annually. It is also available for tablet and smartphone. www.pdrbookstore.com

The Rubins.com—This Web site for seniors offers a complete directory of drug manufacturers. www.therubins.com

RxAssist.org Patient assistance programs run by pharmaceutical companies for those who need temporary financial assistance with their medications. www.rxassist.org

RxList—Drug information, side effects, ingredients, health updates, and alternatives to prescription medications. www.rxlist.com

Hey, Beautiful!

We slather, moisturize, exfoliate, soothe, shave, scrub, soak, shampoo, spray, primp, pluck, and paint. We know firsthand that beauty really *is* skin deep. But some of us break out in a rash just walking past the local Sephora. We make sure there's no gluten in anything that even remotely comes into contact with us and yet we look and feel the opposite of beautiful after using certain beauty products.

Experts insist—some of them get a little snarky about it—that this is all in our pretty heads. Molecules in cosmetics and personal products are too large to be absorbed through our sensitive pores and, in fact, the technology that allows the medicine in skin patches to be delivered and time released is far too complicated and expensive for skin cream and cosmetics formulas.

One can't be too careful.

As you may remember from Chapter 17, there's an intimate gluten-sharing issue. But I am alone in my shower washing my hair. I don't drink shampoo; I'm sure you don't either. Nor do we let it run into our eyes or lick it off our fingers or somebody else's.

Kays Kaidbey, retired University of Pennsylvania adjunct professor of dermatology and one of the independent cosmetics consultants behind the label Dermatologist Tested agrees. Most proteins, including gluten, he explains, are simply too large to penetrate the stratum corneum, the skin's outermost layer.

Even the venerable Mayo Clinic assures us that "gluten can't be absorbed through the skin," and it goes on to say, "The form of celiac disease called dermatitis herpetiformis or DH, which causes an itchy, blistering rash, is caused by ingesting gluten, not by skin contact."

We can't argue with science, but, at the same time, we can't deny our reactions.

My scalp itches so badly after some shampoos, I want to yank my hair out. Not a good idea given we lose forty to one hundred strands a day without lifting a finger. After trying lip plumper, my lips feel like they've been stung by a bee with an anger management problem: not exactly the effect I was after. Are we getting glutenized even though the experts say this is impossible?

Swallowing accounts for part of the problem. According to Huff Post Style, a typical female human downs approximately six pounds or ninety-six tubes of lipstick in her lifetime, which seems like either an excessive amount of licking one's lips or very sloppy technique. You'd have to apply lipstick with a trowel to get that much in your stomach. In the time it takes to think, *They can't mean me*, I discover that lipstick can be absorbed through the lining of the mouth and that the average person will spend two weeks kissing in his or her lifetime. It makes sense to avoid gluten in anything we can accidentally or habitually ingest.

Gluten-sensitive citizens report everything from rashes and redness to stomach upsets and brain fog, blaming gluten osmosis. Every time I use anything containing wheat germ oil, my scalp bursts into flame. The fact is I'm sensitive to wheat germ oil. I hoard my mint shampoo, which is difficult to find now that the company has discontinued it. It contains no chemicals, feels great, and does the job without burning or itchiness. This is good enough for me.

Results of an FDA cosmetics survey show that nearly a quarter of all consumers (they didn't ask who was gluten-free or not) said yes to having suffered an allergic reaction to foundations, moisturizers, and eye shadows.

If you agree, as I do, that those of us with gluten problems aren't quite normal to begin with and that we may be hyperreactors to many substances, it makes sense that we may be affected in larger numbers by personal products containing chemicals, fragrances, and other nonnatural, even toxic ingredients. Gluten may or may not have anything to do with it.

While it's tempting to blame gluten for all of our ills, it's incumbent on all of us to widen our focus. After researching the kinds of chemicals used in personal products, I wonder why we don't all glow in the dark.

Talk about the kiss of death.

Is Gluten the Only Ingredient You Should Worry About?

According to the magazine *Ecologist*, there are a number of toxic ingredients and allergens commonly used in cosmetics and skin care products. The ancient Egyptians stained their lips with henna, a skin irritant, and used mineral clays that contained mercury. This may explain why they looked good and died young.

Ecologist also tells us that many of today's lipsticks and glosses are composed of synthetic oils and petroleum-derived waxes, UV filters, and coal tar dyes that are common irritants. These can cause photosensitivity and dermatitis and may even be neurotoxic.

Mineral oil, found in dozens of products, including baby care lines, is a petrochemical. Long-lasting lipstick formulas require adding a variety of plastics, nylon, and silicone that, literally, glues the color to the lips. Some of these ingredients can cause cheilitis, a painful and unsightly condition of cracked and sore skin at the corners of the mouth, which can make a real dent in that lifetime smooch score.

Dyes like iron oxides and mica add luminescence, but they can also trigger gastrointestinal problems or liver toxicity. This may explain why many of us assume we are having a reaction to gluten.

Tragic Beauty

Getting some of this stuff into your system can cause allergies, dermatitis, nausea, intellectual impairment, memory loss, confusion, gastrointestinal and liver toxicity, and hyperactivity in children. Not pretty.

- ✦ **Dyes**—Coal tar derivatives are suspected carcinogens. They can cause hives, irritation, and photosensitivity. Bismuth compounds are known to cause intellectual impairment, memory loss, and confusion. Carmine has been linked to hyperactivity in children.
- ✦ **Iron oxides, mica**—These add color and luminescence. If ingested, mica poses gastrointestinal or liver toxicity hazards.
- ✦ **Isododecane**—This is a solvent and dispersing agent. Prolonged contact may irritate and cause dermatitis. If swallowed, it can cause nausea.
- ✦ **Nylon 611/dimethicone copolymer**—This film former can irritate eyes, skin, and airways. A related substance, Nylon-6, is considered carcinogenic.
- ✦ **Propylene carbonate**—This is a solvent and plasticizer. It is derived from propylene glycol, a skin irritant.

What's a Gluten-Free Glamour Puss to Do?

- ✦ Read labels and avoid dangerous ingredients.
- ✦ Slog through the *International Cosmetic Ingredient Dictionary and Handbook*, available at public libraries or the Office of the Federal Register.
- ✦ Memorize the partial list of irritants from *Ecologist* above and do some homework before you expose yourself to dangerous chemicals.
- ✦ Go green. Demand full disclosure with your body butter.

Makeup Exam

Yes, I know, it's all about cheek color, lash lengthening, and removing those cobwebs we call the visible signs of aging. But, even in the heat of feigning perfection, a cool head should prevail.

+ Know that the FDA definition of *Natural Ingredients* includes stuff that isn't remotely natural and that an agency that can't seem to keep salmonella and E. coli from the food supply is not going to spend time and money policing your pressed powder.
+ Make use of tester bottles (not those germ-infested tubes and bottles on the counter).
+ Ask for a sample and do a skin test before you purchase an expensive product.
+ Keep track of what you tried on which body part and watch for signs of a reaction.
+ Ask about the shelf life or expiration date of products you already own and those that you are considering.
+ Makeup that has gone off is more likely to cause a reaction than makeup that's fresh.
+ Incidentally, the date on the label refers to conditions and use that are ideal. Two years in a gym bag is not ideal.
+ Frugality is not your friend where the health of your skin is concerned, which, by the way, covers twenty-two square feet of you, according to HowStuffWorks.com.
+ Toss anything that has gotten thick or clumpy, has turned color, has separated, or has otherwise congealed. You'll pay for it one way or another.
+ Buy gluten-free, fragrance-, chemical-, and cruelty-free, and hypoallergenic products. It may cost a little more, but it's better for you and the planet.
+ If you're really, really sensitive, consider using baby products containing none of the above.
+ On the off chance that there really is gluten in something you're using, avoid touching your face or putting your hands in your mouth after use.
+ Ditto for handling bread or wiping off the counter with lotion on your hands.

Bran New Skin

In ancient times Japanese women were called *nuka-bijin*, or bran beauties, because they rubbed their faces with rice bran to cleanse their pores. Rice blotting papers are also very good at taking the shine off a nose. Let us count the ways rice is nice for a modern kabuki girl.

✦ Never use another person's makeup or treatment products. The thought of it should give you hives.
✦ Make your own beauty treatments.

JOJOBA INSTANT SKIN SMOOTHER

This fast and silky soak comes courtesy of beauty expert Bernadette Brescia.

1. Fill a bowl with pure jojoba oil warmed in the microwave for 30 seconds.
2. Soak your hands up to the wrists for 10 minutes.
3. Oil from jojoba is similar to your own sebum, so you'll absorb all of it, leaving you with soft skin minus the goo.
4. Break some hearts.

SENSITIVE BEAUTY LIP BALM

½ teaspoon grated beeswax
1 teaspoon pure cocoa butter
1 teaspoon almond oil

This emollient-rich conditioning balm, also from Bernadette Brescia, is especially great for winter dry lips. For outdoor activities, add a few drops of a good gluten-free sunscreen like Cleure's. For a different taste, substitute coconut oil for cocoa butter. Mix ingredients and heat in microwave for about 10 seconds. Fill a small, clean jar and let cool. Apply and pucker up.

Bone Up on Beauty Terms

Natural—The implication here is that ingredients that come from nature, hence good and pure and safe, don't include anything chemical or produced synthetically. There are plenty of things in nature that could cause a nasty reaction.

Hypoallergenic—The inference here is that this product is less likely to cause an allergic reaction than any other or that it has been formulated to rule out the possibility. Ditto for *dermatologist-tested* or *allergy-tested* or *nonirritating*. There is absolutely no substantiation required for these claims.

Alcohol-free—This means that the product doesn't contain ethyl or grain alcohol, but it doesn't mean you won't find other fatty alcohols like cetyl, stearyl, cetearyl, or lanolin.

Fragrance-free—You'd think this means the product has absolutely no smell. Not so. Fragrance is often added to cover up unattractive odors given off by certain ingredients. The nose may not know, but it's there.

Shelf life or expiration date—Most people think that this is important only in terms of food. Makeup that's gone off is more than likely to cause a reaction. Incidentally, the date on the label refers to storage under ideal conditions. When was the last time you stored your nail polish in the fridge?

Making Up Really *Is* Hard to Do

According to the FDA, cosmetics can be anything from mascara to toothpaste, nail polish to deodorant sprays. Unlike drugs, which are strictly regulated and tested before being marketed for human consumption, cosmetics are not required to undergo approval before being sold to the consumer, though they must display ingredients on any package intended for sale.

The active ingredient or chemical that makes the product effective must be listed first, followed by a list of inactive ingredients in order of decreasing quantity.

By law, cosmetic companies are not required to substantiate claims or conduct product testing, but if safety has not been voluntarily substantiated, the product label must state this with "Warning! The safety of this product has not been determined."

In the secrecy and obfuscation department, cosmetic companies are even worse than the drug companies. You won't see a warning on your Arrest Me Red lipstick any time soon. Believe me, I know.

I wrote cosmetics and fragrance copy at Bergdorf's while moonlighting for Revlon and Lauder, among other companies. To be accurate, the lawyers wrote most of it. If I wanted to say Product X . . . *will erase fine lines and make you look so young, you'll get carded*, the legal department changed it to: *Helps to reduce the surface look of fine lines for the appearance of younger-looking skin.*

If I wanted to say: *Your hair will be so full and thick, it will need a zip code all its own*, the lawyers crossed it off and wrote, *Coats each hair with luminescent bubbles to create the temporary appearance of healthier hair.*

These are loopholes you could drive a truck through.

Still, it's impossible to resist the promise of perfect skin and shining tresses.

There is nothing beautiful about irritation and redness, scaly, flaking, and itchy skin, hives, and, in rare cases, anaphylaxis because peanut oil was used as an ingredient.

You are right to view cosmetic advertising and product claims with a healthy dose of skepticism.

Don't take what these companies say as absolute truth. As with prescription and over-the-counter drugs, call the company. Use the product, by all means, but make no assumptions about its purity. If you use a product regularly—or your lover does and there's a whole lot of smooching going on—check, check, and check again. Ask for their list of gluten-free products and, while you're at it, ask why they always discontinue our favorite shades.

Algenist
www.algenist.com
Almay
www.almay.com
Aveda
www.aveda.com
Aveeno
www.aveeno.com
Avon
www.avon.com
Benefit
www.benefitcosmetics
  .com
Bliss
www.blissworld.com
Blistex
www.blistex.com
Bobbi Brown
www.bobbibrown
  cosmetics.com
Bonne Bell
www.bonnebell.com
Boots
www.boots.com

Burt's Bees
www.burtsbees.com
Chanel
www.chanel.com
Clarins
www.clarinsusa.com
Clinique
www.clinique.com
Covergirl
www.covergirl.com
Dermalogica
www.dermalogica.com
Dr. Hauschka
www.drhauschka.com
Elizabeth Arden
www.elizabetharden
  .com
Estée Lauder
www.esteelauder.com
Kiehl's
www.kiehls.com
Kiss My Face
www.kissmyface.com
Lancôme
www.lancome.com

Laura Mercier
www.lauramercier.com
LORAC
www.loraccosmetics
  .com
L'Oréal
www.loreal.com
M*A*C Cosmetics
www.maccosmetics.com
Mary Kay
www.marykay.com
Maybelline
www.maybelline.com
Merle Norman
www.merlenorman.com
Murad
www.murad.com
NARS
www.narscosmetics.com
Neutrogena
www.neutrogena.com
Origins
www.origins.com

Perricone MD	Shiseido	Tarte
www.perriconemd.com	www.shiseido.com	www.tartccosmetics.com
Revlon	Stila	Urban Decay
www.revlon.com	www.stilacosmetics.com	www.urbandecay.com

Farm Fresh Beauty

What to do with those ripe avocados, kiwis, lemons, yogurt, cucumbers, parsley, leftover bits of oatmeal, and those roses that you-know-who sent? Skip the dyes, chemicals, and synthetics. Whip up natural, organic, and gluten-free skin treatments in your own kitchen. These have been handed down to me by the frugal natural beauties in my family and come from my own kitchen after lots of often hilarious trial and error.

Just don't forget it's on when the UPS guy rings the doorbell.

HONEY LEMON SUGAR SCRUB

Mix ½ cup sugar, ½ cup sweet almond oil, 4 teaspoons lemon juice, 4 tablespoons honey, and 4 drops lemon essential oil. Mix the sugar and almond oil first. Then add other ingredients. Polish skin using gentle pressure. Wipe clean and rinse.

AVOCADO AND OAT FACIAL

Mix 1 ripe avocado with 2 tablespoons raw, organic honey and ¼ cup uncooked oatmeal. (I use certified gluten-free oatmeal just in case.) Apply to a clean face. Think beautiful thoughts for 15 minutes. Wipe off and rinse.

NO HONEY OR OATMEAL?

Mash a quarter of a medium ripe avocado and mix in 1 teaspoon of extra-virgin olive oil. Apply a thin layer to a clean face. Let dry. Rinse well. Done.

CUCUMBER PARSLEY STRESS FIX

Yogurt softens, and cucumber and parsley perk up sunburned or otherwise stressed skin. In the bowl of a blender, purée 1 tablespoon parsley and 1 tablespoon-size chunk of cucumber. Mix in 1 tablespoon plain yogurt until smooth. Apply to the face and clear your mind of obligations for 20 minutes.

ROSE WATER BATH

This was my mother's secret weapon for fatigue, skin smoothing, and getting the rest of us to leave her alone. Pour 1 cup distilled water over 1 cup fresh, organic rose petals. Steep like tea for up to an hour. Strain the petals and reserve the liquid. Let cool completely and pour into a tightly sealed jar. Refrigerate overnight. Add to your bathwater. Optional: Find someone like my father who will keep you in rose petals.

BRIGHTENING AND TIGHTENING FACIAL

Too much work and stress making you a dull girl? Kiwi and citrus are the antioxidant tickets. Peel and purée one ripe kiwi, mix with 1 tablespoon plus 1 teaspoon of freshly squeezed lemon or orange juice. Apply a thin layer, avoiding the eyes. Let dry, rinse. Moisturize. Store in the fridge for the rest of the rough week.

You Glow, Girl!

Knowing that your cheek or lip color is cruelty-free *and* gluten-free, that your foundation and shampoo aren't full of petrochemicals, parabens, dyes, or synthetics is a beautiful thing. Even better is looking positively radiant without using animal by-products or cosmetics that come from a chemistry lab.

Here is a short list of companies that are natural, organic, environmentally friendly, and socially conscious to help you look and feel your best and get your gluten-free game face on:

Afterglow Mineral Cosmetics—Organic Lip Love Lipsticks are about as pure a gluten-free pucker as two lips can get. www.afterglowcosmetics.com

bareMinerals—Gluten-free skin care, treatment products, and makeup. www.bareescentuals.com

California Baby—All products are gluten-free and free of soy, peanuts, and dairy. www.californiababy.com

Desert Essence Organics—Gluten-free products are clearly labeled. www.desertessence.com

Earth Friendly Baby—gluten-free, vegan, natural, and organic baby products. www.earthfriendlybaby.co.uk

Ecco Bella—Gluten-free and preservative-free cosmetics for sensitive skin. www.eccobella.com

Everclen for Sensitive Skin—Cleansers, face and eye creams, toner, body lotion, hand cream. www.everclen.com

Gabriel Cosmetics—100 percent certified gluten-free, vegan, and organic. www.gabrielcosmeticsinc.com

Hamadi Beauty—Gluten-free Healing Scrum, Shea Spray, and Styling Cream. www.hamadibeauty.com

Joelle Cosmetics—A.k.a. My Mineral Glitters—Gluten-free gorgeousness. www.mymineralglitters.com

Juice Beauty—Certified gluten-free skin care and makeup. www.juicebeauty.com

Kathy's Family Personal Care Products—Healing lotions free of all common allergens. www.kathysfamily.com

Monave Mineral Makeup—Gluten-free and cruelty-free, 95 percent vegan and organic lipsticks, concealers, eye shadows, and skin care. www.monave.com

Nourish Organic—No chemicals, no cruelty, no preservatives. www.nourishorganic.com

PeaceKeeper Nail Paint This gluten-free "cause-metics" company donates a portion of its profits for women's urgent human rights issues. www.iamapeacekeeper.com

Pure and Basic—Soaps, body wash, lotions, and hair care. www.pureandbasic.com

Red Apple Lipstick—Free VIP club that includes 20 percent off every month on gluten-free lipstick. www.redapplelipstick.com

Scotch Naturals—All nail polishes are gluten-free. www.scotchnaturals.com

Heartbreak Hotel

If you are a beauty on the go, resist loading up on all of those freebie hotel soaps, shampoos, conditioners, and body lotions. Yes, they smell great. And yes, they give you the sense that you are getting something extra for the ridiculous price you're paying for a bedroom. You have no idea what's in them or who made them for the hotel. Travel with your own beauty essentials or send ahead with your emergency gluten-free food. Ditto for the masseuse: supply your own massage oil with a few drops of lavender in it. You may even get a discount.

Starwest Botanicals—Pure skin-care oils. www.starwest-botanicals.com

Surface Hair Care—All products are gluten-free. www.surfacehair.com

Vermont Soap—Organic, nontoxic soaps and personal products. www.vermontsoap.com

ZuZu Luxe—Vegan, cruelty-free, gluten-free, and corn-free, and eco-friendly packaging. www.gabrielcosmeticsinc.com

Bugs Be Gone

Natural Ingredients That Really Bug Ticks and Mosquitoes

- ✦ Cinnamon
- ✦ Citronella
- ✦ Cloves
- ✦ Coffee
- ✦ Eucalyptus
- ✦ Geranium
- ✦ Mint
- ✦ Orange

Organic, Nontoxic Products to Get Bugs to Buzz Off

BugBand—Sprays, wipes, wristbands. www.bugband.net

Bugs Be Gone—Natural deterrent—Emerson Ecologics. www.emersonecologics.com

Burt's Bees—Natural for you, repellent to them. www.burtsbees.com

LA Fresh—Insect repellent wipes. www.lafreshgroup.com

"No-Bite-Me" Cream—Sallye Ander. www.sallyeander.com

Screen Gems

You want a broad-spectrum sunscreen, which provides UVB *and* UVA protection against melanoma and premature aging. You want a high enough SPF for activity and you don't want to be stingy in slathering it on (two heaping tablespoons to cover the standard-issue body) every twenty to thirty minutes and always after swimming.

Only mad dogs and Englishmen go out in the noonday sun. If you must sunbathe, do it in the morning before 10:00 a.m. and late in the day after 4:00 p.m. when dangerous UV rays are at a minimum. Sunscreen is not something you save for a sunny day. When it's overcast, 80 percent of the sun's rays pass through the clouds. It's not something you save for next season either. Buy new next summer.

Some of you are sensitive to PABA (para-aminobenzoic acid) and other irritants. All of you are gluten-avoidant. What's a sensitive bathing beauty to do?

Cleure—Gluten-free sunscreen, SPF 30. www.cleure.com
TruKid—Sunny Day Mineral sunscreen. www.trukid.com

Learn More

Ecology Magazine—Required reading for those conscious consumers interested in preserving the natural world. www.ecologymagazine.co.uk

Environmental Working Group—The power of information to protect public health and the environment. Database of personal care products ranked by level of hazard. www.ewg.org

International Cosmetic Ingredient Dictionary and Handbook (Cosmetic, Toiletry, and Fragrance Association)—Available at public libraries or at the Office of the Federal Register. www.gpoaccess.gov

Saffron Rouge—This site sells eco-friendly, gluten-free, and cruelty-free cosmetics made with a minimum of preservatives from various companies. Think of it as a Sephora for conscious consumers. www.saffronrouge.com

Part VI

Something Larger Than Ourselves

Food Fights

22

Be the change you wish to see in the world.

—MAHATMA GANDHI

We're finicky about our food and should be.

We have issues, not just about taste and texture and whether or not our food is gluten-free, grain-free, dairy-free, nut-free, or meat-free, but also about where it comes from, who makes it, and what they put in it. We want real food, not food that is boxed, packaged, processed, and otherwise loaded with dyes, additives, chemicals, hormones, preservatives and other dubious ingredients.

We have justifiable complaints about the way our food is grown, raised, labeled, manufactured, marketed, enhanced, and genetically modified. We have questions about why so many of us are no longer tolerating wheat, corn, soy, and sesame and about why there is so much arsenic in the rice.

Call us picky, but we want honest, organic food and produce, not from a petri dish or a chemistry lab, but in season and from local sources, confident that it has been grown sustainably and free of dangerous pesticides.

Alice Waters, food activist, author of *The Art of Simple Food*, and founder of the Edible Schoolyard, which teaches children to see, touch, grow, and value real food, urges us to remember that food is precious.

That precious and finite resource is under assault these days.

Foods free of pesticides, stabilizers, chemical additives, trans fats, high-fructose corn syrup, and other addictive ingredients are seen by some as an elitist choice, something for wealthy food snobs looking for the next big thing. Given the price tag of whole, organic foods versus supermarket brands, that may be a self-fulfilling prophecy.

Why shouldn't we have clean, affordable food that is grown in an environmentally responsible way? Many of us believe that this is not only a health imperative but also an ethical and moral one.

Frankenfoods, or *food-like substances*, as comedian Bill Maher likes to say, beset us. Food makers are addicting our children to high-fat, calorie-dense, sweet food loaded with high-fructose corn syrup, probably the biggest culprit in the ballooning diabetes and obesity epidemic. We are kept in the dark about GMOs, consumer demand for clearly labeled choices blocked by a powerful lobby. Biotech companies like Monsanto are patenting seeds and forcing farmers to abandon the generations-old practices of seed conservation and natural crossbreeding, threatening them with suits if they do not comply.

It's not enough to be glad for gluten-free product labels and go on about our business, never scrutinizing the source of the ingredients in those very products. How can we eat natural gluten-free grains, legumes, and vegetables and turn a blind eye to how they are grown? We of all people—with our delicate plumbing, food allergies, gluten intolerance, chemical sensitivities, and tendency to hyperreact to additives and otherwise chemically altered food—need to be vigilant.

On the following pages, I will present some of the issues affecting the quality of our lives and our precious food supply; draw attention to inequities, unfairness, and downright foul play; and shed some light on those who operate in the dark and without outcry.

Change happens when we take things personally. There is nothing more personal than food.

The FDA Ruling on Gluten-Free Labeling

In *The Gluten-Free Bible*, published on the cusp of the Food Allergen Labeling and Consumer Protection Act of 2004, which promised a standardized definition of gluten-free for the labeling of foods by 2008, I asked a simple question.

How many celiacs does it take to change a food label?

As it turns out, it took more than any of us could imagine.

Though the stakes were certainly higher for those of us with celiac disease, the entire gluten-free community joined in the fight. It was time for full gluten disclosure on food labels. The days of going to the grocery store with a magnifying glass and a dictionary of food additives were over. We wanted the right to shop and eat just like every American.

It took over ten thousand letters and countless phone calls to senators, congressmen, and congresswomen. Petitions were signed and delivered. People like you, dear reader, went to Washington to tell their stories on the Senate floor, testifying to the urgent need for safe, clearly labeled food.

Andrea Levario, executive director of the American Celiac Disease Alliance, and her colleagues launched a massive and many-pronged advocacy campaign and never gave up, no matter how long the wait, partisan the bickering, or uphill the climb. Representative Nita Lowey of New York's Eighteenth District, who authored the 2004 law under which this ruling was required, continued the crusade from the inside, never abandoning her commitment to the gluten-free community. You read about her efforts on behalf of gluten-free labeling for prescription and over-the-counter drugs in the previous chapter.

Some found creative ways to push. Tim Lawson, CEO of New Grains Gluten Free Baker, filed a lawsuit against Utah senator Orrin Hatch for refusing to exert his influence to raise funds for the FDA regulation process.

Galvanized by government foot-dragging, Jules Shepard, a Maryland gluten-free baker with celiac disease (see her recipe for cranberry chutney, page 243), whipped up seven hundred pounds of frosting to ice an eleven-foot cake made of 180 individual sheet cakes. With the help of volunteer activists, she iced and served Washington lawmakers a nineteen-hundred-pound, eleven-foot gluten-free cake that couldn't be ignored.

And we can't forget the decades of activism on the parts of the pioneers of the gluten-free community, without whom the gluten-free label would still be a dream.

In August 2013, a full nine years after its own deadline, the FDA finally ruled on a standardized definition of *gluten-free*. Any product carrying a gluten-free label must contain 20 parts per million of gluten or less. To put this in context, experts say that 50 parts per million can cause intestinal damage in those with celiac disease.

So how many of us changed a label? All of us.

A LITTLE BACKGROUND

According to the FDA Web site (fda.gov), the Food Allergen Labeling and Consumer Protection Act (FALCPA) of 2004 requires food makers to declare the top eight allergens—milk, egg, fish, crustacean shellfish, tree nuts, wheat, peanuts, and soybeans—on their labels. The specific type of nut, fish, and crustacean shellfish must be indicated as well. Mollusks, such as oysters, clams, and mussels, while a type of shellfish some are allergic to, are not considered a major food allergen and do not have to be listed.

✦ Allergens must be listed in parenthesis in the list of ingredients.
✦ For example: Whey (milk), flour (wheat).
✦ The label must use the word *contains* near or after the ingredient list, as in *contains wheat, milk, or soy.*

The law applies to all retail and food service establishments that package, label, and offer products for human consumption, including vending machines and all packages labeled *for individual sale.*

Exempted by the law are fresh fruits and vegetables in their natural state or any highly refined oil derived from the eight common allergens because it is believed that the refining process leaves only minuscule amounts of these allergens and therefore renders the product safe. The law also does not cover prescription drugs or over-the-counter drugs, cosmetics, or health and beauty products (hence Representative Lowey's renewed efforts), but it does cover edible supplements and health products. It does not regulate any restaurant foods that are placed in a wrapper or container in response to a customer request, which lets street vendors, all manner of fairs and festivals, and fast-food restaurants off the hook. Kosher products are not regulated under this law. Nor are pet foods, or animal supplements and supplies.

And finally, FALCPA does not cover any product regulated by the Alcohol and Tobacco Tax and Trade Bureau, which includes alcoholic beverages and spirits, tobacco products, and beer, troubling for the gluten-free imbiber.

WHEN DID THE NEW RULING GO INTO EFFECT?
August 5, 2014.

From that time forward all packaged-food manufacturers making a gluten-free claim must comply with a 20-parts-per-million standard before they can label a food gluten-free. This includes gluten from any source and takes into account any issues of cross-contamination that can occur anywhere in the process.

Under the new guidelines, oats are not allowed in a product unless they contain less than the standard 20 parts per million of gluten. This is good news for those makers of oats grown in dedicated fields, processed in gluten-free facilities, and certified to a higher standard by outside groups.

The downside is that some companies currently labeling their products gluten-free may no longer do so if they feel they cannot meet the stringent new FDA standards, especially those regulations pertaining to cross-contamination issues.

WHY DID IT TAKE SO LONG?
+ Mandatory public comment periods and hearings
+ The inevitable red tape, setbacks, and delays of a large bureaucracy
+ Lawsuits from food producers and supermarkets
+ Corporate lobbyists
+ FDA funding cuts
+ Politics and partisan bickering

DOES THIS MEAN THERE IS ONE GLUTEN-FREE LABEL?
No.

There is no one design or symbol for package labels under the new law, which means consumers must learn to identify different labels on a variety of products.

Certified GF™ Gluten-Free

Gluten-Free Certification Organization

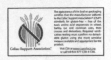

Celiac Support Association

Canadian Celiac Association

National Foundation for Celiac Awareness

Nor are there uniform language standards. Terms like *gluten-free*, *free of gluten*, *no gluten*, and *without gluten* are allowable under the new ruling.

Here's the tricky part:

Companies may still say, *Made with no gluten-containing ingredients* or *Not made with gluten-containing ingredients*, but if these claims are used on a package *without* the gluten-free label, we can't assume these foods meet FDA requirements. In addition, food makers are still allowed to print advisory statements like *Made in a facility that also processes wheat products* on products that bear a gluten-free label. The FDA told Amy Ratner, editor of *Gluten Free Living*, that it will need "to look at foods on a case by case basis to determine whether a specific advisory statement with a gluten-free claim would be misleading."

Naturally gluten-free foods can be labeled gluten-free as well under the final ruling, a change from the proposed rules, which inexplicably banned labeling grains and other products, such as soda and milk, that do not by definition contain gluten. A nod to those jumping on the gluten-free bandwagon, most likely.

The label design and its location on the package will be up to manufacturers. So you can't really pick up a package, scan it for a second or two, and toss it in the cart. Not yet, anyway. Careful scrutiny is still in order, at least until you get the hang of where to look.

WHAT ABOUT CERTIFICATION BY OUTSIDE GROUPS?

Gluten-free seals of certification like those given by the Gluten Intolerance Group, CSA/USA, and the National Foundation for Celiac Awareness are still allowed under the FDA ruling. Companies wanting to meet standards stricter than the FDA's (5- to 10-parts-per-million stringent cross-contamination policies) can continue to use them.

That's great news because we have come to trust products so certified, not by the company that makes the product but by impartial certification agencies.

WHO'S RESPONSIBLE FOR TESTING?

Manufacturers are expected to test their products to prove that they meet requirements under the new ruling, but they are not bound by law to do so. This is not good news.

The FDA ruling says that the agency will make "periodic inspections of food manufacturing facilities; food lab reviews and follow up on customer and industry complaints reported to the agency; and when needed [the key words here are *when needed*] analyze food samples for gluten."

When the FDA does investigate a complaint, it will use ELISA (enzyme-linked immunosorbent assay) testing methods approved by the scientific community. The agency can suggest, but not mandate, the use of the same tests for manufacturers. Clearly, there is still some work to do.

HOW WILL THIS NEW RULING BE POLICED?

I don't mean to sound cynical, but I wouldn't want you to get the impression that you are perfectly safe because there is a gluten-free labeling regulation in place.

In a perfect world, all foods would be routinely inspected and all problems either fixed or recalled. With dwindling resources, you have to ask yourself what is going to get the most attention—the hamburger processing facility or the company that makes gluten-free cake mixes? Even when manufacturers are inspected and found wanting, problems are often not attended to promptly because the chances of the inspector coming back soon are slim.

The FDA promises to recall those products that do not comply with standards and has set up a Consumer Complaint Coordinator to report violations. See "Learn More" at the end of this chapter for the Complaint Coordinator in your area.

WHAT ABOUT GLUTEN-FREE BEER?

It's complicated.

Regulation of alcoholic beverages like beer are the purview of the Alcohol and Tobacco Tax and Trade Bureau and therefore do not come under the FDA ruling. To further confuse matters, there is no approved test for fermented and hydrolyzed products as yet. Beers that originally contained hops and barley and were processed to remove gluten cannot carry the new gluten free label until such time as the FDA issues guidance to ATTTB for testing such products. The FDA has promised these issues will be resolved in a "timely manner," but at this writing this has not happened.

The best thing to do is to continue buying and drinking beers and ales that have been certified as safe by groups such as GIG and CSA/USA.

BOTTOM LINE

This particular food fight is not over by a long shot. There are issues to clarify and lobbying to do for mandated food industry testing and making sure the ruling has teeth. But thanks to a massive effort from the gluten-free community, a huge battle has been won. No law is ever perfect, but this is the start we've all been hoping for. With ever-vigilant advocacy organizations, and with representatives like Nita Lowey and others still committed to safety in labeling, all the kinks will be ironed out.

My best advice is to stay engaged, or to get involved for the first time. Write letters. Vote with your pocketbook. Boycott products that are deceptive and unhealthy. File complaints with your Consumer Complaint Coordinator. Gluten-free companies and food retailers, too, should make use of this whistle-blowing tool. Join one of the national groups and do what you can to keep the ball rolling.

The question before us now is not how many it takes to change a label, but how many to perfect it?

Insurance Coverage for Gluten-Free Food: A Food Fight Worth Having

I read a letter recently, passionate and eloquent, posted on a gluten-free chat site, on the subject of insurance coverage for gluten-free food. The author cited a Canadian study conducted at Dalhousie Medical School in Halifax, Nova Scotia, and published on the NIH site, PubMed, in which the prices of fifty-six gluten-free products and comparable non-gluten-free items were compared to determine if and to what extent gluten-free products are more expensive.

For purposes of comparison, the unit cost of each food—price in dollars per 100 grams of each product—was calculated. Researchers found all fifty-six gluten-free products were more expensive than regular items and, on average, were 242 percent more expensive.

Two hundred and forty-two percent. That's stunning.

With great trepidation at being flamed by those who may be against the Affordable Care Act and other government entitlements, the correspondent urged the gluten-free community to consider what this kind of expense means to someone of limited means, and especially to seniors on Medicare or Medicaid, people who make decisions every day about what drugs they can afford to pay for and what they must do without, more and more of whom are getting diagnosed with celiac disease and non-celiac gluten intolerance well into their old age. This, compounded by the fact that with more and more seniors finding themselves unable to eat gluten at a time when they may not be able to shop for and cook their own food, makes it especially unfair to those who rely heavily on expensive, packaged gluten-free products that are easy to heat and serve.

The writer was so moved by the plight of these gluten-free Americans—whose European counterparts (in Argentina, Italy, Canada, Ireland, the UK, and Finland) are reimbursed, given tax credits, or given monthly stipends or deep discounts for the extra cost of gluten-free food—she wrote to former Health and Human Services secretary Kathleen Sebelius, urging her to consider covering gluten-free food as part of the Affordable Care Act.

Her argument was compelling.

If, under the Americans with Disabilities Act, celiac disease and non-celiac gluten intolerance is considered a disability, albeit a silent one, and if food is the only medicine for this particular condition, why shouldn't the difference in cost be covered the same as any other prescription medicine for everyone, not just seniors?

I couldn't agree more with the letter writer that those in the gluten-free community who teeter on the poverty line need help from the rest of us. If we help the least among us, we help ourselves in important ways.

Our correspondent urged action "now, *before* the Affordable Care Act goes into effect." I endorse the urgency but at this writing the law is in effect. The issue is far from over. Laws, like people, evolve and adapt to their times.

Take the Social Security Act of 1935. When it was enacted, Social Security was not the egalitarian program it is today. It did not include employees of the American Society for the Prevention of Cruelty to Animals. Nor did it cover self-employed doctors, lawyers, and ministers. Excluded were merchant seamen, employees of charitable or educational institutions, and those working for nonprofit organizations. Most perniciously, it overlooked farm and domestic workers, the majority of whom were poor women and African Americans.

If the law had not been amended, broadened, and otherwise brought up to date, many of us, including yours truly, a self-employed writer, would be left out in the cold.

WHY SHOULD I GET INVOLVED?

Unless you are independently wealthy or have up in the attic your own version of the picture of Dorian Gray, there is no way to avoid (1) spending too much money on your food and (2) getting old and ending up on Medicare or Medicaid.

If it's not your issue now, it will be. If you are not now a celiac, you may be in the future. If someone you love is being hurt by this inequity in the system, I don't have to tell you why you should care. It comes down to a matter of unfairness. If the rest of the world understands that food is medicine, isn't it incumbent upon us to make that same case here at home?

We may not be able to change how our society views the old and the poor, but shouldn't we fight for affordable gluten-free food for members of our own community?

WHAT CAN I DO?

Urge advocacy groups like the American Celiac Disease Alliance, Celiac Disease Foundation, Gluten Intolerance Group, Celiac Support Association (CSA), and the National Foundation for Celiac Awareness to take up this issue. Petition and write letters to your congressional representatives. Press them to take up this important matter. Start with Representative Lowey and others friendly to gluten-free issues and concerns. Urge the gluten-free community and the organizations that represent us to push manufacturers to start a discount program for seniors.

As the brave letter writer described here has done, send your letters to the Secretary of Health and Human Services and to the White House.

You've Got a Lot on Your Plate (and It's Not All Food)

In November 2013, as reported by Victoria Shannon for the *New York Times*, Japan and South Korea flat out barred some imports of American wheat from entering their countries. The city of Seoul quarantined US wheat for livestock feed. Thailand put its ports on notice and the European Union urged its twenty-seven member nations to increase testing certain shipments from the United States. This is troubling if you happen to be the world's biggest exporter of wheat.

The "certain shipments" the article refers to contain a strain of genetically engineered wheat developed by Monsanto to resist its Roundup herbicide that was never approved for sale and yet turned up growing in an Oregon field, even though the company ended its field trials in 2004. The article goes on to say that the EU, which has a "zero tolerance" approach to genetically modified food crops, has made it clear that if any US shipment tests positive, they will not be sold.

While other countries are justifiably finicky about GMOs in human food and animal feed, there are no such controls in the United States. According to the Non-GMO Project, in the summer of 2012, large quantities of GMO sweet corn appeared on grocery store shelves and roadside produce stands. In 2011 Monsanto announced its plans to grow genetically modified sweet corn on 250,000 acres, accounting for roughly 40 percent of the sweet corn market. With no warning to consumers, that sweet corn was used for frozen and canned corn products and was available fresh across the country. Like the quarantined wheat, GMO sweet corn is genetically engineered to be herbicide-resistant (Roundup Ready) and to produce its own insecticide. Like all GMOs, genetically modified sweet corn has not been thoroughly tested to ensure that it's safe for human or animal consumption.

WHAT EXACTLY IS A GMO?

GMO stands for "genetically modified organism." These are plants or animals created through the gene-splicing techniques of biotechnology, also called genetic engineering. Unlike crossbreeding, which farmers have done for centuries to improve the genetics of their crops for resistance to drought, disease, and pests, this experimental technology merges DNA from different species, creating combinations of plant, animal, bacterial, and viral genes that cannot occur in nature or in traditional crossbreeding. For example, GMO wheat, soy, flax, and corn seeds contain powerful herbicides. Unlike natural life-forms, GMOs can be patented. For the first time in history, private corporations can own a food source and sue if their seeds end up in a neighboring farm.

ARE GMOS SAFE?

Many developed nations, sixty-four in all according to the watchdog group Non-GMO Project, do not consider GMOs safe and have banned their production and sale or have put serious restrictions on them.

Not so in the United States. The FDA has approved GMOs based on studies conducted by the same corporations that create them and profit from their sale. Despite an increasing public outcry, the FDA does not independently test these products, nor do they require GMO-containing foods to be labeled as such.

While some scientists say GMOs do not contribute to human illness, the American Academy of Environmental Medicine urges doctors to prescribe non-GMO diets for their patients. The academy cites animal studies showing organ damage, gastrointestinal and immune system disorders, accelerated aging, and infertility.

While the debate about human safety rages, and some researchers in the gluten-free community say that engineered wheat has not contributed to the upsurge in gluten intolerance, many of us with food intolerance, sensitivity, and multiple allergies are skeptical.

SHOULD I AVOID GMOS?

The Institute for Responsible Technology lists on their Web site ten compelling reasons to do just that.

1. **People are getting sick**—According to the Institute, numerous health problems increased after GMOs were introduced in 1996. The percentage of Americans with three or more chronic illnesses jumped from 7 to 13 percent in just nine years. Food allergies have skyrocketed. Autism, reproductive disorders, and digestive problems are on the rise. The American Public Health Association and American Nurses Association are among the many medical groups that condemn the use of GM bovine growth hormone because the milk from treated cows has more of the hormone IGF-1 (insulin-like growth factor), which is linked to cancer.

2. **GMOs are forever**—GMOs cross-pollinate and their seeds can travel. It is impossible to fully clean up a contaminated gene pool. Self-propagating GMO pollution can outlast the effects of climate change and nuclear waste, sickening future generations. This threatens organic and non-GMO farmers who struggle to keep their crops untainted.

3. **GMOs increase herbicide use**—Most GM crops are engineered to tolerate deadly weed killers. Monsanto, for example, sells Roundup crops, designed to survive applications of their Roundup herbicide. Between 1996 and 2008 farmers were forced to spray an extra 383 million pounds of herbicide on GMOs, resulting in super weeds resistant to Roundup, a chemical product that has been associated with sterility, hormone disruption, birth defects, and cancer.

4. **You can't put the genie back in the box**—Genetic engineering can be unpredictable. Mixing genes from totally unrelated species can unleash unexpected side effects. The very process of creating a GM plant can produce new toxins, allergens, carcinogens, and nutritional deficiencies. You can't recall a novel life-form.

5. **Government oversight is lax**—The FDA approved GMOs not with impartial independent science but with industry-funded research. To put it as delicately as possible, big money talks. At this writing the GMO lobby has squashed all attempts to require the clear labeling of GMO-derived ingredients.

6. **GMOs are toxic to the environment**—GMO crops and their associated herbicides can harm birds, insects, amphibians, marine ecosystems, and soil organisms. They reduce biodiversity, pollute water resources, and are unsustainable. GMO crops are eliminating habitats for monarch butterflies, whose populations are down by 50 percent. Bees are being affected in even greater numbers. GMO canola has been found growing wild in North Dakota and California, threatening to pass on its herbicide-tolerant genes to weeds.

7. **GMOs won't feed a hungry world**—Sustainable non-GMO agricultural methods used in developing countries have resulted in yield increases of 79 percent and higher. The International Assessment of Agricultural Knowledge, Science, and Technology for Development report, backed by fifty-eight governments and four hundred scientists around the world, concluded that GMO crops were "highly variable," and in some cases "yields declined." The report concluded that GMOs have nothing to offer the goals of reducing hunger and poverty or improving nutrition, health, and rural livelihoods.

8. **GMOs negatively affect American farmers**—Because GMOs are novel life-forms, biotech companies have been able to obtain patents, which restrict their use. As a result, GMO companies have the power to sue farmers whose fields are contaminated with GMOs, even when this is a result of drift from neighboring fields. This is a serious threat to farmer sovereignty and to food security, not just in the developing world but here at home.

9. **GMOs are a direct extension of chemical agriculture**—These are sold, not by food companies, but by the world's largest chemical companies.

10. **GMOs offer no consumer benefits**—At least the companies developing them have offered none. Given the lobbying efforts to keep consumers in the dark, one wonders, why go to such great lengths to conceal?

William Davis, MD, author of *Wheat Belly*, points out that even before the science of genetic engineering dramatically altered the nature of wheat, hybridization experiments did not require the documentation of animal or human testing. "Modern wheat," he writes, "despite all the genetic alterations to modify hundreds, if not thousands, of its genetically determined characteristics, made its way to the worldwide human food supply with nary a question surrounding its suitability for human consumption."

No wonder we all have a bellyache.

WHAT ARE THE MOST COMMON GMO CROPS?

- Alfalfa
- Canola
- Cotton
- Hawaiian papaya
- Soy
- Sugar beets
- Sweet corn
- Zucchini and yellow squash

The Non-GMO Project monitors those crops for which suspected or known incidents of contamination have occurred and those that have genetically altered relatives in commercial production where cross-pollination is possible.

- Acorn squash
- Bok choy
- Chard
- Chinese cabbage
- Delicata squash
- Flax
- Mizuna
- Pattypan squash
- Rapini
- Rice
- Rutabaga
- Siberian kale
- Table beets
- Turnip
- Wheat

Common ingredients derived from GMO risk crops are:

- Amino acids
- Aspartame
- Ascorbic acid
- Citric acid
- Ethanol
- Flavorings—both natural and artificial
- High-fructose corn syrup
- Hydrolyzed vegetable protein
- Lactic acid
- Maltodextrins
- Molasses
- Monosodium glutamate
- Sodium ascorbate
- Sodium citrate
- Sucrose
- Textured vegetable protein
- Vitamin C
- Vitamins
- Xanthan gum
- Yeast products

NOT EVERYONE AGREES

There are some who disagree with those who say GMOs are dangerous, many of them highly regarded scientists. Some researchers studying celiac disease and the connection to engineered wheat and other grain crops say GMOs are not responsible for the uptick in sensitivity to gluten.

Nor do they point to highly glutenized wheat versus the wheat our grand-parents ate as contributing to the epidemic of gluten intolerance.

Clearly, more study is necessary.

In a 2013 article in the *Guardian*, Richard Schiffman, reporting on the failure of a Washington State initiative to pass a GMO labeling law, urged environmental groups to shift their focus from GMOs to the more troubling issue of how industrial agriculture does business. He cites the degradation of soil, the depletion of diminishing groundwater reserves, the destruction of the Amazon forest to grow soybeans to feed beef cattle, and the "chemical treadmill" that forces farmers to use more and more deadly toxins to grow our food as the far more important food fight.

WHAT CAN WE AGREE ON?

According to a 2012 Mellman Group poll, 91 percent of Americans want to see GMOs clearly labeled on the food products and produce they buy. Fifty-three percent of consumers told a recent CBS/*New York Times* poll that they would not buy food that has been genetically modified.

In the spring of 2013, in response to public outcry and a growing demand for clear and mandatory GMO labeling on American products, the FDA posted the following on its Web site:

> We recognize and appreciate the strong interest that many consum-ers may have in knowing whether a food was produced using gene-tic engineering. Recently the FDA has received citizen petitions regarding genetically engineered foods, including the labeling of such foods. The agency is currently considering those petitions, and at this time, has not made a decision.

In 2014, as this book goes to press, three federal judges, hearing sepa-rate civil suits against food manufacturers, asked the FDA to render a ruling as to whether or not products containing GMOs can be labeled all-natural. The FDA respectfully declined to comment.

WHY DO GMOS MATTER TO GLUTEN-FREE CONSUMERS?

We who are sensitive to gluten are on the front line of food sensitivity. Our immune systems are hyperreactive. In spite of giving up gluten, some of us still feel sick.

Many of us no longer eat highly processed foods, whether gluten-free

Sumo Salmon

Nature.com reports that in the remote highlands of Panama, in tanks protected by netting, barbed wire, and guard dogs, swim the world's fattest fish. Salmon, genetically engineered by a company called AquaBounty to grow faster and bigger than their natural siblings, are close to FDA approval and will soon be on American dinner tables, followed by Botero-sized tilapia and trout. The venture is meeting with fierce consumer resistance. I wonder if the security measures are to keep out protesters or to keep the imposters from mating with and contaminating their wild counterparts. Can corpulent shrimp be far behind?

or not. We choose non-GMO products when we can find them and try to eat foods free of all common allergens, not just gluten. We avoid pesticides, buy organic produce, and support sustainable crops here and around the world. But are we really eating as cleanly as we think?

Under the National Organic Program, organic certification does not require GMO testing. Without GMO labeling, we have absolutely no idea if our efforts are successful, or if the kale or bok choy or pattypan squash that looked so good at the farmers' market has been contaminated with GMO crops.

Those of us who do eat commercially processed products may be lulled into a false sense of security, thinking that gluten-free status is enough to make the product safe for us to eat.

Many of the foods and additives we consume in greater quantities than the rest of the population—rice, soy, corn, flax, xanthan gum for gluten-free baking—rank high on the list of crops most likely made from or contaminated with GMOs.

It matters because we are the ones most at risk.

HOW DO I AVOID GMO PRODUCTS?

Voting with your wallet is one of the most effective weapons you have.

Start by shopping at Whole Foods Markets. In March 2013, the *New York Times* reported that Whole Foods Market pledged that by 2018 it would be the first major food retailer in the United States to require labeling of all genetically modified foods in all of its stores, a move that could tip the scales in favor of making it easier to avoid GMOs. As we go to press, *Time* magazine reports that the Chipotle chain has promised to follow suit.

Even more surprising, General Mills announced that Cheerios, their whole-grain oat cereal breakfast cereal (not gluten-free), which isn't made with GMOs, would now ensure that the sugar and cornstarch used in the cereal would come from non-GMO sources, not that the food giant thinks there's anything wrong with GMO ingredients. *Time* quotes VP Tom Forsythe as saying, "We did it because we think consumers might embrace it." This is the power of the purse.

These exceptions aside, it's not as easy to verify GMOs as it is to sniff out gluten. Many of the advocacy organizations have done the homework for us. Like our own gluten-free groups offering certification programs, groups like the Non-GMO Project and Buycott have filled the labeling void by creating smartphone shopping apps with lists of GMO-free verified products and brands.

THE GMO LABEL

Gluten-free labeling efforts have shown that our community embraces the idea of transparency. Let your representatives and our gluten-free advocacy groups know that you are not a science experiment and have zero tolerance for blind consumption. Even if you don't agree with those sounding the alarm, you have the right to know what you and your family are eating and to make informed food choices.

If you think, as I do, that GMOs put our health, organic whole food, and those who grow it at peril, and should be disclosed, check out one of the environmental organizations listed at the end of this chapter.

Arsenic in the Rice, Killer Corn, and Disappearing Honeybees

I know. You've got a lot on your plate.

But there are a few more things we need to talk about before we all sit down to a nice dinner.

ARSENIC IN MY RISOTTO?

I'm afraid so.

And apparently rice is only the tip of the iceberg lettuce. According to the Environmental Protection Agency, and as reported by Rachel Begun in *Gluten-Free Living* magazine, there's even more arsenic in vegetables, fruits and fruit juices, beer and wine, other "unspecified grains," meat, poultry, and eggs, and "others."

That's a lot to swallow, given that rice, rice flour, and rice starch are the gluten-free ingredients found in pretty much everything you and I eat. What's worse, there's more of the stuff on unpolished brown rice, which some of us prefer to white. *Consumer Reports* measured the levels in more than two hundred samples of rice and rice products, called the findings "troubling," and recommended that consumers lay off the paella, cream of rice, and gluten-free brownie mix until further notice.

In the wake of the story, the FDA released the results of its own investigation and, according to Begun, concluded that the "FDA does not currently have adequate scientific basis to recommend changes by consumers regarding their consumption of rice and rice products."

To make matters worse, arsenic, which comes in organic and inorganic forms, as well as from pesticides, is associated with adverse health outcomes. According to the FDA, EPA, and World Health Organization (WHO), it is responsible for higher rates of certain types of cancer.

Noting the opaque language of these agencies, and wanting to give you the specifics, I dug a little deeper. According to MedicineNet.com and the UK site Patient.com.uk, "adverse health outcomes" and "certain types of cancer" associated with arsenic poisoning include the following:

- ✦ Vomiting
- ✦ Abdominal pain
- ✦ Diarrhea
- ✦ Cardiac problems
- ✦ Lymphomas
- ✦ Leukemias
- ✦ Bladder, kidney, and lung cancers
- ✦ Peripheral vascular disease

Furthermore, inorganic arsenic, which is the most toxic kind, occurs in nature in the soil, in copper, and in lead ore deposits. However, it becomes more concentrated when industrial processes use it to make wood preservatives, metal compounds, or organic arsenic-containing compounds, such as insecticides and weed killers. If these compounds are burned, inorganic arsenic can be released into the air and later settle in the ground or in water.

Are you beginning to connect the dots?

WHO'S REGULATING THIS STUFF?

There are no federal limits for arsenic in food. The FDA promised to complete a review of the situation by the end of 2012. As I write this, 2013 is coming to a close. A careful reading of the FDA site shows that the 2012 review deadline has turned into a risk assessment paper report due by the end of 2014. There is no statement as to whether there are plans for federal limits for arsenic in food.

WHAT DO I DO IN THE MEANTIME?

For one thing, understand that your standards are higher than the government's. Will you keel over the next time you order lamb biryani? Not likely. But should you consider the effects of arsenic over the long term? Absolutely.

If you are a baker, experiment with the many non-rice gluten-free flours on the market, in particular high-protein nut and seed flours, such as chia and coconut. Use tapioca, potato, or amaranth flours for dusting and thickening.

Tricia Thompson, the founder of Gluten Free Watchdog, recommends that you:

- ✦ For cooked rice, substitute cooked gluten-free quinoa, millet, and kasha or buckwheat groats.

- Replace rice-based breakfast cereal, pasta, rice cakes, and rice drinks with products made from buckwheat, amaranth, or millet.
- Cook rice in more water than is called for and only until the rice is tender, and then discard the water. The trade-off is a loss of nutrients: a real Hobson's choice here.
- Give children soy, coconut, or almond beverages fortified with calcium and vitamin D instead of rice drinks.

Killer Corn?

Put down that gluten-free tortilla.

Corn is off the charts in terms of being one of the most commonly engineered foods. And so is corn allergy and intolerance. More and more people simply can't digest the stuff.

Robin Bernhoft, MD, medical director of the Bernhoft Center for Advanced Medicine, points to independent animal studies on GMO corn that have found damage to the lining of the animal's gut after ingestion. He advocates for more long-term studies done on GMO corn.

"Here's something that has been dangerous to animals being fed to people anyway," he tells Wendy Mondello for *Living Without* magazine.

The obvious suspects are fresh corn on or off the cob, cornstarch, tortillas made with cornmeal, polenta, grits, corn oil, and corn flour, not to mention popcorn and the all-pervasive high-fructose corn syrup. Corn is everywhere you look and in places you don't.

- Alcohol
- Artificial sweeteners
- Brown sugar
- Caramel and caramel color
- Citric acid
- Food starch
- Fruit coated with wax
- Honey
- Iodized salt
- Paper cups and plates
- Soap
- Sorbitol
- Toothpaste
- Vanilla extract

KERNELS OF TRUTH

Robyn O'Brien, founder of AllergyKids Foundation, is justifiably suspicious. In an interview with *Living Without*, she reports that after genetically modified corn made its way into the food supply in 1996, a 2008 study by the Centers for Disease Control and Prevention showed an increase in hospital discharges of children with any diagnosis related to food allergy—from 2,615 in 1998 to 9,537 by 2006.

While there is no solid proof, we might conclude that maybe some of us are not getting better after giving up gluten because we are still consuming a grain we believe to be safe and is far from it. Like rice, corn is what we turn to when we can't eat gluten.

HOW DO I KNOW IF I'M ALLERGIC TO CORN?

Many of us tend to blame symptoms on hidden gluten. Sometimes that is not the case at all. If you've given up gluten and still have reactions, corn could be the culprit. If you get hives, rash, itchy mouth or ears, nausea, stomach pain, or vomiting, you might want to try giving up corn for a while or consult with an allergist and begin an elimination diet. Rooting out and ridding yourself of corn is not as easy as banishing gluten.

Keep an accurate food journal and share it with your doctor. Make sure it includes:

+ What form of corn you ate
+ What brand
+ How much you ate
+ The time you ate it
+ Drinks that contain corn syrup
+ Your symptoms
+ The time you experienced the symptoms
+ How long the symptoms lasted
+ All medications, if you haven't eaten anything

Everything matters because corn is everywhere—even the dusting inside the rubber gloves the flight attendant or the nurse practitioner used to give you a soda or a flu shot.

Corn Off the Cobbler

+ Replace corn with tapioca or potato starch or flour or sorghum flour in baking.
+ Replace xanthan gum (arsenic and corn) with guar gum.
+ Replace corn syrup with honey, agave nectar, or tapioca syrup.

The Silence of the Bees

The honeybees are dropping like flies.

In March 2013 a *New York Times* article on the inexplicable disappearance of honeybees ran the headline, "Mystery Malady Kills More Bees, Heightening Worry on Farm." According to Michael Wines, the article's author, the unidentified disease, called colony collapse disorder, which surfaced in 2005, has been killing about one-third of all bees, despite beekeepers' best efforts. That toll seems to have escalated dramatically last year, wiping out 40 to 50 percent of the hives needed to pollinate much of the nation's fruits and vegetables.

The owner of Big Sky Honey in Montana, who has been raising bees for thirty years, has never experienced anything like it. The Huffington Post reports that last season it took over 60 percent of all functional honeybees in the country just to pollinate California's almond crop. Wines reports that there is growing evidence that a powerful new class of pesticides, neonicotinoids, engineered directly into the plants themselves, may be responsible for the die-off. What's insidious about neonicotinoids is that they are systemic in the plants and are in the nectar on which the bees feed. "If the death toll continues at the present rate," says scientist Jeff Pettis, who leads bee research at the Federal Agricultural Service in Beltsville, Maryland, "we are one poor weather event or high winter bee loss away from a pollination disaster."

And that's not all.

As farmers plant crop varieties genetically engineered to survive spraying with weed killers, herbicide use has increased. Experts say that some fungicides have been laced with substances that keep insects from maturing.

Eric Mussen, an apiculturist at the University of California, tells the *New York Times* that researchers there have documented about fifty chemical residues in pollen and wax collected from beehives.

This is worrisome because honeybees pollinate pretty much our entire food supply.

It's enough to give you hives.

I'M BUSY—I DON'T HAVE TIME TO SAVE THE BEES

You do, actually. Here are some simple things you can do to help:

+ Buy local honey to support your local bees and beekeepers.
+ Plant bee-friendly plants in your garden, such as aster, cosmos, bee balm, and rosemary.

+ Explore the Xerces Society site, a pollinator conservation organization.
+ When buying from a nursery, ask for plants that have not been treated with neocotinoids.
+ Join the Great Sunflower Project and count the bees in your own backyard.

When I was a baby, something in the eaves of our family cottage left me with a lip so fat, my parents took me to the Board of Health to make sure I had not been bitten by a black widow spider or some equally poisonous insect. It turned out to be a hornet and, to this day, I give these industrious creatures a wide berth. I also carry a card that warns, *No Epinephrine!*

It's their absence now that stops my heart.

I had no idea, when I began to research this chapter, how pervasive the problems were or how connected the issues are that I would stumble upon. I watched the evidence mount. Many human, animal, and insect health problems stem from GMOs, unregulated biotech, agribusinesses, lax regulations, and the presence of ever more powerful herbicides in our food and water. It can't be a coincidence that the huge surge in food allergies corresponds to this growing trend.

We who are so prone to difficulties with gluten and other foods should find these reports troubling. If, as I do, you want full disclosure about what you are eating, you may find this chapter to be a wake-up call.

Michael Pollan, author of *Food Rules: An Eater's Manual*, offers a few simple changes you can make right now.

+ Get out of the supermarket when you can. Farmers' markets are an important part of learning where your food comes from.
+ Eat real food.
+ Don't eat anything your great-grandmother wouldn't recognize as food.
+ Avoid food products containing ingredients a third-grader can't pronounce.

I would add:

+ Talk to the farmers you buy from.
+ Ask how you can help.
+ Fight back at the cash register.

✦ Go to Non-GMO Project and download a list of verified non-GMO products.

Learn More

GLUTEN-FREE LABELING

To read the full text of the Food Allergen Labeling and Consumer Protection Act of 2004 (Public Law 108–282, Title II): www.fda.gov /downloads/food/guidanceregulation/UCM179394.pdf

To read the FDA statement on the final ruling for standardized gluten-free labeling: www.fda.gov/food/guidanceregulation/allergen /UCM362880.htm

For a state-by-state list of FDA Consumer Complaint Coordinators: www.fda.gov/safety/reportaproblem/consumercomplaintcoordinators

American Celiac Disease Alliance. www.americanceliac.org

Celiac Disease Foundation. www.celiac.org

Celiac Support Association. www.csaceliacs.info

Gluten Intolerance Group. www.gluten.net

National Foundation for Celiac Awareness. www.celiaccentral.org

GLUTEN-FREE INSURANCE COVERAGE/MEDICARE/MEDICAID

United States Department of Health and Human Services

200 Independence Avenue SW

Washington, DC 20201

www.hhs.gov

AARP. www.aarp.org

Center for Advocacy for the Rights and Interests of the Elderly. www.carie.org

Feeding America—Nonprofit dealing with senior hunger issues. www.feedingamerica.org

The Senior Source. www.theseniorsource.org

United States Department of Health of Human Services Administration on Aging—Elder Rights. www.aoa.gov

GMOS

Buycott—If you want to support food companies with ethical principles and make sure your money isn't going to companies whose interests are counter to yours, this app traces food items back through the production chain and gives information and contact details for every food maker in the supermarket. www.buycott.com

GMO Checker—This iPhone app will quickly identify products that are organic, vegan, gluten-free, and GMO-free; $3.99. Open iTunes to buy at the Apple App Store.

Green America: Economic Action for a Just Planet. www.greenamerica.org

Just Label It—GMO labeling action group. www.justlabelit.org

Monsanto. www.monsanto.com

Non-GMO Project. www.nongmoproject.org

Non-GMO Project Shopping Guide—Free iPhone app listing all GMO-free brands and products in the project's product verification program. www.nongmoproject.org/find-non-gmo/iphone-app -shopping-guide/

Responsible Technology—A group advocating for the responsible use of biotechnology offers a twenty-five-minute video on GMOs and gluten. www.responsibletechnology.org

True Food—This free app from the Center for Food Safety for iPhone or Android updates in real time with new alerts, news, and tips on how to avoid GMO products and where to find alternatives. www.centerforfoodsafety.org/issues/311/ge-foods/non-gmo -shoppers-guide-325/1847/get-the-app-for-iphone-or-android

Whole Foods Market. www.wholefoodsmarket.com

KILLER CORN, DISAPPEARING BEES, AND ARSENIC IN THE RICE

Consumers Union. www.consumersunion.org

Corn Allergy Girl. www.cornallergygirl.com

Food Allergy Research and Resource Program. www.farrp.uni.edu

BEES/CONSERVATION

The Great Sunflower Project. www.greatsunflower.org

Xerces Society. www.xerces.org

BOOKS

Food, Inc. by Peter Pringle (Simon and Schuster)

Food Rules: An Eater's Manual by Michael Pollan (Penguin Books)

40 Years of Chez Panisse by Alice Waters (Clarkson Potter)

In Defense of Food: An Eater's Manifesto by Michael Pollan (Penguin Books)

Wheat Belly by William Davis (Rodale Books)

The World According to Monsanto: Pollution, Corruption, and the Control of the World's Food Supply by Marie-Monique Robin (The New Press)

DOCUMENTARIES

Fed Up—Katie Couric's film exposes America's epidemic of obesity and food addiction, and a government that has caved to Big Food. Featuring food experts Marion Nestle, Michael Pollan, Deborah Cohen, David Kessler, and President Bill Clinton, among others.

Food Fight—A look at the development of America's agricultural policy and food culture.

Food, Inc.—An examination of the costs of putting value and convenience over nutrition and environmental impact.

Forks over Knives—The argument for rejecting animal-based and processed foods.

Ingredients: The Local Food Movement Takes Root—The genesis of the local food movement; Alice Waters and Peter Hoffman are among the many visionaries.

Supersize Me—While examining the influence of the fast-food industry, Morgan Spurlock eats solely at McDonald's for a month.

23 Community

Community

Oh, I get by with a little help from my friends.
—JOHN LENNON AND PAUL MCCARTNEY

◆ **National Organizations and Local Chapters**
   Celiac Disease Foundation
   CSA
   Gluten Intolerance Group
   Raising Our Celiac Kids (R.O.C.K.)
   Canadian Celiac Association
◆ **Advocacy Community**
   American Celiac Disease Alliance
   National Foundation for Celiac Awareness
◆ **Lobbying Congress Effectively**
◆ **Independent Groups**
◆ **Regional Community**
◆ **Virtual Community**
   Message Boards, Forums, Chats, Collaborative Boards, and Blogs
◆ **Magazines**
◆ **Expos, Festivals, and Conferences**
◆ **Extended Community**
◆ **Books, Cookbooks, and Food References**
◆ **Medical References**
◆ **Essential Equipment**
◆ **Accessories and Novelty Items**
◆ **Testing and Test Kits**
◆ **Additional Resources**

In the early nineties, after my diagnosis, I didn't know another living soul who got sick from gluten. I wanted to meet the tribe I'd just joined, so I headed for Chicago and the annual meeting of the USA Celiac Sprue Association, currently called Celiac Support Association.

What greeted me was a group of sad sacks who were sick and depressed and marginalized by their intolerance to gluten, lack of safe food, the utter disregard of the world in general, and, in some cases, the medical community and even their own families. To give you an idea of the tone, Beano was the buzz of the meeting, as was how to attach a trailer full of food to your car so you wouldn't have to eat in a restaurant. A confusing lecture on halotype associations and genetics left me with the distinct impression that I was at risk for schizophrenia.

How could I be a member of this club? I see the humor in every situation. I am not easily depressed. I bounce back. I wanted out.

I wanted out, that is, until they opened the hotel ballroom to food vendors and I broke into a sweat along with everybody else at the sight of gluten-free peach pies. In retrospect they weren't any good, but they were dough and crust, sugar and sticky fruit, and that's all anybody cared about. As we elbowed one another for the dwindling supply, what propelled me through the aggressively hungry crowd was the belief that I'd never see another pie again.

The point is, the road to the gluten-free revolution started with a handful of people who met around a kitchen table, or in a church or school basement, and finally got big enough for a Chicago airport hotel banquet room.

I stayed.

It wasn't because I was thrilled to be hanging out with a bunch of people who were afraid to walk past a bakery, even though I had been as sick or even sicker than they were. And it wasn't just because of the food, which I hadn't known where to get because Al Gore had not yet invented the Internet.

It was because I sat in that room thinking, *These people are just like me. They need a voice, someone who understands what they are going through. More than anything, they need a good laugh. They need somebody to get the word out and make this all right.*

Then I realized that somebody would be me.

And so, the young woman whose dream was to leave advertising to become a poet and write novels and stories, and who was coping with her new gluten-free diet resourcefully and well, if not a bit eccentrically, even a bit snarkily when the situation warranted it, decided on the spot to be the change she wished to see in the world.

Attending a conference can be a life-changing experience.

But let's face it. Some of us are just not joiners. We need another social network like the proverbial hole in the head. We may be gluten-free but we draw the line at joining a club. The idea of going to a meeting is anathema. Besides, we know what we're doing, don't we?

On the other hand, some of us are pretty sick and need plenty of support. We love nothing more than the physical company of like-minded folks, networking, commiserating, and noshing. We want to learn about the latest research and treatments for associated conditions. We may feel isolated by the diet or our circumstances within it. We look forward to being part of a group, hearing guest speakers, and sampling new gluten-free foods from vendors.

Most of us fall somewhere in the middle. We're dabblers. We're avoiding gluten and want to learn the ropes. Maybe our children have multiple food allergies and we want to know how other parents have coped and discovered what works and what doesn't. We need to know how to negotiate school lunches and overnight playdates. Maybe we're planning a trip and want to know where to eat along the way. We may be looking for an intensive weekend course in nutrition, cooking, and entertaining and are considering a workshop or a gluten-free expo, preferably in a swell resort or city. We want to know what products are worth the money and which ones aren't. We may be moving and need a new doctor.

We drop in and out. We take what we need and forgo the rest.

Some of us thrive in the virtual community. We are citizens of the Twittersphere and Facebook. We are LinkedIn. We are looking for content, a blog or two, and a few sites we can trust to fill us in without our having to make a commitment to attend an actual meeting or a gluten-free event. If possible, we'd prefer a community that shares our worldview as well as our diet. We post our questions and share what we've learned with others in our social network. We like the reciprocity and the anonymity of that. We don't need bricks and mortar and actual eye contact. We do, but for other things.

Then there are the political animals. We join forces. We sign petitions and write checks. We like a good fight. We stand up when we're told to sit down. There's nothing we like more than meeting with others to advocate for positive change, for GMO disclosure on food labels, for humane treatment of animals, for sustainable crops, for codifying gluten-free food as a medical expense. We care about how our food is made and grown, and we like to be around people who share our sense of community and commitment. We believe we can change things.

Some of just can't sit still. We'll walk, run, cycle, and do any number of Herculean things to draw attention to causes we care about, in particular the serious aspects of gluten intolerance, the need for research, even a cure. In the name of our cause, we wear silly T-shirts, get friends to sponsor our races, get interviewed on TV, and commemorate our athletic achievements with photos on our Facebook pages. Afterward, we reward ourselves with a gluten-free beer and a bowl of spaghetti.

The thing is, we all have to eat.

Finding the community that's right for you is the fastest way to the food.

National Community

There are many perks to be had by joining one of the big national groups: monthly newsletters, e-bulletins and blasts, magazines for adults and kids, annual conferences, symposia, kids' camps, events, advocacy, access to the latest research and hot issues, community outreach, gluten-free starter packets and samples, and real grassroots groups close to home.

As in all big families, the various groups do not always agree. For example, there is a difference of opinion about what should be the minimum parts per million of gluten allowable under their certification programs. Some say 5 parts per million max; others say 10. No matter, their standards are higher than the government's, which allows 20. Each group awards qualifying food makers a gluten-free stamp of certification that's standardized and impossible to miss on a package. Different groups focus on different issues. Personalities vary. Where one group is midwestern folksy, another is city slick. Where one is Washington political, another is all business. Others are kid-friendly, family casual.

CELIAC DISEASE FOUNDATION

Founded in 1990 by the dynamic Elaine Monarch, Celiac Disease Foundation is based in L.A.'s San Fernando Valley, with thousands of members and chapters all across the country.

As per its mission statement, CDF is a nonprofit 501(c)(3) public benefit corporation driving diagnosis of celiac disease, dermatitis herpetiformis, and other gluten-related disorders through advocacy, education, and advancing research. Under the guidance of CEO Marilyn Geller, CDF forms a bridge between the scientific community and the improvement in the quality of life for the gluten-intolerant, working hard to make its membership aware of all the newest scientific and clinical advancements and helping to put this information into a practical, actionable context.

CDF is a founding member of the advocacy group American Celiac Disease Alliance and is actively involved with the National Institutes of Health, the National Institutes of Health Celiac Disease Awareness Program, National Digestive Diseases Information Clearinghouse, and the Food and Drug Administration in the furtherance of public awareness of celiac disease and non-celiac gluten sensitivity.

As an organization, CDF uses its considerable clout to press for better food and drug labeling and physician awareness, and works closely with professionals in the pharmaceutical, medical, and research communities. Its advisory board boasts an international roster of the most expert minds in the field. Alessio Fasano, MD, director of the Massachusetts General Hospital's new center for Celiac Research; Ivor D. Hill, MD, director of the Celiac Disease Center at Nationwide Children's Hospital, Columbus, Ohio; Mayo Clinic's Joseph Murray, MD; John Zone, MD, of the University of Utah; and Peter Green, MD, director of the Columbia Celiac Disease Center, are among the notables.

CDF recently launched a comprehensive online directory of reliable health care practitioners familiar with diagnosing and treating celiac disease and other gluten-related disorders.

Insight, its quarterly newsletter, which is available in both digital and paper format, gives subscribers articles on the latest research, clinical trials, product news and warnings, professional conferences, prescription and over-the-counter drug information, dining out, traveling, personal stories, recipes, new products, and other issues pertinent to the gluten-free life.

Through the efforts of its board, CDF hosts professional symposia and conferences, and under its Team Gluten-Free program it sponsors marathons, triathlons, and many other fun events that benefit research, awareness, advocacy efforts, and gluten-free summer camp scholarships.

The annual CDF Gluten-Free Expo is one of the best in the country.

Through CDF Connections and partnership with other groups, the organization sponsors an annual summer camp and has formed an ever-growing grassroots network of chapters all over the country, including groups for parents and kids and teens.

Contributions are tax deductible. Membership is paid in annual dues. www.celiac.org

CDF Chapters

Alabama	Iowa	New York
Alaska	Kansas	North Carolina
Arizona	Kentucky	Ohio
Arkansas	Louisiana	Oregon
California	Maine	Pennsylvania
Colorado	Maryland	Tennessee
Connecticut	Massachusetts	Texas
Florida	Minnesota	Utah
Georgia	Missouri	Vermont
Hawaii	Nevada	Virginia
Idaho	New Hampshire	Washington
Illinois	New Jersey	Wisconsin
Indiana	New Mexico	Wyoming

CSA/USA

Frustrated by the lack of gluten-free food and the barest scraps of information about celiac disease, Celiac Support Association founder Pat Murphy Garst of Des Moines, Iowa, took matters into her own kitchen. When she developed a recipe that pleased her, she photocopied it and added it to the collection that would become the first gluten-free cookbook, a homemade, spiral-bound volume called *Gluten-Free Cooking*.

In December 1977, Garst contacted every person who bought her little book, a total of twelve people, and with a whopping $75 in donations, started the Midwestern Celiac Sprue Association. By the end of 1978, there were forty-one members representing eleven states, forming the basis for what eventually became CSA/USA, the largest and oldest national celiac support organization in the United States.

While patient support and education is still at the heart of its mission—its slogan is *Celiacs Helping Celiacs*—the CSA of today solicits and awards grant money for research and provides its members with the newest scientific and research data and information relating to celiac disease and dermatitis herpetiformis.

As part of its uniquely stringent Recognition Seal Program—no oats allowed—which includes scrutiny of source ingredients as well as product ingredients, CSA offers food companies a chance to offer the gluten-free community quality products verified to be 5 parts per million of gluten or less. Cel-Kids Network supports parents and children with kid-friendly recipes and fun activities, and sponsors several gluten-free summer camps.

The spirit of Pat Murphy Garst lives on in the tone of this organization, decidedly folksy, with essay and photo contests and recipe exchanges. *Lifeline*, its quarterly newsletter in print and downloadable form, is filled with recipes, product news, research, and personal articles.

CSA, a nonprofit 501(c)(3) organization, holds an annual conference; offers its dues paying members discounts on cookbooks, audiotapes, and other educational materials; and publishes an annual list of acceptable gluten-free products. It maintains a referral service and hotline for its members and divides its chapter by region with a director for each.

www.csaceliacs.org

CSA Chapters

REGION I— NORTH-CENTRAL:	REGION II— SOUTH-CENTRAL	REGION III— NORTHEAST
Illinois	Alabama	Connecticut
Indiana	Arkansas	Maine
Iowa	Kansas	Massachusetts
Michigan	Kentucky	New Hampshire
Minnesota	Louisiana	New Jersey
Ohio	Mississippi	New York
Wisconsin	Missouri	Pennsylvania
	Oklahoma	Rhode Island
	Tennessee	Vermont
	Texas	

REGION IV— SOUTHEAST	REGION V— NORTHWEST	REGION VI— SOUTHWEST
Delaware	Montana	Arizona
District of Columbia	Nebraska	California
Florida	North Dakota	Colorado
Georgia	Oregon	Hawaii
Maryland	South Dakota	Nevada
North Carolina	Washington	New Mexico
South Carolina	Wyoming	Utah
Virginia		Guam
West Virginia		Wake Island
Puerto Rico		
Virgin Islands		

GLUTEN INTOLERANCE GROUP

Founded in 1974 by the late Elaine Hartsook, PhD, RD, this Seattle-based national nonprofit organization, also known as GIG, was the first organization to help people diagnosed with gluten reactions to identify safe and appetizing gluten-free foods.

Today's GIG, led by executive director Cynthia Kupper, RD, is certainly more sophisticated, but its mission has remained the same. It supports those with gluten intolerance, celiac disease, dermatitis herpetiformis, and other gluten sensitivities, through consumer and industry services and programs and important work in the dietician community that promote a healthy lifestyle.

Perhaps the most high-profile program is GIG's state-of-the-art Gluten-Free Certification Organization (www.gfco.org), which has awarded more than ten thousand products its GF logo—oats allowed—signifying quality, integrity, and purity to a standard of 10 parts per million or under for gluten-free consumers.

GIG's Gluten-Free Food Service program is a management accreditation course designed to work with large resorts, medical centers, and other types of food service establishments that serve gluten-free consumers, offering training in the proper technique for gluten-free food handling. Its Chef to Plate Gluten-Free Restaurant Awareness Program has had the participation of over thirteen hundred restaurants across the country and was the first of its kind to create industry awareness of the gluten-free diet.

GIG's medical advisory board includes Joseph Murray, MD, Cynthia Rudert, MD, FACP, Alessio Fasano, MD, Ivor Hill, MD, and Michelle Pietzak, MD, with representation in the dental and nutrition community.

With more than eighty branches in thirty-four states, there is plenty of local support. Youth programs include Celiac Kids' Club, GIG Kids Camps, and Teen Advocates for Gluten Sensitivities, a program designed to help teenagers be positive advocates and leaders for themselves as well as for other children following a gluten-free lifestyle. Teens can share stories and provide support for other teens through GIG's *Celiac Kids' Club* magazine.

GIG sponsors Autism Day and Gluten-Free Awareness Night at Seattle Mariners baseball games.

GIG's slick quarterly magazine, which comes with membership, offers articles ranging from health concerns to lifestyle issues, and research updates, with cookbook reviews and recipes regular features. A national conference with top speakers is held every year.

May Is Celiac Awareness Month—So Is October

Both are great times for walks and runs and outdoor events, fund-raising, publicity, and calling attention to the ongoing need for research. National Digestive Diseases Week is in May when medical experts from all over the world get together to discuss the latest developments regarding gluten and human plumbing. In Canada and at CSA, it's been October for over forty years. Until Congress makes it official, you've got twice as much time to get acquainted with the community.

GIG is a 501(c)(3) nonprofit organization funded by private donations. www.gluten.net

GIG Chapters

Alabama	Kansas	Rhode Island
Arizona	Kentucky	South Carolina
Arkansas	Minnesota	South Dakota
California	Missouri	Texas
Colorado	Montana	Utah
Connecticut	New York	Vermont
Delaware	North Carolina	Virginia
Florida	North Dakota	Washington
Georgia	Ohio	West Virginia
Illinois	Oregon	Wisconsin
Indiana	Pennsylvania	Wyoming
Iowa		

RAISING OUR CELIAC KIDS (R.O.C.K.)

In R.O.C.K.'s case, the mother of invention was Danna Korn.

When her son was severely affected by celiac disease and ostracized by the other kids, Korn experienced firsthand the isolation, overwork, and heartbreak so many parents endure trying to help their little ones negotiate the birthday parties, playdates, day care, school snacks, and school lunches, all the while encouraging them to feel as normal as possible.

There was plenty of support for adults, but none addressed the special needs of children.

Raising Our Celiac Kids was born in San Diego. Word spread and now R.O.C.K. is a loosely strung network of groups, some affiliated with the original group, some not, organized around the founder's guiding principles.

Meetings often take place at parks and other venues where kids can picnic and play and members are asked to bring "kid food." There are parties, potlucks, walks, runs, and bike rides for awareness. The idea is to help kids take responsibility for their diets, as well as reading labels and preparing foods for themselves. Education efforts include reaching out to school dieticians, teachers, day care professionals, and family members—all of those entrusted with a child's care and feeding.

Members range in age from one year to preteen, and sharing is encouraged. There are teen groups to help kids (and their parents) cope with the gluten-free lifestyle at this awkward and rebellious age. Children on casein-free diets are welcome, too, as is any family on the gluten-free diet for any reason.

R.O.C.K. is not a nonprofit; rather it is an upbeat club in which membership is free. For a rundown of R.O.C.K. groups in your area and a quick snapshot of its personality, go to www.rockcharlotte.blogspot.com and www.ccliackids.com.

R.O.C.K. Groups

Alaska	Louisiana	North Dakota
Arizona	Maine	Ohio
Arkansas	Maryland	Ontario, Canada
California	Massachusetts	Oregon
Colorado	Michigan	Pennsylvania
Connecticut	Minnesota	South Carolina
District of Columbia/	Mississippi	South Dakota
Metro Area	Missouri	Tennessee
Florida	Montana	Texas
Georgia	Nebraska	Utah
Idaho	Nevada	Vermont
Illinois	New Hampshire	Virginia
Indiana	New Jersey	Washington
Iowa	New Mexico	West Virginia
Kansas	New York	Wisconsin
Kentucky	North Carolina	

CANADIAN CELIAC ASSOCIATION (L'ASSOCIATION CANADIENNE DE LA MALADIE COELIAQUE)

The Canadian Celiac Association, a volunteer-based, federally registered charitable organization, was founded in 1972 by two celiacs from Kitchener, Ontario, probably at a kitchen table, for the sole purpose of providing support and sources for gluten-free food to others in a similar situation. All these many years later, the mission to provide information and support has never wavered, but it has broadened and grown and they've become a national voice for all people who are adversely affected by gluten. Their motto: *The Gluten Problem: Found. Treated. Cured.*

The primary goal of this organization is to educate the general public and health professionals, to encourage medical research, to advise manufacturers and distributors as to what constitutes safe gluten-free foods, and to solicit funds through memberships, private and corporate donations, and estate contributions for the purpose of supporting programs and activities.

To that end, the Gluten-Free Certification Program is the only Canadian voluntary certification program designed for manufacturers of gluten-free food, drugs, and pharmaceutical products that addresses all potential health hazards, as well as gluten. Once a company has gone through this rigorous certification process, which sets the standard at 10 parts per million or under, and involves third-party auditors in order to eliminate any conflicts of interest, they are awarded the Association's trusted Gluten-Free/*Sans Gluten* seal. A list of certified brands appears on their Web site, which is great for Americans and others traveling in Canada to get acquainted with verified products along the way.

Whether in English or *en français*, new members have access to books and products, starter kits, a toll-free member hotline, and all manner of educational materials. In addition to local, face-to-face support, an annual conference is held in host cities all over Canada with seminars, demonstrations, vendor fairs, and a wide range of speakers from inspirational to leading medical and research professionals.

For all of its sophistication and state-of-the-art knowledge, a visit to a Canadian Celiac Association event gives one the feeling that we are sitting at a homey table in Kitchener with its founders. www.celiac.ca

Canadian Celiac Association Chapters

BRITISH COLUMBIA	ALBERTA	SASKATCHEWAN
Kamloops	Calgary	Regina
Kelowna	Edmonton	Saskatoon
Vancouver		
Victoria		

MANITOBA	QUEBEC	NEW BRUNSWICK
Western Manitoba	Quebec City	Fredericton
Winnipeg		Moncton
		Saint John

PRINCE EDWARD ISLAND		NOVA SCOTIA
Charlottetown		Halifax

NEWFOUNDLAND AND LABRADOR

St. John's

ONTARIO

Belleville	Kingston	St. Catherines
Halton-Peel	Kitchener-Waterloo	Toronto
Hamilton	Ottawa	Thunder Bay
London	Peterborough	

Advocacy Community

AMERICAN CELIAC DISEASE ALLIANCE

In 2003 an ad hoc group of fifteen leaders in the celiac community came together to help persuade Congress to require gluten-free food labels and to include information about common allergens. In 2004 the Food Allergen Labeling and Consumer Protection Act came into law and the power of a unified gluten-free community was realized.

Today the ACDA is a permanent nonprofit 501(c)(3) organization whose mission is to represent and advocate for all segments of the celiac community—patients, physicians, researchers, and food manufacturers among them. It provides guidance to food manufacturers on the requirements of the finalized labeling law, as well as assistance to the FDA, USDA, and the Centers for Medicare and Medicaid on issues related to gluten intolerance.

ACDA serves as a watchdog group and publishes alerts on companies that, in an effort to capitalize on the gluten-free market, misrepresent the gluten status of their products, and calls out those organizations that certify products and restaurants whose standards do not conform to what is safe on a gluten-free diet. It also works with related health organizations such as the Arthritis Foundation, Juvenile Diabetes Research Foundation, and the Sjögren's Syndrome Foundation.

A newsletter, available on its Web site, offers news on the latest research and drug testing and offers basic dos and don'ts to those new at the gluten-free diet.

Its members include:

Alvine Pharmaceuticals	*Delight Gluten-Free Magazine*
Celiac Disease Center at Columbia University	Enjoy Life Brands
	Foods By George
Celiac Disease Foundation	*Gluten-Free Living* magazine
Center for Celiac Research	Gluten Intolerance Group

Glutino

Healthy Villi

ImmusanT

Andrea Levario, JD

Living Without magazine

Mary's Gone Crackers

Savory Palate, Inc.

Tricia Thompson, MS, RD

University of Chicago Celiac

Disease Center

Westchester Celiac Sprue Support

Group

www.americanceliac.org

Community Activism: Lobbying Congress Effectively

As it becomes harder and harder to get Congress to enact laws that protect the consumer, we can't sit back and let the associations that represent us get the job done. It is incumbent on all of us to keep up the pressure and to demand mandatory, not voluntary, participation in gluten-free food labeling and full GMO disclosure, and to press for fair medical reimbursement for expensive gluten-free food, especially for the elderly and disadvantaged.

We who are exquisitely sensitive must step up to the plate and let our voices be heard on the subject of how our food is grown and farmed, manufactured and processed, and how this impacts public health and the environment. We must make it clear to our representatives, without rancor, why they need to pay attention to our growing and very vocal community, which means learning how to lobby effectively and unemotionally. We must also let them know that we will make our positions clear at the ballot box.

To find the names of your senators, go to www.senate.gov.

To find the names of your representative, www.house.gov.

For phone calls:

1. Call the Capitol switchboard, 202-224-3121.
2. Ask to be connected to your senator or representative's office.
3. Ask to speak with the aide who handles the issue about which you would like to comment.
4. Identify yourself as a constituent and tell the aide that you would like to leave a brief message, such as "Please tell Senator/Representative _____ that I support/oppose S_____/ H.R._____ because _____."
5. Always give the reasons for your position, and if you don't know, ask

where the senator or representative or agency stands on the bill or issue, and why it is important to you and should be to him or her to support or reject it.

6. Always request a written response to your phone call.

If you'd rather put your views in writing, make your petition as eloquent as you can, but don't rattle on. Be courteous and to the point, include key information, and use examples to support your position. A good rule to follow when writing to a U.S. senator or representative is: one issue/one letter/one page.

Address your letter to:

Office of The Honorable (name of senator or representative)
U.S. Senate, Washington, DC 20515/US House of Representatives, Washington, DC 20510

If you know the name of the Senate subcommittee your representative is sitting on:

The Honorable _____
Name of Subcommittee
Washington, DC 20510

If you are writing to a House subcommittee member:

The Honorable _____
Name of Subcommittee
Washington, DC 20515

The salutation should say:

Dear Senator _____ or Dear Representative _____.

When writing to the secretary or chair of a committee, the salutation is always:

Dear Mr. Secretary, Dear Madame Secretary, Dear Mr. Chairman, or Dear Madame Chairman

Letters to the Speaker should begin:

Dear Mr. or Madame Speaker

Write to the president at The White House, Washington, DC 20500
White House Switchboard: 202-456-1111
president@whitehouse.gov

Whether you send e-mail or snail mail, keep in mind that the same guidelines and courtesies apply, and if you contact the White House, understand that you will have to go through a security screening.

NATIONAL FOUNDATION FOR CELIAC AWARENESS (NFCA)

Founded in 2004 by Alice Bast, mother and activist who suffered the tragic loss of a child due to undiagnosed celiac disease, the mission of this non-profit 501(c)(3) foundation is to empower, educate, advocate, and advance research to improve the quality of life for those on a lifelong gluten-free diet.

NFCA is funded by a National Institutes of Health grant, private donations, corporate sponsorship, banner advertising, and the sale of products and educational resources. To further its goals, it reaches into the business and corporate community, as well as the medical community, for its advisers. Anthony J. DiMarino, MD, Alessio Fasano, MD, Daniel Leffler, MD, Ritu Verma, MD, and Joseph Murray, MD sit on the medical advisory board and there is representation in the fields of nutrition, dentistry, ophthalmology, pharmacology, and research. Fund-raising is an important aspect of NFCA's strategy and they hold many corporate-sponsored benefits a year.

NFCA offers continuing education courses to food service professionals, dieticians, multidisciplinary health professionals, primary care providers, and women's health practitioners. It offers gluten-free food marketers a certification program that essentially endorses the Canadian Celiac Association's standard, certifying products as gluten-free at 10 parts per million or under and offers its own NFCA seal of certification.

While the organization does not provide direct patient support, it does publish a monthly e-mail newsletter with books, products, recipes, event news, and articles on the latest research. On its Web site there are many free printable educational materials and getting-started guides, plus links to additional Web sites as well as free webinars and a blog, *Celiac Central Bits & Bites*. www.celiaccentral.wordpress.com, www.celiaccentral.com

A WORD ABOUT NONPROFITS

The terms *nonprofit* and *not-for-profit* are used interchangeably in many places in our lives. A nonprofit organization designated a 501(c)(3) corporation must report its income to the IRS as such. It's smart to verify the nonprofit status of any organization you are considering supporting through membership and donations. A good place to start is www.guide star.com.

Check the organization's annual report, which must disclose salaries and operating expenses. An organization with high salaries, large staffs, and marketing and public relations budgets may not be the right fit for your donation dollar. If the association states that it funds research, those organizations and institutes it funds should be listed. If you can't find out what a nonprofit gives to, you may want to reserve your gift for another, more transparent association.

Of course, some associations do not have this status, which is fine, but they must fully disclose that they are *for profit*.

We've all seen banners on books and other products declaring that profits go to research. In most cases this is true, and many companies and individuals donate a generous portion of their proceeds to good causes, but bear in mind this has become a popular marketing tool for many businesses. The key word is *profit* or, more specifically, *net profit*, which is what remains after taxes, expenses, capital improvements, overhead, and salaries. If nothing remains after all these matters are settled, there are no profits and, thus, nothing is given to the advertised charity.

Hollywood is famous for this. Movies gross in the millions but show no net profit. This is the substance of many a lawsuit from disgruntled actors and screenwriters, whose salaries and bonuses are tied contractually to a percentage of "the net."

If you want to be absolutely sure your money is going to research or to another cause of your choice, write *For Research Only* on the face of your check.

Regional Community

Most local support groups are chapters of the national organizations described above, but there are independent groups that offer meetings and support in various regions around the country. Many subscribe to one or more of the philosophies espoused by the larger groups but lack affiliation.

CELIAC COMMUNITY FOUNDATION OF NORTHERN CALIFORNIA

This nonprofit Bay Area organization is supported by the Taylor Foundation and offers support and education to individuals and groups, including those affiliated with the Celiac Disease Foundation. CCFNC engages in advocacy and awareness campaigns, runs Camp Celiac, and reaches out to the medical community as well as to those affected by celiac disease and non-celiac disease gluten intolerance. www.celiaccommunity.org

LANCASTER AREA CELIAC SUPPORT GROUP

This nonaffiliated, all-volunteer Pennsylvania support group offers new-member support and a quarterly newsletter—electronic or print—with medical and research articles, restaurant reviews, gluten-free product listings, and R.O.C.K. groups for kids and families. Meetings include expert speakers and a vendor market where new gluten-free companies offer samples of their foods. www.lancasterceliacs.org

WESTCHESTER CELIAC SPRUE SUPPORT GROUP

This independent nonprofit 501 (c)(3) all-volunteer group may be small, but it has accomplished big things, most notably the establishment of the Gluten-Free Restaurant Awareness Program, which grew beyond its original scope and is now run by the Gluten Intolerance Group of North America. They helped establish the Celiac Disease Center at Columbia University and continue to support it, mainly through the Colin Leslie Walk for Celiac Disease. They hold two or three big meetings a year; offer one-on-one counseling for new members; provide a newsletter with medical abstracts, product reviews, and local activities; and run the Gluten-Free Traveling Bears, a child-friendly education/awareness activity. www.westchesterceliacs.org

Virtual Community

A quick search for *gluten-free community* will net many message boards, forums, chat groups, and blogs—too many, actually.

As with all groups, tastes and opinions vary. So, too, does the level of civility and open discourse. Online anonymity can bring out the worst in people. I won't lie. Fights break out. Posters get flamed. Innocent questions can be met with derision. Some are open to all views; others spurn those whose views differ. But just as often, gluten-free veterans buoy newcomers with shortcuts, cooking tips, advice, wisdom, and solidarity.

The key is finding a like-minded community. A good blog should resonate with your issues, share your sensibility, lifestyle, and interests, perhaps even give voice to what you think and feel and might not say. Finding one or two you love is a hit-or-miss operation. But when you do, it's like having a virtual friend.

Bloggers move on and find other interests. What you see here may not be here for the life of this book. But you know how to follow your favorites and find new ones.

As with all things, vet your information carefully. I shouldn't have to tell you not to believe everything you read on the Internet.

Message Boards, Forums, Chats

Canadian Celiac Association List—Support, message board, discussion, product information, and news of interest to the gluten-free community. To subscribe to list: Send e-mail to majordomo@hwcn.org. Leave subject line blank. In body of e-mail: Subscribe Celiac-Canada

Celiac.com—Online support, newsletters, information, and forums. www.celiac.com

Celiac Listserve—Posters ask questions, share information, discuss food, travel, articles, and news items of interest, and, as a courtesy, summarize responses for the archives. Ads are posted once a month.

To subscribe to adult list: Send an e-mail to
LISTSERV@LISTSERV.ICORS.ORG.
SUB: Celiac followed by your name.

To subscribe to children's list: Send e-mail to
LISTSERV@LISTSERV.ICORS.ORG.
SUB: Cel-Kids followed by your name.

To subscribe to celiac/diabetes list: Send e-mail to
LISTSERV@LISTSERV.ICORS.ORG.
SUB: Celiac/Diabetes, followed by your name.

Delphi Forums—Online community support for newcomers to the gluten-free diet as well as those with multiple food allergies. Basic access is free with paid access to certain topics. This forum includes religious discussion groups. www.delphiforums.com

Gluten-Free Faces—Global gluten-free community—social networking, discussion forum, chat, and travel. Kids, teens, and adult groups. www.glutenfreefaces.com

Gluten-Free Forum—One-stop support and shopping. Online support and discussion boards as part of Scott Adams's Celiac.com and Gluten-Free Mall. www.glutenfreeforum.com

GlutenFreeIndy—24/7 online support. www.glutenfreeindy.com

NYC Celiac Meetup—This online group offers diet and product information, support, message boards, and gluten-free meet-ups in and around Brooklyn, Manhattan, and the tristate area. www.meetup.com/celiac

Simply Gluten-Free Magazine—Great site for finding a community in your area, both online and face-to-face. www.simplyglutenfree.com /celiac-support-groups-community

Blogs

Adventures of a Gluten-Free Cultural Heritage Professional—Interesting and beautifully photographed blog for those with non-celiac gluten insensitivity. www.gf-archivist.com

Adventures of a Gluten Free Mom—Kid and parent-friendly issues. www.adventuresofaglutenfreemom.com

Adventures of an Allergic Foodie—Good gluten-free food talk and recipes. www.adventuresofanallergicfoodie.com

Allergy Free and Cheap Like Me—Multiple food sensitivities on a shoestring. allergyfreeandcheaplikeme.blogspot.com

Allergy Sensitive Kitchen—Gluten-free, dairy-free, egg-free, and some nut-free vegan recipes. allergysensitivekitchen.com

Allyson Kramer—Gluten-free, dairy-free, and soy-free vegan recipes from a cookbook writer and food developer. www.allysonkramer.com

Alternative Eating—Gluten-free, paleo, and clean eating. www.alternative-eating.com

Angela's Kitchen—Gluten-free, dairy-free, with a focus on seasonal foods, family favorites, slow cooking, canning, preserving, and fermenting. www.angelaskitchen.com

Baking Backwards—Vegan and gluten-free baking, diabetic-friendly blog. www.bakingbackwards.blogspot.com

Based on a Sprue Story—Silly and serious, literary minded, mostly narrative blog about celiac disease and the gluten-free life. The occasional poem and gluten-free book review. www.spruestory.com

Celiac Chicks—Cheeky, upbeat, fabulous. www.celiacchicks.com

Celiac Teen—Gluten-free straight talk for teens. www.celiacteen.com

Celiac Yoga Momma—Wisdom and recipes from the mother and wife of diagnosed celiacs. www.celiacyogamomma.blogspot.com

Chef Janet—In-home lessons from a gluten-free cooking teacher. www.chefjanetk.com

Daily Forage—Surviving and thriving without gluten, dairy, and many other common allergens. www.dailyforage-glutenfree.com

Elana's Pantry—The focus here is on paleo recipes. www.elanaspantry.com

FrannyCakes—All about baking with recipes easy enough for a beginner. www.frannycakes.com

GF in SF—All about restaurants and bakeries in and around San Francisco. www.gfinsf.com

Gluten Dude—Not for men only. www.glutendude.com

Gluten-Free for Men—Guy food and drink. www.glutenfreeformen.com

Gluten-Free Kid. www.gluten-free-kid.blogspot.com

Gluten Free Philly—Michael Savett is *the* celiac, dad, and man about Philadelphia, New Jersey, and Delaware. www.glutenfreephilly.com

Gluten Free Safari—Gluten-free advice for those interested in great food, good health, and sustainable living. www.glutenfreesafari.com

Goop—Gwyneth Paltrow's weekly publication and shopping site for vegan gluten-free recipes, health, fashion, books, home, travel, and fashion. www.goop.com

Happy Herbivore—Low-fat, gluten-free, vegan. www.happyherbivore.com

Kids With Food Allergies—Family blog from the Kids With Food Allergies Foundation. www.kidswithfoodallergies.org/blog

Kitchen Classroom 4 Kids—Gluten-free and dairy-free cooking with kids. www.kitchenclassroom4kids.com

Naturally Free RD—Gluten-free healing with whole foods from a registered dietician. www.naturallyfreerd.com

No Gluten, No Problem—Amazing gluten-free food from bestselling cookbook authors and foodies Kelli and Peter Bronski. www.noglutennoproblem.blogspot.com

Oh She Glows—And she does. Vegan and gluten-free (not all) recipes from Angela Liddo, founder of Glo Bakery. www.ohsheglows.com

Simply Sugar & Gluten Free—Budget-friendly recipes and wisdom for those who want to lose the gluten and sugar and maintain a healthy weight. www.simplysugarandglutenfree.com

The Gluten Free Vegan—Really good recipes and an e-mail newsletter. www.theglutenfreevegan.com

The Sane Kitchen—Gluten-free, wheatless, meatless, and healthy food. www.thesanekitchen.blogspot.com

The WHOLE Gang—Gluten-free, allergy-free, organic, and eco-friendly choices from a lifestyle coach. www.thewholegang.org

PINTEREST COLLABORATIVE BOARDS

www.pinterest.com/insomniatic/gluten-free-group

www.pinterest.com/explore/vegetarian-gluten-free

Magazines

Allergic Living: Allergies, Asthma, and Gluten-Free. www.allergicliving.com

Delight Gluten-Free Magazine—Digital only. www.delightglutenfree.com

Gluten-Free Living. www.glutenfreeliving.com

Journal of Gluten Sensitivity. www.celiac.com

Living Without magazine. www.livingwithout.com

Simply Gluten-Free. www.simplyglutenfreemag.com

Expos, Festivals, and Conferences

American Vegan Society—Vegetarian congress. www.americanvegan .org/meetingsandconventions.htm

Autism Conferences of America. www.autismconferencesofamerica.com

FARE National Food Allergy Conference. www.foodallergy.org/conference

Gluten and Allergen Free Expo. www.gfafexpo.com

Gluten Free Expo—Canada's largest gluten-free event. www.gluten freeexpo.ca

Gluten-Free for Life Expo. www.glutenfreeforlifeexpo1.blogspot.com

Gluten-Free Living magazine's Annual Conference. www.GFLconference.com

Healthy Lifestyle Expo. www.healthylifestyleexpo.com

Healthy Living and Gluten Free Expo. www.healthylivingandglutenfreeexpo.com

Living Without Magazine conferences.
    www.GlutenFreeFoodAllergyFest.com
National Children with Diabetes Conference. www.childrenwithdiabetes
    .com/activities
National Diabetes Conference. www.tcoyd.org/event/national
    -conferences
Natural Products Expo/East. www.expoeast.com
Natural Products Expo/West. www.expowest.com
Sjögren's Syndrome Foundation National Conference. www.sjogrens.org
World Veg Festival. www.sfvs.org

Extended Community

ADHD Foundation. www.adhdfoundation.org
American Academy of Allergy, Asthma, and Immunology. www.aaaai.org
American Gastroenterological Association. www.gastro.org
Anaphylaxis Canada. www.anaphylaxis.org
Arthritis Foundation. www.arthritis.org
Attention Deficit Disorder Association. www.add.org
Autism Society. www.autism-society.org
Developmental Delay Resources. www.devdelay.org
Diabetic Living. www.diabeticlivingonline.com
Food Allergy and Anaphylaxis Network. www.foodallergy.org
Gluten-Free and Casein-Free. www.gfcfdiet.com
Gluten Free and Sjögren's Information. www.dry.org
IBS, IBD, Crohn's and Colitis Foundation. www.ccfa.org
Juvenile Diabetes Research Foundation. www.jdrf.org
Lupus Foundation of America. www.lupus.org
National Anemia Action Council. www.anemia.org
National Autism Association. www.nationalautismassociation.org
National Down Syndrome Society. www.ndss.org
National Fibromyalgia Association. www.fmaware.org
National Osteoporosis Foundation. www.nof.org
Sjögren's Syndrome Foundation. www.sjogrens.org
Talk About Curing Autism. www.tacanow.org
Wheat Allergy—Asthma and Allergy Foundation. www.aafa.org

Books

Celiac Disease: A Hidden Epidemic, revised and updated, by Peter Green and Rory Jones (William Morrow)

The Complete Low-FODMAP Diet by Sue Shepherd and Peter Gibson (The Experiment)

Dangerous Grains by James Braly and Ron Hoggan (Avery Trade)

Gluten-Free Diet by Shelley Case (Case Nutrition Consulting)

Gluten Freedom by Alessio Fasano (Wiley)

Grain Brain: The Surprising Truth About Wheat, Carbs, and Sugar—Your Brain's Silent Killers by David Perlmutter (Little, Brown and Company)

Nourishing Hope for Autism: Nutrition and Diet Guide for Healing Our Children by Julie Matthews (Healthful Living Media)

Wheat Belly: Lose the Wheat, Lose the Weight, and Find Your Path Back to Health by William Davis, MD (Rodale)

Cookbooks

Almond Flour! Gluten-Free and Paleo Diet Cookbook by Donatella Giordano (CreateSpace Independent Publishing)

Eternally Gluten Free: A Cookbook of Sweets and Inspiration, from a Teen! by Dominick Cura (Amazon Digital Services)

The Everything Organic Cooking for Baby and Toddler Book by Kim Lutz and Megan Hart (Adams Media)

Gluten-Free and Vegan Bread by Jennifer Katzinger (Sasquatch Books)

Gluten-Free and Vegan Pie: More Than 50 Sweet and Savory Pies to Make at Home by Jennifer Katzinger (Sasquatch Books)

The Gluten-Free Asian Kitchen by Laura B. Russell (Celestial Arts)

Gluten-Free Italian: Over 150 Irresistible Recipes Without Wheat—from Crostini to Tiramisu by Jacqueline Mallorca (De Capo Lifelong Books)

Gluten-Free Vegan Comfort Food by Lara Ferroni and Susan O'Brien (Da Capo Lifelong Books)

Great Gluten-Free Whole-Grain Bread Machine Recipes by Donna Washburn and Heather Butt (Robert Rose)

The Heart of the Plate: Vegetarian Recipes for a New Generation by Mollie Katzen (Rux Martin/Houghton Mifflin Harcourt)

The Intolerant Gourmet: Glorious Food Without Gluten and Lactose by Barbara Kafka (Artisan)

The Joy of Gluten-Free Sugar-Free Baking by Peter Reinhart and Denene Wallace (Ten Speed Press)

The Kid Friendly ADHD and Autism Cookbook by Pamela Compart and Dana Laake (Fair Winds Press)

The Longevity Kitchen: Satisfying, Big-Flavor Recipes Featuring the Top 16 Age-Busting Power Foods by Rebecca Katz with Mat Edelson (Ten Speed Press)

1,000 Gluten Free Recipes by Carol Lee Fenster (Houghton Mifflin Harcourt)

Paleo Cooking from Elana's Pantry by Elana Amsterdam (Ten Speed Press)

Sweet Cravings: 50 Seductive Desserts by Kyra Bussanich (Ten Speed Press)

The 30 Day Guide to Paleo Cooking by Hayley Mason and Bill Staley (Victory Belt)

Unbelievably Gluten-Free by Anne Byrn (Workman Publishing)

Vedge: 100 Plates Large and Small That Redefine Vegetable Cooking by Rich Landau and Kate Jacoby (The Experiment)

The Vegetarian and Vegan Gluten-Free Cookbook by Sarah Lee Anniston (CreateSpace Independent Publishing)

Welcoming Kitchen: 200 Delicious Allergen and Gluten-Free Recipes by Kim Lutz (Sterling)

Food References

Librairie Larousse. *Larousse Gastronomique: The World's Greatest Culinary Encyclopedia Completely Revised and Updated* (Clarkson Potter, 2001)

The New Whole Foods Encyclopedia by Rebecca Wood (Penguin Books)

Medical References

Academy of Nutrition and Dietetics. www.eatright.org

Celiac Disease: An Issue of Gastrointestinal Endoscopy Clinics by Benjamin Lebwohl and Peter H. R. Green (Saunders)

The Merck Manual of Diagnosis and Therapy, 19th ed. (Merck). www.merckbooks.com

Physicians' Desk Reference—Prescription drug information (PDR Network)

Essential Equipment

BREAD MAKERS
Breadman. www.breadman.com
Cuisinart. www.cuisinart.com
Oster. www.oster.com

RICE COOKERS
Aroma. www.aroma-housewares.com
Cuisinart. www.cuisinart.com
Sanyo. us.sanyo.com/microcomputerized-rice-cookers
Zojirushi. www.zojirushi.com

PASTA MACHINES
Atlas Marcato Pasta Machine. www.surlatable.com
Imperia Home Pasta Machines. www.imperiapasta.com

BAKING EQUIPMENT
Kerekes Bakery and Restaurant Equipment. www.bakedeco.com

GRINDERS AND GRAIN MILLS
BlendTec Grain Mill. www.blendtec.com
Cuisinart Spice and Nut Grinder. www.cuisinart.com
Nutrimill Grain Mill. www.lequip.com
Roma Multi-Seed Grinder. www.westonproducts.com
Victoria Hand Grain Mill. www.wheatgrasskits.com
WonderMill Grain Mill. www.thewondermill.com

HOME VACUUM SEALERS
www.pleasanthillgrain.com

Gluten-Free Gift Baskets, Gifts, T-Shirts, Accessories, Stationery, Greeting Cards

Beer Lover's Gift Basket—Twelve gluten-free craft beers from Halftime Beverage. www.halftimebeverage.com
Café Press—Gluten-free cards, notebooks, stickers, greeting cards, and business cards. www.cafepress.com

Celiac and the Beast—Gluten-Free T-shirts and hoodies for men and women. www.celiacandthebeast.com

Elegant Medical Alert—Cool, stylish, fun peanut and other food allergy awareness and medical ID bracelets, watches, wristbands, and sports bands for kids, teens, and adults. www.elegantmedicalalert.com

Gluten-Free Food Baskets. www.greatarrivals.com and www.gourmetgiftbaskets.com

Go Nuts!—Gluten-free pomegranate pistachios, maple pecans, and barbecue almonds to send to your favorite nut lover. www.sahale snacks.com

Red Camper—Gluten-free birthday cards. www.redcamper.com

See's Chocolates—Gift boxes. Large gluten-free selection. www.sees.com

Silly Yak Company—Silly T-shirts and accessories for adults and children. www.silly-yak.com

Zazzle—Gluten-free shirts and mugs. www.zazzle.com

Testing and Test Kits

Better Control of Health, USA—Food allergy testing. www.yorkallergyusa.com

Elisa Technologies—Industry and home food test kits. www.elisa-tek.com

Additional Resources

Academy of Nutrition and Dietetics. www.eatright.org

American Diabetes Association. www.diabetes.org

American Health Care Association/Senior Care. www.ahcancal.org

American Medical Association. www.ama.com

American Society for Nutrition. www.nutrition.org

Autism Research Institute. www.autism.com

Council of Better Business Bureaus. www.bbb.com

Eating Locally. www.localharvest.org

Eco-friendly consumer topics. www.care2.com

Environmental Working Group. www.ewg.org

Going Organic. www.organic.org

International Food Information Council Federation—Food safety, healthy eating, and nutrition information. www.foodinsight.org

Journal of the Academy of Nutrition and Dietetics. www.adajournal.org

National Adult Day Services Association. nasda.org

National Association of Child Care Resources and Referral Services. www.naccrra.org

National Digestive Diseases Information Clearinghouse. www.digestive.niddk.nih.gov

National Institute of Diabetes and Digestive and Kidney Disease. www.niddk.nih.gov

Nutrition Services—Administration On Aging. www.aoa.gov

Organic Gardening. www.goingorganic.com

US Food and Drug Administration. www.fda.gov

Epilogue

Grace Note: The Rewards of Doing Without

Forgo, give up, abstain from, avoid, omit, refuse
reject, decline, demur, skip, shun, spurn, steer clear of,
go without, turn down, pass up, eschew,
have nothing to do with

No matter how you say it, going without something as fundamental as bread requires sacrifice, willpower, spine. It takes a willingness to go against spontaneity and impulse, those gratifying moments that make life more satisfying, slightly decadent, and often delicious.

Given the chance, few of us would willingly abstain, even those who have gone gluten-free voluntarily. We would gladly give up the label reading, the constant vigilance, the extra expense of special diets and unprocessed allergy-free living. We would kiss the just-say-no mentality good-bye. Who among us would deny the simple pleasure of tea and toast, or the luxury of a croissant? Even after all of these years gluten-free, the idea of biting into a silky cupcake—that miniature marvel of butter and sugar—without regard for gluten, anytime the spirit moves, is still a pleasure so palpable I can almost taste it.

We refrain for good reasons.

We do it for the sake of our health, not particularly glamorous until it's gone.

We do it for our children, to vote with our wallets against the big food processors and polluters, against the way grain is grown, seeds are altered, animals are raised, and fish are farmed. Sometimes we do it for the planet. Even if gluten-free, dairy-free, nut-free, hormone-free, and antibiotic-free food costs a little more, we do it. We have learned to adjust, to be resourceful, to rein in our impulses.

And isn't restraint the very thing we need more of these days?

No one ever loses something dear without receiving a gift in return. The challenge is seeing it. Ask any painter or poet where inspiration comes from. The answer may hold a deeper understanding of the concept of give-and-take, loss and gain, feast and famine.

Life compensates in breathtaking ways.

So, too, restraint offers unexpected rewards. There is renewed vigor. And there is a fresh capacity for appreciation, taking pleasure in small victories, sweet as stolen kisses.

Harder to see, but there just the same, are moderation, patience, and self-control, qualities in short supply at this moment in time.

Because we can't mindlessly order a casein-laden cheeseburger or a quick slice of pizza, or waste our precious paychecks on products full of high-fructose corn syrup, we have a unique opportunity to consciously decide what we really want. We know that all gluten-free foods are not created equally. We take the time to ask ourselves if the expense and bother are worth the reward or the risk. In a sense, we hunt and gather the way our ancestors did—driven by our needs instead of our desires. We come down on the side of what nourishes, not what numbs.

As America grapples with its habits, we who forgo have already learned the hard lesson of not succumbing to every craving. We are slimmer. We are healthier. Some of us are alive because of it. Genetic makeup and predisposition for certain conditions aside, we have dramatically decreased our chances of acquiring some degenerative diseases by choosing naturally gluten-free foods over those full of excessive fat and sugar and refined carbohydrates.

We have eaten happily ever after.

My young mother, who went through the Great Depression looking like a movie star, prepared me, albeit unwillingly, for the gluten-free life. Her devotion to quality over quantity has never been more relevant. I can still hear her saying, *Buy one beautiful thing and keep it forever. Repair; don't replace.*

She perfected the fine art of forgoing the instant gratification for something worth waiting for. She never purchased food without tasting and smelling it first. She knew where everything came from and what it looked like in its natural state.

As we cut back on expenses, worry about our jobs, and narrow our lives down to the essentials, we know how difficult it is to jettison old habits, how tempting it is to fall back on convenience foods and fast meals. Living without gluten or grain or dairy or soy or corn or animal flesh requires effort.

We find ourselves cooking again, simply and with an understanding of where the ingredients have come from, who has grown or raised our food, and if that process has followed organic and humane principles. We no longer see the garden as decorative, but rather as the center of what is alive, fresh, and green. We do not need supplements when our diet is nutrient dense.

It takes willpower to pass up what is comfortable and easy for what is sustaining and life-giving. We exercise exactitude and are rewarded with delights we never thought we'd enjoy on a zero-gluten diet.

So, too, doing without is to discover our own generosity as well as that of others.

I will remember forever the frigid February night my favorite chef offered me duck cassoulet, neatly checked off on the menu as gluten-free.

I was sure this dish always contained bread crumbs. The chef had produced a safe meal for me so many times before. It was cold, and cassoulet so warm and comforting. I decided to trust him.

"Cassoulet it is," I said, giving my order to the server, who beamed her pleasure at my choice.

"He made one without bread crumbs just in case you ordered it."

Just in case I ordered it.

They did not make a big deal of telling me he went to all that trouble for me, nor did they hint at the waste if I didn't order it. They didn't try to influence my choice. They simply checked it off on the menu, along with other safe meals I might enjoy.

I do not cry easily. But that night, eyes glistening, I looked around the table at my smiling friends, their cast-iron stomachs keeping them from knowing what it's like to be the beneficiary of such generosity.

As children we are taught it's better to give. And that is as it should be. But abstaining forces us to receive, something many of us are not very good at doing. It teaches us to ask for help, to accept that our happiness and well-being depend on and are bound up with the grace and good will of others.

The ability to ask is a kind of intimacy and trust. We look in the mirror of a friend's face and see that suffering in silence honors no one.

There are those who say, *Don't go to any trouble on my account.* Isn't this just another way of saying, albeit unconsciously, *I am not worth the fuss?* Even worse, *I won't trouble myself over you.*

Not taking the gift when it's offered pinches the spirit, cuts off the flow of love. How terrible to have guests at one's table who keep what they need a secret and deny us the bright current of gladness that comes with making a special effort. When we do without, we learn that being a good receiver is another form of generosity.

We who are exquisitely sensitive know something that hardier souls may not. Within our need for special consideration are the seeds of our own reciprocity.

When I visit, one friend takes great pleasure in surprising me with a gluten-free roll or a homemade muffin, the latest gluten-free find in her gourmet market. I, in turn, take equal pride in finding a sugar-free dessert a diabetic friend will love. I render my kitchen a tree nut–free zone for another, and dairy-less for a beloved vegan, a delicious version of pay-it-forward.

We attend to the needs of others not in spite of our own requirements but *because* of them, and we are nourished in more ways than we can imagine. This is what keeps us from feeling sorry for ourselves, isolated; quite the contrary, in fact. "We give," as the poet Mary Oliver so eloquently puts it, "until it feels like receiving."

When one drinks from that river, no one goes thirsty.

Unlike most people who eat on the fly and rarely give a second thought to what they're consuming, we who avoid gluten and other foods must plan our meals and eat them mindfully. We are fully conscious in our choices; we rekindle the lost art of anticipation.

Shared meals are not a race to the finish line but an exercise in mindfulness, a connection to the people who matter most to us. When we slow down and think about the quality of our food, we are more present, more focused, and more alive on every level.

To live with passion, priority, and purpose—this is living with less.

In the best possible sense, couldn't we all do with a little more of less?

This is a good time for those of us who are intolerant of or sensitive to gluten and to many other foods that are often part of the package. We have waited years to be embraced by a food culture that not only understands what gluten is but is fully aware of why so many of us have broken with bread.

But there is something much bigger afoot.

For the first time in history, millions of us are arriving at our own dietary tipping point. We have not only bidden our good-byes to bread but to all but the most natural and freshest foods we can find. In choosing real food over processed, we reject much of what we have been fed for generations. We question our notions about what is healthy and what is not.

Suddenly, we understand that our food is the problem, not our reaction to it.

We find ourselves swept up in a movement far bigger than wheat and gluten. Because we must carefully scrutinize everything on our plates, we have moved beyond those foods that make us sick and avoid those that may not allow us to get well.

We are the new food-conscious consumers.

This truly is revolutionary.

Acknowledgments

I am limp with amazement at the generosity of so many.

Wendy Sherman, whip smart, uncannily wise, a veritable idea factory, walked with me every step of the way. I can't think of anyone I'd rather have in my corner. Allison Adler for her keen insight, deft editing, and smoothing out of every wrinkle. Stephen Rubin, Gillian Blake, Maggie Richards, Pat Eisemann, Carolyn O'Keefe, and the entire Holt marketing, sales, publicity, and design team for their enthusiastic support and for recognizing the importance of this moment. David Shoemaker for his brilliant cover and Meryl Levavi for her elegant type and interior design. Fauzia and John Burke, Jason Liebman, and Phillip Brooks for taking on the impossible and making a social media maven out of me.

It isn't every day you get an e-mail from Alice Waters saying she'd be honored to contribute a recipe to your book. Or that Thomas Keller would be happy to see his name on the cover. So many fine chefs and bakers dropped everything to contribute something scrumptious to the gluten-free lexicon—Katy Sparks, Traci Des Jardins, Aimee Olexy, Bobby Flay, Rick Bayless, Marcie Turney, Steve Di Fillippo, Kristine Kidd, Kelli and Peter Bronski and Dan O'Brien of The Experiment, Katy Taylor, Teensy Beall and the Beall Family of Blackberry Farm, Helmut Newcake's Marie Tagliaferro, Christina Pirello, Shola Olunloyo, Kathleen King, Kriti Seghal, Karen Lynch, Anne Barfield, Jules Shepard, Lisa Stander-Horel, Connie Sarros, Lee Tobin, Jennifer Katzinger, Gwyneth Paltrow and Julia

Turshen, Erin McKenna, Nigella Lawson, the Reverend Michael Alan, Jen Welker, Eileen Plato, The Lagasse Girls (Jilly and Jessie), Glenn Minervini-Zick, Michael Cole, Mary Capone, Bryan Sikora, Lynn Jamison, Rebecca Bunting, Anna Jurinich, Giampaolo Fallai, and Bernadette Brescia, for her natural beauty treatments. A special thanks to Jane Oswaks who rescued the Bleecker Street breadsticks and to Alicia Woodward of *Living Without* magazine for facilitating so much. The honor is entirely mine.

Jay DiMarino, for his friendship, his willingness to answer all of my questions no matter how basic or last-minute, and for his marvelous introduction. Ritu Verma, for her superb piece on pediatric celiac disease and gluten sensitivity. The following experts, so generous with their time, reviewed the sections on conditions related to gluten intolerance, supplied up-to-date information on the newest research, and explained it all to me: Serge Jabbour, Gregory Kane, Frederick Vivino, Kays Kaidbeys, John Zone, and Howard Weitz. I am grateful to Joseph Murray of the Mayo Clinic for his enormous contribution to our understanding of celiac disease and for kindnesses never forgotten.

How do you say thank you in twenty-two languages? Peter Gistelinck, Omer Taffet, Lawrence Mbogoni, Al and Zenola Green, Eduardo Glandt, George Ritchie, Sampeth Kannan, Patrick Coué, Omar Al-Ghazzi, Omer Taffet, Bo Mai, Sharon Black, Christine Parent, Texas Al, Giampaolo Fallai, Anna Jurenich, Maggie Kritsberg, Prawit Thainiyom, and Phillip Le did their best to keep me from getting lost in translation. Theodora Langren, CEO of A2Z Global, and her team gave the international dining cards their final professional polish.

Michael Spain-Smith for his lovely photographs, wonderful art direction and for making a shoot more fun than I ever imagined.

I could not have written this book without the large contributions and dedication of founders and visionaries like Elaine Monarch, Marilyn Geller, Pat Murphy Garst, Diane Eve Paley, Elaine Hartsook, Cynthia Kupper, Janet Rinehart, Phyllis Brogden, and Bette Hagman. I walk in your footsteps.

Jane Kirkwood, Linda Spikol, Michele Mayes, Jane Krensky, Lara, Caroline, and Betsey Rhame, Francesca Costanzo, Jason Cassidy, Tony Lechich, Deborah DiClementi, Kristina Johnson, Kimberly Ekern, Barbara Siegel, Thekla Hammond, Roxanne Panero, Rebecca Bunting, Ray and Barbara Brogliatti, Judy Moon, David Salama, Linda Harris, David Fink, and Karen Carlson surrounded me with their special magic. They listened, read early pages, made suggestions, strategized, networked, encouraged, called in favors, cossetted, calmed, lightened my load, salved my spirit, and kept me upright. You are my earth angels.

For teaching me to be a careful cook, instilling a love of beautiful food, and an anathema of anything packaged, processed and preserved, I will be forever grateful to my finicky French mother and grandmother, Kay Peters and Catherine Petitpain.

And to my beloved John—for your unfailing patience and cheerful acceptance of months of gluten-free takeout and for always rooting for me, listening, counseling, pitching in, and making me laugh, even when it isn't easy. Love is such an insufficient word.

Recipe Acknowledgments and Permissions

My thanks to the editors of *Alimentum: The Literature of Food*, Winter 2010, where "Gluten-Free Poem" was first presented. Essays "The Myth of Perfection," "Live Without," and "Unexpected Grace" first appeared in different form in Food for Thought, *Living Without* magazine. My thanks to Alicia Woodward, editor in chief.

I am grateful to Anthony J. DiMarino Jr., MD, Director, Jefferson Celiac Center, William Rorer Professor of Medicine, Chief, Division of Gastroenterology and Hepatology, Thomas Jefferson University Hospital, Philadelphia, for his excellent foreword, "The Importance of a Well-Informed Patient."

In appreciation of Ritu Verma, MD, Section Chief, Gastroenterology, Associate Professor of Clinical Pediatrics, and Director of the Celiac Center of Children's Hospital of Philadelphia for her thought-provoking essay, "Recognizing, Diagnosing, and Managing Celiac Disease in Children."

The gluten-free dining cards in Chapter 14, "Sprechen Sie Gluten," were translated courtesy of Theodora Landgren, CEO of A2Z Global.

Perfect, Possibly Paleo Pumpkin Pie (page 143) courtesy of Reverend Michael Alan.

A Simple Sponge Cake for Your Repertoire (page 153) from Nigella Lawson, *How to Eat: The Pleasures and Princi-ples of Good Food* (Houghton Mifflin Harcourt), by permission of Nigella Lawson.

Classic Cheese Soufflé (page 154) and Dark Chocolate Soufflé (page 155) courtesy of Shola Olunloyo and Studio Kitchen.

Sweet Potato Rosemary Bread (page 156) from *Flying Apron's Gluten-Free and Vegan Baking Book* by Jennifer Katzinger. Reprinted by permission of Sasquatch Books.

Chickpea Socca (page 157) used by permission of Bryan Sikora, La Fila, Wilmington, Delaware.

Moroccan Braised Eggplant (page 161) by permission of Alice Waters, Chez Panisse.

Grilled Corn and Squash Salad with Chipotle Crema and Lime Vinaigrette and Cotija Cheese (page 162) by permission of Traci Des Jardins, Jardinière, San Francisco.

Bouchon Bakery Gluten-Free Brioche Rolls (page 163) courtesy of Thomas Keller and excerpted from *Bouchon Bakery*, copyright © 2012 by Thomas Keller by permission of Artisan, a division of Workman Publishing Co. Inc., New York. All rights reserved.

Quesadillas Asadas (page 165) from Rick Bayless, *Mexican Kitchen* (Scribner) by permission of Rick Bayless.

Corn and Lobster Pie in a Chili-Polenta Crust (page 167) from *Play It by Ear* by Molly O'Neill, reprinted with permission of The New York Times Company.

Cauliflower with Fontina Mornay, Nutmeg, and Bread Crumbs (page 168), Pan-Roasted Mushrooms Galore with Fine Herbs and Shallots (page 169), and Raw Radish and

Cucumber Salad, Pine Nuts, Feta, Mint, and Sauvignon Blanc Vinaigrette (page 170), by permission of Aimee Olexy, owner, Talulah's Garden, Philadelphia.

Buckwheat Crepes Gratin and Cauliflower, Chanterelles, and Cave-Aged Gruyère (page 171) by permission of Katy Sparks.

Gluten-Free Gnocchi with Wild Mushrooms, Garlic, and White Truffle Oil (page 172) by permission of Steve DiFillippo, Davio's Restaurants, Boston, Atlanta, Philadelphia.

Arctic Char with Kumquat Gremolata, Roasted Fennel, and Potatoes (page 174) by permission of Kristine Kidd.

Crispy Squash Blossoms Barbuzzo (page 176) courtesy of Marcie Turney, executive Chef/owner, Barbuzzo, Philadelphia.

Saffron Risotto Cakes with Shrimp, Red Chili Oil, and Chive Oil (page 178) by permission of Bobby Flay, Gato, New York.

Beau Monde Cider-Brined Berkshire Pork Chops with Pumpkin Sage Risotto, Grilled Pear, Soubise Purée, and Smoked Balsamic Reduction (page 180) courtesy of Crêperie Beau Monde, Philadelphia.

Fresh Strawberry and Blueberry Fruit Tart (page 185) from *Gluten-Free and Vegan Holidays* by Jennifer Katzinger. Reprinted by permission of Sasquatch Books.

Bleecker Street Breadsticks (page 186) adapted by Jane Oswaks from Joseph Pace's Risotteria recipe, which appeared in the *New York Times*. By permission of Jane Oswaks.

Dark Chocolate Fondant, Ginger and Raspberry Coeur (page 188) by permission of Marie Tagliaferro, owner, Helmut Newcake, Paris.

Glenn Minervini-Zick's Raspberry Almond Ravioli Cookie (page 189) by permission of Glenn Minervini-Zick, Zix Cookies.

Cinnamon Almond Cake (page 193) from *Nigellissima: Easy Italian-Inspired Recipes* by Nigella Lawson, copyright © 2012 by Nigella Lawson, Pabulum Productions Limited, by permission of Clarkson Potter Publishers, an imprint of the Crown Publishing Group, a division of Random House, LLC. All rights reserved.

Sweet Potato and Five-Spice Muffins (page 194) from *It's All Good* by Gwyneth Paltrow and Julia Turshen, copyright © 2013 by Gwyneth Paltrow by permission of Grand Central Publishing.

French Toast Pineapple Upside Down Cake (page 195) from executive chef Sarah Ginn by permission of Kriti Sehgal, Pure Fare, Philadelphia.

Meyer Lemon and Bing Cherry Cupcakes with Vanilla Frosting (page 196) from *BabyCakes Covers the Clas-*

sics: Gluten-Free Vegan Recipes from Donuts to Snickerdoodles by Erin McKenna, copyright © 2011 by Erin McKenna. By permission of Clarkson Potter/Publishers, an imprint of the Crown Publishing Group, a division of Random House, LLC. All rights reserved.

Almond Pâte-à-Choux Florentines (page 198) from *Artisanal Gluten-Free Cooking*, copyright © 2009 by Kelli and Peter Bronski, reprinted courtesy of The Experiment, LLC.

Kathleen King's Gluten-Free Chocolate Crinkles (page 199) by permission of Kathleen King, Tate's Bake Shop, Southampton, New York.

Chocolate-Glazed Coconut Macaroons (page 201) from *Glow: A Prescription for Radiant Health and Beauty* by Christina Pirello (HP Trade) by permission of Christina Pirello.

Taffets Mediterranean Focaccia (page 202) by permission of Omer Taffet, Taffets Bakery, Philadelphia.

Vanilla Salted Caramel Cake with Vanilla Buttercream (page 203) by permission of Katie Taylor, Miglet's Cupcake Shop, Danville, California.

Grown-up Macaroni and Cheese (page 208) by permission of Caroline Winge-Bogar.

Pizza Just Like Mama Makes (or Wishes She Could) (page 209) by permission of Glenn Minervini-Zick.

Oh, Mama! Meat Loaf (page 211) by permission of Eileen Plato, owner, Judy's Café.

Kelli and Peter Bronski's Chicken Tikka Masala (page 212) from *Artisanal Gluten-Free Cooking*, copyright © 2009 by Kelli and Peter Bronski, reprinted courtesy of The Experiment, LLC.

Oh, Daddy! Onion Soup (page 213) and Jilly and Jessie's Spiced Carrot Cake with Sweet Mascarpone Frosting (page 215) from *The Gluten-Free Table* by Jilly Lagasse and Jessie Lagasse Swanson, Foreword by Emeril Lagasse, by permission of Grand Central Publishing. All rights reserved.

Old-Fashioned Chicken Potpie (page 216) by permission of Katie Taylor, Miglet's Cupcake Shop, Danville, California.

Mexican Lasagna (page 218) adapted from *The Frog Commissary Cookbook* by permission of Chef Kevin Smith, Ed Baranco, and George Georgiou.

Mother of All Tortes (page 220) by permission of Lynn Jamison.

Reverend Michael Alan's Apple and Fig Crisp (page 221) by permission of Reverend Michael Alan.

Seven Sinful Cheeses and Brandied Sour Cherries (page 226) by permission of Aimee Olexy, Talula's Table, Talula's Daily, and Talula's Garden, Philadelphia.

Irish Soda Bread (page 229) and Lemon-Blueberry Scones (page 229) by permission of Rebecca Bunting.

Chocolate-Dipped Brandy-Soaked Raisin Almond Biscotti (page 230), Chocolate Brandy-Glazed Walnut Cake (page 230), and Spiced Pumpkin Torte (page 232) by permission of Anna Jurinich and Giampaolo Fallai.

Apple Cider–Brined Roast Turkey (page 234), Apple Cider–Bourbon Gravy (page 235), and Pear Ginger Cranberry Relish (page 235) by permission of Mary Capone, author of *The Gluten Free Italian Cookbook: Classic Cuisine from the Italian Countryside* and creator of Bella Gluten-Free Baking Mixes, and Alicia Woodward, editor in chief, *Living Without* magazine.

Banana Split Cake (page 236) from *Gluten-Free and Vegan Holidays* by Jennifer Katzinger. Reprinted by permission of Sasquatch Books.

Sweet Potato, Pumpkin, and Sage Latkes (page 238) and Harvest Tsimmes (page 239) by permission of Lisa Stander-Horel, author of *Nosh on This: Gluten-Free Baking from a Jewish-American Kitchen* (The Experiment), and Alicia Woodward, editor in chief, *Living Without* magazine.

Nigella Lawson's *Proper English Trifle* (page 240) from Nigella Lawson, *How to Eat: The Pleasures and Principles of Good Food* (Houghton Mifflin Harcourt) by permission of Nigella Lawson.

Cranberry Chutney (page 243) by permission of Jules Shepard, Jules Gluten Free mixes, and Alicia Woodward, editor in chief, *Living Without* magazine.

Ethiopian Injera (page 294) by permission of Yeworkwoha "Workeye" Ephrem, Ghenet Restaurant, Brooklyn, New York.

Caipirinha (page 295) courtesy of the advertising team at FCB, São Paolo, Brazil.

A Trio of Authentic Stir Fry Sauces (page 297) adapted from *The Frog-Commissary Cookbook* (Doubleday) by Steven Poses, Anne Clark, and Becky Roller.

Garlic Naan (page 302) from *Artisanal Gluten-Free Cooking*, copyright © 2009 by Kelli and Peter Bronski, reprinted by permission of The Experiment, LLC.

Sweet and Spicy Chutney (page 303) and Cucumber Raita (page 304) by Sara J. Pluta, reprinted by permission of *Living Without* magazine.

Panna Cotta (page 305) with Amber Caramel (page 305) by permission of Steve DiFillippo, owner of Davio's Restaurants.

Miso Soup (page 307) adapted from *Cooking the Whole Foods Way* (HP Trade) by Christina Pirello courtesy of Christina Pirello.

Traditional Russian Borscht (page 311) in memory of Jerzy Kosinski.

Thai Grapefruit Salad with Toasted Coconut and Fresh Mint (page 314) from *Quick and Easy Thai* by Nancie McDermott, reprinted by permission of Chronicle Books, San Francisco.

Blackberry Farm's Truly Southern Waffles with Sorghum and Moonshine Cherries (page 355) by permission of Sarah Elder Cabot, Blackberry Farm, Walland, Tennessee.

Hilton Head Health Gluten-Free Blueberry Pancakes (page 357) by permission of executive chef Jen Welker.

Inn on Randolph Gluten-Free Granola (page 359) by permission of Karen Lynch, owner, Inn on Randolph, Napa, California.

Joe's Chicken Paradise French Toast Bananas Foster (361) by permission of Anne Barfield, owner, Chicken Paradise, San Antonio, Texas.

Roasted Chili Polenta with Shiitake Tomatillo Sauce (page 362) by permission of Chef Bill Wavrin, Glen Ivy Hot Springs Resort, Corona, California.

A Twice-Baked Teething Biscuit (page 417) by permission of Joe Garrera.

Cornmeal Porridge for Baby and Me (page 418) by permission of Gourmet, Condé Nast Publications.

Rice Pudding (page 418) from *Christina Cooks* (HP Trade) by permission of Christina Pirello.

Playdate Play Dough (page 419) by Connie Sarros from *Wheat-Free, Gluten-Free Cookbook for Kids and Busy Adults* (McGraw-Hill) by permission of Connie Sarros.

Bubbles (page 420) by Connie Sarros from *Wheat-Free, Gluten-Free Cookbook for Kids and Busy Adults* (McGraw-Hill) by permission of Connie Sarros.

Bathtub Paint (page 420) from *CDF Newsletter* by permission of Elaine Monarch, Founder, Celiac Disease Foundation.

No More Tummy Aches Cupcakes with Raspberry Frosting (page 428) from *No More Cupcakes & Tummy Aches* by Jax Peters Lowell, courtesy of Chef Lee Tobin, creator of title cupcake.

Face Paint (page 440) by Connie Sarros from *Wheat-Free, Gluten-Free Cookbook for Kids and Busy Adults* (McGraw-Hill) by permission of Connie Sarros.

Jojoba Instant Skin Smoother (page 524) and Sensitive Beauty Lip Balm (page 524) courtesy of Bernadette Brescia, Brescia Spa.

Honey Lemon Sugar Scrub (page 527), Avocado and Oat Facial (page 527), Cucumber Parsley Stress Fix (page 528), Rose Water Bath (page 528), and Brightening and Tightening Facial (page 528) updated and adapted from Peters family beauty secrets with love and thanks to Catherine Petitpain and Kay Peters.

References

Introduction: The Gluten-Free Revolution

Gupta, Ruchi, Ann Lurie, and Robert H. Lurie, Children's Hospital of Chicago, and the Northwestern University Feinberg School of Medicine. "Study of Overall Cost of Childhood Food Allergies." *JAMA Pediatrics* (September 16, 2013).

Report on the Gluten-Free Market in the U.S. Packaged Facts Market Research as reported by *Huffington Post*, October 22, 2012.

Strom, Stephanie. "A Big Bet on Gluten-Free." *New York Times*, February 17, 2014.

Fasano, A., I. Berti, T. Gerarduzzi, T. Not, R. B. Colletti, S. Drago, et al. "Prevalence of Celiac Disease in At-Risk and Not-at-Risk Groups in the United States: A Large Multi-Center Study." *Archives of Internal Medicine* 163, no. 3 (February 10, 2003).

NPD Group. "Is Gluten-Free Eating a Trend Worth Noting?" NPD Group, 2012.

NPD Group. "Percentage of U.S. Adults Trying to Cut Down or Avoid Gluten in Their Diets." NPD Group, March 2013.

Statistic Brain. "Gluten/Celiac Statistics." University of Chicago Celiac Disease Center and National Institutes of Health, May, 2013.

Beck, Melinda. "Clues to Gluten Sensitivity." *Wall Street Journal*, March 15, 2011.

"Top Ten Food Trends of 2012." *Time*, December 4, 2012.

"Gluten Goodbye: One-Third of Americans Say They're Trying to Shun It." NPR, March 9, 2013.

"Celiac Disease Rising Four-Fold in Last 50 Years." University of Chicago Celiac Disease Center.

Wines, Michael. "Mystery Malady Kills More Bees." *New York Times*, March 28, 2013.

1. Gluten-Free Nation

"Celiac Disease Facts and Figures." University of Chicago Celiac Disease Center.

Duffy, Brigid. "Non-Celiac Gluten Sensitivity: Gastrointestinal Hip or Hype." *Gastroenterology and Endoscopy News* 64, no. 6 (June 2013).

Celiac Disease and Non-Celiac Gluten Intolerance. Celiac Community Foundation of Northern California.

Wyrick, Julianne. "Gluten Sensitivity: What Does It Really Mean?" *Scientific American*, March 4, 2013.

Green, Peter (lecture). *Celiac Disease vs. Gluten Sensitivity: How Common?* Columbia University Celiac Disease Center Intestinal Immune-Based Inflammatory Diseases Symposium, Columbia University Medical Center, March 2012.

"Following a Gluten-Free Diet." Beth Israel Deaconess Medical Center.

"Gluten-Free Diet: What's Allowed, What's Not." Mayo Clinic.

Raymond, Nixie, Jenny Heap, and Shelley Case. "The Gluten-Free Diet: An Update for Health Professionals." *Practical Gastroenterology*, September 2006.

"Processed Foods and Ingredients That May Contain Wheat, Rye and Barley." Academy of Nutrition and Dietetics.

Porter, Robert S. *The Merck Manual of Diagnosis and Therapy*. 19th ed. John Wiley and Sons, 2011.

"Gluten-Free Diet Quick Start Guide." *Living Without* magazine.

Biesiekierski, J., E. D. Newnham, P. M. Irving, J. S. Barrett, M. Haines, J. D. Doecke, et al. "Gluten Causes Gastrointestinal Symptoms in Subjects Without Celiac Disease: A Double-Blind Randomized Placebo-Controlled Trial." *American Journal of Gastroenterology* 106, no. 3 (March 2011): 508–14.

Baum, James. "A Scientific Explanation of Gluten Intolerance." DrJamesBrown.com.

Gluten-Intolerance Group. "Can I Use Oats?" *Gluten-Free Living*.

"Oats/The Gluten-Free Diet." MassachusettsGeneralHospital.org.

The Academy of Nutrition and Dietetics, *Manual of Clinical Dietetics*. 6th ed. October 2000.

Thompson, Tricia. "Gluten Contamination of Commercial Oat Products in the United States." *New England Journal of Medicine* 351 (November 4, 2004): 2021–22.

"Definition of Gluten-Free for Food Labeling." FDA ruling, August 2, 2013. www.fda.gov.

"Grains and Glossary." CSA/USA Library of Resource Materials.

Guandalini, Stefano, and Michelle Melin-Rogovin. *The History of Celiac Disease and of Its Diagnostic Practices*. University of Chicago Celiac Disease Center.

Rubin, Emily. "Celiac Disease and the Gluten-Free Diet" (presentation). Thomas Jefferson Digestive Disease Institute, September 2013.

Agatston, Arthur. "Gluten: 5 Things You Need to Know." CNN Health, April 5, 2013.

2. The New Food Hyphenate

Kolata, Gina. "Mediterranean Diet Shown to Ward Off Heart Attack and Stroke." *New York Times,* February 25, 2013.

Estruch, Ramon, et al. "Primary Prevention of Cardiovascular Disease with a Mediterranean Diet." *New England Journal of Medicine* 368 (April 4, 2013): 1279–90.

"Mediterranean Diet: A Heart-Healthy Eating Plan." Mayo Clinic. August 2013.

Bittman, Mark. "When Diet Meets Delicious: The Mediterranean Approach." *New York Times*, February 26, 2013.

Amidor, Toby. "Mediterranean Diet 101." Food Network.

"Dr. Oz's Mediterranean Diet Shopping List." www.doctoroz.com

Paturel, Amy. "The Ultimate Arthritis Diet: Stock Your Fridge and Pantry with Mediterranean Staples to Fight Pain and Inflammation." *Arthritis Today*, January–February 2013.

Challaway, Ewen. "Ancient Bones Show Signs of Struggle with Coeliac Disease." Nature.com, April 2014.

"Paleo Diet—What You Need to Know." *US News Best Diets*. December 2013.

Lee, Janet. "The Paleo Diet: The Trend, Explained." *Real Simple*, October 2012.

Telis, Gisela. "The Truth About Gluten-Free, Paleo and Other Diet Books." *Washington Post*, August 5, 2013.

Wolf, Robb. *The Paleo Solution: The Original Human Diet*. Victory Belt Publishing, 2010.

Davis, William. *Wheat Belly: Lose the Wheat, Lose the Weight, and Find Your Way Back to Health*. Rodale Books, 2011.

"Essential Facts and Figures—Guidelines for a Vegetarian Lifestyle." *Vegetarian Living*.

"Vegetarian & Vegan Alternatives & Substitutions." *Vegetarian Living*.

"Substitution Solutions and Simple Substitutions." *Simply Gluten-Free* and *Living Without*, August 2013.

"Vegan Diet: What You Need to Know." *US News Best Diets*. December 2013.

"What Is a Vegetarian?" Vegetarian Society.

"Vegetarian Basics 101." VegetariansinParadise.com

"Food Allergy and Intolerance Fact Sheet." Vegetarian Society.

"Vegging Out: Eva MacSweeney on Turning Her Family Vegetarian." *Vogue*, June 2013.

"Types of Vegetarian Diets." Mayo Clinic.

"Veganism in a Nutshell." Vegetarian Resource Group.

"Dairy-Free and Non-Dairy: Milk Allergic Consumers?" Food Allergy Resource and Research Program, University of Nebraska.

"Cow's Milk Allergy Versus Lactose Intolerance." National Dairy Council.

Northrup, Laura. "Why Non-Dairy Creamer Has Dairy in It." Consumerist.com, June 2013.

Wakim-Fleming, Jamilé. "Celiac Disease and Malabsorptive Disorders." In *Mosby's Medical Dictionary*. 6th ed. Mosby, 2002.

"Symptoms of Lactose Intolerance." WebMD and MayoClinic.com.

"Lactase Deficiency." In *Charles B. Clayman*, ed., *The American Medical Association Encyclopedia of Medicine*. Random House, 2006.

Pennesi, C. M. and L. C. Klein. "Effectiveness of the Gluten-Free, Casein-Free Diet for Children Diagnosed with Autism Spectrum Disorder: Based on Parental Report." *Journal of Nutritional Neuroscience* 15, no. 2 (March, 2012): 85–91.

Alaedini, Armin. "Elevated Gluten Antibodies Found in Children with Autism, but No Link to Celiac Disease." PhD, Assistant Professor of Medical Sciences, Department of Medicine and Institute of Human Nutrition, et al, Columbia Medical Center, New York, *PLOS ONE*, June 20, 2013.

"Casein-Free Diet, A Quick Start Guide." *Living Without*.

Silberberg, Barrie. *The Autism and ADHD Diet: A Step-by-Step Guide to Hope and Healing by Living Gluten Free and Casein Free*. Sourcebooks, 2009.

Silberberg, Barrie. "Autism and the Miracle of a Life Free of Gluten and Casein." *Living Without*, June–July 2008.

"A Parent's Guide to Autism Spectrum Disorders." *AutismWeb*, May 2013.

Lewis, Lisa. *Special Diets for Special Kids: Understanding and Implementing a Gluten and Casein Free Diet to Aid in the Treatment of Autism and Related Developmental Disorders*. Rev. ed. Future Horizons, 2011.

"Elimination Diet." MayoClinic.com.

"What's Elimination Diet?" WebMD.

Bradley, Jeanette. "Is Your Food Making You Sick? Using Elimination Diets to Discover Food Sensitivities and Intolerances." About.com, October 2012.

Clean Program. "Clean 21-Day Elimination Diet." Goop .com.

"Elimination Diet." Arizona Center for Integrative Medicine.

"Elimination Diet." *The Dr. Oz Show*, November 12, 2013.

4. Gluten-Free Thinking

"Internal Revenue Service Publication #502, Amended Beginning After December 31, 2012." Guidelines for deducting medically mandated gluten-free food.

Kass, Howard J. "The Celiac Tax Deduction: What's New?" Celiac.com, March 2012.

Canada Revenue Agency. "Canadian Tax Regulations."

Federal Emergency Management Agency. "Basic Disaster Supplies Kit."

American Red Cross. "Prepare for a Disaster."

Mondello, Wendy. "Disaster Relief." *Living Without*, February–March 2014.

"Top 4 Most Dangerous Artificial Sweeteners." *Fit Day*.

Tepper, Rachel. "12 Sweeteners You Should Know." *Healthy Living*, July 2013.

Girdwain, Jessica. "Superfood Fight." Oprah.com, August 2013.

Doherty, Christine. "The Top 10 Super Foods." *Living Without*, February–March 2009.

"Best Superfoods for Weight Loss." Health.com.

"The 40 Best Age-Erasing Superfoods." MensHealth.com.

"Learn How Celiac Disease Is Diagnosed: Only a Biopsy Lets You Know for Sure." University of Chicago Celiac Disease Center.

Petersen, Vikki. "Is Gluten Making You Fat?" *Simply Gluten-Free*, January–February 2013.

Anca, Alex. "Blue Cheese in the Gluten-Free Diet—A Research Update." *Celiac News* 23, no. 1 (March 2009).

Forrest, Jamie. "Serious Cheese: Is Blue Cheese Gluten-Free?" SeriousCheese.com, 2009.

Goodman, Brenda. "Scientists Working Toward Pill for Celiac Disease." WebMD, December 21, 2012.

Anderson, Jane. "Celiac Disease Drugs in Development." About.com, February 15, 2013.

Clevenger, Jason. "Progress on Celiac Vaccine, but Clinical Trial for Pill Disappointing." *Gluten Free Living*, March–April 2013.

"Facts and Fallacies About Digestive Diseases—Frequency of Bowel Movements." National Digestive Diseases Information Clearinghouse.

"Celiac Disease Myths Debunked." *Insight*, Winter 2013.

Ungar, Laura. "Gluten-Free Diet Depends on What's Eating You." *Louisville Courier-Journal*, USA Today, August 27, 2013.

"Standards of Medical Fitness." Department of Defense, Army Regulation 40-501.

Andrasik, B. Donald. *Gluten Free in Afghanistan*. CreateSpace Independent Publishing platform, 2012.

Boyd, Christine. "Soldier On: A Special Diet in War-Torn Afghanistan." *Living Without*, October–November 2013.

Inmate Information Handbook. Federal Bureau of Prisons.

6. Essential Skills

Librairie Larousse. *Larousse Gastronomique: The World's Greatest Culinary Encyclopedia, Completely Revised and Updated*. Clarkson Potter, 2009.

MacMillan, Norma, and Carole Clements. *The Encyclopedia of Cooking Skills and Techniques: A Comprehensive Visual Guide to Cookery Processes*. Anness, 2011.

Elliot, Jeffrey, and James DeWan. *Zwilling J. A. Henckels Complete Book of Knife Skills: The Essential Guide to Use, Techniques and Care*. Robert Rose, 2010.

Le Cordon Bleu Kitchen Essentials: The Complete Illustrated Reference to the Ingredients, Equipment, Terms, and Techniques Used by Le Cordon Bleu. John Wiley and Sons, 2001.

"Guide to Rice Varieties." *Fine Cooking*, Issue 31.

Bittman, Mark. "Brown Rice: Not Just for Hippies Anymore." *New York Times Magazine*, November 10, 2011.

"A Cook's Guide to Rice Varieties." *Huffington Post*, January 2012.

Rhodes, Phillip. "Good For You and the Planet, New Dietary Guidelines Recommend Fish Twice Per Week." *Cooking Light*, April 2011.

"Green Is Good." *Real Simple*, February 2013.

Mowbray, Scott, and Ann Taylor Pittman. "7 Simple Ways to Become a Better Cook." *Cooking Light*, November 2013.

"Test-Kitchen Wisdom." MarthaStewart.com.

Mattox, Charlyne. "Kitchen Skills." *Real Simple*, October 2013.

12. Dining Out with No Reservations

Librairie Larousse. *Larousse Gastronomique: The World's Greatest Culinary Encyclopedia, Completely Revised and Updated*. Clarkson Potter, 2009.

Le Cordon Bleu Kitchen Essentials: The Complete Illustrated Reference to the Ingredients, Equipment, Terms, and Techniques Used by Le Cordon Bleu. John Wiley and Sons, 2001.

Child, Julia, Simone Beck, and Louisette Bertholle. *Mastering the Art of French Cooking*. Vol. 1. Alfred A. Knopf, 1961.

Escoffier, Auguste. *The Escoffier Cookbook and Guide to the Fine Art of Cookery: For Connoisseurs, Chefs, Epicures*. Crown Publishers, 2000.

Scourboutakos, Mary J., Zhila Semnani-Azad, and Mary R. L'Abbe. "Restaurant Meals: Almost a Full Day's Worth of Calories, Fats, and Sodium." *JAMA Internal Medicine* 173, no. 14 (July 22, 2013): 1373–74.

Urban, Lorien E. "Accuracy of Stated Energy Contents of Restaurant Foods." Megan A. McCrory, Gerard E. Dallai, Sai Krupa Das, Edward Saltzman, Judith L. Weber, et al. *JAMA* 306, no. 3 (July 20, 2011): 287–93.

Miller, Tracy. "Worse Than Fast Food." *New York Daily News*, May 13, 2013.

Wu, Helen, and Roland Sturm. "Changes in the Energy and Sodium Content of Main Entrées in US Chain Restaurants from 2010 to 2011." *Journal of the Academy of Nutrition and Dietetics* 114, no. 2 (February 2014): 209–19. October 2013.

"We make our omelets extra fluffy by adding a splash of our buttermilk and wheat pancake batter to the mix." IHOP Restaurant Web site.

Bittman, Mark. "Why Won't McDonald's Really Lead?" *New York Times*, October 8, 2013.

15. Get Outta Here

Pawlowski, A. "Airline Considers Fee for Lavatory Use." *CNN*, April 7, 2010.

Brown, Genevieve Shaw. "Most Outrageous, Non-Existent Airline Fees." *Good Morning America*, September 19, 2012.

Roglieri, Maria Ann. *The Gluten-Free Guide to France*. 2nd ed. Mari Productions, 2013.

L'Association Française Des Interolants Au Gluten.

Lebovitz, David. *Living the Sweet Life in Paris* (blog). www.davidlebovitz.com.

Cooban, Jane. *Gluten Free for Tea: My Gluten Free Life in London* (blog). glutenfreefortea.wordpress.com.

Coeliac UK.

Minchilli, Elizabeth. *Elizabeth Minchilli in Rome* (blog). www.elizabethminchilliinrome.com.

Roglieri, Maria Ann. *The Gluten-Free Guide to Italy*. 6th ed. Mari Productions, 2013.

Associazione Italiano Celiachia.

16. Your Cheating Heart

Marcason, Wendy. "Is There Evidence to Support the Claim That a Gluten-Free Diet Should Be Used for Weight Loss?" *Journal of the American Dietetic Association* 111, no. 11 (November 2011): 1786.

Merdian, Mark J. "Celiac Disease and Holy Communion: A Medical and Spiritual Dilemma." *Homiletic and Pastoral Review*, June 24, 2013.

Adams, Jefferson. "More Churches Offering Gluten-Free Communion Bread Options." Celiac.com, June 11, 2012.

Gellman, Marc, and Thomas Hartman. "If You Can't Eat Bread, Drink Only the Wine." *Newsday*, May 22, 2004.

Section 504/Americans with Disabilities Act.

Full Text of the Settlement Agreement Between the United States of America and Lesley University, DJ 202-36-231.

17. Sex and the Celiac

Simmons, Deborah S. "Celiac Disease, Gluten Sensitivity, and Your Fertility." American Fertility Association.

Kuczynski, Alex. "The Nine Months of Living Anxiously." *New York Times*, May 23, 2004.

"Food to Avoid During Pregnancy." American Pregnancy Association.

Szajewska, H. A. Chemielewska, M. Piescik-Lech, A. Ivarsson, S. Kolacek, S. Koletzko, et al. "Systematic Review: Early Infant Feeding and the Prevention of Coeliac Disease." *Alimentary Pharmacology and Therapeutics* 36, no. 7 (October 2012): 607–18.

Velasquez-Manoff, Moises. "Who Has the Guts for Gluten?" *New York Times*, February 23, 2013.

Velasquez-Manoff, Moises. *An Epidemic of Absence: A New Way of Understanding Allergies and Autoimmune Diseases*. Reprint ed. Scribner, 2013.

Petersen, Vikki. "A Real Cause of Infertility and Miscarriage Has Been Identified." Health Now Medical Center, January 2013.

Boyd, Christine. "Why Can't We Have a Baby?" *Living Without*, February–March 2013.

Johnston, E. B., G. T. Fossum, J. B. Palascak, M. B. Awsare, C. Chouldhary, and A. J. Di Marino, "Reported Rates of Recurrent Spontaneous Abortion and Infertility in Patients with Celiac Disease." *Fertility and Sterility* 84, Supp. 1 (September 2005): S160.

Choi, Janet M., Jefferey Wang, Susie K. Lee, Joseph A. Murray, and Peter H. R. Green. "Increased Prevalence of Celiac Disease with Unexplained Fertility in the United States: A Prospective Study." *Journal of Reproductive Medicine* 56, no. 5–6 (May–June 2011): 199–203.

Collin, P., S. Vilska, P. K. Heinonen, O. Hällström, P. Pikkarainen. "Infertility and Coeliac Disease." *Gut* 39, no. 3 (1996): 382–84.

Freeman, Hugh James. "Reproductive Changes Associated with Celiac Disease." *World Journal of Gastroenterology* 16, no. 46 (December 14, 2010): 5810–14.

Ludvigsson, J. F., and J. Ludvigsoon, "Coeliac Disease in the Father Affects the Newborn." *Gut* 49 (2001): 169–75.

Green, Peter H. R., and Bana Jabri. "Coeliac Disease." *Lancet* 362, no. 9381 (August 2, 2003): 383–91.

Martinelli, P., R. Troncon, F. Paparo, P. Torre, E. Trapanes, C. Fasano, et al. "Coeliac Disease and Unfavourable Outcome of Pregnancy." Gut 46, no. 3 (March 2000): 332–35.

Simmons, Deborah S. "Celiac Disease, Gluten Sensitivity, and Your Fertility." American Fertility Association.

Bast, Alice. "Alice's Story." BAST, *Greater Philadelphia Support Group Newsletter*.

Hozyasz, K. K. "Coeliac Disease and Birth Defects in Offspring." Letter to the Editor. *Gut* 49, no. 5 (2001): 738.

Scarparo, Gloria. "Stay in Shape While You're Expecting." Gluten-Free Trading Co., August 2003.

"Foods to Avoid During Pregnancy." American Pregnancy Association.

Hess, Mary Abbott, Anne Elise Hunt, and Roy Pitkin. *Eating for Two: The Complete Guide to Nutrition During Pregnancy*. Wiley, 1992.

Kuczynski, Alex. "The Nine Months of Living Anxiously." *New York Times*, May 23, 2004.

Williams, R. D. "Breast-Feeding Best Bet for Babies." US Food and Drug Administration Statement.

Shaw, Gary M., Thu Quach, Verne Nelson, Suzan L. Carmichael, Donna Schaffer, Steve Selvin, and Wei Young. "Neural Tube Defects Associated with Maternal Periconceptional Dietary Intake of Simple Sugars and Glycemic Index." *American Journal of Clinical Nutrition* 78, no. 5 (November 2003): 972–78.

18. And Baby Makes Three

Perlmutler, David, and Kristin Loberg. *Grain Brain: The Surprising Truth about Wheat, Carbs, and Sugar—Your Brain's Silent Killers*. New York: Little Brown, 2013.

Genuis, Stephen J., and Thomas P. Bouchard. "Celiac Disease Presenting as Autism." *Journal of Child Neurology* 25, no. 1 (January 2010): 114–19.

de Magistris, Laura, Valeria Familiari, Antono Pascotto, Anna Sapone, Alessandro Frolli, Patrizia Iardino, et al. "Alterations of the Intestinal Barrier in Patients with Autism Spectrum Disorders and in Their First-Degree Relatives." *Journal of Pediatric Gastroenterology and Nutrition* 51, no. 4 (October 2010): 418–24.

Dorfman, Kelly. "Is Gluten Intolerance Making Your Child Act Out?" *Living Without*, September 2013.

Vader, W., Y. Kooy, P. Van Veelen, A. De Ru, D. Harris, W. Benckhuijsen, et al. "The Gluten Response in Children with Celiac Disease Is Directed Toward Multiple Gliadin and Glutenin Peptides." *Gastroenterology* 122, no. 7 (June 2002): 1729–37.

Lieberman, Jay A., Christopher Weiss, Terrence J. Furlong, Mati Sicherer, and Scott H. Sicherer. "Bullying Among Pediatric Patients with Food Allergy." *Annals of Allergy, Asthma & Immunology* 105, no. 4 (October 2010): 282–86.

Interview with Ritu Verma, MD, director of the Center for Celiac Disease at Children's Hospital of Philadelphia on bullying children with food allergies. December 2013.

"Filing 504 School Plans." Section 504 of the Rehabilitation Act of 1973, National Lunch Program, Americans with Disabilities Act.

Moore, Tim. "Facts About Celiac Disease and Filing for Disability." Social Security Disability and SSI Resource Center.

Thernstrom, Melanie. "The Allergy Buster." *New York Times Magazine*, March 7, 2013.

Bittman, Mark. "Kitchen Little." *New York Times*, May 7, 2013.

Merryman, Ashley. "Losing Is Good for You." *New York Times*, September 24, 2013.

Zou, Jie Jenny. "Gluten Danger Puts Schools to the Test." *Wall Street Journal*, August 1, 2012.

"Trick-or-Treat but Hold the Wheat." ABC News, October 26, 2009.

"Tips for Trick-or-Treating Safely on Halloween." Food Allergy Network.

"Halloween Health and Safety Tips." Center for Disease Control and Prevention.

"Trick or Treat! Tips for Halloween Safety." *Consumer Reports*, October 25, 2013.

19. The Seven-Year Itch and Other Associated Conditions
I am grateful to the following physicians for their careful review and suggestions for the presentation of the conditions associated with celiac disease and gluten intolerance: John J. Zone, MD, chair, Department of Dermatology, University of Utah Healthcare; Gregory Kane, MD, Pulmonology, Allergy, Immunology, Jane and Leonard Korman Professor of Pulmonary Medicine, vice chair, Education, Department of Medicine, Thomas Jefferson University Hospital; Howard Weitz, MD, Bernard L. Segal Professor of Clinical Cardiology, Director, Division of Cardiology, Jefferson Heart Institute, Thomas Jefferson University Hospital; Frederick Vivino, MD, Chief, Rheumatology, Associate Professor of Clinical Medicine, Director, Penn Sjögren's Syndrome Center, Penn Presbyterian Medical Center; Serge A. Jabbor, MD, FACP, FACE, Professor, Director, Division of Endocrinology, Diabetes and Metabolic Diseases, Jefferson Medical College of Thomas Jefferson University; Anthony J. DiMarino Jr., Codirector, Jefferson Celiac Center, William Rorer Professor of Medicine, Chief, Division of Gastroenterology and Hepatology, Thomas Jefferson University Hospital; Joseph A. Murray, MD, Professor of Medicine, Division of Gastroenterology and Hepatology, Celiac Disease Clinic, Mayo Clinic, Rochester, Minnesota.

Ludvigsson, Jonas F., Kari Hemminki, Jan Wahlström, and Catarina Almqvist, "Celiac Disease Confers a 1.6-Fold Increased Risk of Asthma: A Nationwide Population-Based Study." *Journal of Allergy and Clinical Immunology* 127, no. 4 (April 2011): 1071–73.

Green, Peter H. R. "Was JFK the Victim of an Undiagnosed Disease Common to the Irish?" History News Network.

Sapone, Anna, Julio C. Bai, Carolina Ciacci, Jernej Dolinsek, Peter H. R. Green, Marios Hadjivassiliou, et al. "Spectrum of Gluten-Related Disorders: Consensus on New Nomenclature and Classification." *BMC Medicine* 10 (2012).

"Dermatitis Herpetiformis." Celiac Awareness Campaign of the National Institutes of Health.

Zone, John J. "Skin Manifestations of Celiac Disease." *Gastroenterology* 128, no. 4, Suppl. 1 (April 2005): 587–91.

Riches, Philip L., Euan McRorie, William D. Fraser, Catherine Determann, Rob van't Hof, and Stuart H. Ralston. "Osteoporosis Associated with Neutralizing Autoantibodies Against Osteoprotegerin." *New England Journal of Medicine* 361 (October 8, 2009): 1459–65.

Shane, Elizabeth, David Burr, Peter R. Ebeling, B. Abrahamsen, Robert A. Adler, et al. "Atypical Subtrochanteric and Diaphyseal Femoral Fractures: Report of a Task Force of the American Society for Bone and Mineral Health Research." *Journal of Bone and Mineral Research* 25, no. 11 (November 2010): 2267–94.

West, Joe, Richard F. A. Logan, Tim R. Card, Chris Smith, and Richard Hubbard. "Fracture Risk in People with Celiac Disease: A Population-Based Cohort Study." *Gastroenterology* 25, no. 2 (August 2003): 429–36.

"Osteomalacia." In *Medline Plus Medical Encyclopedia.* U.S. National Library of Medicine, National Institutes of Health.

"Osteomalacia." Orthopaedics-Rheumatology/Diseases and Conditions. Cleveland Clinic.org.

"Osteomalacia." Mayo Clinic.

Dreifus, Claudia. "Focus on Vitamin D: A Need That Doesn't Change with the Seasons." *New York Times,* January 28, 2003.

Dreifus, Claudia. Shining a Light on the Health Benefits of Vitamin D." *New York Times,* January 28, 2003.

Ventura, Allessandro, Giuseppe Magazzù, and Luigi Greco. "Duration of Exposure to Gluten and Risk for Autoimmune Disorders in Patients with Celiac Disease." *Gastroenterology* 117, no. 2 (August 1999): 297–303.

Melamed, Farhad. "Aphthous Stomatitis: Brief Clinical Update." UCLA Department of Medicine, April 17, 2001.

Shakeri, Ramin, Farhad Zamani, Rasoul Sotoudehmanesh, Afsaneh Amiri, Mehdi Mohamadnejad, Fereydoun Davatchi, et al. "Gluten Sensitivity Enteropathy in Patients with Recurrent Aphthous Stomatitis." *BMC Gastroenterology* 9 (2009).

Not, T., A. Tommasini, G. Tonini, E. Buratti, M. Pocecco, C. Tortul, et al. "Undiagnosed Coeliac Disease and Risk of Autoimmune Disorders in Subjects with Type I Diabetes Mellitus." *Diabetologia* 44, no. 2 (February 2001): 151–55.

"Rheumatoid Arthritis." Centers for Disease Control and Prevention.

"Rheumatoid Arthritis." American College of Rheumatology.

Wallace, Daniel J., ed. *The Sjögren's Book.* Oxford University Press, 2011.

Johnsen, S. J., J. G. Brun, L. G. Gøransson, M. C. Småstuen, T. B. Johannesen, K. Haldorsen, et al. "Risk of Non-Hodgkin's Lymphoma in Primary Sjögren's Syndrome: A Population-Based Study." *Arthritis Care and Research* (Hoboken) 65, no. 5 (May 2013): 816–21.

Mosby's Medical Dictionary. 6th ed. Mosby, 2002.

Clayman, Charles B., ed. *The American Medical Association Encyclopedia of Medicine.* Random House, 2006.

"Asthma." American Lung Association.

Porter, Robert S. *The Merck Manual of Diagnosis and Therapy.* 19th ed. John Wiley and Sons, 2011.

Carper, Jean. *Food—Your Miracle Medicine.* Harper Collins, 1993.

Aletaha, Donald, Tuhina Neogi, Alan J. Silman, Julia Funovits, Donald T. Felson, Clifton O. Bingham III, et al. "2010 Rheumatoid Arthritis Classification Criteria." *Arthritis and Rheumatism* 62, no. 9 (September 2010): 2569–81.

"Systemic Lupus Erythematosus," National Library of Medicine, National Institutes of Health, MedlinePlus .com.

Virilli, C., G. Bassotti, M. G. Santaguida, R. Iuorio, S. C. Del Duca V. Mercuri, et al. "Atypical Celiac Disease as Cause of Increased Need for Thyroxine: A Systematic Study." *Journal of Clinical Endocrinology and Metabolism* 97, no. 3 (March 2012): E419–22.

"Non-Hodgkin Lymphoma." Lymphoma Research Foundation.

"Lymphoma." Lymphoma Research Foundation.

Green, Peter H. R., A. T. Fleischauer, G. Bhagat, R. Goyal, B. Jabri, and A. I. Neugut. "Risk of Malignancy in Patients with Celiac Disease." *American Journal of Medicine* 115, no. 3 (August 2003): 191–95.

Lebwohl, Benjamin, Fredrik Granath, Anders Ekbom, Karin E. Smedby, Joseph A. Murray, Alfred I. Neugut, et al. "Mucosal Healing and Risk for Lymphoproliferative Malignancy in Celiac Disease: A Population-Based Cohort Study." *Annals of Internal Medicine* 159, no. 3 (August 6, 2013): 169–75.

20. The Doctor Will See You Now

Mayer, Caroline E. "Is It Time to Find a New Doctor?" *AARP The Magazine,* August–September 2013.

Burling, Stacey. "Yogurt a Solution to Hospital Infection?" *Philadelphia Inquirer,* December 8, 2013.

Falchuk, Evan. "Why Diagnoses Go Wrong and What You Can Do About It." *Philadelphia Life,* March 2013.

Woodward, Alicia. "Historic Health Care Bill and Celiac Disease." *Living Without,* March 26, 2010.

The Affordable Care Act and Reconciliation Act. United States Department of Health and Human Services, March 23, 2010.

Goodman, Brenda. "Hospital-Acquired Infection Cost $10 Billion a Year: Study." *U.S. News and World Reports,* September 3, 2013.

Walsh, Bryan. "Happy Clean Your Hands Day!" *Time,* May 5, 2011.

Pronovost, Peter, and Eric Vohn. *Safe Patients, Safe Hospitals: How One Doctor's Checklist Can Help Us Change Health Care from the Inside Out.* Plume, 2011.

Mosby's Medical Dictionary. 6th ed. Mosby, 2002.

Kohn, Linda T., Janet M. Corrigan, and Molla S. Donaldson. *To Err Is Human: Building a Safer Health System.* National Academy Press, 2000.

James, John T. "A New, Evidence-Based Estimate of Patient Harms Associated with Hospital Care." *Journal of Patient Safety* 9, no. 3 (September 2013): 122–28.

"Gluten Antibody Testing, Genetic Testing, and Small Bowel Biopsy." Interview with Anthony J. DiMarino Jr. and Ritu Verma, November 2013.

"Diagnosing Celiac Disease." National Digestive Diseases Information Clearinghouse.

Tammaro, A., A. Narcisi, G. De Marco, and S. Persechino. "Cutaneous Hypersensitivity to Gluten." *Dermatitis* 23, no. 5 (September–October 2012): 220–21.

21. Winning the Drug War

Gluten in Medication Identification Act of 2012. H.R. 4972. 112th Cong. [2012].

Gluten in Medicine Act of 2013. Ryan (D) Ohio and Lowrey (D) New York, not yet enacted.

Plogsted, Steve. "Medications and Celiac Disease—Tips from a Pharmacist. *Practical Gastroenterology,* January 2007.

"Gluten in Medications Guide." American Society of Health System Pharmacists.

Crowe, Jeanne, and Nancy Patin Falini. "Gluten in Pharmaceutical Products." *American Journal of Health-System Pharmacy* 58, no. 5 (March 1, 2001): 396–400.

Drug and Medical Abbreviations. RxList.com, MedicineNet .com, MediLexicon.com.

Bittman, Mark. "The Cosmetics Wars." *New York Times,* March 2, 2013.

Lowell, Jax Peters. "What Price Beauty?" *Living Without,* February–March 2009.

Lowell, Jax Peters. "Sensitive to Sunscreen?" *Living Without,* August–September 2009.

"Regulatory Requirements for Marketing Cosmetics in the United States." U.S. Food and Drug Administration.

"Cosmetic Labeling and Label Claims." U.S. Food and Drug Administration.

Hampton, Aubrey. "Ten Synthetic Cosmetic Ingredients to Avoid." Organic Consumers Association.

Workingboxwalla, Dinyar. "Do You Know About These Harmful Ingredients in Your Cosmetics?" Health.India .com.

Thomas, Pat. "Behind the Label: Nivea Moisturising Lotion." *Ecologist,* June 1, 2005.

"Environmental Working Group's Skin Deep Cosmetics Database." EWG.org.

"Makeup Ingredients You Might Want to Avoid." *Huffington Post*, October 2013.

The International Cosmetic Ingredient Dictionary and Handbook. 11th ed. 4 vols. CTFA, 2006.

Burke, Sheila. "Rice Bran Oil. A Wonderful Gift from Nature." *Zen-Sational Living Blog*.

22. Food Fights

Full text of the Food Allergen Labeling and Consumer Protection Act of 2004.

FDA Final Ruling for Standardized Gluten-Free Labeling. August 2, 2013.

"FDA Defines 'Gluten-Free' for Food Labeling." FDA News Release, August 2, 2013.

Edney, Anna. "Gluten-Free Labels Defined Under New U.S. FDA Standard." *Bloomberg*, August 2, 2013.

Leger, Amy. "GF Congressional Crusader: An Interview with Congresswoman Nita Lowey." *Gluten-Free Living*, September–October 2013.

"An Interview with Jules Shepard, Activist Baker." *Gluten-Free Living*, Fall 2012.

Myers, Gryphon. "New Grains CEO Sues Utah Senator over Inaction on Gluten-Free Labeling." Celiac.com, June 5, 2012.

"Facts About the FDA Gluten-Free Food Labeling Rule." Celiac Disease Foundation *Insight*, Fall 2013.

"Frequently Asked Questions About the Food Allergen Labeling and Consumer Protection Act of 2004 (FALCPA)." KidsWithFoodAllergies.org, May 2013.

"Questions and Answers on the Gluten-Free Labeling Proposed Rule." FDA, January 23, 2007.

Boyd, Christine. "A Closer Look at Gluten-Free Labeling." *Living Without*, April–May 2010.

Stevens, L., and M. Rashid. "Gluten-Free and Regular Foods: A Cost Comparison." *Canadian Journal of Dietetic Practice and Research* 69, no. 3 (Fall 2008): 147–50.

Schweigert, Mary Beth. "When CD Comes with Age: How Seniors Deal with Unique Challenges of Diagnosis Later in Life." *Gluten-Free Living*, May–June 2013.

Gilliland, Ayn. "Open Letter to Celiac Listserv and to Secretary of Health and Human Services Sibelius on the Urgency of Covering Expensive Gluten-Free Food Under the Affordable Care Act for Those on Medicare and Medicaid." August 6, 2013.

Shannon, Victoria. "Japan and South Korea Bar Imports of U.S. Wheat." *New York Times*, May 31, 2013.

Ledford, Heidi. "Transgenic Salmon Nears Approval." *Nature*, May 1, 2013.

"GMO Facts." Non-GMO Project.

Walsh, Bryan. "Hunger Games: Cheerios Has Ditched GMOs. Does It Matter?" *Time*, January 20, 2014.

Dorfman, Kelly. "GMO Ingredients: A Case for Choosing Organic." *Living Without*, February–March 2014.

Strom, Stephanie. "Seeking Food Ingredients That Aren't Gene-Altered." *New York Times*, May 26, 2013.

Smith, Jeffrey. "10 Reasons to Avoid GMOs." ResponsibleTechnology.org.

Schweigert, Mary Beth. "How GMOs Impact the GF Diet." *Gluten-Free Living*, January–February 2014.

Davis, William. *Wheat Belly: Lose the Wheat, Lose the Weight, and Find Your Path Back to Health*. Rodale Books, 2011.

"65 Health Risks of GMO Foods." ResponsibleTechnology.org.

Amster, Randall. "Monsanto's Death Patents." *Counterpunch*, March 22, 2013.

Strom, Stephanie. "Major Grocer to Label Foods with Gene-Modified Content." *New York Times*, March 8, 2013.

Schiffman, Richard. "GMOs Aren't the Problem. Our Industrial Food System Is." TheGuardian.com, November 6, 2013.

Kasarda, Donald. "Can an Increase in Celiac Disease Be Attributed to an Increase in the Gluten Content of Wheat as a Consequence of Wheat Breeding?" *Journal of Agricultural and Food Chemistry* 61, no. 6 (February 13, 2013): 1155–59.

"Arsenic in Your Food." *Consumer Reports*, November 2012.

"Arsenic Facts." USA Rice Federation.

Pollack, Andrew. "Unease in Hawaii's Cornfields." *New York Times*, March 10, 2013.

Mondello, Wendy. "Corn Fed." *Living Without*, October–November 2013.

Begun, Rachel. "Rice Rules: What You Need to Know About Arsenic in Rice." *Gluten-Free Living*, January–February 2013.

"Arsenic Poisoning." MedicineNet.com.

"Save America's Pollinators Act of 2013." Save the Bees Action, The Peace Team.

Walsh, Bryan. "The Plight of the Honey Bee: Mass Deaths in Bee Colonies May Mean Disaster for Farmers—and Your Favorite Foods." *Time*, August 19, 2013.

Schwartz, John. "Program Looks to Give Bees a Leg (or Six) Up." *New York Times*, April 2, 2014.

Wines, Michael. "Mystery Malady Kills More Bees, Heightening Worry on Farms." *New York Times*, March 28, 2013.

Bauers, Sandy. "Best to Be Your Bees' Keeper." *Philadelphia Inquirer*, August 4, 2013.

"Food 101 with Michael Pollan." Oprah.com, January 21, 2010.

"The Most Terrifying Foods in the World." Huffpost *Taste*, May 2014.

Bellatti, Andy. "Seeking Longevity? Eat Real Food." Huffpost *Healthy Living*, August 22, 2013.

O'Brien, Robyn. "Organic Food vs. Conventional: What the Stanford Study Missed." *Huffington Post*, September 6, 2012.

"Why Your 'Natural' Foods Might Not Be So Healthy." GreenAmerica.org.

23. Community

MISSION STATEMENTS, CHAPTERS, ACTIVITIES:
American Celiac Disease Alliance
Canadian Celiac Association
Celiac Disease Foundation
Celiac Support Association
Gluten Intolerance Group
National Foundation for Celiac Awareness

General Index

Recipe Index

About the Author

JAX PETERS LOWELL, diagnosed with celiac disease more than twenty years ago, was the first to bring national attention to the gluten-free diet. In addition to writing bestselling books on living well without wheat, she is an award-winning poet and the author of the novel *Mothers*. She is a recipient of the Leeway Foundation Transformation Award in fiction and poetry and for her pioneering efforts in bringing public awareness to gluten intolerance. She lives in Philadelphia in a restored bread factory.